Fundamentals in Gynaecologic Malignancy

Amal Chandra Kataki
Debabrata Barmon
Editors

Fundamentals in Gynaecologic Malignancy

Springer

Editors
Amal Chandra Kataki
Department of Gynaecologic Oncology
Dr Bhubaneswar Borooah Cancer Institute (A unit of Tata Memorial Centre, Mumbai)
Guwahati, Assam, India

Debabrata Barmon
Department of Gynaecologic Oncology
Dr Bhubaneswar Borooah Cancer Institute (A unit of Tata Memorial Centre, Mumbai)
Guwahati, Assam, India

ISBN 978-981-19-5862-5 ISBN 978-981-19-5860-1 (eBook)
https://doi.org/10.1007/978-981-19-5860-1

This Springer imprint is published by the registered company Springer Nature Singapore Pte Ltd.
The registered company address is: 152 Beach Road, #21-01/04 Gateway East, Singapore 189721, Singapore

Contents

Epidemiology of Gynaecological Cancers

Amal Chandra Kataki, Parmita Tiwari, R. Thilagavthi, and Manigreeva Krishnatreya

Gynaecological cancers refer to the malignancies of the female reproductive system that includes cancer of vulva (C51), vagina (C52), cervix uteri (C53), corpus uteri and uterus part unspecified (C54–C55), ovary(C56), fallopian tube (C57), and placenta (C58) [1, 2]. Global burden of gynaecological cancer is rising exponentially. Forecasts show an increasing trend in burden for the next 20 years [3, 4]. Globally, 1.4 million females were estimated to be newly diagnosed with gynaecological cancers in 2020 and there were 6.8 lakh deaths [3]. One in 20 women develop gynaecological cancer in their lifetime and one in 33 women die from it [1]. Disability adjusted life years (DALYS)[1] for gynaecological cancers were estimated to be 17 million approximately, contributing one-sixth of the DALYs of all cancers among women [5]. Carcinoma cervix uteri is the most common among gynaecological cancers, accounting to 43.2% cases worldwide [6] (Fig. 1).

National and sub-national level cancer burden estimates are essential and offer valuable information to policymakers and advocacy groups for planning tailored cancer prevention strategies and early detection programmes. In the year 1981, the Indian Council of Medical Research (ICMR) established the National Cancer Registry Programme (NCRP) of National Centre for Disease Informatics and Research (NCDIR) in India to systematically collect reliable data on magnitude and patterns of cancer [7, 8]. The initiative included two types of registries: Population Based Cancer Registries (PBCRs) that keeps track of all new cancer cases and deaths from the defined population within a certain geographic area and Hospital Based Cancer Registries (HBCRs) that collects data on cancer patients visiting a certain hospital, with an emphasis on clinical care, treatment, and outcome. There are

[1]Disability adjusted life years is a time-based measure of cancer burden that takes into account years of life lost due to premature mortality (YLLs) and years of life lost due to time lived in states of less than full health, or years of healthy life lost due to disability (YLDs). One DALY represents the loss of the equivalent of 1 year of full health.

A. C. Kataki (✉)
Department of Gynaecologic Oncology, Dr. Bhubaneswar Borooah Cancer Institute (A Unit of Tata Memorial Centre, Mumbai), Guwahati, Assam, India

P. Tiwari
Department of Gynaecologic Oncology, AIIMS, Rishikesh, Uttarakhand, India

R. Thilagavthi
National Centre for Disease Informatics and Research, Bangalore, Karnataka, India
e-mail: ncdir@ncdirindia.org

M. Krishnatreya
Department of Epidemiology and Cancer Registry, Dr. Bhubaneswar Borooah Cancer Institute, Guwahati, Assam, India

A. C. Kataki, D. Barmon (eds.), *Fundamentals in Gynaecologic Malignancy*,
https://doi.org/10.1007/978-981-19-5860-1_1

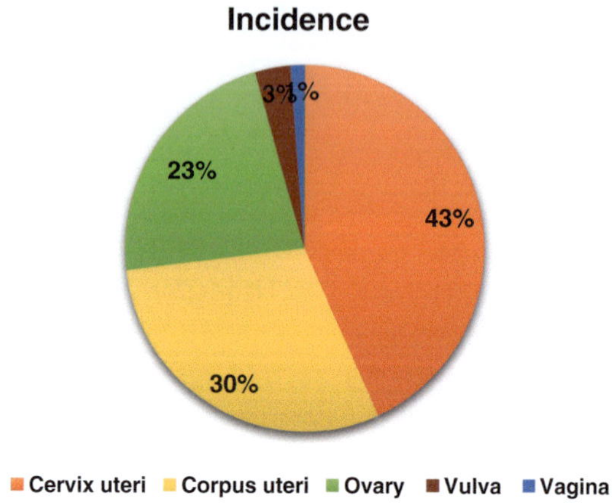

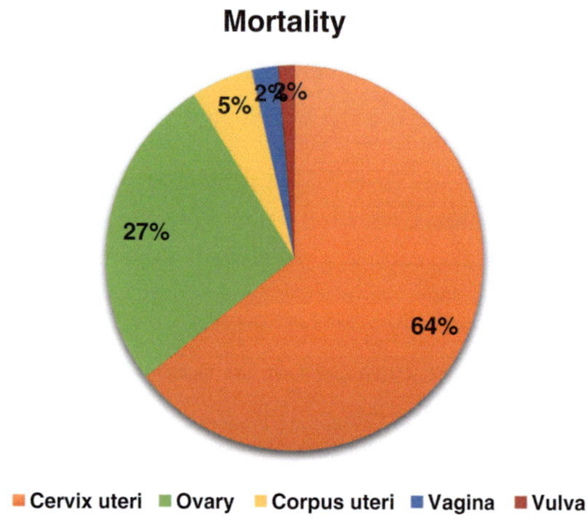

Fig. 1 Distribution of cases and deaths for gynaecological cancers in 2020. (Source: GLOBOCAN 2020)

38 PBCRs and more than 250 HBCRs registered under NCRP network, as of December 2021. They together serve as India's "health intelligence" for cancer control.

In India, 2 lakh new gynaecological cancer cases were diagnosed in 2020 and 1.2 lakh deaths occurred due to it among females [3]. Every 1 in 30 Indian women develops gynaecological cancer in their lifetime and one in 48 women die from it [3]. Among Indian females, occurrence of cancer was observed mainly in the age group of 35–64 years, which is also the most productive age group [7]. The estimated number of patients is expected to be influenced by factors such as risk behaviours, prevention strategies, screening programmes, and improved diagnostic procedures.

Three of the ten most common cancers among Indian women are gynaecological cancers, with cervix uteri (10.6% of total women cancer) being the most prevalent, followed by ovary (6.2%) and corpus uteri (3.7%) [8]. These malignancies are on the increasing trend [9] and research is essential for improving survival outcomes.

1 Carcinoma Cervix

Cervical cancer is the most common cancer among gynaecological cancers as well as leading cause of death globally [3]. It ranks fourth in most common cancers among women followed by breast, colorectal, and lung cancer. It was estimated that 604,127 women were newly diagnosed with cervical cancer and 341,831 women died from it in 2020 [3]. One in 72 women developed the disease and one in 122 died from it [3]. Global burden estimates showed an age standardized DALY rate of

210.6 for 2019 which was 4.8% lower than DALYs observed in 2010 [5]. Incidence and mortality was high in low/medium Human Development Index (HDI) countries compared to high/very high HDI countries, where the rates were 40–50% lower [3]. The disproportionately high burden of cervical cancer in developing countries and elsewhere in medically underserved populations is largely due to a lack of screening programmes detecting pre-cancerous and early stage cervical cancers. Sub-Saharan Africa has the highest regional incidence and mortality followed by South-eastern Asia [3]. Kyadondo, Uganda, had the world's highest incidence rate of cervical cancer (49.1 per 100,000) [7]. The age standardized incidence rate for Indian women was 18 per 100,000 women in 2020 [3]. India accounts for one-fifth of world's cervical cancer incidence and deaths with an estimated 123,907 incident cases and 77,348 deaths [3]. The age standardized DALY rate for Indian women was estimated as 229 per 100,000 in 2019 [9]. Papumpare district of Arunachal Pradesh has the highest cervical cancer incidence rate in Asia (27.7 per 100,000) [6].

The natural history of cervical cancer is well understood. Persistent infection with one of thirteen high-risk types of human papillomavirus (HPV) is the most leading cause for cervical cancer. Globally, HPV (especially type 16 and 18) accounts for over 70% of invasive cervical cancers [10]. Other co-factors that facilitate initiation and progression are early age at intercourse, multiple sexual partners, sexually transmitted infections, smoking, multiparity and prolonged use of oral contraceptives. In India, over 80% of cervical cancer are linked with infection due to HPV, which is greater than the global average [10].

Availability of highly effective primary (HPV vaccine) and secondary (screening) prevention measures makes cervical cancer highly preventable [11]. HPV vaccination programmes have the potential to decrease the long-term future burden of the disease. High-quality screening programmes are necessary to prevent cervical cancer among unvaccinated population and for early detection of disease. Evidence shows that national level HPV vaccination programmes had been implemented in one-third of the low-middle income countries (LMICs) compared to three-fourth of high-income countries [12]. This inadequate screening for cervical cancer contributed to its high prevalence in LMICs [13]. However, this cancer has better outcome and survival when diagnosed and treated at early stage.

Given the significant global burden of cervical cancer and increasing inequity, the World Health Organization called for global action in 2018 to eliminate cervical cancer (elimination threshold: ≤4 per 100,000 women worldwide) through the triple-intervention strategy that includes (1) vaccinating 90% of all girls by age 15 years, (2) screening 70% of women twice in the age range of 35–45 years, and (3) treating at least 90% of all precancerous lesions detected during screening [10].

Cervical cancer prevention and control necessitate a coordinated effort to raise knowledge of primary and secondary prevention techniques among target population, as well as access to treatment and palliative care. A targeted multi-sectoral approach is required to meet the World Health Organization's cervical cancer elimination by 2030 [14].

2 Carcinoma Ovary

Ovarian cancer accounts for 3.4% of new cancer cases (313,959 newly diagnosed cases) and 4.7% of cancer deaths (207,252 deaths) among women in 2020, acquiring eighth position globally [3]. By the year 2040, global incidence will rise by 37% leading to a total of 428,966 new cases, with much greater increase in the number of deaths [3]. In terms of overall burden, ovarian cancer is the sixth leading cause of cancer-related DALYs globally, with an age standardized rate (ASR) of 124.7 per 100,000 in 2019. Increasing trend in DALYs were observed in 2019 from 2010 which sum up to 2.9% [5]. Ovarian cancer is a silent killer and most lethal among gynaecological cancers with highest mortality rate [15]. This is mainly due to the asymptomatic growth of the tumour, with delayed onset of symptoms. Hence, majority of the patients are diagnosed at an advanced stage due to ambiguous symptoms and lack of screening methods. Advanced stage ovarian cancer has a dismal prognosis 5-year survival rates of less than 30%.

Ovarian cancer is more common in high-income countries, although its incidence is rising in lower-income countries as well. However, mortality due to ovarian cancer remains the same in both high and low income countries [3]. It was estimated to be the third most common cancer among Indian women [16]. It is also a leading cause of death from cancer in Indian women, with a cumulative risk of 1.3 and an estimated age-adjusted incidence rate of 6.7 per 100,000 women [3]. The highest incidence was reported from Papumpare district, Arunachal Pradesh (AAR: 13.7), followed by Kamrup urban, Assam (AAR: 9.8) and Delhi (AAR: 9.5). The incidence of ovarian cancer increases with age. The age specific incidence rate increases from age 35 years and peaks between the ages of 55 and 64 years [17]. Epithelial ovarian cancer is the most predominant type of histology, majorly contributed by adenocarcinoma - serous adenocarcinoma, mucinous adenocarcinoma, and papillary carcinoma [18].

A variety of biological, hormonal, behavioural, and geographic factors influence the risk of ovarian cancer. Epidemiological studies have firmly linked hormonal and reproductive variables to the development of ovarian cancer. Early menarche, late menopause, nulliparity, lactation, older age at first childbirth (more than 35 years) and obesity confer an increased risk of developing ovarian cancer. Ovarian cancer has a strong genetic propensity and having a family history of the disease is one of the most significant risk factors [17]. Carriers of the BRCA1 mutation have a lifetime risk of developing ovarian cancer of 26–54%, while carriers of the BRCA2 mutation have a risk of 10–23% [1]. Hereditary nonpolyposis colorectal cancer (HNPCC) or Lynch syndrome, which is caused by mutations in mismatch repair (MMR) genes, is associated with a 12% lifetime risk of developing epithelial ovarian cancer [16]. BRCA1 and BRCA2 gene mutations have been linked to high-grade serous histology, and HNPCC syndrome has a proclivity for endometrioid and clear cell histology [19].

Factors found to be protective against ovarian cancer include younger age at pregnancy and first childbirth (30–60% decreased risk of cancer), high parity, use of combined oral contraceptives for more than 5 years, lactation, and tubal ligation [16].

3 Carcinoma Corpus Uteri

Uterine corpus cancer is the sixth most common cancer in women globally, accounting for 417,367 new cases and 97,370 deaths in 2020 [3]. With a global age standardized incidence rate of 8.7 per 100,000 women and lifetime cumulative risk of 1.05%, it is the most common gynaecological cancer in developed nations [3]. Absolute DALYs of uterine cancer in 2019 has seen 11.6% increase from 2010 and occupies 13th rank globally. Incidence rates vary ten-folds across the globe, highest rates are seen in the countries with a very high HDI include Northern America, Europe, Micronesia/Polynesia, and Australia/New Zealand, where nearly two-thirds of all cases occur, whereas most African regions and South Central Asia have the lowest incidence rates.

In developing nations like India, though cervical cancer remains the third most common gynaecological cancer, recently there has been an upsurge in the incidence of endometrial cancer [3]. The number of estimated new cases of uterine cancer among Indian women in 2020 was 16,413 with 6385 deaths [3]. In India, the ASR of endometrial cancer was 2.3/100,000 women. The estimated DALYs for 2019 was 1.8 million, accounting 0.2% to the total all cause DALYs [9]. The top five PBCRs in which high incidence for cancer corpus uteri were found in Hyderabad district (ASR: 8.0), Chennai (ASR: 6.3), Bangalore (ASR: 5.9), Thiruvananthapuram district (ASR: 5.8), and Delhi (ASR: 5.8) [6]. Eight out of ten uterine cancers are of endometrial epithelial histology type [18].

The surge in endometrial cancer in India is primarily due to changing patterns of lifestyle and reproductive profile of women, particularly in metropolitan regions. The majority of cases occur in the sixth and seventh decades of life, with the average age at diagnosis being 60 years [20]. There is insufficient evidence that screening with endometrial sampling reduces mortality from endometrial cancer. Routine mass screening for endometrial cancer is not recommended since it is not cost-effective and promotes unwarranted anxiety and invasive procedures.

Hormones play a major role in the development of endometrial cancer. Each of the identified risk factors is primarily caused by excessive unopposed exogenous or endogenous oestrogen exposure including nulliparity, early menarche, late menopause, anovulation, polycystic ovarian syndrome, and hormone replacement therapy. Obesity, diabetes, and high blood pressure are further risk factors. On the contrary, use of oral contraceptive pills, increased age at menarche, having high parity and smoking were all attributed to a reduced risk of endometrial cancer [21]. Tamoxifen, a selective oestrogen-receptor modulator used for the treatment of oestrogen-receptor positive breast cancer, has also been shown to be associated with a two- to seven-fold increased risk of developing endometrial cancer. This occurs after prolonged use (>2 years), particularly in postmenopausal women with pre-existing uterine disease, usually has more aggressive histology with poor prognosis [22]. Hereditary non-polyposis colorectal cancer (Lynch syndrome) caused by a mismatch repair gene defect accounts for less than 5% of endometrial cancer cases, with a 30–60% lifetime risk of developing endometrial cancer [20].

4 Carcinoma Vulva

Carcinoma vulva is a rare malignancy of the female genital system. It accounts for 4% of all gynaecologic malignancies worldwide, with more than half of all cases occurring in higher-income countries [3, 23]. This accounts to an estimated 45,240 new cases and 17,427 deaths among women worldwide [3]. Globally, one in 1111 women developed the disease and 1 in 3333 died from it [3]. Over the last three decades, changing sexual behaviour, smoking, and human papillomavirus infections have resulted in a 20% increase in incidence and increasing prevalence in younger women from 11% to 41% over the past three decades [24, 25].

GLOBOCAN estimated 3447 women in India were diagnosed with vulval cancer and 1694 deaths in 2020 [3]. Indian women have a 1 in 1667 chance of developing vulvar cancer and 1 in 1429 chance of dying due to disease at any point during their life time.

It is mainly seen in postmenopausal women, with the median age being 67 years, although it is also becoming more common in younger women [25]. These tumours share numerous risk factors for cervical cancer. Vulval cancer diagnosed in younger women is often associated with HPV infection, while in older women, these tumours are caused by persistent vulvar dermatosis, such as lichen sclerosis, and are not linked to HPV infection.

In developing countries majority of the patients are diagnosed at an advanced stage due to social stigma, low to middle socioeconomic status, low literacy rate, logistic challenges, poor screening programmes, and lack of understanding about the disease.

5 Carcinoma Vagina

Cancer of the vagina is a rare malignancy that accounts for 0.2% of cancers among women and 0.5% of cancers in the female genital tract. It accounted for an estimated 17,908 cases and 7995 deaths worldwide in 2020. The age standardized incidence rate is 0.4 per 100,000 women worldwide. Every 1 out of 2500 women developed the disease and one in 5000 died from it. In India, 5518 women were diagnosed with vaginal cancer in 2020, and 2723 died of the disease [3]. There is one in 1111 chance of developing vaginal cancer and 1 in 909 chance of dying due to disease for Indian women [3]. Due to the rarity of the disease, most of the epidemiological data is based mainly on studies of small numbers of cases.

It occurs mainly in older and postmenopausal women, with an average age of diagnosis of 67 years [26, 27]. Vaginal cancer has many of the same risk factors as cervical cancer, including multiple sexual partners, early age at first intercourse, smoking, and immunosuppressed state [28]. It has a close correlation with persistent human papillomavirus infection. HPV has been associated with 40% of vaginal malignancies, while HPV type 16 was detected in 50–64% of high-grade vaginal intraepithelial lesions [29, 30]. A known precursor lesion is vaginal intraepithelial neoplasia (VAIN). Previous history of anogenital cancer (especially cervical cancer), immunocompromised status, diethylstilboestrol (DES) exposure, and chronic vaginal irritation induced by prolonged pessary use are all risk factors [31, 32].

6 Gestational Trophoblastic Disease

The term "Gestational Trophoblastic Disease" (GTD) refers to a group of interrelated disease processes originating from the placental trophoblastic tissues. A huge discrepancy in incidence has been reported around the world. GTD is less common in the European and American continents (0.2–1.5/1000 deliveries) in comparison to Southeast Asian countries (2–12/1000 deliveries) [32]. GTD is more common among Japanese, Chinese, Indonesians, Filipinos, Africans, and Indian women. Indonesia has the highest number of cases in Asia (1 in 77 pregnancies and 1 in 57 deliveries) [33].

Unlike western countries, India does not have a disease-specific registry for gestational trophoblastic disease. All of the studies are hospital-based studies and are from tertiary care centres. In India, the incidence is estimated to be between 1 in 160 and 500 pregnancies [34]. Prevalence differs not just among countries and continents, but even within the country. The northern states in India have shown a lower prevalence of GTD (1.31 per 1000 deliveries) compared to that in Kerala, a southern state (4.8 per 1000 deliveries) [32].

Geographical location, genetic, demographic, environmental, and host-related factors all have a role in the prevalence of GTD. The possibility of a molar pregnancy strongly correlates with maternal age. A higher frequency of molar pregnancy is seen in the upper and lower extremes of maternal age, that is, younger than 13–18 years or older than 45–50 years [35]. Regular follow-up of the patients is critically important to prevent relapse or persistence and to ensure complete remission of the disease.

7 Conclusion

Gynaecological cancer burden is steadily rising in India and worldwide. The ICMR-NCDIR National Cancer Registry Programme anticipates a 12% increase in cancer cases in India by 2025 [4]. According to geographical distribution trends, high incidence has been detected in the northeast region of the country. As cancer is a complex disease with numerous treatment options, there is no one-size-fits-all solution regarding treatment or screening.

Cancer registries are the foundation of cancer prevention and control programmes. Study of gynaecological cancer trends is essential for developing and accessing cancer control initiatives. Cancer registration in India is confronted with a number of obstacles. As cancer is not a notifiable disease in many states of India, data collection is challenging. Data linkage between cancer registry data with Ayushman Bharat, mortality databases, and hospital information system would improve cancer registration, follow-up, and outcome statistics.

A multidisciplinary approach to cancer prevention, control, and care, including cancer awareness initiatives, preventive measures, early detection screening programmes, vaccination, and prompt personalized treatment is crucial to reduce gynaecological cancer burden in the coming decades. Strengthening these efforts along with cancer research shall change the trajectory of cancer and support in achieving national non-communicable disease targets as well as the sustainable development goals [36, 37].

References

1. CDC – National Center for Health Statistics. https://www.cdc.gov/cancer/gynecologic/basic_info/what-is-gynecologic-cancer.htm. Accessed 7 Jan 2022.
2. Sankaranarayanan R, Ferlay J. Worldwide burden of gynecological cancer. In: Handbook of disease burdens and quality of life measures; 2010. p. 803–23. https://doi.org/10.1007/978-0-387-78665-0_46.
3. Sung H, Ferlay J, Siegel RL, Laversanne M, Soerjomataram I, Jemal A, Bray F. Global cancer statistics 2020: GLOBOCAN estimates of incidence and mortality worldwide for 36 cancers in 185 countries. CA Cancer J Clin. 2021;71(3):209–49.
4. Foreman KJ, Marquez N, Dolgert A, et al. Forecasting life expectancy, years of life lost, and all-cause and cause-specific mortality for 250 causes of death: reference and alternative scenarios for2016-40 for195 countries and territories. Lancet. 2018;392(10159):2052–90. https://doi.org/10.1016/S0140-6736(18)31694-5.
5. Global Burden of Disease 2019 Cancer Collaboration. Cancer incidence, mortality, years of life lost, years lived with disability, and disability-adjusted life years for 29 cancer groups from 2010 to 2019: a systematic analysis for the Global Burden of Disease Study 2019, JAMA Oncol. 8(3):2021, 420–444. https://doi.org/10.1001/jamaoncol.2021.6987.
6. Sung H, Ferlay J, Siegel RL, Laversanne M, Soerjomataram I, Jemal A, Bray F. Global cancer statistics 2020: GLOBOCAN estimates of incidence and mortality worldwide for 36 cancers in 185 countries. CA Cancer J Clin. 2021;71(3):209–49. https://doi.org/10.3322/caac.21660.
7. Report of National Cancer Registry Programme (ICMR-NCDIR), Bengaluru, India; 2020. https://www.ncdirindia.org/All_Reports/Report_2020/default.aspx.
8. Mathur P, Sathishkumar K, Chaturvedi M, Das P, Sudarshan KL, Santhappan S, Nallasamy V, John A, Narasimhan S, Roselind FS, ICMR-NCDIR-NCRP Investigator Group. Cancer statistics, 2020: report from national cancer registry programme, India. JCO Glob Oncol. 2020 Jul;6:1063–75.
9. Institute for Health Metrics and Evaluation (IHME). GBD compare. Seattle, WA: IHME, University of Washington; 2015. https://vizhub.healthdata.org/gbd-compare/. Accessed 6 Jan 2022.
10. Bhatla N, Meena J, Kumari S, Banerjee D, Singh P, Natarajan J. Cervical cancer prevention efforts in India. Indian J Gynecol Oncol. 2021;19(3):1–6.
11. Sankaranarayanan R, Basu P, Kaur P, Bhaskar R, Singh GB, Denzongpa P, et al. Current status of human papillomavirus vaccination in India's cervical cancer prevention efforts. Lancet Oncol. 2019;20(11):e637–44. https://doi.org/10.1016/s1470-2045(19)30531-5.
12. PATH. Global HPV vaccine introduction overview: projected and current national introductions, demonstration/pilot projects, gender-neutral vaccination programs, and global HPV vaccine introduction maps (2006-2023). PATH; 2020. path.org/resources/global-hpv-vaccine-introduction-overview/. Accessed 23 Nov 2020.
13. Lemp JM, De Neve JW, Bussmann H, et al. Lifetime prevalence of cervical cancer screening in 55 low- and middle-income countries. JAMA. 2020;324:1532–42.
14. Global strategy to accelerate the elimination of cervical cancer as a public health problem. Geneva: World Health Organization; 2020. Licence: CC BY-NC-SA 3.0 IGO.
15. Coburn SB, Bray F, Sherman ME, Trabert B. International patterns and trends in ovarian cancer incidence, overall and by histologic subtype. Int J Cancer. 2017;140(11):2451–60.
16. Zayyan MS. Risk factors for ovarian cancer. In: Tumor progression and metastasis; 2020. IntechOpen.
17. Puri S, Chadha V, Pandey AK. Epidemiology of ovarian tumours in Northern India—a tertiary hospital based study. Indian J Community Fam Med. 2018;4(2):37.
18. ICMR-NCDIR. Clinicopathological profile of cancers in India: a report of the hospital based cancer registries, 2021, Bengaluru, India.
19. Zheng G, Yu H, Kanerva A, Försti A, Sundquist K, Hemminki K. Familial risks of ovarian cancer by age at diagnosis, proband type and histology. PLoS One. 2018;13(10):e0205000.
20. Vălu MV, Toma O. Endometrial cancer. A review and evaluation of risk factors. Analele Stiintifice ale Universitatii Alexandru Ioan Cuza din Iasi. Sectiunea II A, Genetica si Biologie Moleculara. 2017;18(3).
21. Raglan O, Kalliala I, Markozannes G, Cividini S, Gunter MJ, Nautiyal J, Gabra H, Paraskevaidis E, Martin-Hirsch P, Tsilidis KK, Kyrgiou M. Risk factors for endometrial cancer: an umbrella review of the literature. Int J Cancer. 2019;145(7):1719–30.
22. Emons G, Mustea A, Tempfer C. Tamoxifen and endometrial cancer: a janus-headed drug. Cancers. 2020;12(9):2535.
23. De Martel C, Ferlay J, Franceschi S, Vignat J, Bray F, Forman D, Plummer M. Global burden of cancers attributable to infections in 2008: a review and synthetic analysis. Lancet Oncol. 2012;13(6):607–15.
24. Schuurman MS, Van Den Einden LC, Massuger LF, Kiemeney LA, van der Aa MA, de Hullu JA. Trends in incidence and survival of Dutch women with vulvar squamous cell carcinoma. Eur J Cancer. 2013;49(18):3872–80.
25. Hampl M, Deckers-Figiel S, Hampl JA, Rein D, Bender HG. New aspects of vulvar cancer: changes in localization and age of onset. Gynecol Oncol. 2008;109(3):340–5.
26. Adams TS, Rogers LJ, Cuello MA. Cancer of the vagina: 2021 update. Int J Gynecol Obstet. 2021;155:19–27.
27. Adhikari P, Vietje P, Mount S. Premalignant and malignant lesions of the vagina. Diagn Histopathol. 2017;23(1):28–34.

28. Deshpande A. Vaginal cancer trends in women of low resources settings. J Univ Surg. 2016;4(3):54.
29. Srodon M, Stoler MH, Baber GB, Kurman RJ. The distribution of low and high-risk HPV types in vulvar and vaginal intraepithelial neoplasia (VIN and VaIN). Am J Surg Pathol. 2006;30(12):1513–8.
30. Hampl M, Sarajuuri H, Wentzensen N, Bender HG, Kueppers V. Effect of human papillomavirus vaccines on vulvar, vaginal, and anal intraepithelial lesions and vulvar cancer. Obstet Gynecol. 2006;108(6):1361–8.
31. Akino N, Wada-Hiraike O, Matsumoto Y, Arimoto T, Oda K, Kawana K, Osuga Y, Fujii T. Vaginal cancer possibly caused by pessary and immunocompromised condition: multiple risk factors may influence vaginal cancer development. J Obstet Gynaecol Res. 2016;42(6):748–51.
32. Ballal PK, Kushtagi P, Shetty N, Polnaya R. Variation in prevalence of gestational trophoblastic disease in India. Indian J Gynecol Oncol. 2016;14(3):1–5.
33. Smith HO, Qualls CR, Prairie BA, Padilla LA, Rayburn WF, Key CR. Trends in gestational choriocarcinoma: a 27-year perspective. Obstet Gynecol. 2003;102(5):978–87.
34. Padubidri VG, Daftary SN. Shaw's textbook of gynecology E-book. Elsevier Health Sciences; 2014.
35. Savage PM, Sita-Lumsden A, Dickson S, Iyer R, Everard J, Coleman R, Fisher RA, Short D, Casalboni S, Catalano K, Seckl MJ. The relationship of maternal age to molar pregnancy incidence, risks for chemotherapy and subsequent pregnancy outcome. J Obstet Gynaecol. 2013;33(4):406–11.
36. WHO: NCD Global Monitoring Framework. https://www.who.int/nmh/global_monitoring_framework/2013-11-06-who-dc-c268-whp-gap-ncds-techdoc-def3.pdf?ua=1. Accessed 7 Jan 2022.
37. United Nations: transforming our world: the 2030 agenda for sustainable development. https://sustainabledevelopment.un.org/content/documents/21252030%20Agenda%20for%20Sustainable%20Development%20web.pdf. Accessed 8 Jan -2022.

Molecular Profiling of Gynaecological Cancer and Breast Cancer

Avdhesh Kumar Rai, Pankaj Borah, and Amal Chandra Kataki

1 Introduction

Gynaecological cancer accounts for 10% of women cancer cases incidence worldwide and they are also leading cause of death among women. Anatomical sites of these cancer are ovary, vulva cervix, uterus, and vagina [1]. Breast carcinoma is also one of the most frequent cancers among women. Globally, 2,300,000 new cancer cases and more than 600,000 death due to breast cancer were reported in 2020 and 5-year prevalence was 7,800,000 cases [1].

In the last few years, experimental studies have focused on molecular profiling of tumours from patients with a wide range of cancers. Molecular pathology and medicine have now been evolving as efficient practice not only for tumour diagnosis and prognosis but also to develop targeted therapeutic decisions. This has resulted in new field called "personalized" or "precision" or "systems" medicine [2]. There is rapid evolution in molecular profiling and molecular classification of cancers [3]. Most patients with advanced cancer undergo molecular profiling as a routine part of their treatment strategy because it is replacing the traditional model of treating them based on their origin of tumour, tumour histology, and stage. Oncologists can now reorganize their perception of cancer by looking at the genomics of tumorigenesis and recommend treatment based upon that knowledge. This has led to dramatic and sometimes successful results, such as cures [4].

Instead of a few small, disease-specific, predictive tests, we are now shifting our focus into multiple gene panel testing for wider coverage of multiple gene level modulations. Depending on the genomic alterations, they can serve as predictive biomarkers for both the specific therapy response and the prognosis of the patient. Therefore, for the better treatment response, it is necessary to differentiate between the germline and somatic aberrations. Pancreatic cancer patients are now being offered BRCA gene (BReast CAncer gene) germline testing. Currently, BRCA gene testing in germlines covers the entire gene, while somatic testing in a limited number of regions. Genomic and somatic mutation analysis will be similarly covered as whole exome sequencing progresses [4].

A. K. Rai (✉)
DBT Centre for Molecular Biology and Cancer Research (DCMBCR), Dr. Bhubaneswar Borooah Cancer Institute (A Unit of Tata Memorial Centre, Mumbai), Guwahati, Assam, India

P. Borah
Department of Molecular Biology and Biotechnology, Tezpur University, Tezpur, India

A. C. Kataki
Department of Gynaecologic Oncology, Dr. Bhubaneswar Borooah Cancer Institute (A Unit of Tata Memorial Centre, Mumbai), Guwahati, Assam, India

A. C. Kataki, D. Barmon (eds.), *Fundamentals in Gynaecologic Malignancy*,
https://doi.org/10.1007/978-981-19-5860-1_2

2 Molecular Profiling Techniques

Molecular profiling is a way to determine the molecular profile (DNA/RNA) for a cancer patient by taking samples from a tumour biopsy or by sampling circulating tumour cells, the latter being less well-established as a method of cancer diagnosis. It was originally used to describe DNA analysis, but technological advancements have expanded its scope to analyze protein and RNA. Changes at DNA level are not sufficient to directly correlate with physiological/ biological changes, thus making examination at the "multiomic" (whole genome, transcriptomes, exome, proteome, and methylome) manner necessary. Changes at the DNA level do not necessarily result in biological changes. Therefore, multiomic examinations gives a holistic understanding of the disease etiology, progression, and therapy response [4].

Large amount of multidimensional data (Big data) is generated by the integrated omics analysis. This requires sophisticated computer hardware and software methods [5]. Bioinformaticians construct robust computer facility that enables the analysis and interpretation of biological data using artificial intelligence and machine learning (AI/ML) based approaches [6]. Such integrative systems biology-based approaches has paved the way for the identification of crucial molecular events linked with oncogenesis, risk prediction, therapy monitoring, and development of precision therapies [7]. The Cancer Genome Atlas (TCGA), the International Cancer Genome Consortium (ICGC) are the most pioneering and successful cancer genomics programs developed to date [8].

2.1 Polymerase Chain Reaction (PCR)

Due to tissue heterogeneity and the scarcity of nucleic acids, detecting nucleic acid biomarkers was difficult prior to the invention of polymerase chain reaction (PCR). PCR is an in vitro amplification techniques which is utilized for amplification and detection of target nucleotide sequence of DNA and RNA. PCR amplification help in creating millions of copies of a specific DNA sequence which can be easily detected and analyzed.

2.2 Real-Time PCR

Real-time PCR, which was developed almost three decades ago, is now widely applied in diagnostic testing facilities for quantitative and semi-quantitative analysis of DNA/RNA. Starting number of target template DNA/RNA sequence determines the efficiency of PCR product amplification which will reflect in target sequence bound fluorescent signal increase in proportional fashion [9].

In comparison with endpoint PCR, this quantitative technology proved to be significantly more accurate but lacked specificity because DNA product of any double stranded nature can bind to the intercalating dye such as primer dimers from PCRs without targets). By using fluorescent reporter DNA probes that had an absorbance wavelength that overlapped the fluorescent molecule's wavelength, however, this limitation has been overcome. The fluorescent molecule is complementary to the region that is being amplified, whereas the quencher molecule has an opposite absorbance wavelength. Because the quencher is near the tag (intact probe), the tag fluorescence is suppressed during PCR. The exonuclease within the polymerase cleaves the bound probe, releasing both tag and quencher, improving the fluorescent signal. As a result of this, genetic mutations can be detected (ASPCR) through the dual specificity generated by the primers and the probe binding [9, 10].

Modifications of probe design have helped further improve the detection sensitivity, specificity, and design flexibility of molecular beacon or scorpion probes, which have an internal hairpin loop. Also, sophisticated modifications of the real-time PCR method have dramatically improved detection sensitivity, such as co-amplification at lower denaturation temperatures [11].

Studies suggest that real-time PCR-based assays have an overall limit of detection of 1–2 target molecules and a limit of quantitation of up to 20 targets. Variant detection limits of detection are set at 2×10^{-4} to 8×10^{-4} [12, 13].

A variety of genomic variants can be detected using fluorescent probe-based, real-time PCR. The more sensitive quantitative PCR (qPCR), as well as quantitative reverse transcription PCR (RT-qPCR), can be used now to detect tumour-specific DNA and to detect RNA-based biomarkers, such as miRNAs [14, 15]. The use of digital PCR and NGS, along with qPCR, is gaining strength in detecting scarce biomarkers. Digital PCR is the newest variation of PCR that has recently gained popularity for the diagnosis of very rare events and gene variants in patients' samples that are difficult to detect using standard qPCR methods [10].

2.3 Droplet Digital PCR (ddPCR)

Input DNA is partitioned for each droplet so that a copy of the template DNA and all of the components needed for PCR, wild-type, and mutation-specific primers and probes (for variant detection) are present. This approach can be used to partition the PCR into millions of microreactors made of emulsion droplets. A PCR reaction is followed by individual scanning of the droplets for a fluorescent signal specific to the mutant or wild type, which allows a high degree of sensitivity and specificity when quantifying the mutation levels [16].

ddPCR has reported LOD of 0.1% but it can be increased up to 0.001% by increasing input DNA. Due to higher sensitivity and precise mutation detection and quantification ddPCR utilization is increasing in cancer research and diagnostics. BEAMing techniques increases the number of copies of each template DNA on magnetic beads to millions of microdroplets [17–19].

By hybridizing fluorescently labeled, sequence-specific oligonucleotide probes to the beads after amplification, amplified DNA on the beads is labeled by flow cytometry. A ddPCR is combined with a flow cytometer with high detection sensitivity to achieve a clonal amplification method. The LOD of the beads has been reported to range between 0.01% and 0.02% VAF. Using modifications such as rolling-circle amplification, the LOD can be improved even further to levels upto 0.01% [20–22].

2.4 Next-Generation Sequencing (NGS)

For routine use of cancer biomakers in molecular diagnostic laboratories, NGS platforms have gained considerable traction in the past decade. They have had a dramatic impact in a relatively short period of time on the quality, scale, and variation of clinical genome sequencing. It was reported by the National Survey of Precision Medicine in Cancer Treatment, 75.5% of oncologists used NGS results to guide treatment decisions in 2017, demonstrating how important and valuable NGS has become to oncology. This revolutionary massively parallel sequencing technology is what has made NGS so popular, because it is capable of detecting many genomic changes (such as mutations, gene amplifications, and gene fusions and expression) at the same time in multiple samples [23].

As part of clinical sequencing tests, the lower limit of detection (LOD) is an important factor to consider. This measure defines the lowest levels of genomic variants that the platform has the ability to detect consistently in the background of wild-type sequences. Depending on the NGS method, LOD can be defined as the minor allele frequency at which 95% of the samples will be reliably detected. Depending on the type of genetic change detected and the NGS workflow, this can range from 2% to 15% for most validated clinical NGS platforms [13–20]. There are currently few routine NGS workflows geared towards consistently identifying LODs that are sufficient for specialized applications such as testing of samples with limited tumour content, clonal heterogeneity, and treatment response monitoring. This means that the majority of these applications are implemented using non-NGS high-sensitivity technologies such as droplet digital PCR (ddPCR), BEAMing, and allele-specific real-time PCR (ASPCR) [24–31].

2.5 NGS Workflow

2.5.1 PCR Amplification

In NGS workflows, at least one PCR amplification step usually takes place. This process is crucial in determining the presence of tumour-associated genes, especially when using DNA of limited quantity and quality. To prepare sequencing-ready libraries, the NGS workflow consists largely of two methods. First method uses sequence-specific primers and generally a high number of PCR cycles to amplify sequences of interest from the whole genomic background, then a second PCR step using a sequencing adapter-specific primers for less number of cycles. Second, target enrichment technique utilizes hybridization probe for separation of target DNA sequence and PCR amplification helps in enrichment of target DNA sequence by using adapter primers. Due to the reliance of both of these methods on PCR, the accuracy of the final sequence depends on DNA quality and quantity, the PCR cycle count, and the polymerases' fidelity to handle the nucleic acid artifacts. Studies addressing the role of polymerase fidelity have demonstrated that higher-fidelity polymerases can improve the accuracy of NGS, although to varying degrees, depending on the target sequence and applications examined. PCR-dependent workflows can also underrepresent the genomic regions rich in GC and AT, resulting in low sequence coverage and suboptimal variant detection, particularly for gene copy number changes [12, 32–34].

2.5.2 Massive Parallel Sequencing

NGS platforms use massively parallel sequencing technology, but the fundamental sequencing technologies are different, resulting in differences in timing, output, read length, errors, and run time. Sequencing by synthesis is performed with Illumina platforms (San Diego, CA), on glass flowcell surface target DNA sequence is amplified to create clusters, these clusters used for synthesis of complimentary strand. Although Illumina platforms provide high sequencing accuracy, errors still occur. These mistakes often occur because of the strands running out of sync during sequencing cycles (GGC sequence pattern or inverted repeat). It has been estimated for the Illumina platforms that there is a sequencing error rate between 0.25% and 0.8%, posing a challenge for routine detection of low-level variants [35].

Today, a second NGS technology widely employed in clinical laboratories is Ion Torrent sequencing (Life Technologies, San Francisco, CA),a revolutionary nonoptimal, semiconductor-based technology. An array of millions of wells attached to a semiconductor chip houses cloned DNA fragments amplified by amplification on beads. As templates, DNA is transferred onto these beads and sequencing is performed with regulated pattern release of nucleotides. Incorporation of nucleotides lead to formation of phosphodiester bonds, a flood of protons is released. The semiconductor chips are then able to detect pH changes and electric potential changes [36].

In Ion Torrent sequencing during homopolymer stretches, nucleotides are incorporated simultaneously into the sequence, resulting in spurious indels. Therefore, it has been demonstrated that indel sequencing errors are 1.1–2%, whereas substitution errors are negligible (0.04–0.1%) [37, 38].

Other NGS platforms available on the market utilize distinctly different and novel sequencing methods, such as those offered by Oxford Nanopore Technologies (Oxford, UK) and Pacific Biosciences (PacBio; Menlo Park, CA). They have relatively high error rates (estimated at >5%), and they have yet to gain significant ground in mainstream clinical applications [39, 40].

2.5.3 Sequencing Data Analysis

The digital processing of the sequencer-generated voluminous sequencing information is an essential part of the NGS workflow that allows the generation of meaningful genomic profiles and the detection of variants. Combining base calling with raw signal information from the sequencer, low-quality base calls elimination, aligning sequences to a reference sequence to identify potential sequence variants, and aligning reads to the reference sequence are all included in this process. Among the crucial elements of genomic analysis is sequence alignment, where repetitive sequences and complex insertions or deletions may cause misalignments that adversely affect variant detection. In data processing, filtering the variants depending on the sequencing quality and variant allelic frequency (VAFs), is another critical step. A contributing factor is the relatively short read lengths of popular sequence platforms (300–400 bp). Predetermined parameters are required, which when too lax can result in sequencing artifacts (false positives) or when too stringent can result in filters that exclude true mutations (false negatives). In order to minimize errors, it is crucial that these parameters are carefully set and validated in relation to the nature of NGS technology, sequencing read lengths, and type of variants [35, 36].

3 Criteria for Evidence-Based Classification of Molecular Biomarkers

National Comprehensive Cancer Network (NCCN) panel of experts and other experts classify conditions for "evidence" available and its relevance in cancer patient's therapy management. The evidences are classified as follows:

1. Evidence from large, well-designed, randomized controlled trials
2. (a) Evidence from phase 2 or nonrandomized trials, multiple smaller trials, indirect comparisons among randomized trials). (b) Evidence from retrospective studies, clinical experience alone.

4 Microsatellite Instability-High Tumours and DNA Mismatch Repair Molecular Biomarkers

Microsatellite instability (MSI) occurs when DNA mismatch repair system is inactivated, and is characterized by an inordinate number of frameshift mutations in microsatellite DNA. MSI occurs in certain tumours such as hereditary lynch syndrome is associated with germline mutations in any of the mismatch repair genes (PMS2, MSH2, MLH1, MSH6). However, most MSI cases (80%) arise sporadically from hypermethylation of the MLH1 gene promoter rather than from a familial condition [41, 42]. There have been reports of MSI-high (MSI-H) in many primary cancer types and it has been estimated to influence 4% of all cancers in adults [43, 44]. Patients with tumours that are MSI-H at an early stage show better prognosis than those with microsatellite stable tumours, and many MSI-H tumours are highly sensitive to PD-1/PD-L1 inhibitors. A PD-1 inhibitor called pembrolizumab has been approved by the FDA for non-resectable/metastatic, solid tumours who are MSI-H or MMR-deficient (dMMR) [45, 46].

5 Germline Mutations Molecular Biomarkers

A gene mutation can either be germline or somatic; the somatic mutations occur spontaneously after birth, whereas germline is inherited (i.e., inherited from birth). A genetic test can uncover germline mutations which may be relevant to cancer treatment and prevention. Genetic testing (somatic) can identify mutations that may be in fact germline alterations, but they need to be confirmed in matched normal samples from the tumour bearing host (e.g., white blood cells, buccal swabs, and cultured skin fibroblasts) [4].

Genetic modifications in tumours can fall into three main categories with various expectations related to whether or not they represent germline changes. The first category comprises genes associated with common tumour mutations and rare germline mutations. Unless a family or personal history suggests a genetic disorder, germline testing is not needed. TP53 mutations can occur as familial syndromes like Li-Fraumeni, but such inheritance is extremely rare. More than 60% of lung cancers have TP53 mutations [47].

In the second category, you will discover the most common somatic mutations, which may be linked to familial syndromes. dMMR is found in about 12% of colon cancers when MSI or IHC testing is routinely performed. The majority of the dMMR alterations are inherited according to molecular germline testing. Germline mutation confirmatory testing in patients and members of their family need to be done [48].

In the third category, we find novel mutations in tumour that are commonly germline mutations. BRCA1 and BRCA2 gene mutations testing in breast and ovarian cancer patients should routinely be done, particularly if the personal history of cancer in family is found. BRCA1/ BRCA2 mutations are being identified on routine molecular genetic testing in patients with other tumours where they are less likely to be found. Detection of BRCA1 and BRCA2 gene mutations may aid in treatment selection for such tumours. Germline BRCA1 and BRCA2 gene mutation confirmation is recommended for providing genetic counseling to the family member of the patient [49].

It is important to note that all inherited breast and ovarian cancer cases may not necessarily BRCA1/ BRCA2 mutations, it may occur due to absence of coverage of that mutations in the somatic panel, or where large-scale deletions and duplications are present. Despite a lack of accompanying clinical history, multigene panel profiling may actually detect previously unknown and clinically relevant germline mutations that are inherited from the parents or that are acquired de novo [45].

6 Molecular Profile of Gynaecologic Cancers

6.1 Endometrial Cancers Molecular Profile

Molecular tumour testing should be performed in all patients with uterine cancer to determine if they have MSI or not. It is estimated that between 2% and 5% of all uterine cancers are caused by genes linked to Lynch syndrome, such as MLH1, MSH2, MSH6, or PMS2. Hypermethylation should also be tested for abnormalities in MLH1, since this can lead to MSI-H tumours even when no germline mutation is present. A germline mutation or hypermethylation of MSI-H causes recurrent uterine cancer to be a candidate for pembrolizumab, according to a 2017 FDA approval granted site-agnostic use of the drug [50]. The prognosis for women with POLE-aberrant endometrial cancer is good, and they may need less aggressive treatment in the future, although this is still merely a theory. In Phase 2 trials, mTOR inhibitors were found to be active against endometrioid carcinoma of the uterus, but assays are not used to verify that molecular screening can effectively select for potential effectiveness [46].

6.2 Ovarian Cancers Molecular Profile

A subgroup of high-grade serous epithelial ovarian cancers, characterized by pathogenic mutations in BRCA-related genes, has a distinct biology, family history, and sensitivity to platinum and PARP inhibitors. Here are the mutations which fall into this category: BRCA1, BRCA2, STK11, BRIP1, PALB2, MLH1, RAD51C, RAD51D, PMS2, BARD1, MSH6, and MSH2. These mutations will improve the prognosis for the patient, increase platinum sensitivity, and create a more favorable possibility of better overall survival. In homologous recombination (HR)-deficient (HRD) cancers molecular profiling for BRCA associated mutation may act as biomarkers for platinum sensitivity [51–53].

In patients with ovarian cancer that is recurrent or had BRCA1/BRCA2 mutations or HRD, PARP inhibitors were first approved as monotherapy (olaparib or rucaparib). Olaparib, rucaparib, and niraparib have now been approved for use as switch maintenance therapy for platinum-sensitive ovarian cancer patients following platinum treatment in the second-line or third-line setting. The initial platinum and taxane therapy followed by the maintenance bevacizumab therapy may serve better for patients without BRCA-related mutations compared to those with the mutations (Gynaecologic Oncology Group Study 0218 [GOG-7]) [54–57].

Identifying mutations in BRCA-related genes is also necessary to identify family members at risk of subsequent ovarian, tubal, peritoneal, and breast cancer with risk-reducing surgery and surveillance. Pembrolizumab is approved by the FDA for patients with MSI-H tumours, which makes PD-1 and PD-L1 evaluation important in patients with ovarian cancer [12].

6.3 Cervical Cancers Molecular Profile

Patients with recurrent cervical cancer have a poor prognosis because of treatment difficulties. There are no molecular markers that can predict patient response to bevacizumab treatment; however, it has been approved for recurrent disease in combination with platinum, taxanes, and topotecan. A 2018 FDA approval of pembrolizumab was given on the basis of KEYNOTE 158 study evidence (14% success) (ClinicalTrials.gov identifier NCT02628067) in recurrent/metastatic cervical cancer patient on or post-chemotherapy with PD-L expression. Furthermore, nivolumab, when used as a single agent, demonstrates a 26% response rate in patients with recurrent cervical cancer. Trials are currently being conducted to evaluate combinations of nivolumab and ipilimumab [4].

6.4 Breast Cancer Molecular Profile

In breast cancer patients, well-established biomarkers determine treatment decisions. These include estrogen receptor (ER) expression, progesterone receptor (PR) expression, and HER2 overexpression or amplification. All the newly diagnosed invasive breast cancers as well as recurrences should be evaluated for their ER, PR, and HER2 status. These three markers are routinely assessed to predict treatment response and guide treatment planning for breast cancer patients. The androgen receptor (AR), ESR1, and PD-L1 may be useful markers for future breast cancer treatment. The overexpression of AR is observed in subset of triple-negative breast cancers (TNBCs). Patients with metastatic, AR-positive TNBC have shown promising preliminary results in clinical trials with AR-targeted treatments [58, 59].

ESR1 mutations affect the ER's ligand-binding domain, leading to a constitutively active, ligand-independent form of the ER; this could position the ER for resistance to aromatase inhibitors. In cases of hormone receptor-positive breast cancer, ESR1 mutations are most commonly observed during or after treatment with aromatase inhibitors. The treatment recommendation is to consider direct targeting of the ER directly in the presence of a de novo ESR1 mutation [60].

Multiple trials evaluating immune checkpoint blockade in the treatment of breast cancer will provide a better understanding of PD-L1's role as a predictive biomarker for the use of checkpoint inhibitors for breast cancer treatment. In early stage breast cancer, multigene genomic tests such as Oncotype DX, MammaPrint, and Prosigna (formerly PAM 50) are routinely used to guide treatment decisions [60].

7 Oncology Basket Trials and Precision Medicine

Up to a few years ago, approved genetic testing was limited to a few tests conducted on patients with specific cancers in order to target a specific therapy. In patients with CRC, pan-RAS testing (KRAS, NRAS, and HRAS) to determine the needed anti-EGFR therapy cetuximab and panitumumab have been identified as examples of mutational status being key to treatment recommendations. The anti-HER2-targeted therapy trastuzumab, and the tyrosine kinase inhibitor lapatinib may be administered to patients with breast cancer based on HER2 testing. Before pan-RAS and HER2 tests became a standard diagnostic approach for predicting response to treatment, many different clinical trials involving large number of patients were conducted for many years [61–63].

As part of current oncology basket trials, biomarker-driven designs are used to test a range of therapies across different populations. The biomarkers that are selected must be clinically feasible assays that can be used to enrich responses to the targeted therapy. These Trials involving broad-panel molecular profiling are large and small-scale trials which include the European Organization for Research and Treatment of Cancer–Screening Patients for Efficient Clinical Trial Access (EORTC-SPECTA) program, the American Society of Clinical Oncology (ASCO) Targeted Agent and Profiling Utilization Registry (TAPUR) study, the National Cancer Institute's Molecular Analysis for Therapy Choice (NCI-MATCH) trial. Molecularly tailored therapies are being investigated in these studies in order to expand the boundaries of precision medicine.

NCI-MATCH (Molecular Analysis for Therapy Choice), a novel phase 2 trial, was initiated in August 2015. According to individual tumour genomic profiling, NCI-MATCH aims to measure the proportion of patients who exhibit objective responses (ORs) to targeted therapies. Whenever a mutation-matched therapy has a response rate of at least 25%, this match will go into larger phase 2 trials. The U.S. has well over 1000 study sites, and pharmaceutical and biotechnology companies provide targeted agents to patients across those sites. It does not matter what the patients' tissue origin or cancer is, they receive treatment according to their molecular profile. In "master" trial, investigator can be allowed to add drugs of interest at any time point. The trial can be accessed at ClinicalTrials.gov under the identifier NCT02465060, where you will find the most up to date information [64].

TAPUR is a multicenter, nonrandomized clinical trial that opened in 2016 and is ongoing. In this trial, FDA-approved medications will be used to treat advanced cancer patients outside of the approved indications of the medication, which will target a specific mutation in tumours. Enrollment is open to patients with having solid tumours as well as lymphomas and multiple myelomas. It aims to observe the real-world use of targeted therapies among patients who have cancers with known genomic changes with a specific drug target or with identified sensitivity to a drug offered in the study. Over 2500 patients are expected to be enrolled for TAPUR. The clinical trial is registered in ClinicalTrials.gov under NCT02693535, where current information about it can be found [65].

The EORTC-SPECTA project is a collaborative European molecular screening program that coordinates various disease-specific platforms and aims to offer targeted therapy to patients who show actionable mutations (ClinicalTrials.gov identifier NCT02834884). Using one entry point, this large-scale basket allows researchers to access multiple studies and high-quality, annotated material for research. Patients are followed longitudinally to understand disease progression pattern [66–68].

8 Multiomics and Systems Medicine Approach in Gynaecological Cancer and Breast Cancer

In cancer research and therapeutics, the translation of traditional single-factor treatment modalities such as radiotherapy and chemotherapy into real-time clinical practice is challenging. It is comparatively ineffective in preventing cancer and predicting the accurate therapy response rate of cancer patients [69]. These limitations of single-factor treatment strategies have resulted in the development of predictive, preventive, participatory, and personalized medicine (P4 medicine) which aid in accurate prediction of patients' survival outcome, prevent tumour recurrence, stratify patients, and personalize effective treatment strategies for individual patients [70]. Due to advancement of high throughput sequencing technologies and big data analytics, MultiOmics based analysis (genome and exome sequencing (genomics), RNA-sequencing (transcriptomics), DNA methylation (epigenomics) proteomics, and metabolomics have gained popular attention in oncology particularly in cancer with high occurrence rate such as breast cancer, cervical cancer, and other gastrointestinal and gynaecological cancer. The multidimensional omics-based approaches have increased our knowledge

Table 1 Summary of MultiOmics dataset for breast and gynaecological cancer

Cancer type	Cases	Genomics (files)			Transcriptomics (files)	Epigenomics (files)	Proteomics (files)
		SNV	CNV	SSV			
Breast cancer	9111	25,363	10,627	460	8013	1241	920
Gynaecological cancer MultiOmics data							
Ovary	3399	9706	4808	–	2637	624	433
Cervix	914	4731	2225	319	2911	312	172
Vagina	72	83	46	1	–	–	–
Vulvar	10	21	–	–	–	–	–
Ureter	15	31	–	–	–	–	–

The information regarding MultiOmics datasets on breast and gynaecological cancers has been summarized from TCGA portal [71] (https://portal.gdc.cancer.gov/)

on cancer biology research and identified key gene mutations and metabolic pathways through bioinformatics analysis which can be used as a potential target gene for development of diagnostic, prognostic, and therapeutic models [69].

The development of NGS technologies and large-scale collaborative cancer research projects has facilitated the generation of huge multidimensional cancer datasets that are publicly accessible in cancer databases. The Cancer Genome Atlas (TCGA) [71] and The International Cancer Genome Consortium (ICGC) [72] are the most well-known, largest, and distinguished collaborative cancer projects that includes 50 different cancer type MultiOmics datasets that are of high clinical significance [73].

- The ICGC portal is one of the most prominent cancer databases that contains well annotated structured cancer dataset. The dataset information and storage in ICGC portal is based on the BioMart data management platform that uses advanced and seamless data models for maintaining the uniformity of different cancer datasets [74–76]. The ICGC Data Portal contains data from other large-scale cancer genome projects, including TCGA, Johns Hopkins University (Baltimore, MD, USA), and Tumour Sequencing Project (TSP). The cancer projects interface contains data available in the 49 ICGC member projects, as well as additional filters and a selection of attributes. The Data Repository of the ICGC portal provides access to all ICGC cancer project datasets in the form of processed and annotated files [77]. The datasets can be downloaded and exported for further downstream analysis.
- TCGA is a collaborative joint project between the National Cancer Institute (NCI) and the National Human Genome Research Institute (NHGRI) (both from Bethesda, MD, USA) which provides a complete map of the major genetic changes that occur in various cancer types and subtypes [71]. TCGA includes clinical information of cancer patients, characterization of genomic data, and high-level sequenced data of the tumour genomes. The TCGA Data Portal also allows investigators to explore, download, and analyze datasets generated by TCGA. The data types stored in TCGA mainly includes gene expression datasets, copy number variations, somatic mutations, single nucleotide polymorphisms (SNPs), microRNAs, clinical outcomes, and tissue slide images [77]. The TCGA Roadmap has been developed for indexing and file annotations in the TCGA open access HTTP through advanced web technology, Web 3.0 [78] (Table 1).

8.1 MultiOmics Studies on Breast Cancer (BRCA)

BRCA is one of the most common cancer types in female population worldwide. The development multiomics-based breast cancer dataset has helped to identify crucial molecular marker genes related to breast cancer. In last few years, several

MultiOmics analysis-based studies in BRCA were performed to determine the potential molecular determinants associated with breast cancer. MultiOmics data integration of transcriptomics, genomics, and epigenomics in breast cancer identified pathophysiological system linked to BRCA development and also identified clinically important subtypes of BRCA patient [79]. In another study, genomic heterogeneity in triple-negative breast cancer (TNBC) was reported for the first time by analyzing BRCA omics dataset derived from TCGA [80]. A recent study was conducted on one of the largest TNBC MultiOmics dataset using immunogenomic approaches which revealed the crucial immune escape mechanism that is related to tumour heterogeneity. This study has paved the pathway for development of personalized immunotherapy in TNBC [81]. MultiOmics analysis of BRCA PMC42 cell line reported that PMC42 is a significant MET model and regulates the phenotypic plasticity in BRCA. The integrated omics study on BRCA also identified important marker genes which are associated with drug resistance that will help to stratify patient groups and thereby improve the drug response rate and survival outcome of BRCA treatment [82].

8.2 MultiOmics Studies on Gynaecological Cancer

1. **Ovarian Cancer (OC)**

   OC is the fifth leading cause of cancer related death in women and is known to be one of the most lethal gynaecological malignancy. The integrated omics-based analysis on ovarian cancer and other gynaecological cancer has identified novel targets and aid in development of personalized therapy in for ovarian cancer patients. The integrated transcriptomics and proteomics analysis on ovarian cancer identified STAT3 signaling pathway as a crucial signaling molecule that acts as a multifaceted sword and found to be involved in important regulatory functions EMT, cell cycle progression, and cancer stemness in several ovarian cancer model systems [83]. A recent study identified novel biomarkers in serous ovarian cancer (SOC) using integrated transcriptomics, proteomics, and epigenomics approach [84]. The immune characteristics, genomic. and clinical features of the three subtypes of ovarian cancer were analyzed computationally, and the molecular basis of the immunosuppressive microenvironment of ovarian cancer was characterized through integration of multiomics analyses, that includes methylation and genome variation, providing a new perspective for improved immunotherapeutic response in OC [85]. A recent study reported the role of circadian clock genes in ovarian cancer. The study through MultiOmics analysis demonstrated that circadian clock genes are highly dysregulated in cancer and are strongly correlated with the cancer prognosis [86].

2. **Cervical Cancer (CC)**

   Globally, cervical cancer (CC) is the fourth most common female malignancy and which is responsible for high mortality rates worldwide, especially in developing countries [87]. MultiOmics studies on CC has identified key immunological and genetic signatures and further evaluation of this signatures are urgently needed for development of personalized treatment strategies for CC patients. In a recent study, a novel immune classification system was developed using MultiOmics CC dataset from TCGA database. The immune classification system will help clinicians to select patients for induvial personalized immunotherapy/combination therapies [88]. In another study, using RNAseq and somatic mutation integrative data analysis, a panel of immune related prognostic genes (IRPGs) were identified that can act as a prognostic biomarker for CC patients [89]. MultiOmics analysis on CC dataset has identified several target genes that are important for development of targeted therapeutics for CC patients [90, 91].

3. **Other gynaecological cancers (vaginal, vulva, and uterine cancers)**

   The malignancy of the female sex organs is rare compared to that of other gynaecological cancers. Due to rarity of these cancers, the

MultiOmics based dataset are limited. The overall incidence and mortality rate of gynaecological cancers has declined globally due to HPV vaccines and early detection and advanced treatment modalities. However, incidence of vagina and vulva have risen [92]. Recent studies have demonstrated the involvement of microbial composition in cancers of the female lower reproductive tract. In several studies, it has been reported that there is significant correlation between vaginal microbial profile, HPV infection, and cancers of the female reproductive tract particularly the female lower reproductive tract [93, 94]. However, further MultiOmics and system biology-based studies are required for understanding the basis of such cancers and subsequent development of predictive and personalized treatment strategies.

A study reported genetic alterations in m6A regulatory genes through MultiOmics analysis of uterine cancer dataset. It is predicted that m6A RNA methylation facilitates malignant progression and thereby can act as a potential biomarker for uterine cancer [95]. More systems biology and big data based MultiOmics analysis are needed to develop diagnostic/prognostic and therapeutic biomarkers for these rare type of cancers

9 Challenges of Molecular Profiling of Cancer

9.1 Lack of Randomized, Controlled Clinical Trials

In the absence of randomized clinical trials demonstrating the effectiveness of large panels or whole genome sequencing is challenging. Considering the high cost of drugs and genomic testing, as well as potential risks associated with exposing patients to toxicity of drugs without proof of effectiveness, the field requires more evidence. There is no question that Overall Survival (OS) is the gold standard, but it depends on whether multiple lines of therapy are used and if targeted therapy is used beyond the conditions of the study. Although progression free survival (PFS) is a reasonable endpoint, the impact of molecularly targeted therapy may be underestimated if the randomization occurs when appropriate standard therapies are available. With Molecularly Assigned Therapy, there is a chance to break new ground in trial design. Von Hoff's PFS ratio remains a good metric to predict outcome in molecularly assigned therapies [4].

9.2 Unavailability to Suitable Molecular Target Drugs

It is also crucial to address the fact that there are currently no approved drugs to address the many drivers of various types of cancer. These include mutated β-catenin, mutated P53, or mutated RAS, among others. A positive aspect is the possibility of offering drugs to patients with actionable mutations in retrospective manner. A similar challenge may be the non-availability of drugs which can effectively target evolving resistance against targeted therapies. EGFR, ALK, and BCR-ABL mutations are exceptions [4].

9.3 Challenge of Tumour Heterogeneity

Various forms of tumour heterogeneity are evident in treated advanced stage cancers. These include heterogeneity at intralesion, interlesion, and interpatient level. These heterogeneities leads to complication in treatment and outcome recommendations [4].

9.4 Molecular Profiling Platform Variations

For molecular profiling in clinical settings, there are several different platforms that are available; each of them has its own degree of specificity and sensitivity. Various commercial and academic platforms continually evolve, making it more difficult to pool data from multiple platforms. This heterogeneity contributes to the difficulty of pooling data from different platforms. Furthermore, no studies have been conducted that have shown that larger panels are worth the expense over smaller targeted gene panels used frequently in cancer care (e.g., KRAS, NRAS, BRAF, and MSI in CRC) [4].

9.5 Challenges of Quality Control Measures for Molecular Profiling

In the USA, The Clinical Laboratory Improvement Amendments (CLIA) create definition for laboratories involved in performing test on clinical specimen derived from humans for the purpose of diagnosing, preventing, or treating disease or impairment. The rigorous laboratory quality control procedures for molecular profiling tests can be challenging in many developing countries. Additionally, high costs make it difficult for cancer patients to afford molecular profiling tests, and these tests are not covered by insurance companies [4].

Clinical laboratory test offerings must continually evolve to provide advanced testing facilities in cancer care. In deciding which tests or customized solutions will be most effective for a lab, clinician, and patient population, various factors are taken into consideration. Comparing assay systems is greatly simplified by using a reference material that is highly multiplexed, consistent, and well-characterized [4].

However, specificity, sensitivity, and reproducibility of the molecular profiling assays are the most important factors for determining effective, personalized treatment for patients, and these parameters can be difficult to critically assess, but need to be rigorously validated.

9.6 Appropriate Condition for Molecular Profiling of Cancer

The evidence-based on which to make recommendations regarding when to perform genomic testing remains in flux, and there is disagreement about the optimal time for the procedure to maximize its therapeutic value to individual cancer patients. The tumour genome continues to evolve in patients with advanced cancer as time passes, as well as with the continuous pressure exerted by several therapeutics which ultimately promote the growth of tumour subclones that are resistant to therapies. In patients with refractory disease, investigators often recommend performing a rebiopsy to for genomic analysis can accurately create the tumours recent genetic composition ensure the genomic analysis used to make informed decisions about clinical trials with targeted agents reflects the tumour's current genetic makeup [4].

10 Future Perspective

The best cancer care begins with advanced cutting edge molecular diagnostics, employing very efficient know-how to interpret and application of the results in clinical setting, and staying in tune with current developments. Phase 3 trials are no longer the sole basis for the approval of drugs; these late-stage trials have been replaced by "basket" and "umbrella" trials, which can lead to the best suited drug being administered faster to the most suitable patient. Using "liquid biopsies" or cell-free DNA to evaluate the tumour genome without needing to repeat invasive biopsy has been hailed as a new method for assessing the tumour genome. Does liquid biopsy replace tissue-based biopsy adequately in dealing with tumour heterogeneity? Does testing a large number of patients justify and is it feasible to test a large number of patients, knowing that we are very unlikely to find the "needle in the haystack"? Is it possible for newly developed expensive targeted therapies to be affordable when they only target a decreasing number of patients? Management of patient's expectations in today's information flooded world with multifold increase of hype and publicity our new discoveries with limited rigorous clinical trial data?

Now that precision medicine is a part of our standard practice, many new challenges are emerging.

References

1. Yi M, Li T, Niu M, Luo S, Chu Q, Wu K. Epidemiological trends of women's cancers from 1990 to 2019 at the global, regional, and national levels: a population-based study. Biomark Res. 2021;9:1–12.
2. Flores M, Glusman G, Brogaard K, Price ND, Hood L. P4 medicine: how systems medicine will transform the healthcare sector and society. Per Med. 2013;10:565–76.
3. Eliyatkın N, Yalçın E, Zengel B, Aktaş S, Vardar E. Molecular classification of breast carcinoma: from traditional, old-fashioned way to a new age, and a new way. J Breast Health. 2015;11:59.
4. El-Deiry WS, Goldberg RM, Lenz HJ, et al. The current state of molecular testing in the treatment of patients with solid tumors, 2019. CA Cancer J Clin. 2019;69:305–43.
5. Dlamini Z, Francies FZ, Hull R, Marima R. Artificial intelligence (AI) and big data in cancer and precision oncology. Comput Struct Biotechnol J. 2020;18:2300–11.
6. Barah P, Bhattacharyya DK, Kalita JK. Gene expression data analysis: a statistical and machine learning perspective. CRC Press; 2021.
7. Tomczak K, Czerwińska P, Wiznerowicz M. The Cancer Genome Atlas (TCGA): an immeasurable source of knowledge. Contemp Oncol. 2015;19:A68.
8. Jennings JL, Stein LD, Calvo F. International cancer genome consortium (ICGC). Cancer Research. 2017;77(13):377-.
9. Higuchi R, Fockler C, Dollinger G, Watson R. Kinetic PCR analysis: real-time monitoring of DNA amplification reactions. Biotechnology. 1993;11:1026.
10. Singh RR. Next-generation sequencing in high-sensitive detection of mutations in tumors: challenges, advances, and applications. J Mol Diagn. 2020;22:994–1007.
11. Li J, Wang L, Mamon H, Kulke MH, Berbeco R, Makrigiorgos GM. Replacing PCR with COLD-PCR enriches variant DNA sequences and redefines the sensitivity of genetic testing. Nat Med. 2008;14:579e584.
12. Filges S, Yamada E, Styaahlberg A, Godfrey TE. Impact of polymerase fidelity on background error rates in next-generation sequencing with unique molecular identifiers/barcodes. Sci Rep. 2019;9:3503.
13. Schwarz G, Bäumler S, Block A, Felsenstein FG, Wenzel G. Determination of detection and quantification limits for SNP allele frequency estimation in DNA pools using real time PCR. Nucleic Acids Res. 2004;32:e24.
14. Cree IA. Diagnostic RAS mutation analysis by polymerase chain reaction (PCR). Biomol Detect Quantif. 2016;8:29–32.
15. Chen E, Li Q, Wang H, Yang F, Min L, Yang J. MiR-92a promotes tumorigenesis of colorectal cancer, a transcriptomic and functional based study. Biomed Pharmacother. 2018;106:1370–7.
16. Hatch AC, Fisher JS, Tovar AR, et al. 1-Million droplet array with wide-field fluorescence imaging for digital PCR. Lab Chip. 2011;11:3838–45.
17. Milbury CA, Zhong Q, Lin J, et al. Determining lower limits of detection of digital PCR assays for cancer-related gene mutations. Biomol Detect Quantif. 2014;1:8–22.
18. Dong L, Wang S, Fu B, Wang J. Evaluation of droplet digital PCR and next generation sequencing for characterizing DNA reference material for KRAS mutation detection. Sci Rep. 2018;8:9650.
19. Fitarelli-Kiehl M, Yu F, Ashtaputre R, et al. Denaturation-enhanced droplet digital PCR for liquid biopsies. Clin Chem. 2018;64:1762–71.
20. Diehl F, Schmidt K, Choti MA, et al. Circulating mutant DNA to assess tumor dynamics. Nat Med. 2008;14:985–90.
21. Garcia J, Forestier J, Dusserre E, et al. Cross-platform comparison for the detection of RAS mutations in CfDNA (DdPCR biorad detection assay, BEAMing assay, and NGS strategy). Oncotarget. 2018;9:21122–31.
22. Li M, Diehl F, Dressman D, Vogelstein B, Kinzler KW. BEAMing up for detection and quantification of rare sequence variants. Nat Methods. 2006;3:95.
23. Freedman AN, Klabunde CN, Wiant K, et al. Use of next-generation sequencing tests to guide cancer treatment: results from a nationally representative survey of oncologists in the United States. JCO Precis Oncologia. 2018;2:1–13.
24. Lin M-T, Mosier SL, Thiess M, et al. Clinical validation of KRAS, BRAF, and EGFR mutation detection using next-generation sequencing. Am J Clin Pathol. 2014;141:856–66.
25. Cheng DT, Mitchell TN, Zehir A, et al. Memorial Sloan Kettering-integrated mutation profiling of actionable cancer targets (MSK-IMPACT): a hybridization capture-based next-generation sequencing clinical assay for solid tumor molecular oncology. J Mol Diagn. 2015;17:251–64.
26. Kadri S, Long BC, Mujacic I, et al. Clinical validation of a next-generation sequencing genomic oncology panel via crossplatform benchmarking against established amplicon sequencing assays. J Mol Diagn. 2017;19:43–56.
27. Lih C-J, Harrington RD, Sims DJ, et al. Analytical validation of the next-generation sequencing assay for a nationwide signal-finding clinical trial: molecular analysis for therapy choice clinical trial. J Mol Diagn. 2017;19:313–27.
28. Luthra R, Patel KP, Reddy NG, et al. Next-generation sequencing-based multigene mutational screening for acute myeloid leukemia using miseq: applicability for diagnostics and disease monitoring. Haematologica. 2014;99:465–73.
29. Froyen G, Broekmans A, Hillen F, et al. Validation and application of a custom-designed targeted next-generation sequencing panel for the diagnos-

tic mutational profiling of solid tumors. PLoS One. 2016;11:e0154038.
30. Bonfiglio S, Vanni I, Rossella V, et al. Performance comparison of two commercial human whole-exome capture systems on formalin-fixed paraffin-embedded lung adenocarcinoma samples. BMC Cancer. 2016;16:692.
31. Wrzeszczynski KO, Felice V, Abhyankar A, et al. Analytical validation of clinical wholegenome and transcriptome sequencing of patient-derived tumors for reporting targetable variants in cancer. J Mol Diagn. 2018;20:822–35.
32. Goldstein A, Toro PV, Lee J, et al. Detection fidelity of AR mutations in plasma derived cell-free DNA. Oncotarget. 2017;8:15651–62.
33. Ma X, Shao Y, Tian L, et al. Analysis of error profiles in deep next-generation sequencing data. Genome Biol. 2019;20:50.
34. Benjamini Y, Speed TP. Summarizing and correcting the GC content bias in high-throughput sequencing. Nucleic Acids Res. 2012;40:e72.
35. Quail MA, Smith M, Coupland P, et al. A tale of three next generation sequencing platforms: comparison of ion torrent, pacific biosciences and illumina MiSeq sequencers. BMC Genomics. 2012;13:341.
36. Rothberg JM, Hinz W, Rearick TM, et al. An integrated semiconductor device enabling non-optical genome sequencing. Nature. 2011;475:348–52.
37. Loman NJ, Misra RV, Dallman TJ, et al. Performance comparison of benchtop highthroughput sequencing platforms. Nat Biotechnol. 2012;30:434–9.
38. Fox EJ, Reid-Bayliss KS, Emond MJ, Loeb LA. Accuracy of next generation sequencing platforms. Next Gener Seq Appl. 2014;1:1000106.
39. Mikheyev AS, Tin MM. A first look at the Oxford nanopore MinION sequencer. Mol Ecol Resour. 2014;14:1097–102.
40. Boland CR, Goel A. Microsatellite instability in colorectal cancer. Gastroenterology. 2010;138:2073–2087.e3.
41. Lynch HT, de la Chapelle A. Hereditary colorectal cancer. N Engl J Med. 2003;348:919–32.
42. Vanderwalde A, Spetzler D, Xiao N, Gatalica Z, Marshall J. Microsatellite instability status determined by nextgeneration sequencing and compared with PD-L1 and tumor mutational burden in 11,348 patients. Cancer Med. 2018;7:746–56.
43. Bonneville R, Krook MA, Kautto EA, et al. Landscape of microsatellite instability across 39 cancer types. JCO Precis Oncol. 2017;1:1–15.
44. Chang L, Chang M, Kautto HM, et al. Microsatellite instability: a predictive biomarker for cancer immunotherapy. Appl Immunohistochem Mol Morphol. 2018;26:e15–21.
45. Ott PA, Bang YJ, Berton-Rigaud D, et al. Safety and antitumor activity of pembrolizumab in advanced programmed death ligand 1-positive endometrial cancer: results from the KEYNOTE-028 Study. J Clin Oncol. 2017;35:2535–41.
46. Ding L, Getz G, Wheeler DA, et al. Somatic mutations affect key pathways in lung adenocarcinoma. Nature. 2008;455:1069–75.
47. Yurgelun MB, Kulke MH, Fuchs CS, et al. Cancer susceptibility gene mutations in individuals with colorectal cancer. J Clin Oncol. 2017;35:1086–95.
48. Waddell N, Pajic M, Patch AM, et al. Whole genomes redefine the mutational landscape of pancreatic cancer. Nature. 2015;518:495–501.
49. Schrader KA, Cheng DT, Joseph V, et al. Germline variants in targeted tumor sequencing using matched normal DNA. JAMA Oncol. 2016;2:104–11.
50. Slomovitz BM, Jiang Y, Yates MS, et al. Phase II study of everolimus and letrozole in patients with recurrent endometrial carcinoma. J Clin Oncol. 2015;33:930–6.
51. Coleman RL, Oza AM, Lorusso D, et al. Rucaparib maintenance treatment for recurrent ovarian carcinoma after response to platinum therapy (ARIEL3): a randomised, double-blind, placebo controlled, phase 3 trial. Lancet. 2017;390:1949–61.
52. Ledermann J, Harter P, Gourley C, et al. Olaparib maintenance therapy in platinum-sensitive relapsed ovarian cancer. N Engl J Med. 2012;366:1382–92.
53. Moore K, Colombo N, Scambia G, et al. Maintenance olaparib in patients with newly diagnosed advanced ovarian cancer. N Engl J Med. 2018;27:2495–505.
54. Burger RA, Brady MF, Bookman MA, et al. Incorporation of bevacizumab in the primary treatment of ovarian cancer. N Engl J Med. 2011;365:2473–83.
55. Oza AM, Cook AD, Pfisterer J, et al. Standard chemotherapy with or without bevacizumab for women with newly diagnosed ovarian cancer (ICON7): overall survival results of a phase 3 randomised trial. Lancet Oncol. 2015;16:928–36.
56. Ledermann J, Harter P, Gourley C, et al. Olaparib maintenance therapy in patients with platinum-sensitive relapsed serous ovarian cancer: a preplanned retrospective analysis of outcomes by BRCA status in a randomised phase 2 trial. Lancet Oncol. 2014;15:852–61.
57. Niemeier LA, Dabbs DJ, Beriwal S, Striebel JM, Bhargava R. Androgen receptor in breast cancer: expression in estrogen receptor-positive tumors and in estrogen receptor-negative tumors with apocrine differentiation. Mod Pathol. 2010;23:205–12.
58. Gucalp A, Tolaney S, Isakoff SJ, et al. Phase II trial of bicalutamide in patients with androgen receptor-positive, estrogen receptor-negative metastatic breast cancer. Clin Cancer Res. 2013;19:5505–12.
59. Schiavon G, Hrebien S, Garcia-Murillas I, et al. Analysis of ESR1 mutation in circulating tumor DNA demonstrates evolution during therapy for metastatic breast cancer. Sci Transl Med. 2015;7:313ra182.
60. Karnoub AE, Weinberg RA. Ras oncogenes: split personalities. Nat Rev Mol Cell Biol. 2008;9:517–31.
61. Gianni L, Dafni U, Gelber RD, et al. Treatment with trastuzumab for 1 year after adjuvant chemotherapy in patientswith HER2-positive early breast cancer:

a 4-year follow-up of a randomised controlled trial. Lancet Oncol. 2011;12:236–44.
62. Baselga J, Bradbury I, Eidtmann H, et al. Lapatinib with trastuzumab for HER2-positive early breast cancer (NeoALTTO): a randomised, open-label, multicentre, phase 3 trial. Lancet. 2012;379:633–40.
63. McNeil C. NCI-MATCH launch highlights new trial design in precision medicine era. J Natl Cancer Inst. 2015;107:djv193.
64. Mangat PK, Halabi S, Bruinooge SS, et al. Rationale and design of the Targeted Agent and Profiling Utilization Registry (TAPUR) study. JCO Precis Oncologia. 2018;2018.
65. European Organization for Research and Treatment of Cancer (EORTC). SPECTA (Screening Patients for Efficient Clinical Trial Access). Recent developments of the EORTC collaborative program towards precision medicine. https://eortc.org/app/uploads/2017/05/SPECTA-flyer-2015.pdf. Accessed 20 Oct 2021.
66. Lacombe D, Tejpar S, Salgado R, et al. European perspective for effective cancer drug development. Nat Rev Clin Oncol. 2014;11:492–8.
67. European Organization for Research and Treatment of Cancer. The European Organization for Research and Treatment of Cancer Screening Patients for Efficient Clinical Trial Access (EORTCSPECTA) program. http://eortc.org/spect. Accessed 20 Oct 2021.
68. Thierry AR, Pastor B, Jiang ZQ, et al. Circulating DNA demonstrates convergent evolution and common resistance mechanisms during treatment of colorectal cancer. Clin Cancer Res. 2017;23:4578–91.
69. Yoo BC, Kim KH, Woo SM, Myung JK. Clinical multi-omics strategies for the effective cancer management. J Proteome. 2018;188:97–106.
70. Hu R, Wang X, Zhan X. Multi-parameter systematic strategies for predictive, preventive and personalised medicine in cancer. EPMA J. 2013;4:1–2.
71. Weinstein JN, TCGAR Network, Collisson EA, et al. The Cancer Genome Atlas Pan-cancer analysis project. Nat Genet. 2013;45:1113–20.
72. Anderson W, Aretz A, Barker AD, Bell C, Bernabé RR, Bhan MK, Calvo F, Eerola I, Gerhard DS, Guttmacher A, Guyer M. International network of cancer genome projects. Nature. 2010;464:993–8.
73. Vasaikar SV, Straub P, Wang J, Zhang B. LinkedOmics: analyzing multi-omics data within and across 32 cancer types. Nucleic Acids Res. 2018;46:D956–63.
74. Zhang J, Baran J, Cros A, Guberman JM, Haider S, Hsu J, Liang Y, Rivkin E, Wang J, Whitty B, Wong-Erasmus M. International Cancer Genome Consortium Data Portal—a one-stop shop for cancer genomics data. Database. 2011.
75. Guberman JM, Ai J, Arnaiz O, Baran J, Blake A, Baldock R, Chelala C, Croft D, Cros A, Cutts RJ, Di Génova A. BioMart Central Portal: an open database network for the biological community. Database. 2011.
76. Haider S, Ballester B, Smedley D, Zhang J, Rice P, Kasprzyk A. BioMart Central Portal—unified access to biological data. Nucleic Acids Res. 2009;37:W23–7.
77. Pavlopoulou A, Spandidos DA, Michalopoulos I. Human cancer databases. Oncol Rep. 2015;33:3–18.
78. Robbins DE, Grüneberg A, Deus HF, Tanik MM, Almeida JS. A self-updating road map of The Cancer Genome Atlas. Bioinformatics. 2013;29:1333–40.
79. Nguyen QH, Nguyen H, Nguyen T, Le DH. Multi-omics analysis detects novel prognostic subgroups of breast cancer. Front Genet. 2020;11:1265.
80. Bareche Y, Venet D, Ignatiadis M, Aftimos P, Piccart M, Rothe F, Sotiriou C. Unravelling triple-negative breast cancer molecular heterogeneity using an integrative multiomic analysis. Ann Oncol. 2018;29:895–902.
81. Xiao Y, Ma D, Zhao S, Suo C, Shi J, Xue MZ, Ruan M, Wang H, Zhao J, Li Q, Wang P. Multi-omics profiling reveals distinct microenvironment characterization and suggests immune escape mechanisms of triple-negative breast cancer. Clin Cancer Res. 2019;25:5002–14.
82. Bhatia S, Monkman J, Blick T, Duijf PH, Nagaraj SH, Thompson EW. Multi-omics characterization of the spontaneous mesenchymal–epithelial transition in the PMC42 breast cancer cell lines. J Clin Med. 2019;8:1253.
83. Lu T, Bankhead A III, Ljungman M, Neamati N. Multi-omics profiling reveals key signaling pathways in ovarian cancer controlled by STAT3. Theranostics. 2019;9:5478.
84. Zhang Z, Huang K, Gu C, Zhao L, Wang N, Wang X, Zhao D, Zhang C, Lu Y, Meng Y. Molecular subtyping of serous ovarian cancer based on multi-omics data. Sci Rep. 2016;6:26001.
85. Shen J, Liu T, Bei Q, Xu S. Comprehensive landscape of ovarian cancer immune microenvironment based on integrated multi-omics analysis. Front Oncol. 2021;11:685065.
86. Zhu J, Zhou Q, Pan M, Zhou C. Multi-omics analysis of the prognosis and therapeutic significance of circadian clock in ovarian cancer. Gene. 2021;788:145644.
87. Torre LA, Bray F, Siegel RL, Ferlay J, Lortet-Tieulent J, Jemal A. Global cancer statistics, 2012. CA Cancer J Clin. 2015;65:87–108.
88. Lyu X, Li G, Qiao Q. Identification of an immune classification for cervical cancer and integrative analysis of multiomics data. J Transl Med. 2021;19:1–9.
89. Nie H, Bu F, Xu J, Li T, Huang J. 29 immune-related genes pairs signature predict the prognosis of cervical cancer patients. Sci Rep. 2020;10:1–6.
90. Wu Y, Zhao J, Dong S, Wang Y, Li A, Jiang Y, Chen Z, Li C, Wang W, Zhang Z. Whole-exome and RNA sequencing reveal novel insights into the pathogenesis of HPV associated cervical cancer. Cancer Biomark. 2019;25:341–50.
91. Zhong Q, Lu M, Yuan W, Cui Y, Ouyang H, Fan Y, Wang Z, Wu C, Qiao J, Hang J. Eight-lncRNA signature of cervical cancer were identified by integrating DNA methylation, copy number variation and transcriptome data. J Transl Med. 2021;19:1–6.

92. Ledford LR, Lockwood S. Scope and epidemiology of gynecologic cancers: an overview. Semin Oncol Nurs. 2019;35:147–50.
93. Shannon B, Yi TJ, Perusini S, Gajer P, Ma B, Humphrys MS, Thomas-Pavanel J, Chieza L, Janakiram P, Saunders M, Tharao W. Association of HPV infection and clearance with cervicovaginal immunology and the vaginal microbiota. Mucosal Immunol. 2017;10:1310–9.
94. Rizzo AE, Gordon JC, Berard AR, Burgener AD, Avril S. The female reproductive tract microbiome—implications for gynecologic cancers and personalized medicine. J Pers Med. 2021;11:546.
95. Wang Y, Ren F, Song Z, Wang X, Ma X. Multiomics profile and prognostic gene signature of m6A regulators in uterine corpus endometrial carcinoma. J Cancer. 2020;11:6390.

Tumour Biomarkers in Gynaecologic Oncology

Lopa Mudra Kakoti, Debabrata Barmon, Amal Chandra Kataki, and Zirsangliana Chhangte

1 Introduction

Biomarkers are defined as any biological substance or molecules that can be measured easily to provide any information regarding the ongoing disease process [1]. Tumour markers are the substances either produced by the cancer cells or by any other cells in the body in response to the cancer. They can be cell surface antigens, cytoplasmic proteins, enzymes, hormone, and proteomics [2].

Tumour markers are used as screening test for early detection of malignancy in asymptomatic patients, whereas in symptomatic patients, biomarkers help to differentiate benign from malignant disease. Following diagnosis and appropriate treatment, these markers may be used as post-treatment surveillance tool for assessing treatment response, prognosis, therapy prediction, and early detection of recurrence.

An ideal tumour biomarker exhibit the following characteristic features [3]:

- They should possess a high positive predictive and negative predictive value
- They should be acceptable to subjects undergoing the test
- They should have cost-effective, simple, 'standardized' and automated assay with clearly defined reference limits
- They should have its clinical value validated in a large prospective trial.

There are no, the so-called ideal biomarkers exists currently, because of their lack of sensitivity for premalignant lesions or early invasive disease and lack of specificity for malignancy.

Owing to the molecular studies that have recently widened the opportunity for testing new possible markers, but only few markers has got practical applicability in clinic. With the advent of targeted therapy and newer modalities in cancer patient management, the clinicians are inclined to adapt the personalized therapy offering new tools to estimate the possibility of cure, i.e., the overall outcome of patient.

L. M. Kakoti (✉)
Department of Pathology, Dr. Bhubaneswar Borooah Cancer Institute (A Unit of Tata Memorial Centre, Mumbai), Guwahati, Assam, India

D. Barmon · A. C. Kataki
Department of Gynaecologic Oncology, Dr. Bhubaneswar Borooah Cancer Institute (A Unit of Tata Memorial Centre, Mumbai), Guwahati, Assam, India
e-mail: dydiracademic@bbci.tmc.gov.in

Z. Chhangte
Department of Medical and Gynaecological Oncology, Mizoram State Cancer Institute, Zemabawk, Aizawl, Mizoram, India

A. C. Kataki, D. Barmon (eds.), *Fundamentals in Gynaecologic Malignancy*,
https://doi.org/10.1007/978-981-19-5860-1_3

There are various types of tumour markers based on their biochemical characteristic either tissue or serum based. Serum based biomarkers are commonly used and measured in biological fluids such as blood or any other body fluid including urine that can be obtained with minimal inconvenience to subjects undergoing screening. Tissue based biomarkers are mainly used for confirmation of tumour from their mimickers and for performing predictive markers. Immunohistochemistry (IHC) is useful modality to perform the predictive markers.

2 Tumour Markers in Gynaecological Cancers

Gynaecological cancers comprise a heterogenous group of cancers with varying etiopathogenesis to management and varying survival pattern. According to Globocan 2020, cervical cancer is the most common gynaecological malignancy in female in most of the developing countries, whereas endometrial cancer is the most common in developed country [4]. In developed countries, most malignancies present in earlier stages compared with developing countries except ovarian carcinomas which has the highest mortality due to their late presentation [5].

This genomic era has identified many novel genes and pathways of many malignancies and with improved technical advances has fostered many potential biomarkers in gynaecological malignancies. But most of them require replication and individual validation to be used in the clinical practice. There are few regularly utilized serum markers in gynaecologic malignancies are—CA125, CA19.9, CEA, and beta-HCG. They lack sensitivity and specificity. Routine screening tests are used in ovarian malignancies, germ cell tumour, and gestational trophoblastic diseases, however, they are used for disease monitoring during therapy and to identify relapse in most of the other female genital tract malignancies.

This chapter focuses on the different routinely used biomarkers of different gynaecologic malignancies with a comprehensive update in recent potential markers.

3 Tumour Biomarkers in Ovarian Malignancies

Almost 80% of ovarian tumours are of epithelial origin and rest are non-epithelial. There are different tumour markers indicated for specific tumour types (Table 1).

Table 1 Commonly indicated tumour markers for various ovarian tumour types [5]

Tumour type	Screening test	Disease monitoring/ follow-up tests
Ovarian epithelial tumour	CA125, CA19.9	CA125
Granulosa theca cell tumour	Inhibin	Inhibin
Germ cell tumour	Beta-HCG, AFP	Beta-HCG, AFP
Gestational trophoblastic disease	Beta-HCG	Beta-HCG

3.1 Epithelial Ovarian Cancers

Epithelial ovarian cancer (EOC) is the highest mortality gynaecological cancer worldwide because of their late presentation. Due to the critical necessity of the biomarkers, the ongoing various genomic and proteomic profiling experiments could provide an insight into the pathogenesis of ovarian malignancy and help in identifying the newer ovarian cancer biomarkers. The capacity of these recently emerging biomarkers might improve early detection as well as therapeutic efficacy in ovarian cancer management. Hereby we summarize various biomarkers, currently in use and mentioning also, the potential emerging markets with their utilities (Table 2).

Table 2 List of current ovarian cancer biomarkers and potential emerging biomarkers [6]

Current ovarian cancer biomarkers	Potential newly emerging biomarkers
CA125, osteopontin, Kallikreins, Bikunins, Human epididymis protein, Vascular endothelial growth factor, Prostasin, Creatinine kinase B, Mesothelin, Apolipoprotein A1, Transthyretin, Transferrin	Cu isotope, Exosomes, lnc., RNA and mRNA, Aldehyde dehydrogenase 1, Folate receptor alpha, Glutathione S transferase, Polymorphisms (GSTP)

3.1.1 Carbohydrate Antigen or Carcinoma Antigen (CA125)

Serum Ca125 is indispensable in the management of patients with EOC. It is a mucin glycoprotein (MUC16) that was identified using monoclonal antibody OC 125, originally identified by Bast et al. [7]. It is secreted by mesothelial cells of the pleura, pericardium, peritoneum, and mullerian derived tubal, endometrial, and endocervical epithelial cells. A serum value of 35 IU/mL is accepted as upper normal limits. However, in postmenopausal and post-hysterectomy women, the level of CA125 is lower than 35IU/L [8, 9].

3.1.2 CA125 as Screening Marker for Ovarian Cancers

CA125 is raised (>35 U/mL) in about 85% of EOC patients and only 50% of stage I tumour show raised CA125 in contrast to advanced stage disease (raised in >90% of patients).

CA125 is infrequently elevated in mucinous, clear cell, and borderline tumour. But, it is commonly elevated in Serous adenocarcinoma as well as many other benign conditions [5]. Because of its low sensitivity and specificity, the European Group on Tumour Marker (EGTM) guidelines do not recommend CA 125 either alone or as composite marker, as screening test in asymptomatic ovarian cancer women outside the context of a randomized controlled trial [8]. However, EGTM recommends CA 125 to be used as an additional test in differential diagnosis of benign and malignant pelvic masses in post-menopausal women [8, 10].

In genetically predisposed high risk patients (such as Lynch syndrome, BRCA gene mutations or a strong family history of breast and ovarian cancer), trans vaginal ultrasonogram and CA-125 may suffice to screen the ovarian cancer. However, even in these women, no studies have proven that using these screening modalities would reduce the mortality of ovarian cancer [9, 11].

3.1.3 CA125 as Marker for Disease Monitoring in Ovarian Cancers

Serum CA125 is a useful predictor of chemotherapy response. After the two cycles of chemotherapy, CA125 value reduction by 50% predicts achieving a good response [10]. On the contrary, a rising CA125 may indicate chemoresistance necessitating an alternative chemotherapeutic regimen. After completion of the therapy, CA125 is commonly used in the follow-up of patients for recurrence [12]. Gynaecologic Cancer Intergroup (GCIG) recommends the first sample to be taken within 2 weeks before treatment and subsequent samples at 2–4 weeks during treatment. During follow-up, CA125 test should be done at intervals of 2–3 weeks [9].

3.1.4 CA125 as Prognostic Marker in Ovarian Cancers

Pre-operative CA125 value correlate well with prognosis, especially in stage I disease. If elevated, the risk of death is sixfold. There can be transient rise of CA125 in the immediate post-operative period due to surgery induced inflammation; thus, for monitoring, it is advisable to start CA125 test 4 weeks after surgery. Pre-operative CA125 levels also reflect progression or regression of disease in 90% of ovarian cancer cases. Sometimes, despite being CA125 within normal limit, around 12–38% of patients may have an active disease on second look laparotomy. Therefore, the trend of CA125 is more important than absolute value or cut-off point. CA125 level after second cycle of chemotherapy, before third cycle has been used successfully to assess response to therapy. CA125 declining in exponential regression pattern is more useful in assessing response [11].

3.1.5 Human Epididymis Protein 4 (HE4)

HE4 is another promising biomarker after CA125 for malignant ovarian tumours. It is a glycoprotein, member of the large family called WAP(whey acidic protein). The alternate name is whey acidic four-disulphide core proteins (WFDC2) [13]. These proteins are composed of 50 amino acids and their biological function has not yet been established [14].

HE4 was initially isolated in the epididymis indicating their role in spermatogenesis and sperm maturation. HE4 is over expressed in malignant epithelial ovarian tumours, but is not elevated in non-malignant ovarian conditions. They have higher sensitivity and specificity for detection of serous and endometrioid subtypes [5]. They are rarely expressed in clear cell ovarian carcinoma [15].

Many recent studies showed that HE4 is more reliable to diagnose ovarian epithelial cancer than CA125 [15, 16]. There are various methods used to measure this biomarker, out of which, electro-chemiluminescent (ECLIA) or chemiluminescent microparticle immunoassay (CMIA) are referred methods.

While interpreting HE4 results, methods of assay to be considered as suggested by all the meta-analysis. The cut-off value of HE4 is 70 pmol/L for pre-menopause patients and 140 pmol/L for menopause patients using CMIA method [17].

The advantage over CA125 is that HE4 is not elevated in benign ovarian conditions like endometriotic cyst and not modified by body mass index (BMI) like Ca125; whereas HE4 is influenced by smoking and oral contraceptive methods in contrast to CA125 [5]. HE4 level is increased in smokers compared to non-smokers [16, 18]. Therefore, it is worth to measure both the markers to confirm a cases of suspected ovarian neoplasm as malignant ones when both the values are raised.

3.1.6 Evaluation of Women with Pelvic Masses

Around 13–21% of pelvic masses are ovarian epithelial carcinoma. It is essential to predict the nature of pelvic masses pre-operatively to plan for appropriate management as patients with pelvic mass likely to be malignant will be referred to gynaecologic oncologist.

3.1.7 Risk of malignancy index (RMI)

Risk of malignancy index (RMI) is a scoring system based on menopausal status, CA125, and pelvic ultrasound. The score will predict the probability of malignancy. RMI score of 200 or greater provides a sensitivity of 85% and specificity of 97% for ovarian malignancy. The various studies evaluating the role of RMI have reported sensitivity and specificity ranging from 71–88.5% and 74.3–97%, respectively [5, 17].

$$\mathrm{RMI} = M \times U \times C$$

where

M = menopausal state (1 for pre and 3 for post)
U = ultrasound findings (0 for normal 1 for each of; multilocular cysts, bilateral cysts, solid components, ascites, metastatic disease, maximum score of 3)
C = serum CA125 level
If RMI >200, high probability ovarian carcinoma

3.1.8 Risk of Ovarian Malignancy Algorithm (ROMA)

ROMA, proposed by Moore, incorporates CA125, HE4 and menopausal status of the women to assign the adnexal mass into a high risk or low risk group for an ovarian malignancy. ROMA score corresponds to predicted probability [PP] and is expressed by a percentage rate. For pre-menopausal and post-menopausal women, cut-off levels are different [17, 19].

$$\begin{aligned}
&\text{Pre-menopausal Predictive Index}(\mathrm{PI}) && = -12.0 + 2.38 \times \mathrm{LN}(\mathrm{HE4}) + 0.0626 \times \mathrm{LN}(\mathrm{CA125}) \\
&\text{Post-menopausal Predictive Index}(\mathrm{PI}) && = -8.09 + 1.04 \times \mathrm{LN}(\mathrm{HE4}) + 0.732 \times \mathrm{LN}(\mathrm{CA125}) \\
&\text{Predicted Probability}(\mathrm{PP}) && = \exp(\mathrm{PI}) / \left[1 + \exp(\mathrm{PI})\right] \times 100
\end{aligned}$$

3.1.9 OVA1 Test

OVA1 test, approved by FDA (2009) is used to aid in presurgical evaluation of pelvic mass for ovarian cancers. This test uses a blood sample to measure the levels of five different biomarkers liver proteins that are altered in ovarian cancer. Five proteins whose values are altered in ovarian cancer: apolipoprotein A1, prealbumin, transferrin (decrease in cancer),beta-2 microglobulin, and CA125 (increase in cancer) are measured in the serum. The individual biomarker results are then transformed by computer software analysis to generate a single numerical score between 0 and 10. Higher the score higher the likelihood of malignant ovarian tumour. This test is meant for women above 18 years of age undergoing surgery for pelvic mass. The accuracy was 92% when combined with radiological test. However, false positive rate is 64% [20].

3.1.10 Carcinoembryonic Antigen (CEA)

CEA is a complex glycoprotein, consists of single polypeptide chains with varying carbohydrate components. They are associated with the plasma membrane of tumour cells and developing foetus, from which they may be released into the blood. First detected in colon cancer, now found to be raised in many other cancers and benign conditions (hepatic diseases, including extrahepatic biliary obstruction, intrahepatic cholestasis and hepatocellular disease), where there is altered clearance rate [12]. CEA is can be used in gynaecology to see the treatment response in mucinous tumour with pseudomyxoma peritonei [21]. Immunohistochemical expression of CEA was found to be specific for endometrioid carcinomas, brenner tumours, and mucinous tumours with intestinal differentiation [22].

3.1.11 Cancer Antigen 19-9 (CA 19-9)

Carbohydrate antigen 19-9, also called as sialylated Lewis antigen, is a member of the Lewis blood group antigens. Although, the elevated serum levels of CA19.9 are found mainly in pancreatic malignancy, they are also found to be elevated in 76% of mucinous ovarian tumours and in 27% of serous ovarian tumours [23]. It can be used to monitor therapy response or detect cancer recurrences of various cancers (mucinous ovarian neoplasm, cholangiocarcinoma gastric cancer, gallbladder cancer, pancreatic cancer, or adenocarcinoma of the ampulla of Vater). The combination of CA19-9 with CA125 are proven to be useful in borderline ovarian tumour [24].

3.2 Markers of Non-epithelial Ovarian Cancers (Non-EOC)

Around 10% of the ovarian tumours are of non-epithelial origin which includes germ cell, sex cord stromal cell, metastatic carcinomas to the ovary, and the rare sarcomas. Contrary to EOC, non-EOC are usually found in young patients [22]. Germ cell tumours are detected and monitored by serum HCG and AFP that have significant effects on the treatment plan [22].

3.2.1 Human Chorionic Gonadotropin (hCG)

The Human Chorionic Gonadotropin (hCG) hormone is glycoprotein composed of 244 amino acids normally produced during pregnancy by the syncytiotrophoblast, and it consists of two non-covalently linked, alpha and beta subunits as with other glycoproteins luteinizing hormone (LH), follicle-stimulating hormone (FSH), and thyroid-stimulating hormone (TSH).The α (alpha) subunit is identical in these glycoproteins, the β (beta) subunit is unique which is elevated in serum as well as in urine of patients with gestational trophoblastic neoplasm (GTN) and germ cell tumours with chorionic component [22, 25].

In GTN, there is a close correlation of HCG and tumour burden [26].

3.2.2 Serum Alpha-Fetoprotein (sAFP)

sAFP is a glycoprotein, physiologically produced by the foetal yolk sac, liver, and upper gastrointestinal tract [22]. Physiologically it is elevated during pregnancy, specially reaching peak concentration during 12 weeks of gestation. This oncofoetal protein raised in pathological conditions like cancers of GI tract(liver, pancreas, stomach, and colon) and germ cell tumour like (a) endodermal sinus tumour, (b) immature teratoma, and (c) dysgerminoma [22]. In germ cell tumour management, sAFP is reliably used for monitoring therapeutic responses and detecting recurrences. In mixed germ cell tumours, elevated sAFP reflect a yolk sac component in the tumour [27] sAFP is also rarely raised in EOC [17, 27].

3.2.3 Inhibin and Activin

Inhibin and activin are member of transforming growth factor-β (TGF-β) superfamily composed of dimeric glycoproteins. They have opposing biological effects like inhibin down regulates pituitary synthesis and secretion of follicle-stimulating hormone (FSH) whereas activin enhances it [17, 22]. Elevated serum Inhibin levels are found in granulosa cell tumour and ovarian sex cord stromal tumour and 5–31% EOC. Inhibin is useful to monitor the therapeutic responses and predict recurrence of ovarian granulosa cell tumours. Activin is found to be significantly elevated in undifferentiated EOC [28, 29].

3.2.4 Osteopontin (OPN)

Osteopontin is an extracellular calcium-binding phosphorylated glycoprotein secreted by activated T lymphocytes, osteoblasts, and many other organ tissues, found in all bodily fluids. It was initially isolated from bone matrix. OPN predominantly functions as immune modulator, contributes as a cytokine in many biological functions such as in inflammation, cell adhesion, cell migration, macrophage regulation, and wound healing [30]. OPN helps in many solid tumour progression and metastasis, independently correlates with poor prognosis [31]. It is found that higher level of OPN (isoform C-terminal fragment of OPN) of mainly positively associated with ovarian cancers, specially clear cell carcinoma of ovary [17, 32–34].

3.2.5 Kallikreins (KLK)

Kallikreins are members of serine proteases with different physiological roles. They are formed by 15 kallikrein genes (ch 19q13.4), being identified as the largest uninterrupted gene cluster in the human genome [34]. Researchers have demonstrated rise of different kallikreins in body fluids of patients with ovarian, breast, and prostate cancers as compared to normal situation [34, 35]. They are promised to be useful serum biomarkers in these cancers.

Recent study showed that combined panel of KLK6, KLK13 along with CA125 is more sensitive to detect early stage ovarian cancer than CA125 alone [17].

This serum elevation of hK10 significantly correlated with unfavourable prognosis, serous subtype, advanced stage disease, and resistance to chemotherapy [36].

3.2.6 Bikunin

Bikunin is a glycosylated, Kunitz-type protease inhibitor which is known to inhibit invasion and metastasis. That is why, high pre-operative plasma bikunin found to have to favourable prognosis in ovarian cancer compared to low serum bikunin levels [34, 37, 38].

3.2.7 Mesothelin

Mesothelin, a GPI-anchored glycoprotein and a differentiation antigen found in mesothelial pleura, peritoneum, and pericardium. Mesothelin is an epithelial marker highly expressed by adenocarcinoma of ovary, gastric, pancreas, lung, cholangiocarcinoma, and mesotheliomas [39]. Mesothelin tissue expression is associated with poor survival and chemoresistance of ovarian cancer patients in recent studies [17].

Many therapy targeting the mesothelin have been in clinical trials, including antimesothelin immunotoxins and antibody-drug conjugates (ADC). Anetumab ravtansine is an ADC exhibits improved potency in combination with carboplatin, compared to either drug alone in animal model of ovarian cancer [6, 17].

3.2.8 Vascular Endothelial Growth Factor (VEGF)

VEGF is a cytokine, contributing to tumorigenesis by becoming the key regulator of angiogenesis. VEGF levels are found to be elevated in patients with ovarian cancer especially with ascites [39]. Studies have revealed that higher serum VEGF levels independently correlate with shorter survival time [40]. Bevacizumab, VEGFR inhibitor when used as maintenance therapy in ovarian cancer following debulking surgery and first-line chemotherapy, there is improvements in the progression-free survival of patients, however, no significant change in the overall survival [6].

3.2.9 Human Prostasin (PSN)

PSN is a trypsin-like proteinase, plays a major role in the activation of epithelial sodium channels [6]. Microarray gene expression analysis identified that PSN was overexpressed in ovarian cancer (>100 times greater) compared to benign ovarian neoplasms. This was specially found in the early stages of ovarian cancer, maintained in the higher stages and higher grades [41].

3.2.10 Apolipoprotein A-I (apoA-I)

ApoA-I is a high-density lipoprotein (HDL), found in plasma. Serum Apo A-I levels decrease in ovarian cancer patients. A fluorescence spectroscopic based system called multiplexed magnetic nanoparticle-antibody conjugates (MNPs-Abs) analysis combines three biomarkers, namely CA125, 2-M, and ApoA1 for the early detection of ovarian cancer. It was performed by Pal et al. that showed "CA125 is elevated in 50–60% of early stage ovarian cancer, while the three biomarkers combined achieve sensitivity of 94% and specificity 98% for detecting early stage ovarian cancer [29, 42].

3.2.11 Transthyretin (TTR)

TTR is a prealbumin protein synthesized mostly in the liver and responsible for transportation of thyroid hormones and retinol protein binding to the retinal complex. TTR was found to be elevated in stage I–II ovarian cancer, with a sensitivity of 78.6% and specificity of 68.8%, respectively [29]. TTR serum levels were found to be decreased in ovarian cancer and this value combined with other biomarkers can be used for ovarian cancer diagnosis [29, 43].

3.2.12 Transferrin

Transferrin is blood plasma glycoprotein, synthesized by hepatocytes and is responsible for plasma ferric-iron delivery to the cells. It has a significant role in cell division and proliferation. Because of its low sensitivity and specificity, transferrin needs to be used in combination with other biomarkers to achieve clinical significance [29].

3.2.13 Creatine Kinase B (CKB)

Creatine kinase is essential in the energy homeostasis of cells and its overexpression is found in many cancers. Recently, CKB is found to be highly expressed in early stages of ovarian cancer and may be a potential candidate marker for early detection of ovarian cancer [44].

3.2.14 Lysophosphatidic Acid (LPA)

Lysophosphatidic acid (LPA, 1-acyl-2-lyso-snglycero-3-phosphate) is found to be raised in body fluids of ovarian cancer patients [22]. LPA has biological role in ovarian cancer cell growth by promoting actions of proteases and the invasiveness of ovarian cancer cells. Hence, they are one of the contributors of ovarian cancer spread [45]. Lysophosphatidic acid is a promising marker for screening of ovarian cancer.

4 Cervical Cancer

Exfoliative cytology remains the main screening and diagnostic tool for cervical cancer recurrence, but not useful for monitoring therapeutic response. In cervical cancer, suitable tumour markers are necessary to monitor the disease response and to differentiate cervical adenocarcinoma from endometrial adenocarcinoma. There are very few available handful of the serum markers that can be of some help, for e.g., CA-125, CA-19.9, SCC-Ag, CYFRA 21-1, CEA, etc. [22, 46].

Another novel potential group of biomarkers includes serum based microRNAS (miRNAs) based on epigenetic modifiers [45]. Differential expression of miRNAs is compared in serum of healthy controls and in patients of cervical cancer by using solexa sequencing and recent available literature has showed a promising results of miRNA as disease monitoring tool after treatment [46].

Raised CA-125 either in serum and cervical or vaginal secretions can be used for detection of precancerous lesions of the cervix [46]. CA125 is more sensitive in detecting cervical adenocarcinoma and can be used as prognostic and tumour virulence indicator when used in combination with CA19.9 or CEA or SCC-Ag. During treatment, gradual decline of CA125 levels correlates well with chemosensitivity [22].

CA-19.9 is elevated in cervical adenocarcinoma than cervical SCC. It is even raised in early relapse of cervical cancer patients undergoing radiotherapy and who has negative CA-125 value [46].

4.1 Squamous Cell Carcinoma Antigen (SCC-Ag)

SCC-Ag is a marker of squamous cell differentiation with low specificity and high sensitivity [46]. It is raised in 64% cervical SCC patients and 25% of cervical adenocarcinoma [46]. The serum level of SCC-Ag correlates well with the tumour differentiation, tumour volume, and stage of the disease [46, 47]. Post-treatment elevated serum levels of SCC-Ag reflects treatment response and tumour relapse.

4.2 CYFRA 21-1

CYFRA 21-1 is a cytokeratin 19 fragment, soluble in serum. It has specificity comparable to SCC-Ag. Elevated levels of CYFRA 21-1 correlate with tumour size and FIGO staging of cervical squamous cancer. Serial monitoring of CYFRA 21-1 during post-treatment, can predict tumour response and recurrence, but fail to provide survival benefit [22, 48].

5 Endometrial Cancer

Patients with endometrial cancer (EC) usually have early onset of symptoms and most of them are diagnosed at an early stage. As such screening requirement is essential for high risk groups (patients with hereditary syndromes like Lynch, PTEN gene defect, patients on Tamoxifen therapy, morbidly obese and diabetic patients) for early detection. Several biomarkers have been tested for endometrial cancer screening such as HE4, CA-125, CA-72.4, CA-19.9, CA-15.3, OVXI, CEA, Dickkopf-1 (DKK-1), DJ-1, etc. [22, 49]. Amongst them, HE4 has the highest sensitivity for both early and late stage endometrial cancer [49]. Usually CA125 level parallels with the clinical course of the disease, correlating with lymph node metastasis, peritoneal seeding, deep myometrial invasion, and extrauterine disease spread. But as a screening marker for early detection, the individual role of CA-125 is limited [22]. Overall, the most promising serum markers till date is the combination of CA125 and HE4 compared to individual markers alone, as combined markers shows a clinically significant statistical correlation [22].

For post-treatment surveillance of patients with endometrial carcinoma, serial measurements of HE4 and CA125 can indicate disease activity and normalization of their value may indicate cure despite radiologic evidence of persistent disease in the form of nonviable tumour [50].

Another recent potential markers are—macrophage colony-stimulating factor (M-CSF) and YKL-40. Both are found to be raised in endometrial cancer patients specially predicting the high risk patients with aggressive clinical course [51].

In case of patients with uterine papillary serous carcinoma, a few markers like human kallikreins (subset K-10, 6) and Serum Amyloid A (SAA) levels are found to be significantly higher than healthy control and benign group. They might be potential biomarkers for monitoring early disease recurrence and response to treatment [22].

6 Vulval Cancer

Vulval cancer though rare has high mortality rate. No reliable serum markers have been identified except a few studies showing serum SCC-ag found to be elevated in vulval cancer, more so in patients with pT2 compared to pT1 vulval cancer, however, it did not correlate with lymph node involvement, tumour grade and patient's age [50]. Although it does not correlate well with prognosis, its elevation indicates relapsed disease [22]. Recently robust molecular analysis have identified many potential novel prognostic biomarkers in vulvar cancer, e.g., GNB3 with favourable prognosis and PLXDC2 with unfavourable prognosis [51].

To conclude, numerous molecular biomarkers are currently under study. Yet, based on stable value of these markers in healthy controls over time, the recommendations to utilize these biomarkers are divided into either negative or mildly positive categories only. There is an inevitable desire to enhance the strategies for early detection biomarkers to reduce the both mortality and morbidity from cancers.

References

1. Duffy MJ. Clinical uses of tumor markers: a critical review. Crit Rev Clin Lab Sci. 2001;38:225–62.
2. Nagpal M, Singh S, Singh P, Chauhan P, Zaidi MA. Tumor markers: a diagnostic tool. Natl J Maxillofac Surg. 2016;7:17–20.
3. Duffy MJ. Use of biomarkers in screening for cancer. Adv Exp Med Biol. 2015;867:27–39.
4. Sung H, Ferlay J, Siegel RL, Laversanne M, Soerjomataram I, Jemal A, et al. Global Cancer Statistics 2020: GLOBOCAN estimates of incidence and mortality worldwide for 36 cancers in 185 countries. CA Cancer J Clin. 2021;71(3):209–49.
5. Aggarwal P, Kehoe S. Serum tumour markers in gynaecological cancers. Maturitas. 2010;67(1):46–53.
6. Atallah GA, Abd. Aziz NH, Teik CK, Shafiee MN, Kampan NC. New predictive biomarkers for ovarian cancer. Diagnostics. 2021;11(3):465.
7. Bast RC, Feeney M, Lazarus HE, Nadler LM, Colvin RB, Knapp RC. Reactivity of a monoclonal antibody with human ovarian carcinoma. J Clin Investig. 1981;68(5):1331–7.
8. Petricoin EF, Ardekani AM, Hitt BA, Levine PJ, Fusaro VA, Steinberg SM, et al. Use of proteomic patterns in serum to identify ovarian cancer. Lancet Lond Engl. 2002;359(9306):572–7.
9. Morrow DA, Cannon CP, Jesse RL, et al. National Academy of Clinical Biochemistry Laboratory Medicine Practice Guidelines: clinical characteristics and utilization of biochemical markers in acute coronary syndromes. Clin Chem. 2007;53(4):552–74. https://doi.org/10.1373/clinchem.2006.084194. PMID: 17384001.
10. Buamah P. Benign conditions associated with raised serum CA-125 concentration. J Surg Oncol. 2000;75(4):264–5.
11. Barakat RR. Principles and practice of gynecologic oncology. Philadelphia: Wolters Kluwer Health/ Lippincott Williams & Wilkins; 2013.
12. Voorzanger-Rousselot N, Garnero P. Biochemical markers in oncology. Part I: molecular basis. Part II: clinical uses. Cancer Treat Rev. 2007;33(3):230–83.
13. Bouchard D, Morisset D, Bourbonnais Y, Tremblay GM. Proteins with whey-acidic-protein motifs and cancer. Lancet Oncol. 2006;7(2):167–74.
14. Kirchhoff C, Habben I, Ivell R, Krull N. A major human epididymis-specific cDNA encodes a protein with sequence homology to extracellular proteinase inhibitors. Biol Reprod. 1991;45(2):350–7.
15. Yanaranop M, Anakrat V, Siricharoenthai S, Nakrangsee S, Thinkhamrop B. Is the risk of ovarian malignancy algorithm better than other tests for predicting ovarian malignancy in women with pelvic masses? Gynecol Obstet Invest. 2017;82(1):47–53.
16. Romagnolo C, Leon AE, Fabricio ASC, Taborelli M, Polesel J, Del Pup L, et al. HE4, CA125 and risk of ovarian malignancy algorithm (ROMA) as diagnostic tools for ovarian cancer in patients with a pelvic mass: An Italian multicenter study. Gynecol Oncol. 2016;141(2):303–11.
17. Dochez V, Caillon H, Vaucel E, Dimet J, Winer N, Ducarme G. Biomarkers and algorithms for diagnosis of ovarian cancer: CA125, HE4, RMI and ROMA, a review. J Ovarian Res. 2019;12(1):28.
18. Urban N, Thorpe J, Karlan BY, McIntosh MW, Palomares MR, Daly MB, et al. Interpretation of single and serial measures of HE4 and CA125 in asymptomatic women at high risk for ovarian cancer. Cancer Epidemiol Biomark Prev. 2012;21(11):2087–94.
19. Sölétormos G, Duffy MJ, Othman Abu Hassan S, Verheijen RHM, Tholander B, Bast RC, et al. Clinical use of cancer biomarkers in epithelial ovarian cancer. Int J Gynecol Cancer. 2016;26(1):43–51.
20. Rein BJD, Gupta S, Dada R, Safi J, Michener C, Agarwal A. Potential markers for detection and monitoring of ovarian cancer. J Oncol. 2011;2011:475983.
21. Lin W, Cao D, Shen K. Prognostic significance of preoperative serum CEA in primary mucinous ovarian carcinoma: a retrospective cohort study. Cancer Manag Res. 2018;10:6913–20.
22. Tanyi JL, Scholler N. Oncology biomarkers for gynecologic malignancies. Front Biosci Elite Ed. 2012;4:1097–110.
23. Gocze PM, Szabo DG, Than GN, Csaba IF, Krommer KF. Occurrence of CA 125 and CA 19-9 tumor-associated antigens in sera of patients with gynecologic, trophoblastic, and colorectal tumors. Gynecol Obstet Invest. 1988;25(4):268–72.
24. Tamakoshi K, Kikkawa F, Shibata K, Tomoda K, Obata NH, Wakahara F, Tokuhashi Y, Ishikawa H, Kawai M, Tomoda Y. Clinical value of CA125, CA19-9, CEA, CA72-4, and TPA in borderline ovarian tumor. Gynecol Oncol. 1996;62(1):67–72.
25. Cole LA. New discoveries on the biology and detection of human chorionic gonadotropin. Reprod Biol Endocrinol RBE. 2009;7:8.
26. Muller CY, Cole LA. The quagmire of hCG and hCG testing in gynecologic oncology. Gynecol Oncol. 2009;112(3):663–72.
27. Chow SN, Yang JH, Lin YH, Chen YP, Lai JI, Chen RJ, et al. Malignant ovarian germ cell tumors. Int J Gynaecol Obstet. 1996;53(2):151–8.
28. Menon U, Riley SC, Thomas J, Bose C, Dawnay A, Evans LW, et al. Serum inhibin, activin and follistatin in postmenopausal women with epithelial ovarian carcinoma. BJOG Int J Obstet Gynaecol. 2000;107(9):1069–74.
29. Lambert-Messerlian GM, Steinhoff M, Zheng W, Canick JA, Gajewski WH, Seifer DB, et al. Multiple immunoreactive inhibin proteins in serum from post-

menopausal women with epithelial ovarian cancer. Gynecol Oncol. 1997;65(3):512–6.
30. https://www.scribd.com/book/519193478/Handbook-of-Hormones-Comparative-Endocrinology-for-Basic-and-Clinical-Research.
31. Zhao H, Chen Q, Alam A, et al. The role of osteopontin in the progression of solid organ tumour. Cell Death Dis. 2018;9:356. https://doi.org/10.1038/s41419-018-0391-6.
32. Diagnostic markers for early detection of ovarian cancer | Clinical Cancer Research. [cited 2021 Aug 31]. https://clincancerres.aacrjournals.org/content/14/4/1065.figures-only.
33. Ye B, Skates S, Mok SC, Horick NK, Rosenberg HF, Vitonis A, et al. Proteomic-based discovery and characterization of glycosylated eosinophil-derived neurotoxin and COOH-terminal osteopontin fragments for ovarian cancer in urine. Clin Cancer Res. 2006;12(2):432–41.
34. Coticchia CM, Yang J, Moses MA. Ovarian cancer biomarkers: current options and future promise. J Natl Compr Canc Netw. 2008;6(8):795–802.
35. Diamandis EP, Yousef GM. Human tissue kallikreins: a family of new cancer biomarkers. Clin Chem. 2002;48(8):1198–205.
36. Yousef GM, Scorilas A, Katsaros D, Fracchioli S, Iskander L, Borgono C, et al. Prognostic value of the human kallikrein gene 15 expression in ovarian cancer. J Clin Oncol. 2003;21(16):3119–26.
37. Matsuzaki H, Kobayashi H, Yagyu T, Wakahara K, Kondo T, Kurita N, et al. Plasma bikunin as a favorable prognostic factor in ovarian cancer. J Clin Oncol. 2005;23(7):1463–72.
38. King SM, Burdette JE. Evaluating the progenitor cells of ovarian cancer: analysis of current animal models. BMB Rep. 2011;44(7):435–45.
39. Chang K, Pastan I. Molecular cloning of mesothelin, a differentiation antigen present on mesothelium, mesotheliomas, and ovarian cancers. Proc Natl Acad Sci U S A. 1996;93(1):136–40.
40. Hefler LA, Zeillinger R, Grimm C, Sood AK, Cheng WF, Gadducci A, et al. Preoperative serum vascular endothelial growth factor as a prognostic parameter in ovarian cancer. Gynecol Oncol. 2006;103(2):512–7.
41. Ahmed N, Oliva KT, Barker G, Hoffmann P, Reeve S, Smith IA, et al. Proteomic tracking of serum protein isoforms as screening biomarkers of ovarian cancer. Proteomics. 2005;5(17):4625–36.
42. Kiechle M, Jacobsen A, Schwarz-Boeger U, Hedderich J, Pfisterer J, Arnold N. Comparative genomic hybridization detects genetic imbalances in primary ovarian carcinomas as correlated with grade of differentiation. Cancer. 2001;91(3):534–40.
43. Garzon R, Fabbri M, Cimmino A, Calin GA, Croce CM. MicroRNA expression and function in cancer. Trends Mol Med. 2006;12(12):580–7.
44. Farley J, Brady WE, Vathipadiekal V, Lankes HA, Coleman R, Morgan MA, et al. Selumetinib in women with recurrent low-grade serous carcinoma of the ovary or peritoneum: an open-label, single-arm, phase 2 study. Lancet Oncol. 2013;14(2):134–40.
45. Laengsri V, Kerdpin U, Plabplueng C, Treeratanapiboon L, Nuchnoi P. Cervical cancer markers: epigenetics and microRNAs. Lab Med. 2018;49(2):97–111. https://doi.org/10.1093/labmed/lmx080. Erratum in: Lab Med. 2018 Mar 21;49(2):190. PMID: 29378033.
46. Kato H, Torigoe T. Radioimmunoassay for tumor antigen of human cervical squamous cell carcinoma. Cancer. 1977;40(4):1621–8.
47. Maruo T, Yoshida S, Samoto T, Tateiwa Y, Peng X, Takeuchi S, Motoyama S. Factors regulating SCC antigen expression in squamous cell carcinoma of the uterine cervix. Tumour Biol. 1998;19(6):494–504.
48. Bonfrer JM, Gaarenstroom KN, Kenter GG, Korse CM, Hart AA, Gallee MP, et al. Prognostic significance of serum fragments of cytokeratin 19 measured by Cyfra 21-1 in cervical cancer. Gynecol Oncol. 1994;55(3 Pt 1):371–5.
49. Hutt S, Tailor A, Ellis P, Michael A, ButlerManuel S, Chatterjee J. The role of biomarkers in endometrial cancer and hyperplasia: a literature review. Acta Oncol. 2019;58(3):342–52.
50. Gadducci A, Cosio S, Carpi A, Nicolini A, Genazzani AR. Serum tumor markers in the management of ovarian, endometrial and cervical cancer. Biomed Pharmacother. 2004;58(1):24–38.
51. Lavorato-Rocha AM, Akagi EM, de Melo Maia B, Rodrigues IS, Botelho MCS, Marchi FA, et al. An integrative approach uncovers biomarkers that associate with clinically relevant disease outcomes in vulvar carcinoma. Mol Cancer Res MCR. 2016;14(8):720–9.

Cancer: Infection and Vaccines

Amrita Talukdar, Amal Chandra Kataki,
Shripad Banavali, and Jaya Ghosh

1 Introduction

Microbial infection by viruses, bacteria and parasites are known to be an important cause of cancers in various organ systems of the human body. According to the International Agency for Research on Cancer (IARC), 15.4% of all cancers have an infective aetiology [1]. That roughly translates to around 2.2 million cancers worldwide in a year. However, the incidence of such infection-attributable cancers is not the same in all parts of the world, with more incidence noted in the less developed nations (23.4%) compared to less incidence in the developed regions (9.2%). The other remarkable fact is that although around 20 distinct cancers have been identified to have association with such infective oncogenic agents, only three such cancers (non-cardia gastric cancer, liver cancer and cervical cancer) account for more than 4/5th of the entire burden [2]. The knowledge of the life cycles, infectivity, infective mechanism, pathogenicity and putative and proven carcinogenesis pathways is important for oncologists, epidemiologists and researchers to develop effective strategies to diminish their adverse impact specifically in terms of cancer burden and on human health at large.

IARC has labelled 12 micro-organisms as carcinogenic agents and this includes eight viruses, three parasites and one bacterium [3] (Table 1). These pathogenic organisms have been known for a long time to mankind but their association with cancers took time to discover. For an example, even though the parasites mentioned below have been known to humankind since the nineteenth century, it was only in 2009 that IARC declared them as carcinogens [4].

A. Talukdar (✉)
Department of Microbiology, Dr. Bhubaneswar Borooah Cancer Institute (A Unit of Tata Memorial Centre, Mumbai), Guwahati, Assam, India

A. C. Kataki
Department of Gynaecologic Oncology, Dr. Bhubaneswar Borooah Cancer Institute (A Unit of Tata Memorial Centre, Mumbai), Guwahati, Assam, India

S. Banavali
Tata Memorial Centre, Dr Ernest Borges Marg, Mumbai, India

J. Ghosh
Department of Medical Oncology, Tata Memorial Centre and Homi Bhabha National Institute, Mumbai, India

A. C. Kataki, D. Barmon (eds.), *Fundamentals in Gynaecologic Malignancy*,
https://doi.org/10.1007/978-981-19-5860-1_4

Table 1 List of infective pathogens causing cancer

Pathogen	Year of discovery	Malignancy
Virus		
Epstein–Barr virus (EBV)	1964	Burkitt's lymphoma Diffuse large B-cell lymphoma Hodgkin lymphoma Undifferentiated nasopharyngeal carcinoma Gastric adenocarcinoma Leiomyosarcoma Post-transplant lymphoproliferative disease
Hepatitis B virus (HBV)	1965	Hepatocellular carcinoma
Human T-lymphotropic virus-1 (HTLV-1)	1980	Adult T-cell leukaemia (ATL)
Human genital papillomavirus (HPV) (Subtypes 16, 18, 31, 33, 35, 39, 45, 51, 52, 56, 59 and 59)	1983	Cervical carcinoma Squamous cell head and neck carcinoma Squamous cell anal cancer, penile cancer and vulvar cancer
Hepatitis C virus (HCV)	1989	Hepatocellular carcinoma
Kaposi sarcoma herpesvirus (KSHV/HHV8)	1994	Kaposi's sarcoma Primary effusion lymphoma Multicentric Castleman disease
Merkel cell polyomavirus (MCV)	2008	Merkel cell carcinoma
Bacterium		
Helicobacter pylori	1982	Gastric mucosa associated lymphoid tissue (MALT) lymphoma Gastric non-Hodgkin lymphoma (NHL) Gastric adenocarcinoma
Parasites		
Schistosoma haematobium	1851	Urinary bladder carcinoma
Clonorchis sinensis	1875	Cholangiocarcinoma
Opisthorchis viverrini	1886	Cholangiocarcinoma

2 Mechanism of Action

All the above-mentioned organisms are believed to exert direct carcinogenic effect with one exception, which is HIV-1. The retrovirus HIV-1, by virtue of immunosuppression, indirectly potentiates carcinogenesis by creating favourable conditions for persistent infections by other oncogenic pathogens [5–7]. Examples of direct oncogenicity include cellular gene products such as HPV E6 and E7, EBV LMP1, MCPyV T antigen and HTLV-1 Tax, which influence proliferative and anti-apoptotic activities [8]. The other mechanism is by propagation of chronic tissue injury and a consequent chronic inflammatory response that acts as a fertile ground for development of cancer. Organisms such as HBV, HCV and helicobacter pylori are well-known to do that [9].

3 Oncogenic Viruses

3.1 Papillomaviruses

In the mid-nineteenth century, Dominico Rigonni-Stern observed that nuns rarely contracted cervical cancer whereas prostitutes had more incidence of the disease than other females and linked uterine cancer with sexual behaviour [10]. A century later, subtypes of human papillomavirus (HPV) were linked with cervical cancer. A majority of HPV-induced cancers arise in the zones of transition between stratified squamous epithelia and the single layer (columnar) epithelia of the endocervix, anal canal and the tonsillar crypts. The theory is that there may be dysregulation of the normal coupling of the HPV life cycle to keratinocyte differentiation [11].

The high-risk HPV subtypes include 16, 18, 31, 33, 35, 45, 52 and 58 and these are implicated in the causation of several cancers in the human body including cervical cancer, vaginal and vulvar cancers in females and penile cancer in males and anal and oropharyngeal cancer in both sexes. The lifetime risk of sexual exposure to a high-risk HPV type has been estimated to be more than 70% and individuals who are unable to clear the infection resulting in chronic or persistent infection are at high risk of developing precursor lesions and cancer [12].

The HPVs encode L1 and L2 capsid proteins and six key early region genes (E1, E2, E4, E5, E6 and E7). E6 protein of high-risk HPVs caused ubiquitin-protein ligase mediated destruction of the guardian of the genome, the tumour suppressor gene p53. It also caused activation of cellular telomerase. On the other hand, E7 proteins interact with the proto-oncogene pRB gene [13–16].

3.2 Polyomaviruses

In 2008, Chang and Moore discovered the fifth known human polyomavirus and named it MCV (Human Polyoma virus 5 or HPyV5) by virtue of its presence in Merkel cell carcinoma (MCC) [17]. Merkel cell carcinoma is a rare but highly aggressive cutaneous malignancy occurring in sun-exposed areas of the body. MCV DNA is present in approximately 80% of MCC cases [18]. The other polyoma virus that is implicated in the causation of cancer is the BK Polyoma virus with association being linked with a small percentage of bladder cancer [19].

3.3 Epstein–Barr Virus (Human Herpesvirus 4 or HHV4)

Nearly all cases of endemic Burkitt lymphoma are EBV-positive and one-fifth of sporadic cases of Burkitt lymphoma that occur in immunocompetent individuals outside of malaria-prone regions have EBV positivity. Half of HIV-associated lymphomas also contain EBV. In addition to these, EBV is also associated with a histologically diverse range of lymphoid cancers such as post-transplant lymphoproliferative disease (PTLD), mixed-cellularity and lymphocyte-depletion subsets of Hodgkin's lymphoma and natural killer (NK)/ T-cell lymphoma [20–22].

The other malignancy with almost universal EBV presence is nasopharyngeal carcinoma, irrespective of whether it occurs in endemic or non-endemic regions. In fact, individuals with rising or relatively high immunoglobulin A (IgA) antibody responses to EBNA1, EBV DNase and/or capsid antigens are at increased risk of developing nasopharyngeal carcinoma. This is one of the early detection methods for high-risk individuals [23–25].

EBV is present in 5 to 15% of gastric adenocarcinomas and more than 90% of gastric lymphoepithelioma-like carcinomas [26].

3.4 Kaposi Sarcoma Herpesvirus (KSHV or Human Herpesvirus 8 or HHV8)

It was in the nineteenth century that dermatologist Moritz Kaposi identified a rare type of indolent cutaneous sarcoma in older men and that was named Kaposi sarcoma. One century later, in the 1980s, with the onset AIDS pandemic, an aggressive counterpart of this sarcoma was reported among younger gay men and an association was established with this type of herpes virus. HHV8 or KSHV is responsible for all types of Kaposi sarcoma (KS), including the classical KS seen in elderly men, AIDS-associated (epidemic) KS, transplantation-associated KS and endemic KS which is seen in sub-Saharan Africa [27–32].

Apart from these, KSHV is also responsible for two forms of B-cell proliferative disorders, namely, multicentric Castleman disease (MCD) and primary effusion lymphoma (PEL).

3.5 Retroviruses

Human T-cell leukaemia virus (HTLV) subtype 1 (HTLV-1), which was identified in 1980, was the first human retrovirus discovered to have association with cancer. Only 2–5% of HTLV-1 infected individuals develop disease [33]. It is associated with various inflammatory disorders [uveitis, polymyositis, pneumonitis, Sjogren syndrome, myelopathy apart from adult T-cell leukaemia/lymphoma (ATLL)].

HIV-1 is another retrovirus which is associated with a variety of malignancies but these occur through indirect effects of immunosuppression which gives the advantage to several oncoviruses like high-risk human papillomaviruses, polyomaviruses and herpesviruses [34].

3.6 Hepatitis Viruses

It was in 1966 that Blumberg discovered the Australia antigen which is now known to be hepatitis B surface antigen (HBsAg) and 4 years later, Dane discovered the virus. Hepatitis B virus is an enveloped DNA virus and even though HBV replication in the human body per se is not cytotoxic, it is the host immune response in the form of T-cell mediated and proinflammatory cytokine milieu that causes hepatocyte damage. About 5% infections in adults and approximately 90% of infections in neonates result in a chronic infection and one-fifth of those who have persistent infection go on to develop liver cirrhosis, in the background of which hepatocellular carcinoma is seen to arise [35, 36]. On the other hand, hepatitis C virus is a single-stranded RNA virus and although 30% of those who get exposed to this virus, will clear the infection on their own, the remainder will go on to develop chronic infection and subsequent cirrhosis, if left untreated. The risk of hepatocellular cancer is about 1% per year in patients with cirrhosis even after successful sustained virologic response to antiviral treatment [37].

4 Oncogenic Bacteria

4.1 Helicobacter pylori

It is associated with non-cardia gastric adenocarcinoma and lymphoma of the stomach. It is a spiral shaped bacterium that grows in the mucus layer over the epithelial lining of the stomach and is able to survive the harsh acidic environment by secreting an enzyme called urease that converts chemical urea to ammonia and locally neutralizes the acidity [38, 39]. H. pylori infection is widespread all around the world and caused well-tolerated gastritis in most people. In a small fraction of infected people, it induces gastric mucosal atrophy, metaplasia and eventually, cancer (a well-defined sequence of events and elucidated by Correa) [40]. Even then, it is estimated that approximately 75% of the global gastric cancer burden is attributable to this bacterium induced inflammation [41]. Two toxin-encoding genes cytotoxin associated gene A (cagA) and vacuolating gene (vacA) are present in virulent strains of H. pylori [42]. The use of eradication protocols with antibiotics targeting this infection (anti H pylori regimens) and improved hygiene have decreased the incidence of significant H. pylori infections in developed countries. The flipside to this is the increased risk of gastric cardia and oesophageal carcinoma seen with people in whom H. pylori is eradicated related to gastroesophageal reflux of acidic gastric content.

5 Parasites Causing Cancer

5.1 Schistosoma haematobium

This was the first blood fluke discovered by Theodor Bilharz in Cairo (Egypt) in 1851 and hence the terminology bilharziasis applied to infections caused by this parasite [43]. Humans are the definitive hosts and freshwater snails are the intermediate hosts for this trematode. Schistosomiasis causes chronic granulomatous cystitis leading to squamous metaplasia of the transitional epithelium and subsequently, development of squamous cell carcinoma of the urinary bladder.

5.2 Opisthorchis viverrini and Clonorchis sinensis

These liver flukes are seen to cause infections mostly limited to the South-east Asian nations (like Thailand, Laos, Cambodia and Vietnam).

The freshwater snails are the first intermediate hosts and certain varieties of freshwater fish become the second intermediate host and thereafter, the metacercarial stage of these flukes become infective to humans and other fish-eating mammals like dogs and cats. These parasites are implicated in causation of intrahepatic cholangiocarcinoma by effecting bile duct chronic inflammation, periductal fibrosis and epithelial hyperplasia and goblet cell metaplasia [44].

6 The Microbiome and Carcinogenesis

An interesting development in cancer research is the increasing importance attributed to the microbiological flora (microbiome) within the body. There is growing evidence to support a function of the microbiome in cancer development in human beings. Studies have shown that enrichment and depletion of particular bacterial taxa were associated with colonic adenomas and carcinomas. There is also suggestion that the faecal microbiome may itself become a screening tool for colorectal cancer. On the other hand, the oral microbiome may harbour potential risk markers for oral and oesophageal cancers. The intactness of the intestinal barrier function is also vital to keep in check bacterial translocation and consequent chronic inflammation at various body sites. Dietary components do play an important role in modifying this barrier function. Future research is destined to unravel the secrets of the microbiome and its association with cancer [45, 46].

7 Infection Control and Prevention in Cancer Patients

Cancer patients are particularly susceptible to community-acquired and hospital-acquired infections (HAI). The basic infection control measures such as hand hygiene, transmission-based precautions, environmental hygiene, aseptic techniques, HAI "bundles" and antimicrobial stewardship are essential components of any hospital infection prevention programme, and the same applies for cancer treatment hospitals with heightened importance. The key components of the infection prevention and control programmes can be discussed under the following headings:

7.1 Hygiene

Personal and environmental hygiene is important in preventing infections in patients, and this is even so more important in the cancer patients who are immunocompromised. Routine inspection of the skin, especially at the sites which are more to infection like intravascular catheter sites, drain sites and areas prone to maceration like the axilla and the perineum is important. Digital rectal examinations, rectal thermometers, enemas and suppositories must be avoided during periods of neutropenia to avoid mucosal breakdown. Chlorhexidine bathing is recommended to reduce transmission of multidrug-resistant organisms (MDROs) and prevent infections. The oral cavity and the gut microbiota are important sources of infections and so stringent periodontal health and healthy diet are important. Especially in the management of head and neck cancers, complete periodontal examination followed by necessary treatment is recommended, especially in patients receiving high-dose chemotherapy, stem cell transplantation and any cancer regimen that is expected to lead to significant immunosuppression. To minimize the risk of mucositis and pneumonia, oral rinses with sterile water or normal saline are recommended 4–6 times per day. Neutropenic patients should routinely brush their teeth with soft bristles, taking care to minimize gingival trauma. Antivirals and antifungals are included in the prophylactic regimen according to the institutional protocols and are often given to patients considered at high risk for serious infection.

7.2 Device Associated Infection

In cancer patients, there is an increased use of intravascular catheters, implantable ports and peripherally inserted central catheter (PICC) lines and these are often kept in the body for a long duration of time. These predisposes these patients to catheter related infection and complications. Central line associated blood stream infection (CLABSI) prevention “bundle” strategies are aimed to counter such infections by frequently training nursing staff and care givers in these procedures with full barrier precautions, rigorous exit site care with daily assessment and infection control audit [47].

7.3 Environmental Hygiene

The overall environmental hygiene has an important impact in infection prevention. Surveillance of air, water and food quality and prompt corrective action is crucial in preventing infection in cancer patients.

7.4 Education and Awareness of Health Care Personals

Special care should be given to educate patients and healthcare workers regarding measures to reduce risk of exposure to infectious pathogens, such as common bacteria, community respiratory viruses and fungi. In addition, hospital infection control team, clinicians should be aware of the local epidemiology and devise an antibiotic stewardship programme and implement measures to reduce the exposure and spread of antibiotic-resistant pathogens in the institute.

8 Cancer Vaccines

The infectious aetiology of certain cancers provides us an opportunity to take preventive measures to counter the burden of these cancers by means that prevent these infections. One such potent method is development and use of prophylactic vaccines.

8.1 Hepatitis B Vaccines

Hepatitis B vaccine was the first licenced prophylactic vaccine against an infectious cause of cancer [48]. The commercial vaccines available in the 1980s were based on sub virion 22-nm HBV surface antigen (HBsAg) particles purified from the blood of chronically infected people. These were made safe for use by inactivation and absence of the 42-nm virion particles

The second-generation vaccines used recombinant DNA technology and produced HBsAg vaccines in genetically engineered yeast like *Saccharomyces cerevisiae.* These contain HBs protein spikes embedded in 22-nm lipid particles and they closely resemble the HBsAg particles produced during human infections. The method of delivery of this vaccine is by intramuscular injection at 0, 1 and 6 months. A recent development is an HBsAg containing CpG adjuvant (a Toll-like receptor 9 agonist) which is delivered as a two-dose regimen in adults [49].

In 1992, World Health Organization (WHO) recommended universal vaccination programmes targeting infants, with the first dose optimally delivered within 24 h of birth. This is very important because of the fact that the earlier age of infection, the more the chances of chronic infection and hepatocellular carcinoma eventually. A reduction of chronic HBV infection rates of more than 90% have been seen in countries with successful infant vaccination programmes [36]. An example of the effectiveness of HBV vaccination in preventing hepatocellular carcinoma (HCC) is seen from Taiwan. In that country, universal infant vaccination was started in the year 1984 and the observed incidence of HCC in 6- and 26-year-old cohorts born before and after initiation of the programme were 9.2 and 2.3 cases per ten million person-years, respectively, with a striking relative risk (RR) of 0.24 (Confidence interval 0.21–0.29) [50].

8.2 Human Papillomavirus Vaccines (HPV Vaccines)

The overwhelming importance of these particular vaccines is due to the fact that essentially all cervical cancer occurs from HPV infection. Whereas HPV16 and18 are responsible for 70% of cases of cervical cancer, other subtypes, namely HPV31, 33, 35, 45, 52 and 58, cause most of the remaining cancers [51]. Apart from cervical cancers, a vast majority of anogenital cancers (anal cancer, vaginal and vulvar cancer, penile cancer) and a good proportion of oropharyngeal cancers are attributable to HPV infections. HPV16 and 18 are responsible for the lion's share of these cases.

The HPV prophylactic vaccines [52–56] are based on VLPs or non-enveloped virus-like particles, which are composed of copies of the L1 major virion protein in the shape of an icosahedron, mimicking the outer shell of HPV. Cervarix (GlaxoSmithKline, Brentford, United Kingdom) is a bivalent vaccine containing VLPs of subtypes 16 and 18. Gardasil (Merck, Kenilworth, New Jersey) is a quadrivalent vaccine containing the VLPs of subtypes 6, 11, 16 and 18. The HPV subtypes 6 and 11 cause genital warts and are never implicated in cancer. Gardasil-9 offers protection against HPV 6, 11, 16, 18, 31, 33, 45, 52 and 58.

The current CDC (Centres for Disease Control and Prevention, USA) recommendation is for HPV vaccination for all boys and girls at ages 11–12 years to protect against HPV-related infections and cancers. Anyone starting the series before the age of 15 years should receive two doses of the vaccine, with at least 6 months between the first and second doses. Adolescents who receive the two doses less than 5 months apart, need a third dose. The recommendation is for HPV vaccination of all through the age 26 years. Those who start their doses at ages 15–26 years, still need three doses. Three doses are recommended for those who have immunocompromised conditions, between age 9 and 26 years. Adults aged 27–45 years, who are not vaccinated, may opt to get the vaccine after discussion with a physician about their risk of acquiring infection and possible benefit of vaccination [57].

The Indian Academy of Paediatrics Committee on Immunization (IAPCOI) recommends offering HPV vaccine to all females who can afford the vaccine. Vaccination can be given to females as young as 9 years as well as in those aged 13–26 years who have not previously completed vaccination [58].

The impact of HPV vaccination can be understood from the example of Scotland which has high coverage rate of 80% of adolescent girls having completed the complete three doses of Cervarix and approximately 90% having received at least one dose. Decrease was noted in the incidence of cervical intraepithelial neoplasia (CIN) type 3 at the first cervical screening between the 1988 birth cohort and the 1994 birth cohort with values of 11.9 per 100,000 and 2.9 per 100,000, respectively, with the former cohort being the one before the launch of national vaccination programme [59]. However, it should be noted that even after vaccination, girls should get PAP smear done as per guidelines.

9 Therapeutic Vaccines

It is believed that cancer cells arise in the body from time to time but are scavenged or destroyed by the immune system. This process is known as immunosurveillance and it is when the immune system fails to destroy such aberrant cells that a tumour may arise [60]. This idea is not a new concept. In 1890, an American surgeon William Coley reported about the complete regression of a sarcoma in a patient with high fever due to bacterial infection and he put this observation into clinical practice by trying to treat cancer patients with bacteria (Coley's toxin) to induce immune reaction [61]. His approach was highly criticized at that time. In the early 21st century significant response rates were to high dose interleukin 2 against malignant melanoma and renal cell carcinoma [62]. Since then, there has been tremendous development in the immunologic therapies for cancer. In this perspective the immunogenicity of oncogenic microbial agents deserves special mention.

9.1 Bacillus Calmette Guerin (BCG)

It is a vaccine primarily used against tuberculosis but it also has an approved oncologic use. It is used by intravesical route to prevent recurrences in the treatment of non-muscle invasive bladder cancer.

9.2 Sipuleucel-T

It is a cellular vaccine composed of dendritic cells presenting the fusion protein PA2024, which is expressed in prostate cancer cells. Full-length prostatic acid phosphatase is co-expressed with the cytokine GM-CSF to form PA2024. This is then loaded on to autologous dendritic cells isolated from individual patients by leukapheresis. This vaccine was approved in 2010 for the treatment of patients with metastatic castrate-resistant prostate cancer (mCRPC) with minimal or no symptoms [63].

9.3 Talimogene Laherparepvec (T-VEC)

It is an oncolytic, genetically modified herpesvirus that generates an "in situ vaccine" effect. This genetically engineered herpes simplex virus (HSV) is only capable of replicating in cancer cells, where it generates the cytokine GM-CSF. The high levels of local GM-CSF recruit dendritic cells and macrophages and make them antigen-presenting cells (APCs) leading to priming of tumour-specific T cells in the tumour microenvironment after direct intra-tumoral injection. It is approved to treat stage III and IV malignant melanoma patients for whom surgical intervention is not appropriate and with tumours which can be directly injected [64].

10 Conclusion

The world of microbiology is intricately related to the various processes of cancer in the human body, right from the evolution to the existing and future therapies and a detailed knowledge of the same is paramount for the entire community involved in cancer care. Indeed, it is undeniable that a good medical microbiology team is an indispensable component in the multidisciplinary management of cancer.

References

1. Plummer M, de Martel C, Vignat J, Ferlay J, Bray F, Franceschi S. Global burden of cancers attributable to infections in 2012: a synthetic analysis. Lancet Glob Healt. 2016;4:e609–16. https://doi.org/10.1016/S2214-109X(16)30143-7.
2. Thun MJ, DeLancey JO, Center MM, Jemal A, Ward EM. The global burden of cancer: priorities for prevention. Carcinogenesis. 2010;31(1):100–10. https://doi.org/10.1093/carcin/bgp263.
3. IARC. Monographs on the identification of carcinogenic hazards to humans. Lyon (FR): International Agency for Research on Cancer; 1987. https://www.ncbi.nlm.nih.gov/books/NBK294452/. Last Accessed 15 Oct 2021.
4. Bouvard V, Baan R, Straif K, Grosse Y, Secretan B, El Ghissassi F. A review of human carcinogens–part B: biological agents. Lancet Oncol. 2009;10(4):321–2.
5. Zur Hausen H, Villiers ED. Cancer 'causation' by infections—individual contributions and synergistic networks. Semin Oncol. 2015;41:860–75.
6. Grivennikov SI, Greten FR, Karin M. Immunity, inflammation, and cancer. Cell. 2010;140:883–99.
7. Hanahan D, Weinberg RA. Review hallmarks of cancer: the next generation. Cell. 2011;144:646–74.
8. Krump NA, You J. Molecular mechanisms of viral oncogenesis in humans. Nat Rev Microbiol. 2018;16(11):684–98. https://doi.org/10.1038/s41579-018-0064-6.
9. Coussens LM, Werb Z. Inflammation and cancer. Nature. 2002;420(6917):860–7. https://doi.org/10.1038/nature01322.
10. Aviles NB. The little death: Rigoni-Stern and the problem of sex and cancer in 20th-century biomedical research. Soc Stud Sci. 2015;45(3):394–415.
11. Münger K, Basile J, Duensing S, et al. Biological activities and molecular targets of the human papil-

lomavirus E7 oncoprotein. Oncogene. 2001;20:7888–98. https://doi.org/10.1038/sj.onc.1204860.
12. Chesson HW, Dunne EF, Hariri S, Markowitz LE. The estimated lifetime probability of acquiring human papillomavirus in the United States. Sex Transm Dis. 2014;41(11):660–4.
13. Aguilar-Lemarroy A, Gariglio P, Whitaker NJ, Eichhorst ST, Zur HH, Krammer PH, et al. Restoration of p53 expression sensitizes human papillomavirus type 16 immortalized human keratinocytes to CD95-mediated apoptosis. Oncogene. 2002;21:165–75. https://doi.org/10.1038/sj.onc.1204979.
14. Doorbar J, Egawa N, Griffin H, Kranjec C, Murakami I. Human papillomavirus molecular biology and disease association. Rev Med Virol. 2016;25:2–23. https://doi.org/10.1002/rmv.1822.
15. Hellner K, Mar J, Fang F, Quackenbush J, Munger K. HPV 16 E7 oncogene expression in normal human epithelial cells causes molecular changes indicative of an epithelial to mesenchymal transition. Virology. 2009;391:57–63. https://doi.org/10.1016/j.virol.2009.05.036.
16. Jabbar SF, Abrams L, Glick A, Lambert PF. Persistence of high-grade cervical dysplasia and cervical cancer requires the continuous expression of the human papillomavirus type 16 E7 oncogene. Cancer Res. 2009;69:4407–14. https://doi.org/10.1158/0008-5472.CAN-09-0023.
17. Merkel F. Tastzellen and Tastkoerperchenbei den Hausthieren und beim Menschen. Arch Mikr Anat. 1875;11:636–52.
18. DeCaprio JA. Merkel cell polyomavirus and Merkel cell carcinoma. Philos Trans R Soc Lond B Biol Sci. 2017;372(1732):20160276. https://doi.org/10.1098/rstb.2016.0276.
19. Starrett GJ, Buck CB. The case for BK polyomavirus as a cause of bladder cancer. Curr Opin Virol. 2019;39:8–15. https://doi.org/10.1016/j.coviro.2019.06.009.
20. Young L, Yap L, Murray P. Epstein–Barr virus: more than 50 years old and still providing surprises. Nat Rev Cancer. 2016;16:789–802.
21. Epstein MA. On the discovery of Epstein–Barr virus: a memoir. Epstein–Barr Virus Rep. 1999;6:58–63.
22. Thorley-Lawson DA, Allday MJ. The curious case of the tumour virus: 50 years of Burkitt's lymphoma. Nat Rev Microbiol. 2008;6:913–24.
23. Tsao SW, Tsang CM, To KF, Lo KW. The role of Epstein–Barr virus in epithelial malignancies. J Pathol. 2015;235:323–33.
24. Tsao SW, Tsang CM, Lo KW. Epstein-Barr virus infection and nasopharyngeal carcinoma. Philos Trans R Soc Lond B Biol Sci. 2017;372:20160270. https://doi.org/10.1098/rstb.2016.0270.
25. Hutajulu SH, Fachiroh J, Argy G, et al. Seroprevalence of IgA anti Epstein-Barr virus is high among family members of nasopharyngeal cancer patients and individuals presenting with chronic complaints in head and neck area. PLoS One. 2017;12(8):e0180683. Published 2017 Aug 11. https://doi.org/10.1371/journal.pone.0180683.
26. Murphy G, Pfeiffer R, Camargo MC, Rabkin CS. Meta-analysis shows that prevalence of Epstein-Barr virus-positive gastric cancer differs based on sex and anatomic location [published correction appears in Gastroenterology. 2011 Mar;140(3):1109]. Gastroenterology. 2009;137(3):824–33.
27. Mesri EA, Cesarman E, Boshoff C. Kaposi's sarcoma and its associated herpesvirus. Nat Rev Cancer. 2010;10(10):707–19. https://doi.org/10.1038/nrc2888.
28. Kaposi M. Idiopathisches multiples Pigmentsarkom der Haut. Arch Dermatol Syph. 1872;4 (Original description of KS).
29. Centers for Disease Control. Kaposi's sarcoma and Pneumocystis pneumonia among homosexual men—New York City and California. MMWR Morb Mortal Wkly Rep. 1981;30:305–8.
30. Gottlieb GJ, et al. A preliminary communication on extensively disseminated Kaposi's sarcoma in young homosexual men. Am J Dermatopathol. 1981;3:111–4.
31. Chang Y, et al. Identification of herpesvirus-like DNA sequences in AIDS-associated Kaposi's sarcoma. Science. 1994;266:1865–9.
32. Gallo RC. The enigmas of Kaposi's sarcoma. Science. 1998;282:1837–9.
33. Gonçalves DU, Proietti FA, Ribas JG, et al. Epidemiology, treatment, and prevention of human T-cell leukemia virus type 1-associated diseases. Clin Microbiol Rev. 2010;23(3):577–89. https://doi.org/10.1128/CMR.00063-09.
34. Yarchoan R, Uldrick TS. HIV-associated cancers and related diseases. N Engl J Med. 2018;378(11):1029–41. https://doi.org/10.1056/NEJMra1615896.
35. Fung J, Lai CL, Yuen MF. Hepatitis B and C virus-related carcinogenesis. Clin Microbiol Infect. 2009;15(11):964–70. https://doi.org/10.1111/j.1469--0691.2009.03035.x. PMID: 19874379.
36. Nelson NP, Easterbrook PJ, McMahon BJ. Epidemiology of hepatitis B virus infection and impact of vaccination on disease [published correction appears in Clin Liver Dis. 2017 May;21(2):xiii]. Clin Liver Dis. 2016;20(4):607–28. https://doi.org/10.1016/j.cld.2016.06.006.
37. Di Bisceglie AM. Hepatitis C and hepatocellular carcinoma. Hepatology. 1997;26(3 Suppl 1):34S–8S.

https://doi.org/10.1002/hep.510260706. PMID: 9305661.
38. Wroblewski LE, Peek RM Jr, Wilson KT. Helicobacter pylori and gastric cancer: factors that modulate disease risk. Clin Microbiol Rev. 2010;23(4):713–39. https://doi.org/10.1128/CMR.00011-10.
39. Amieva MR, Vogelmann R, Covacci A, Tompkins LS, Nelson WJ, Falkow S. Disruption of the epithelial apical-junctional complex by Helicobacter pylori CagA. Science. 2003;300:1430–4.
40. Kusters JG, van Vliet AH, Kuipers EJ. Pathogenesis of Helicobacter pylori infection. Clin Microbiol Rev. 2006;19(3):449–90. https://doi.org/10.1128/CMR.00054-05.
41. Herrera V, Parsonnet J. Helicobacter pylori and gastric adenocarcinoma. J Clin Microbiol Infect. 2009;15(11):971–6.
42. Rudi J, Kolb C, Maiwald M, et al. Diversity of Helicobacter pylori vacA and cagA genes and relationship to VacA and CagA protein expression, cytotoxin production, and associated diseases. J Clin Microbiol. 1998;36(4):944–8. https://doi.org/10.1128/JCM.36.4.944-948.1998.
43. Di Bella S, Riccardi N, Giacobbe DR, Luzzati R. History of schistosomiasis (bilharziasis) in humans: from Egyptian medical papyri to molecular biology on mummies. Pathog Glob Health. 2018;112(5):268–73. https://doi.org/10.1080/20477724.2018.1495357.
44. Schwartz DA. Helminths in the induction of cancer: Opisthorchis viverrini, Clonorchis sinensis and cholangiocarcinoma. Trop Geogr Med. 1980;32(2):95–100. PMID: 6252671.
45. Irfan M, Delgado RZR, Frias-Lopez J. The oral microbiome and cancer. Front Immunol. 2020;11:591088. Published 2020 Oct 23. https://doi.org/10.3389/fimmu.2020.591088.
46. Vivarelli S, Salemi R, Candido S, et al. Gut microbiota and cancer: from pathogenesis to therapy. Cancers (Basel). 2019;11(1):38. Published 2019 Jan 3. https://doi.org/10.3390/cancers11010038.
47. Bell T, O'Grady NP. Prevention of central line-associated bloodstream infections. Infect Dis Clin North Am. 2017;31(3):551–9. https://doi.org/10.1016/j.idc.2017.05.007. Epub 2017 Jul 5. PMID: 28687213; PMCID: PMC5666696.
48. Chang MH. Hepatitis B virus and cancer prevention. Recent Results Cancer Res. 2011;188:75–84. https://doi.org/10.1007/978-3-642-10858-7_6. PMID: 21253790.
49. Bode C, Zhao G, Steinhagen F, Kinjo T, Klinman DM. CpG DNA as a vaccine adjuvant. Expert Rev Vaccines. 2011;10(4):499–511. https://doi.org/10.1586/erv.10.174.
50. Chang MH, You SL, Chen CJ, Liu CJ, Lee CM, Lin SM, Chu HC, Wu TC, Yang SS, Kuo HS, Chen DS, Taiwan Hepatoma Study Group. Decreased incidence of hepatocellular carcinoma in hepatitis B vaccinees: a 20-year follow-up study. J Natl Cancer Inst. 2009;101(19):1348–55. https://doi.org/10.1093/jnci/djp288. Epub 2009 Sep 16. PMID: 19759364.
51. Braaten KP, Laufer MR. Human papillomavirus (HPV), HPV-related disease, and the HPV vaccine. Rev Obstet Gynecol. 2008;1(1):2–10.
52. Stanley M. Prophylactic HPV vaccines. J Clin Pathol. 2007;60(9):961–5. https://doi.org/10.1136/jcp.2006.040568.
53. Crosbie EJ, Einstein MH, Franceschi S, Kitchener HC. Human papillomavirus and cervical cancer. Lancet. 2013;382:889–99. https://doi.org/10.1016/S0140-6736(13)60022-7.
54. Moscicki AB, Schiffman M, Kjaer S, Villa LL. Chapter 5: updating the natural history of HPV and anogenital cancer. Vaccine. 2006;24(Suppl. 3):S3/42–51. https://doi.org/10.1016/j.vaccine.2006.06.018.
55. Cutts FT, Franceschi S, Goldie S, Castellsague X, de Sanjose S, Garnett G, et al. Human papillomavirus and HPV vaccines: a review. Bull World Health Organ. 2007;85:719–26. https://doi.org/10.2471/BLT.06.038414.
56. Arbyn M, Xu L, Simoens C, Martin-Hirsch PPL. Prophylactic vaccination against human papillomaviruses to prevent cervical cancer and its precursors. Cochrane Database Syst Rev. 2018;5(5):CD009069. https://doi.org/10.1002/14651858.CD009069.pub3.
57. Meites E, Szilagyi PG, Chesson HW, Unger ER, Romero JR, Markowitz LE. Human papillomavirus vaccination for adults: updated recommendations of the Advisory Committee on Immunization Practices. MMWR Morb Mortal Wkly Rep. 2019;68:698–702.
58. Singhal T. Indian Academy of Pediatrics Committee on Immunisation (IAPCOI)-consensus recommendations on immunization 2008. Indian Pediatr. 2008;45:635–48.
59. Drolet M, Benard E, Boily MC, Ali H, Baandrup L, Bauer H, et al. Population level impact and herd effects following human papillomavirus vaccination programmes: a systematic review and meta-analysis. Lancet Infect Dis. 2015;15(5):565–80.
60. Fulop T, et al. Potential role of immunosenescence in cancer development. Ann N Y Acad Sci. 2010;1197:158–65.
61. McCarthy EF. The toxins of William B. Coley and the treatment of bone and soft-tissue sarcomas. Iowa Orthop J. 2006;26:154–8.
62. Jiang T, Zhou C, Ren S. Role of IL-2 in cancer immunotherapy. Oncoimmunology. 2016;5(6):e1163462. Published 2016 Apr 25. https://doi.org/10.1080/2162402X.2016.1163462.
63. Kantoff PW, Higano CS, Shore ND, Berger ER, Small EJ, Penson DF, Redfern CH, Ferrari AC, Dreicer R, Sims RB, Xu Y, Frohlich MW, Schellhammer PF, IMPACT Study Investigators. Sipuleucel-T immunotherapy for castration-resistant prostate cancer. N Engl J Med. 2010;363(5):411–22. https://doi.org/10.1056/NEJMoa1001294. PMID: 20818862.
64. Bommareddy PK, Patel A, Hossain S, Kaufman HL. Talimogene laherparepvec (T-VEC) and other oncolytic viruses for the treatment of melanoma. Am J Clin Dermatol. 2017;18(1):1–15. https://doi.org/10.1007/s40257-016-0238-9. PMID: 27988837.

Imaging in Gynaecological Malignancies

Binoy Kumar Choudhury, Geetanjali Barman, and Amal Chandra Kataki

Imaging plays an important role in the management of gynaecological malignancy. Most of the imaging modalities are utilized to investigate suspected gynaecological malignancy and these include ultrasound (US), computed tomography (CT), magnetic resonance imaging (MRI) and positron emission tomography (PET). These modalities have essential role in diagnosis, staging, management, post-treatment follow-up, detection of recurrence and in predicting prognosis. More recently, hybrid imaging of positron emission tomography and computed tomography (PET-CT) is increasingly utilized to supplement conventional imaging in assessing gynaecological malignancies.

1 Ultrasound

Ultrasound (US) is the primary imaging modality for initial assessment of suspected gynaecological malignant lesions. It is an easily available, relatively cheap and reliable initial screening modality for suspected gynaecological malignancy. Both transabdominal and transvaginal ultrasound (TVS) are widely utilized in the assessment of endometrial thickness, characterization of adnexal masses and detection of recurrent diseases. Colour Doppler sonography have allowed the assessment of vascularity of tumour. Combined with morphological features, colour Doppler has increased the accuracy of determining benign from malignant adnexal masses. Recent advances such as dynamic contrast enhanced TVS using microbubbles allow detection of microvascular tumour networks and it has been shown to have higher sensitivity and specificity than conventional TVS.

2 Computed Tomography (CT)

Computed tomography (CT) has an extremely important role in the preoperative staging of gynaecological malignancy. Contrast enhanced CT (CECT) helps to differentiate malignant lesions from normal tissue. It plays an essential role in identifying distant metastases, enlarged lymph nodes and peritoneal deposits. It is also useful in detecting recurrent pelvic tumours following treatment. Peritoneal deposits smaller than 1 cm in size can be difficult to detect, particularly in the absence of ascites. When lymph nodes measure greater than 1 cm in short axis, or when there are morphologic changes, such as rounded shape or necrosis, tumour involvement is suspected [1].

B. K. Choudhury (✉) · G. Barman
Department of Radiology, Dr. Bhubaneswar Borooah Cancer Institute, Guwahati, Assam, India

A. C. Kataki
Department of Gynaecologic Oncology, Dr. Bhubaneswar Borooah Cancer Institute (A Unit of Tata Memorial Centre, Mumbai), Guwahati, Assam, India

A. C. Kataki, D. Barmon (eds.), *Fundamentals in Gynaecologic Malignancy*,
https://doi.org/10.1007/978-981-19-5860-1_5

Modern CT scanners using 128 or 256 detectors allow rapid acquisition of scan and facilitates multiplanar reconstruction in axial, sagittal and coronal dimension with high resolution. Though CT scan is widely used in gynaecological malignancy it has disadvantages like exposure to ionizing radiation, adverse reactions to iodinated contrast material and lower soft tissue resolution as compared with MRI.

3 Magnetic Resonance Imaging (MRI)

MRI is the imaging modality of choice for diagnosis and staging of cervical and uterine malignancies and is widely used for characterization of adnexal masses. It provides excellent soft tissue resolution in multiple planes. It is helpful for determining metastatic disease, especially if liver lesions on CT scan are indeterminate [1]. T2 weighted MRI (T2W MRI) are helpful for demonstrating the pathological lesion as presence of tumour causes distortion of the normal anatomy with associated altered signal intensity. T1 weighted MRI (T1W MRI) are helpful for identification of blood and proteinaceous product inside a tumour. These two components show high signal intensity on T1W MR images. Fat suppressed imaging sequences are required for detection of fat within the lesion. Fat suppressed post-contrast T1W MRI allows detection of peritoneal tumour deposits. Contrast enhanced MR images demonstrate the differentiation of neoplastic from normal tissue. Conventional MRI plays an important role in evaluation of morphology and extent of tumour because of better soft tissue resolution, but cannot accurately detect metastatic lymph nodes. Functional MR imaging techniques allow functional assessment of tumours. It consists of dynamic multiphase contrast enhanced magnetic resonance imaging (DCE-MRI) and diffusion weighted magnetic resonance imaging (DW-MRI) with ADC (apparent diffusion coefficient). These techniques have emerged as a very helpful tool not only in lymph node metastases, but also depicting residual tumours and differentiating tumour recurrence from radiation fibrosis in treated cases. They also improve characterization of cystic adnexal lesions and detection of small peritoneal implants in patients with ovarian cancer [2]. DW-MRI detects extra-uterine disease and thus helps in preoperative staging of cervical and endometrial cancer. Limitations of MRI include higher cost, its limited availability, long image acquisition times leading to motion artifact, decreased patient compliance and safety issues related to MRI.

4 PET-CT

PET-CT fuses anatomical and metabolic information about a tumour. In gynaecological cancers, PET-CT allows complete assessment of locoregional tumour extent, whole body evaluation for nodal peritoneal and skeletal metastases [3]. PET-CT has been widely adopted in gynaecology for staging of advanced malignant tumours, detection of suspected recurrence, post-treatment response evaluation and to determine prognosis [4]. PET-CT is not free from pitfalls. False positive results are encountered in areas that show normal physiological uptakes like endometrium and ovaries in premenopausal patients. Multiple benign conditions like fibroid, pelvic inflammatory disease and endometriotic cyst also show FDG uptake. Serosal and peritoneal disease may be masked by physiological activity in bladder and bowel [4]. PET-CT shows false negative results in cases of necrotic, cystic, mucinous and low grade tumours due to low FDG uptake.

5 Cervical Cancer

Cervical cancer is a major cause of cancer mortality in women. Cervical cancer is a public health problem in developing nations like India and India alone accounts for one quarter of the cervical cancer cases worldwide [5]. FIGO staging is clinically based, however, the revised FIGO staging system encourages imaging as an adjunct to clinical staging.

In order to be visible by imaging, cervical tumour should be at least stage Ib [6]. MRI is the imaging modality of choice for evaluation of primary tumour and local extent. Distant metastases can be best assessed with CT or PET-CT.

Ultrasound is the initial imaging modality and shows heterogenous hypoechoic mass involving cervix and may show increased vascularity on colour Doppler. US is also helpful in showing size of the tumour, vaginal and parametrial invasion and involvement of adjacent organs. Transvaginal US may be used to measure the primary tumour and also to assess the local spread into the cervical stroma or parametrium in patients suspected of having early disease. Mass may occlude the endocervical canal resulting in hydro or pyometra. In case of isoechoic mass, cervical enlargement may be the only finding. Transabdominal US can be used to evaluate complications like hydronephrosis in advanced cases.

CT is not very helpful in evaluation of primary tumour. Primary tumour may be isodense or hypodense to normal cervical stroma on CT (Fig. 1). It is useful in advanced disease (Figs. 2, 3, 4, and 5). CT can improve clinical FIGO staging as it can detect urinary obstruction, help to assess lymphadenopathy and distant metastases [7] (Fig. 5). CT can demonstrate details of the ureteric involvement (Fig. 4) and functional status of the kidneys and has replaced conventional radiological technique like intravenous urography (IVU). It helps in planning the placement of radiation ports and guiding percutaneous biopsy.

MRI is the primary imaging modality to assess the primary tumour and local extent. T2 is the key sequence for visualization of primary tumour and local staging [8]. Sagittal T2WI is useful to assess the depth of cervical stromal invasion, invasion of vagina, uterine body (Figs. 6, 7, and 8) and urinary bladder. Axial T2WI is helpful for parametrial invasion, pelvic sidewall invasion and rectal invasion. Coronal T2WI also useful for evaluation of depth of cervical stromal invasion and parametrial invasion. Usually T1WI reveals the lesion as isointense compared to pelvic muscles. T1 Contrast (T1C) is not required routinely, but it may be useful to depict small tumours considered for trachelectomy. In addition to assessing the presence of parametrial extension (stage IIB), MRI is also useful for evidence of pelvic nodal disease. Parametrial invasion (Figs. 9 and 10) is demonstrated as disruption of the cervical stromal ring, spiculated mass or soft tissue exten-

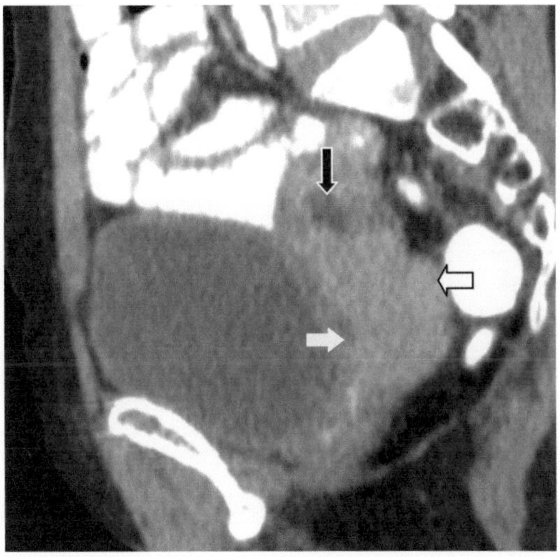

Fig. 1 Sagittal CT scan of pelvis showing a soft tissue mass in the uterine cervix (thick horizontal white arrows), extending to the lower uterine body and upper vagina. There is mild endocavity collection (vertical black arrow)

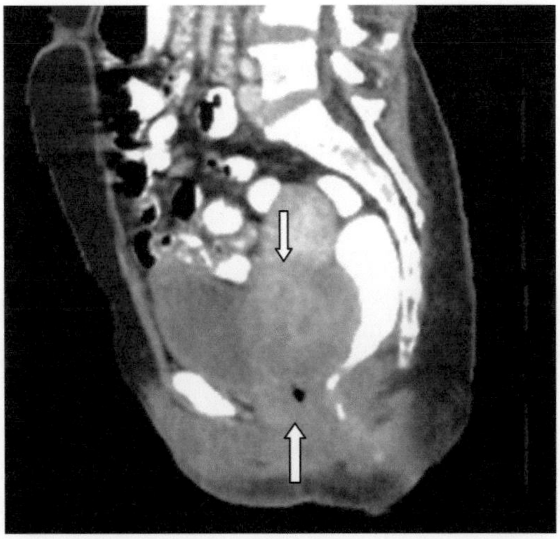

Fig. 2 Cervical cancer. Sagittal CECT scan of pelvis showing a bulky cervical growth (white arrows) extending to lower uterine body and upper vagina with involvement of endocervix

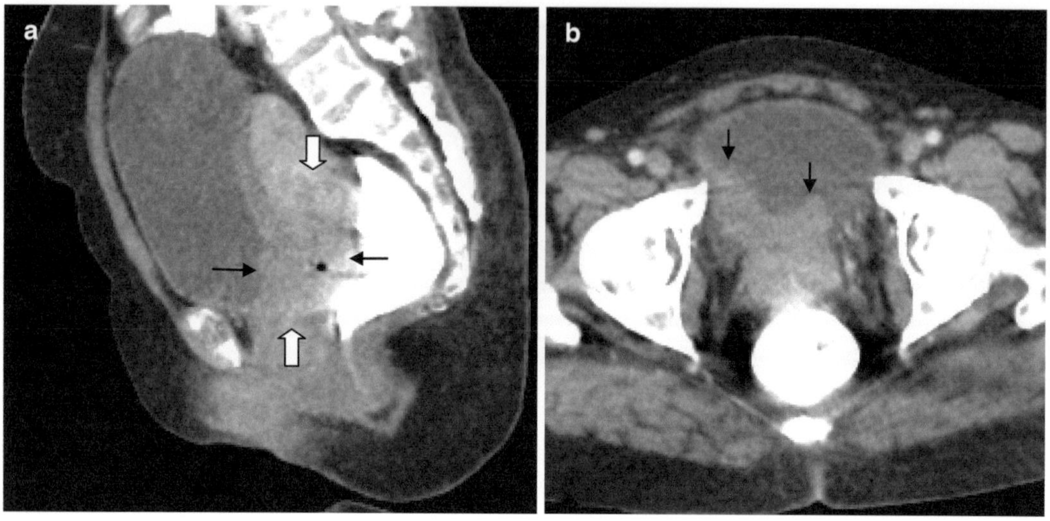

Fig. 3 Cervical cancer infiltrating uterine body, vagina, bladder and rectum. (**a**) Sagittal CECT scan of pelvis showing cervical growth (vertical white arrows) extending to lower uterine body and upper vagina. The lesion infiltrates posterior wall of urinary bladder and anterior wall of rectum (thin black arrows). (**b**) Axial CECT showing the mass infiltrating the posterior wall of the urinary bladder (thin black arrows)

sion into the parametria or encasement of the periuterine vessels. Later stages of cervical carcinoma is demonstrated as extension of the tumour into the lower third of the vagina (IIIa), to the pelvic side wall (Fig. 11) or presence of hydronephrosis (IIIb). Invasion into the bladder or rectum represents stage IV disease and is identified as intermediate signal intensity tumour on T2WI images infiltrating the bladder or rectal wall.

Diffusion weighted imaging (DWI) combined with conventional MRI improves lesion detection. Tumour shows diffusion restriction and appears more distinct against normal tissue. DWI is also helpful in cases where MR contrast agent cannot be administered. In early post-treatment period it may be difficult to distinguish residual tumour from post-treatment and inflammatory changes. DWI is considered to be the best modality for monitoring treatment response and evaluation of recurrent disease. Cervical cancer shows lower ADC in comparison with normal cervix and the ADC increases after chemoradiation.

MRI is also useful in evaluation of young patients, willing to preserve fertility and with small invasive tumours where conservative surgical procedures like trachelectomy can be performed. MRI can be used to confirm the correct positioning of insertion of MR compatible brachytherapy applicators. This helps in accurate calculation of radiotherapy dosage to the tumour.

PET-CT may be considered as imaging modality of choice for staging, for detection of nodal and distant metastases in advanced cervical cancer. It is not good enough to replace the performance of laparoscopic nodal dissection. It has greatest role in detection of distant recurrent disease and is essential in patients who are selected for extenterative surgery. PET-CT can also perform functional evaluation of the primary tumour by measuring the standard uptake value (SUVmax). The mean SUV of pelvic nodes helps in functional evaluation that can be used in future as a marker for response evaluation and for prediction of disease recurrence.

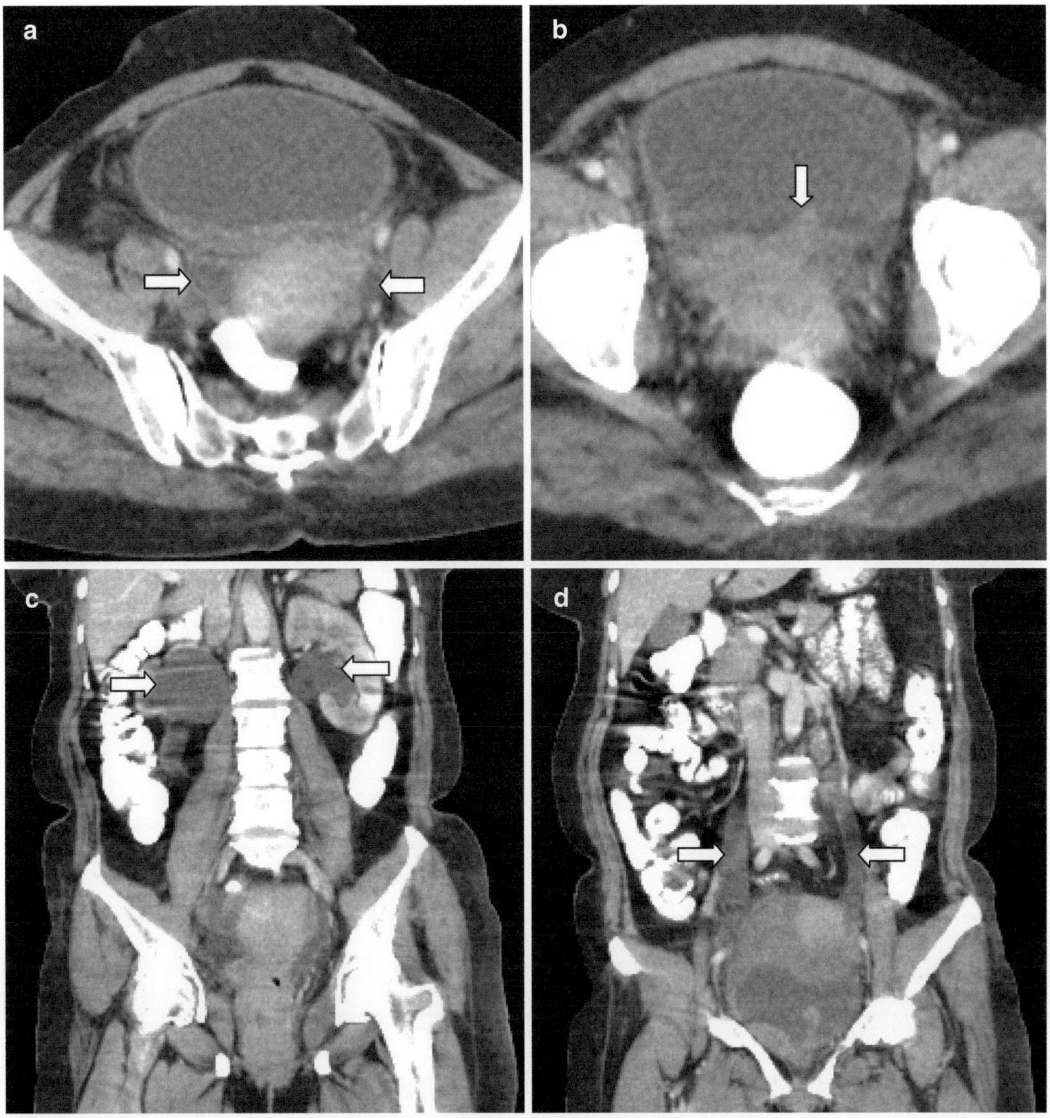

Fig. 4 Cervical cancer causing bilateral hydroureteronephrosis. (**a**, **b**) Axial CECT scan showing cervical growth with bilateral hydroureter (horizontal white arrows) due to infiltration of bilateral vesicoureteric junction at lower sections. The growth has infiltrated the posterior wall of the urinary bladder (vertical white arrow) as well. (**c**, **d**) Coronal CECT showing bilateral hydronephrosis and hydroureter (horizontal white arrows)

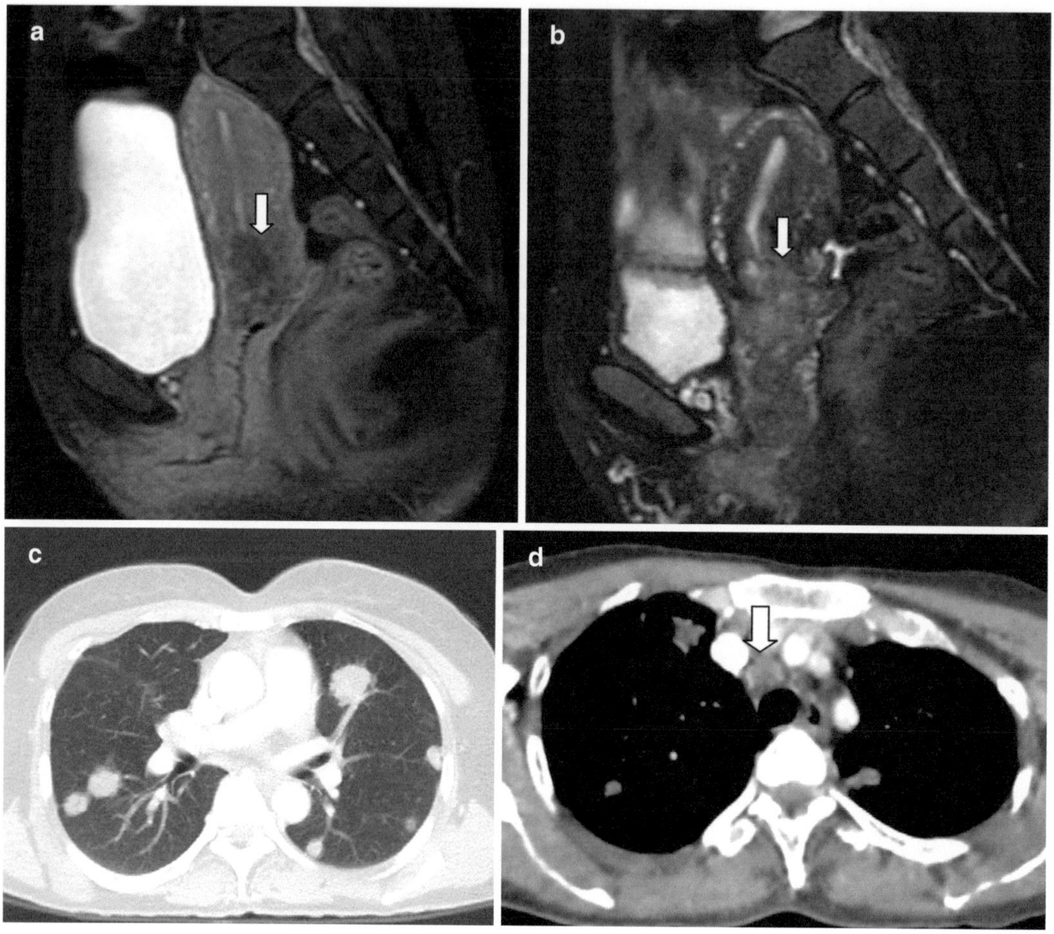

Fig. 5 Cervical cancer with pulmonary and mediastinal nodal metastases. (**a**, **b**) Sagittal T2W and T1W contrast MRI scan showing cervical growth (white vertical arrows). (**c**) CT Thorax showing multiple pulmonary metastases. (**d**) CECT Thorax shows mediastinal lymphadenopathy in pretracheal location (vertical arrow)

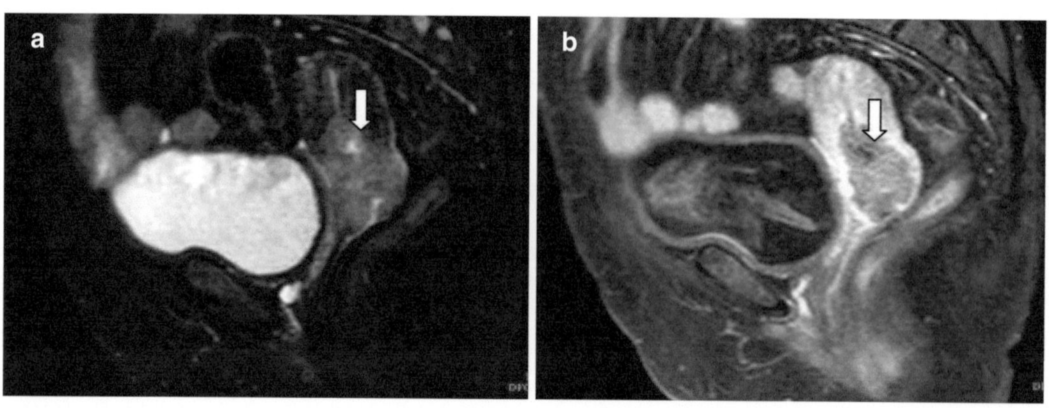

Fig. 6 Cervical cancer. (**a**) Sagittal T2W MRI of pelvis showing an irregular mass (vertical arrow) in the cervix extending to lower uterine body and upper vagina. (**b**) On contrast enhanced image the mass is clearly seen (vertical arrow)

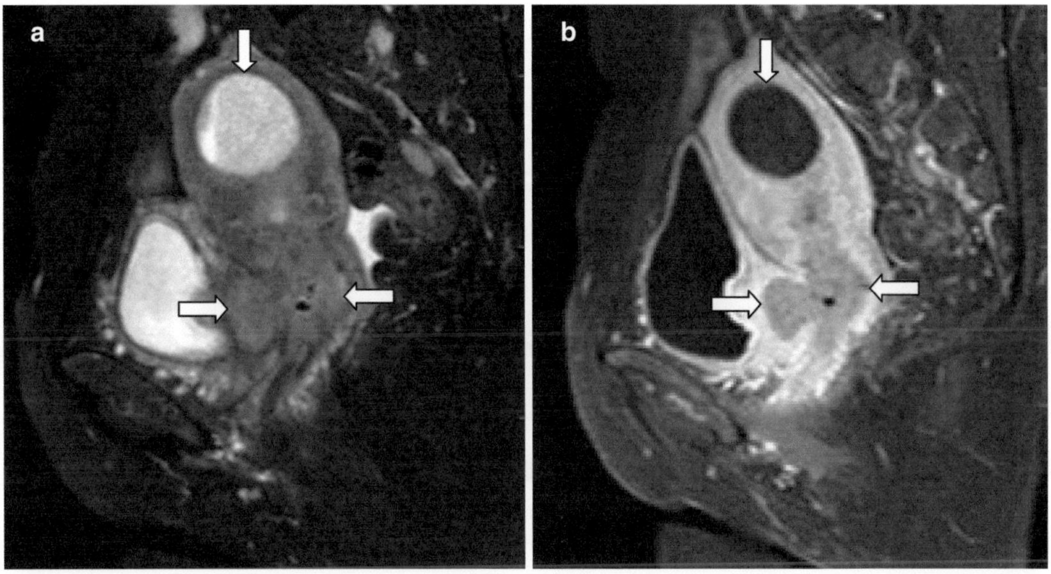

Fig. 7 Cervical cancer. (**a**, **b**) Sagittal MRI (T2 and T1 contrast) showing a soft tissue mass in the cervix involving both anterior and posterior lip (white horizontal arrows) as well as extending to upper vagina and lower uterine body with moderate endocavity collection (vertical arrows)

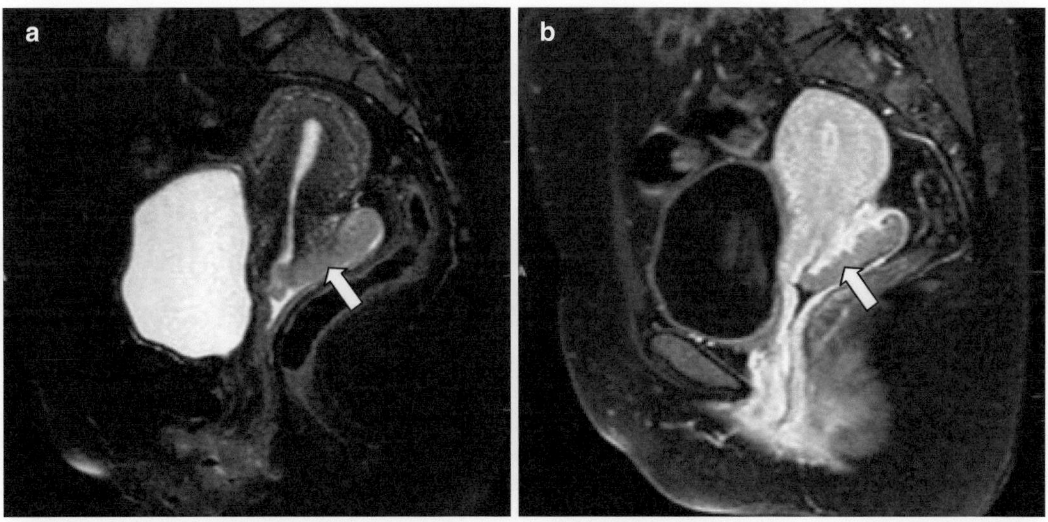

Fig. 8 Cervical cancer. (**a**, **b**) T2W and T1 contrast MRI in sagittal sections showing a cervical mass involving the posterior lip of the cervix and extending towards the posterior vaginal fornix (arrows)

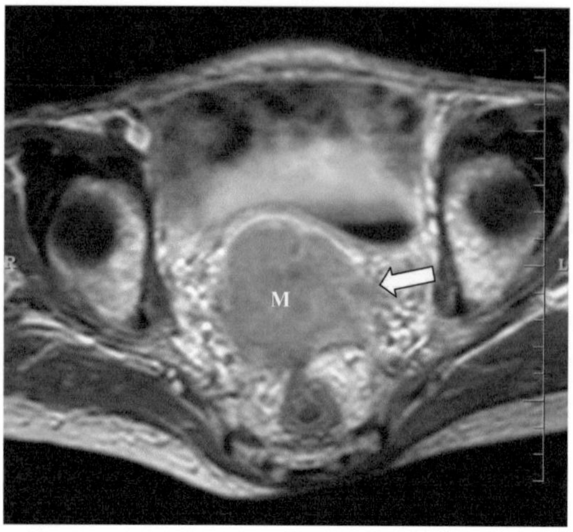

Fig. 9 Cervical cancer with parametrial invasion. Axial T1 contrast MRI showing an enhancing cervical mass (M) with bilateral parametrial infiltration (more on left) (arrow)

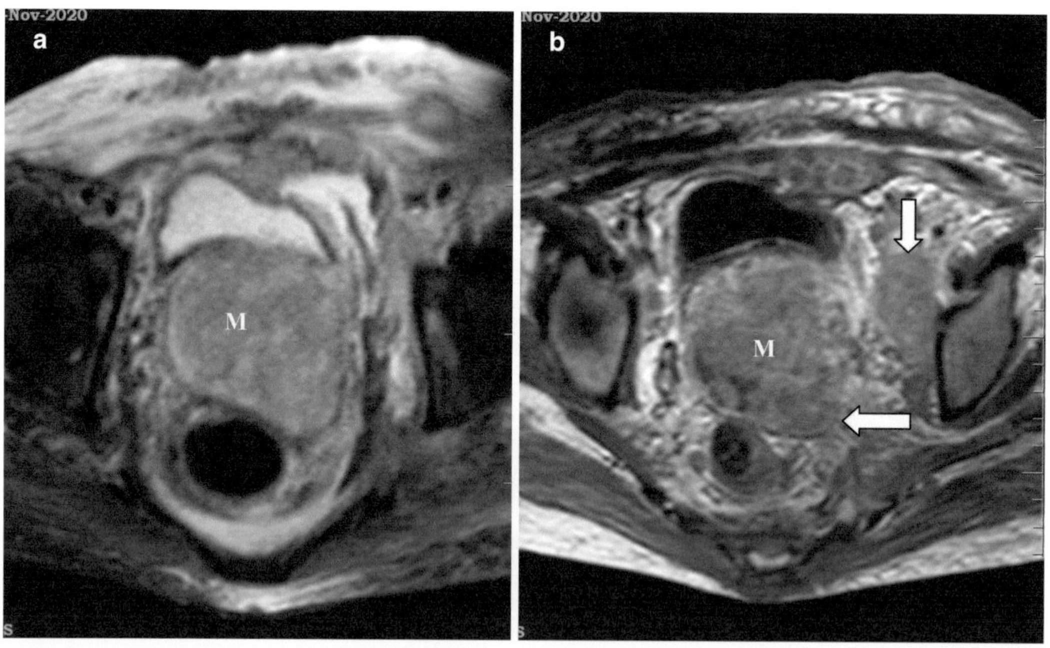

Fig. 10 Cervical cancer (M) with parametrial invasion and enlarged iliac node. (**a**) T2 axial MRI showing a bulky cervical mass. (**b**) T1 contrast axial MRI showing cervical mass infiltrating bilateral parametrium (more on the left) (horizontal white arrow) with enlarged left iliac node (vertical white arrow). (**c**, **d**) T1 and T1 contrast sagittal MR images showing a bulky mass in the cervix extending to upper vagina and lower uterine body with endocavity collection (arrows)

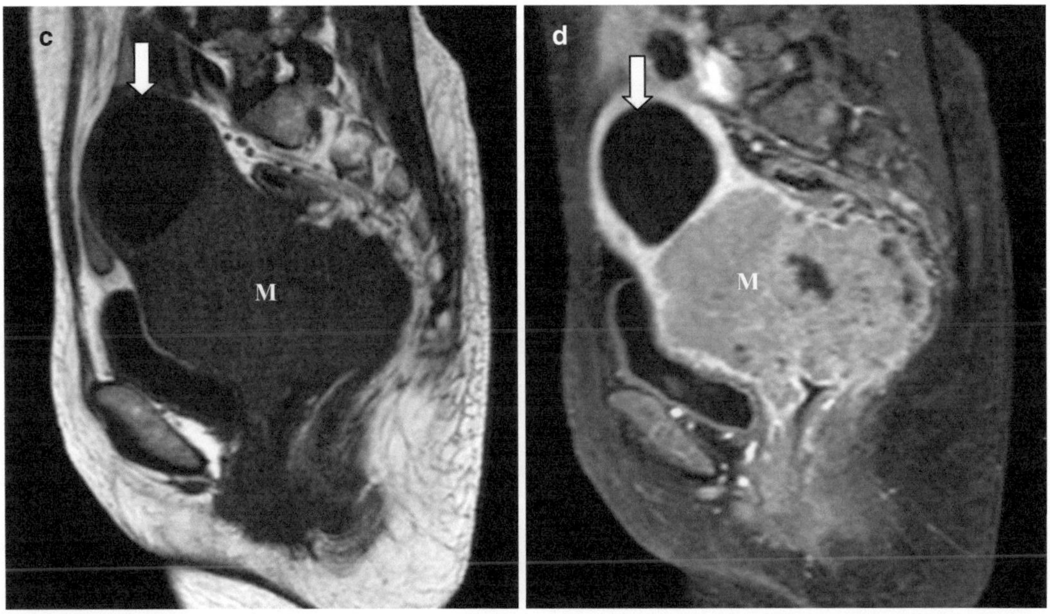

Fig. 10 (continued)

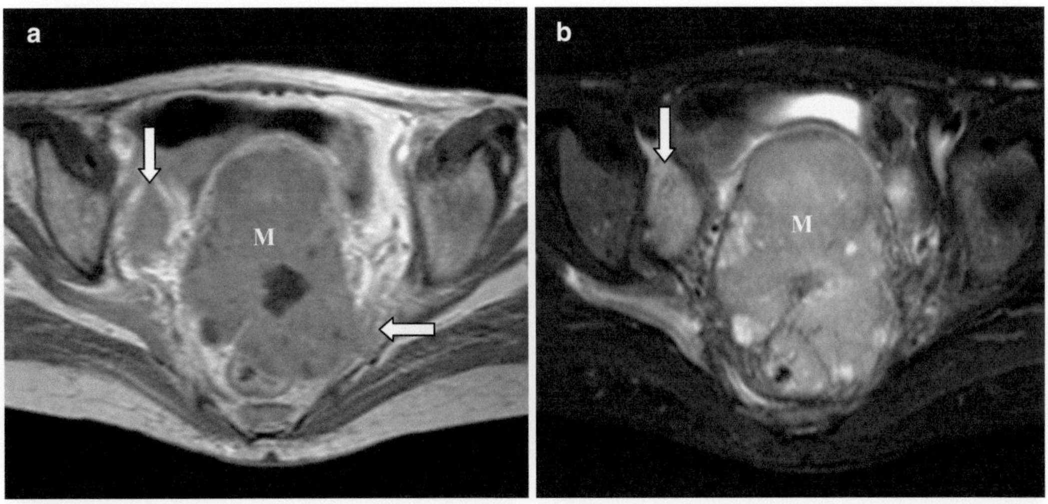

Fig. 11 Cervical cancer with pelvic side wall invasion. (**a**, **b**) Axial T1W and T2W MR images showing a large lobulated cervical mass (M) with areas of necrosis. Mass infiltrates bilateral parametrium, left pelvic side wall (horizontal arrow) and also infiltrates the anterior rectal wall. There is associated right iliac lymphadenopathy (vertical arrows)

6 Endometrial Cancer

Endometrial cancer is the most common malignancy of the uterine corpus [9]. It is the most common female genital cancer in the developed countries [10].

However, the incidence of endometrial cancer cases are low in India [11]. Both ultrasound and pelvic MRI are useful imaging modalities for evaluation of endometrial cancer. Transvaginal ultrasound (TVS) is the initial imaging modality of choice to assess endometrial thickness in women presenting with postmenopausal bleeding [12]. Endometrial thickness greater than 4–5 mm in these patients (more than 8 mm if on hormone replacement therapy or tamoxifen) should be considered suspicious. Sonographic features are nonspecific. It is often not possible to distinguish between endometrial lesions like endometrial polyps, endometrial hyperplasia from stage Ia endometrial carcinoma using US. A thickened endometrium requires endometrial biopsy. US features that may be suggestive of endometrial carcinoma include heterogenous and irregular thickened endometrium (Fig. 12), polypoid lesion and frank myometrial invasion. Disruption of subendometrial halo is suggestive of myometrial invasion. Sonohysterography may be performed in cases where endometrial evaluation is not sufficient on TVS. Here uterus is distended with sterile saline and adequate sonographic evaluation of endometrium may be done.

CT is generally not used for initial diagnosis or local staging as CT lacks contrast between tumour and myometrium (Fig. 13). CT is useful in detecting nodal status and distant metastases. It is difficult to differentiate tumour from normal uterus on non-contrast CT. Post-contrast CT may show diffuse thickening or mass within the endometrial cavity and these lesions may be hypoenhancing (Fig. 14). In cases of endometrial cancers, TVS has an overall accuracy of 60–76% in assessing the degree of myometrial invasion [13]. It can also evaluate the involvement of cervix by endometrial mass.

MRI pelvis is recommended for assessment of extension of the disease and is superior to CT. Contrast enhanced MRI shows better accuracy in detecting myometrial invasion (Fig. 15). In T1 MRI, the lesion appears hypo to isointense to normal endometrium. T1 contrast MRI will demonstrate less enhancement of tumour tissue than normal endometrium. DCE-MRI sequences are useful in assessment of depth of myometrial invasion. Delayed phase images show cervical stromal invasion. T2WI demonstrate iso to hypointense mass lesion relative to normal endo-

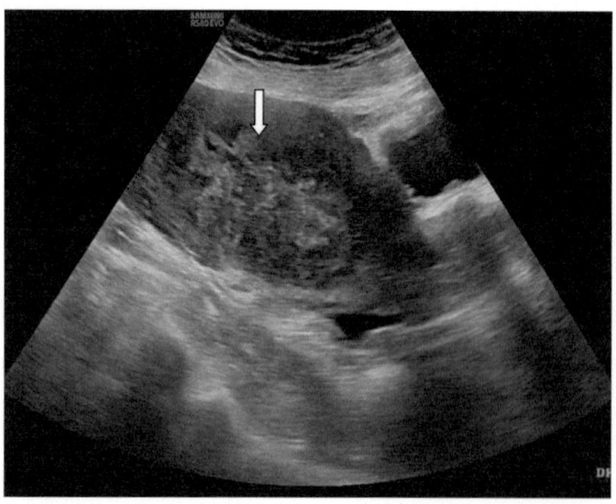

Fig. 12 Endometrial cancer. Ultrasonography of pelvis showing a soft tissue mass of heterogenous echotexture replacing the normal endometrium with evidence of myometrial infiltration (arrow)

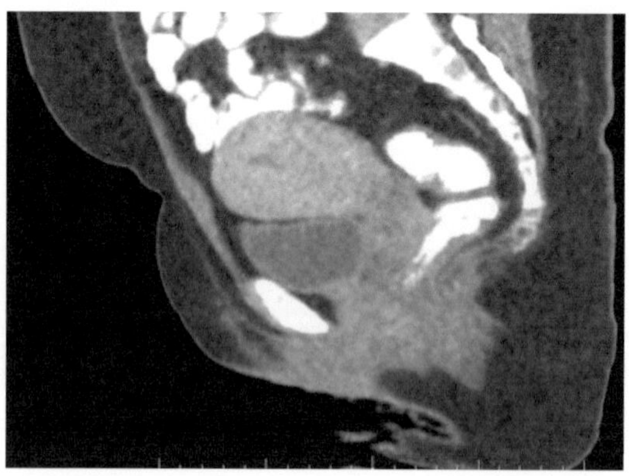

Fig. 13 CECT scan (sagittal section) of the same patient of Fig. 12. The mass cannot be clearly delineated. CT lacks contrast between tumour and myometrium

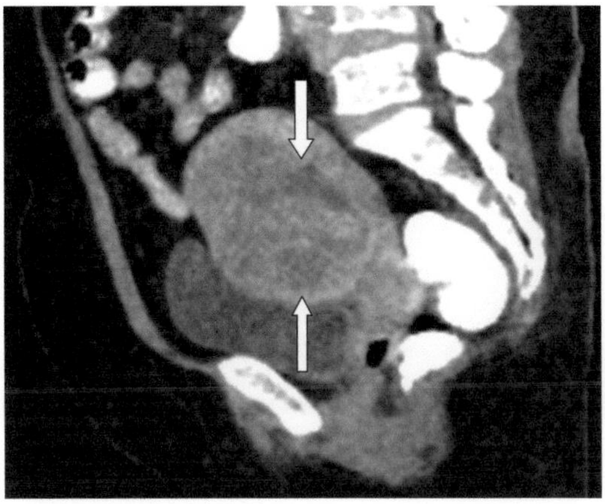

Fig. 14 Endometrial cancer. CECT scan (sagittal section) of pelvis showing a bulky hypodense mass involving the endometrium with myometrial infiltration (arrows)

metrium, often heterogenous, DWI shows restricted diffusion.

Endometrial cancer mainly affects the postmenopausal age group where the zonal anatomy of the uterus disappears and the junctional zone increases in signal intensity. In these cases, outlining the depth of myometrial invasion by tumour is difficult to assess on T2W imaging. Therefore, MR contrast agent is often used to highlight a poorly vascular tumour against a much more avidly enhancing myometrium (Fig. 16). DCE-MRI is useful in the evaluation of myometrial extension.

However, diffusion weighted imaging (DWI) has also been shown to accurately delineate the depth of myometrial invasion (Fig. 17),

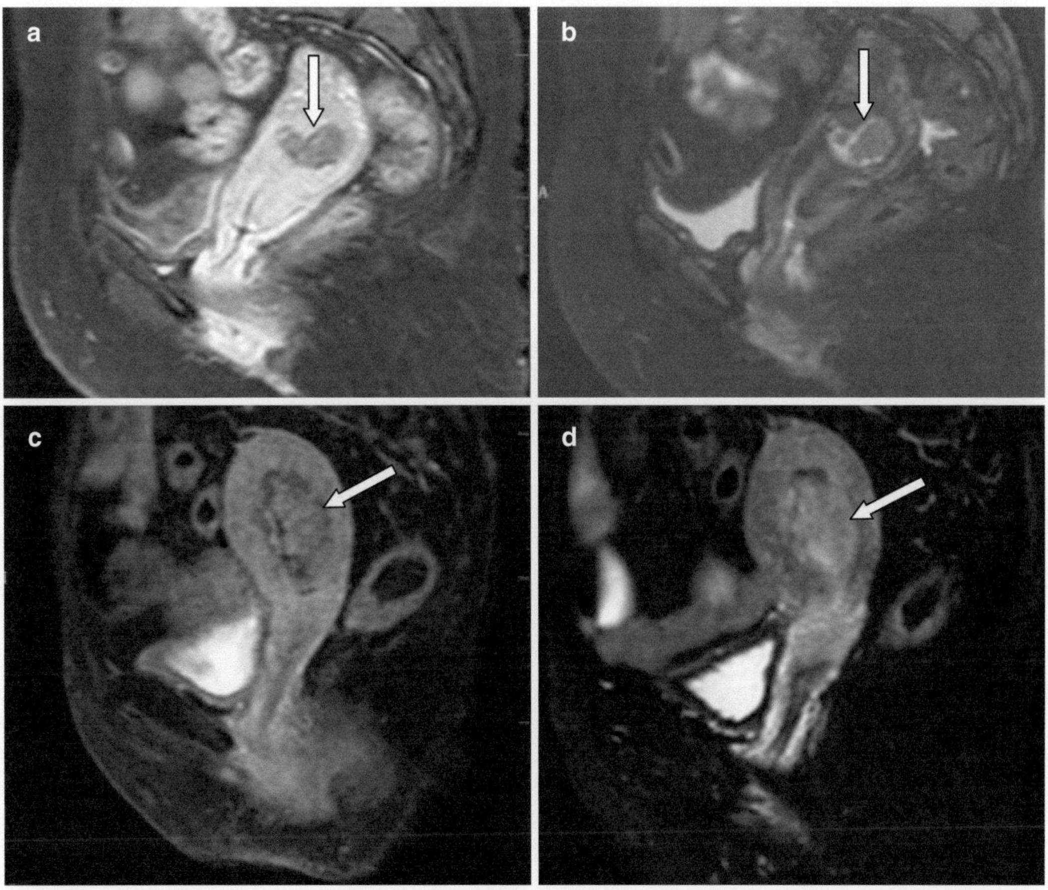

Fig. 15 Endometrial cancer infiltrating myometrium in two different cases. (**a**, **b**) T1 contrast and T2 sagittal MRI showing polypoidal endometrial cancer infiltrating myometrium (arrows). (**c**, **d**) Another patient. Sagittal T1 contrast & T2 MRI showing endometrial mass with infiltration of inner myometrium (arrows)

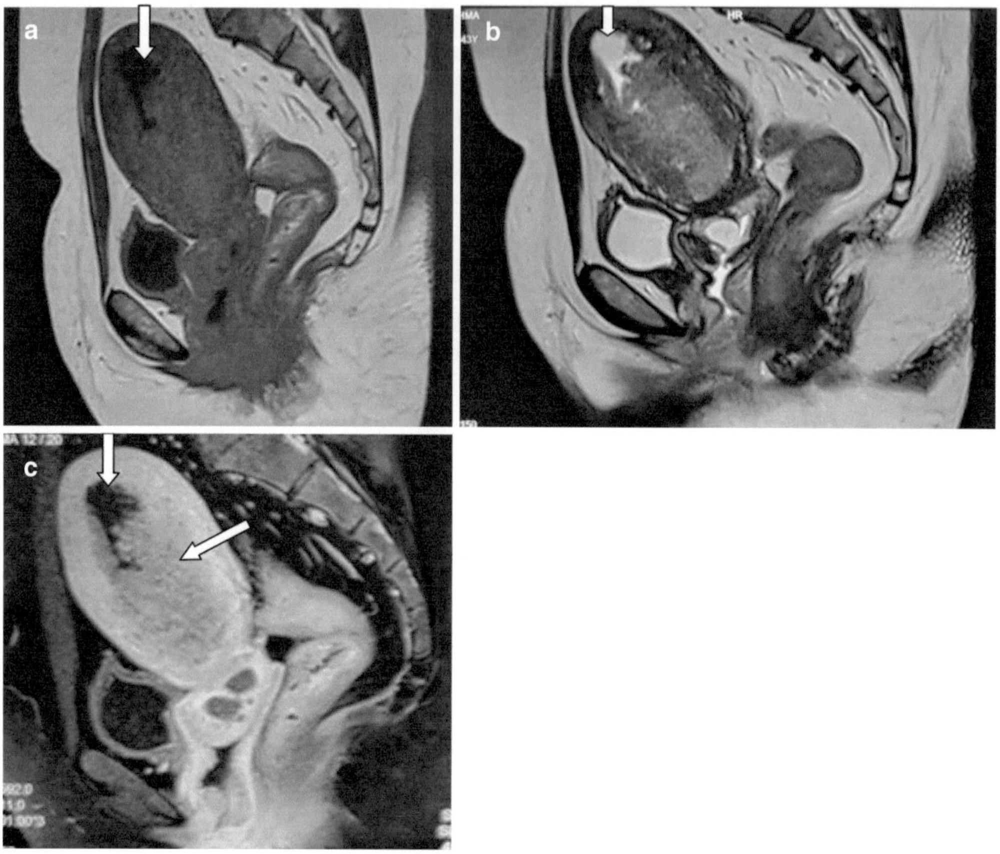

Fig. 16 Endometrial cancer. (**a–c**) Sagittal T1, T2 and T1 contrast MR images of the pelvis showing an enhancing endometrial mass with loss of junctional zone (oblique arrow) and myometrial invasion. There is endocavity fluid collection in the fundal region (vertical arrows)

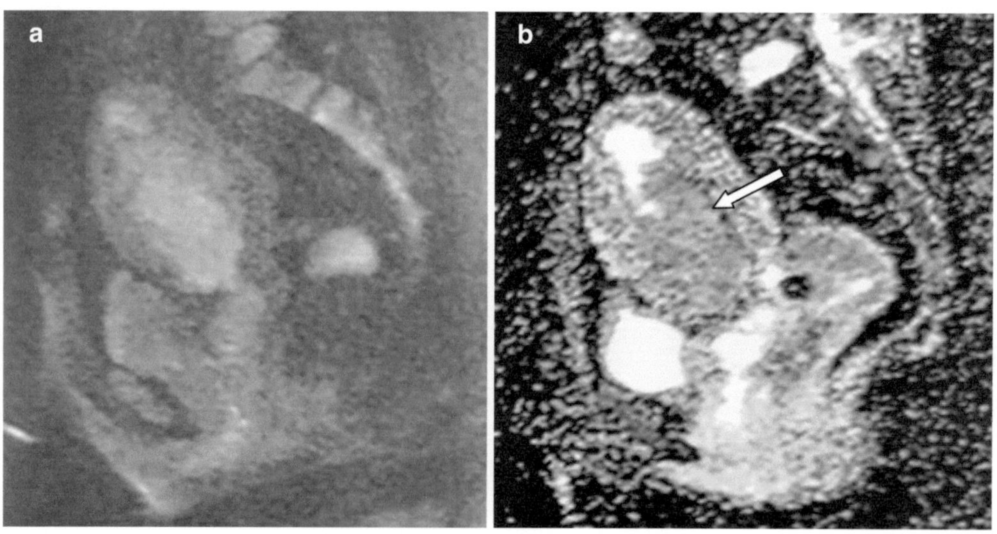

Fig. 17 Endometrial cancer. (**a**, **b**) Diffusion weighted sagittal MRI with ADC mapping of an endometrial mass showing restricted diffusion (arrow)

without the need for intravenous gadolinium [14].

On T2WI, if the junctional zone is intact, deep myometrial invasion is excluded.

PET-CT is useful in identifying nodal metastases. In endometrial cancer the greatest role of PET-CT is for detection of extrauterine disease. It has an established role in detection of recurrent disease. It is recommended in patients considered for exenterative surgery to exclude unsuspected distant metastases.

7 Ovarian Cancer

Ovarian neoplasms are relatively common and account for 6% of female malignancies [15].

Ovarian cancer is usually diagnosed late because of lack of symptoms. By the time women present with abdominal distension and discomfort, there may be widespread peritoneal dissemination with ascites.

US is useful in the detection and characterisation of adnexal lesions but not useful in staging. However, US guided biopsy of adnexal or peritoneal masses are required in patients who are not suitable for primary surgery.

International ovarian tumour analysis (IOTA) simple rules, for ovarian mass states that if an ovarian lesion has at least one of these features and no benign features it can be confidently considered malignant. These features include irregular solid tumour, irregular multilocular-solid mass >10 cm in diameter, ≥4 papillary structures, ascites marked vascularity within the mass on Colour Doppler [16].

Ovarian cancer is recognized by complex solid cystic masses (partly solid, partly cystic) within one or both ovaries. The solid components may be seen in the form of nodules, septations or papilliform fronds and when detected in these patterns are characteristic of epithelial ovarian cancer (Fig. 18).

MRI is a problem-solving modality in evaluating indeterminate adnexal masses on US. There is evidence that DW-MRI and DCE-MRI can help in characterisation of ovarian masses, distinguishing benign from malignant and in detection of peritoneal deposits.

MRI is useful when fertility preserving surgery is being considered specifically to diagnose other non-malignant lesions. MRI features most predictive of malignancy correlate with US findings which include irregular solid mass, an enhancing solid component or papillary projections within a cystic lesion, irregular/thickened septa >3 mm, ascites and peritoneal deposits. DWI combined with T2WI can be useful in detecting peritoneal metastases and helps predict the likelihood of optimal debulking at surgery.

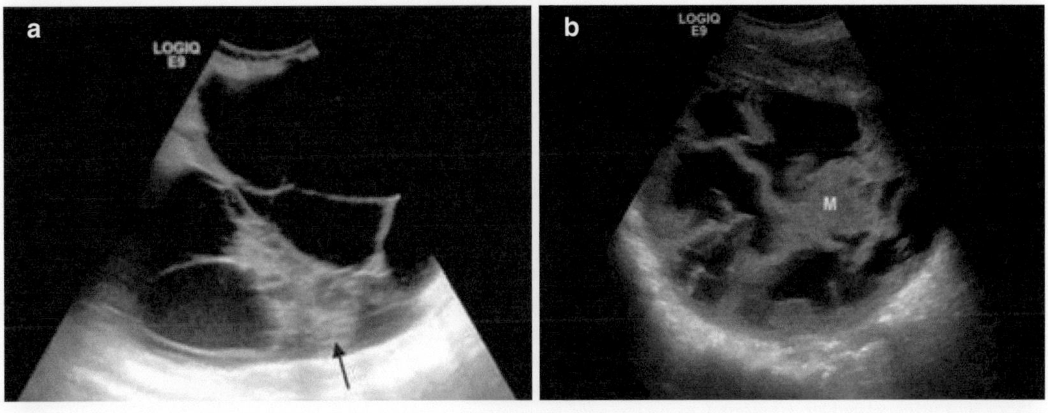

Fig. 18 Ovarian cancer. (**a**, **b**) Ultrasonography of pelvis showing a complex cystic adnexal mass with thick internal septations and irregular solid components (black arrow)

CT is currently the modality of choice in staging ovarian cancer. It may be used to guide biopsy of peritoneal, nodal or adnexal disease. CT helps in evaluating primary tumour (Figs. 19 and 20), peritoneal deposits and in detection of enlarged lymph nodes and ascites. This information classifies those patients with non-resectable disease from those patients who should undergo primary cytoreductive surgery.

CT is also useful to identify associated complications such as hydronephrosis and bowel obstruction. The extent of peritoneal disease is best evaluated on CT as it can scan the abdomen from the dome of the diaphragms to the pelvic floor within a few seconds.

Peritoneal deposits can be seen as discrete enhancing soft tissue nodules specially in the background of ascites.

Liver, lung and renal metastases and malignant pleural effusion (Fig. 21) are seen in advanced disease.

MRI is a problem-solving modality in evaluating indeterminate adnexal masses on US or CT because of its excellent soft tissue resolution (Fig. 22). There is evidence that DW MRI and DCE MRI can help in characterisation of ovarian masses, distinguishing benign from malignant and in detection of peritoneal deposits.

PET-CT has an important role in the ovarian cancer patients who are considered for salvage therapy due to relapse (either with documented or

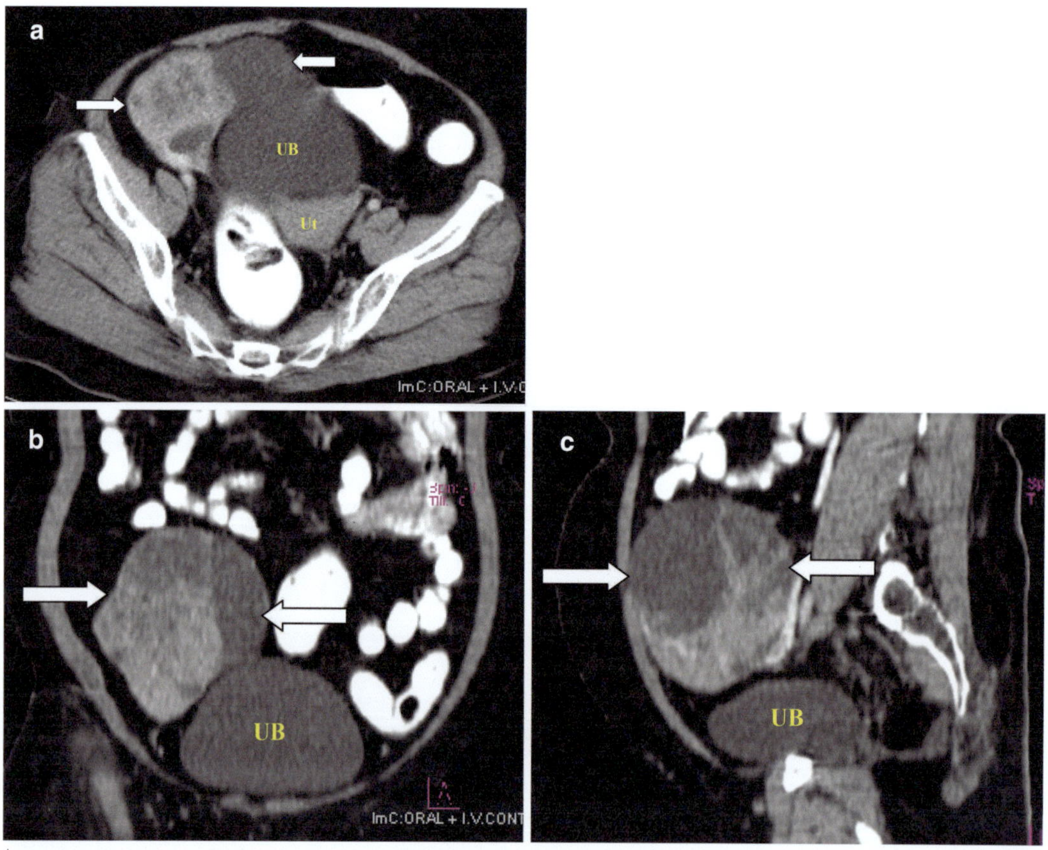

Fig. 19 Ovarian cancer. (**a–c**) CECT axial, coronal and sagittal images showing a solid cystic mass (arrows) in right adnexa (*UB* urinary bladder, *Ut* uterus)

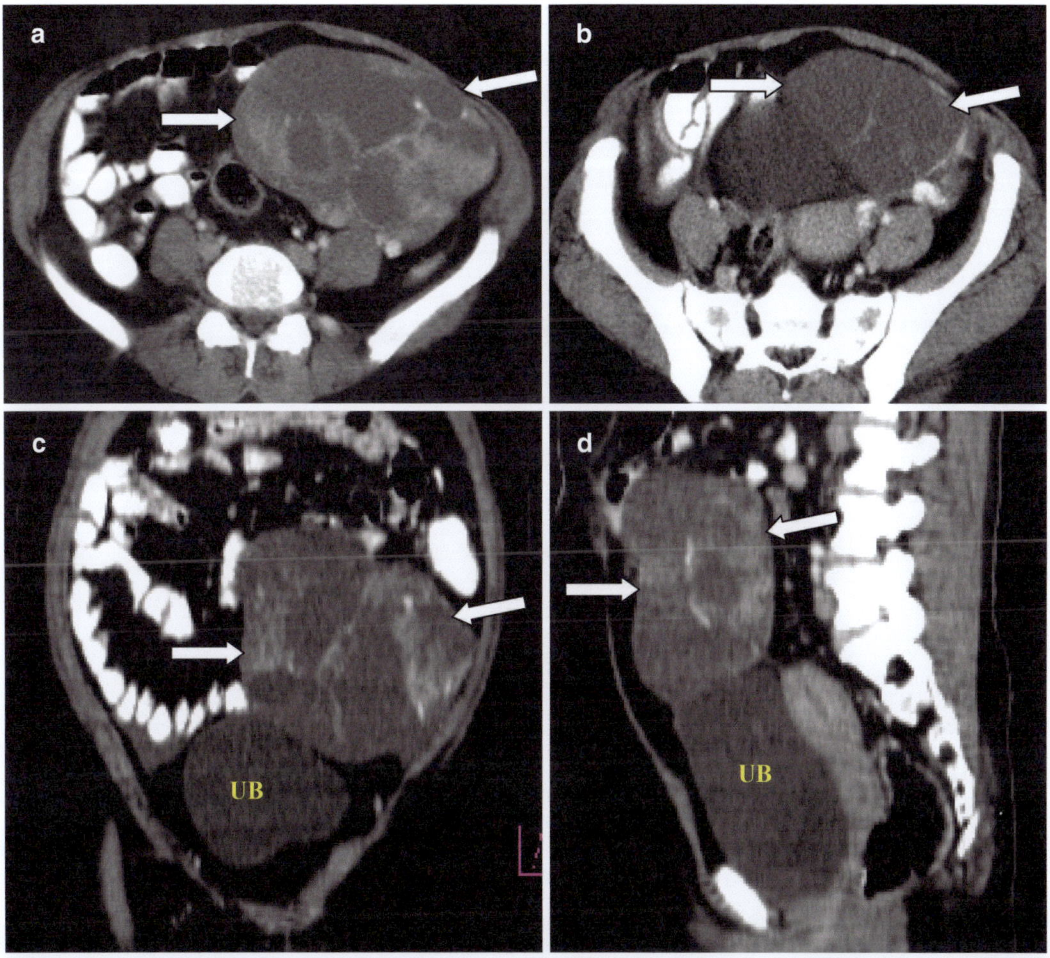

Fig. 20 Ovarian cancer. Axial (**a**, **b**), coronal (**c**) and sagittal (**d**) CECT showing a complex cystic mass in left adnexa (arrows) with multiple enhancing internal septations and solid components (*UB* urinary bladder)

suspected relapse with increased level of CA125). Though PET-CT is superior to CT alone in characterization of adnexal masses but inferior to combination of US and MRI [3]. For response evaluation of patients undergoing neoadjuvant chemotherapy, it shows promising role.

Diagnosis of a primary ovarian malignant tumour is generally made with open or laparoscopic surgery as there is potential risk of peritoneal seeding with image-guided biopsy. However, patients having advanced disease or poor clinical condition may not be able to undergo radical cytoreductive surgery, and in these cases image-guided biopsy (Fig. 23) is performed for a histologic diagnosis prior to chemotherapy.

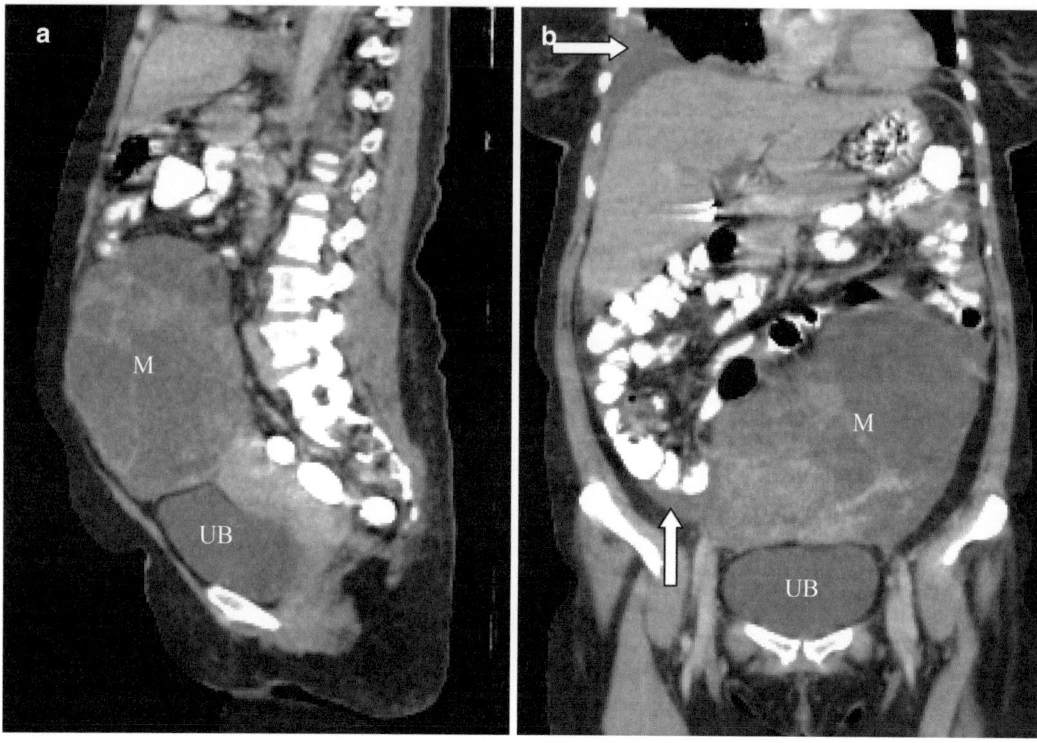

Fig. 21 Ovarian cancer. CECT in sagittal (**a**) and coronal (**b**) sections showing complex cystic left adnexal mass (M) with mild right pleural effusion (horizontal arrow) and minimal pelvic ascites (vertical arrow) (*UB* urinary bladder)

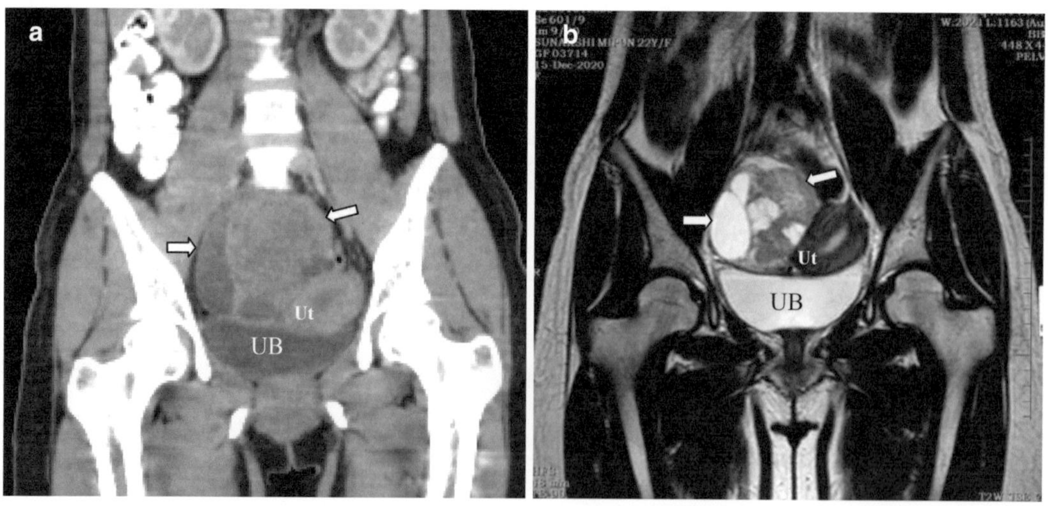

Fig. 22 Ovarian cancer. (**a**, **b**) Coronal CT scan and T2W MR images showing a solid cystic right adnexal mass (arrows) compressing and displacing the uterus towards left. The details of the pelvic organs and the right adnexal mass are more clearly visualized on MRI (*Ut* uterus, *UB* urinary bladder)

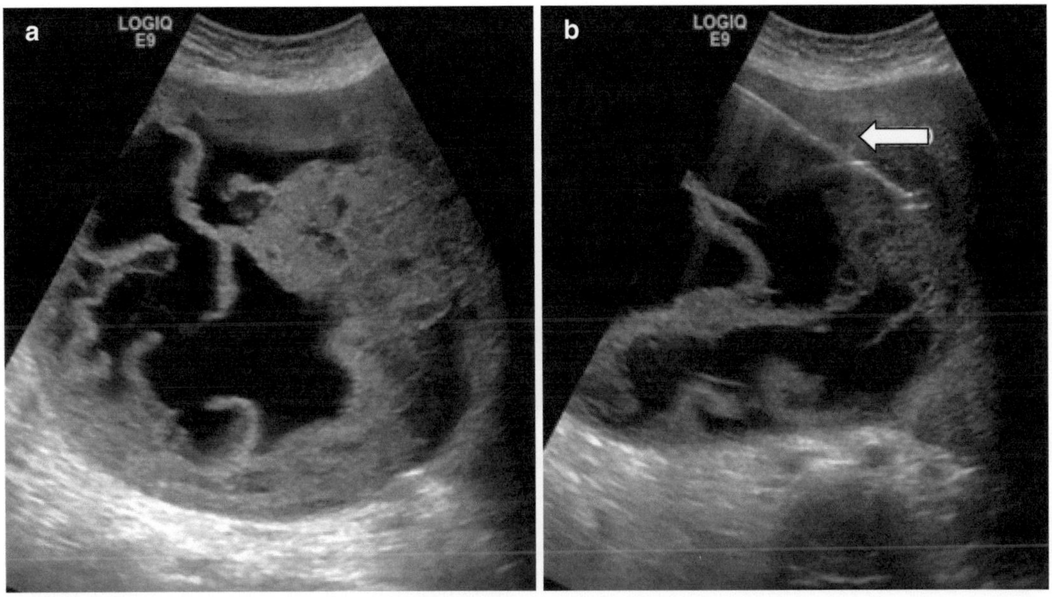

Fig. 23 Ovarian cancer. (**a**) Ultrasound showing a solid cystic adnexal mass with irregular, thick internal septations and solid components. (**b**) US guided biopsy was performed. Biopsy needle is seen as bright line (thick white arrow) with its tip inside the solid component of the mass

8 Vaginal Cancer

Primary vaginal carcinoma is a rare cancer. A primary vaginal carcinoma is defined as a neoplasm that arises solely from the vagina without involvement of the external os superiorly or the vulva inferiorly [17]. MRI is superior to CT for evaluation of primary tumour. For lymph node evaluation both CT and MRI may be used.

9 Vulval Malignancies

Vulval cancer accounts for 3–5% of female genital tract malignancies [18]. It tends to affect women less than 50 years or older than 70 years. Squamous cell vulval carcinoma is associated with human papilloma virus infection.

The size and depth of the tumour, involvement of inguinal lymph nodes and distal spread are prognostic factors and are incorporated into the FIGO staging.

Local staging is performed by MRI, due to its excellent soft tissue resolution. On T2 MRI, the tumour shows intermediate signal intensity and demonstrates restricted diffusion on DWI Variable enhancement is seen with gadolinium contrast medium.

CT is useful for assessment of nodal disease and distant metastases. CT has limitations for local staging. Sometimes contrast enhanced CT may detect primary disease (Fig. 24). PET/CT is helpful in assessing equivocal lymph node involvement. MRI and US can be used in recurrent disease.

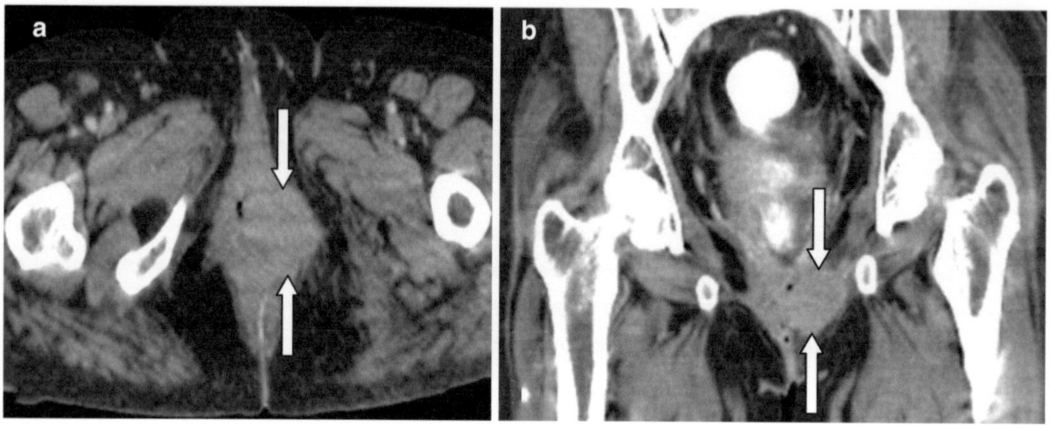

Fig. 24 Vulval cancer. CECT scan in axial (**a**) and coronal (**b**) sections showing a vulval mass (arrows) on the left side with compression and displacement of the urethra towards right

10 Leiomyosarcoma

Leiomyosarcoma is a rare tumour arising from uterine smooth muscle. On MRI it appears as a soft tissue mass with irregular margin, peripheral enhancement and shows rapid growth on interval imaging. MRI cannot reliably differentiate leiomyomas from leiomyosarcomas, as both are intermediate signal intensity on T2WI and both show restricted diffusion on DWI. Leiomyosarcomas may present with lymphadenopathy and bone metastases.

11 Gestational Trophoblastic Neoplasia (GTN)

GTN refers to gestational trophoblastic disease (GTD) that is almost always malignant and includes invasive mole, choriocarcinoma, placental site trophoblastic tumour and epithelioid trophoblastic tumour.

On ultrasonography invasive GTD are seen as echogenic, hypoechoic, complex, or multicystic focal masses within the myometrium with a variable endometrial component. Anechoic spaces may be seen and these represent haemorrhage, necrosis, cysts or vascular spaces. In extensive disease there may be invasion through the myometrium and beyond the uterus into the parametrium, vagina and other pelvic organs.

On colour Doppler US, there is usually high vascularity within the mass due to intralesional arteriovenous shunts. On spectral Doppler US, trophoblastic vessels demonstrate a high-velocity low resistance waveform.

CT is generally used for detection of metastatic disease. Uterine disease is seen as an enlarged uterus with focal irregular lesions with low attenuation, and these lesions may be associated with bilateral ovarian enlargement with multiple theca lutein cysts. CT can also identify vascular malformations resulting from GTN.

MRI is a problem-solving tool to assess the depth of myometrial invasion and extrauterine disease spread. On MRI there is uterine enlargement with distension of the endometrial cavity indistinct endomyometrial junction with obliteration of the normal zonal anatomy. On T1WI, haemorrhage is seen as focal signal hyperintensity. MRI is useful for identification of parametrial invasion.

Approximately 30% of patients with GTN have metastases at the time of diagnosis, most commonly to the lungs (80% of cases), vagina , liver and brain [19]. Other sites include the skin, gastrointestinal tract, kidney, breast and bones. Therefore, imaging of the lungs is recommended for all patients with GTN. CT scan is more sensitive than chest radiograph for diagnosing lung metastases.

Patients with known lung or vaginal metastases are at significant risk of central nervous system involvement and should be screened with MRI or CT to exclude brain metastases.

12 Imaging Nodal Disease (N-Staging)

In cervical cancer, lymph node status is the most important prognostic factor. The 5-year survival rate without nodal metastases is estimated at 85%, this reduces to 71% with the presence of pelvic lymph nodes [20]. Cervical cancer spreads to paracervical and parametrial nodes. Obturator nodes are common sites of metastases. It can also spread to iliac chains, para-aortic and retroperitoneal nodes.

Lymphadenectomy is part of the surgicopathological staging of endometrial cancer. In low FIGO stage disease (<IB) lymphadenectomy may not be performed. So preoperative imaging is essential in optimal surgical planning. Pelvic nodes >8 mm in short axis are generally considered enlarged and likely to be metastatic. The middle and lower uterus drain to regional lymph nodes in the paracervical, parametrium and obturator nodes, while the upper uterus drains to para-aortic and common iliac chains. The presence of enlarged para-aortic lymph nodes indicates poor prognosis.

Lymph node metastases from the ovaries occur to obturator, internal and external iliac inguinal and para-aortic lymph nodes.

PET-CT is the most sensitive investigation for detection of metastatic nodes. The high sensitivity, specificity and accuracy of PET-CT in detection of lymph node metastases is due to increased FDG uptake by the lymph node independent of the size.

If PET-CT is not available, then CT or MRI is a second line alternative. Morphological features which suggest involved lymph nodes include round shape, irregular outline and size greater than 10 mm. Metastatic lymph nodes show restricted diffusion on DW MRI.

13 Imaging Metastatic Spread (M-Staging)

The lungs are the commonest site of metastases in endometrial cancer. Sometimes peritoneal deposits are also seen.

Similarly, in cervical cancer distant spread to the lungs (Fig. 5c), liver and bones can occur but is uncommon at presentation.

Due to the non-specific nature of associated symptoms, majority of patients with ovarian cancer often present with advanced disease. Regional lymph node metastases and peritoneal metastases outside the pelvis including subcapsular liver deposits and are common at presentation. When metastatic deposits are identified beyond the peritoneal cavity or within liver parenchyma advanced disease is recognized.

Surgical staging is considered to be the gold-standard. A staging CT is commonly used in cases where treatment is with primary chemotherapy followed by interval debulking surgery and has a quoted accuracy of 70–90% [20].

CT detects peritoneal disease, ascites, nodal, visceral and bone lesions which helps in surgical planning. Detection of peritoneal deposits depends on factors including size (over one cm), presence of ascites. CT can easily detect calcified metastases.

Image-guided biopsy may be necessary if likelihood of suboptimal surgical debulking is high and primary chemotherapy is given.

Additional roles of CT are in diagnosing primary peritoneal carcinoma which may be indistinguishable from ovarian cancer pathologically as well as in identifying ovarian metastases [20].

Newer imaging techniques such as DWI are now being increasingly used in whole body protocols for identifying metastases. DWI has proved to be useful in detection of small peritoneal, serosal, subdiaphragmatic and subcapsular liver deposits which are seen as bright signal intensity areas.

For recurrence of gynaecological malignancies, morphological methods such as CT scan and MRI are still the norm, but functional imaging techniques like PET-CT, DCE-MRI and DW-MRI are increasing used.

14 Image-Guided Biopsy

Very often a definite diagnosis of a pelvic mass is not possible with non-invasive imaging alone. Image-guided biopsy may be necessary for undiagnosed pelvic tumours or enlarged pelvic lymph nodes. There is potential risk of peritoneal seeding in image-guided biopsy and that is why diagnosis of primary malignant ovarian tumour is made with surgery. However, in some situations image-guided biopsy is required. Some patients may not be able to undergo radical surgery because of advanced disease or poor clinical status and image-guided biopsy is used in these cases for definitive diagnosis prior to chemotherapy. Biopsy is necessary for suspicious recurrent tumour (Fig. 25) and newly appearing nodal mass (Fig. 26) in follow-up cases prior to chemotherapy. Image-guided biopsy is also used in patients with history of primary cancer elsewhere and known to metastasize to ovaries and present as ovarian masses mimicking primary ovarian cancers.

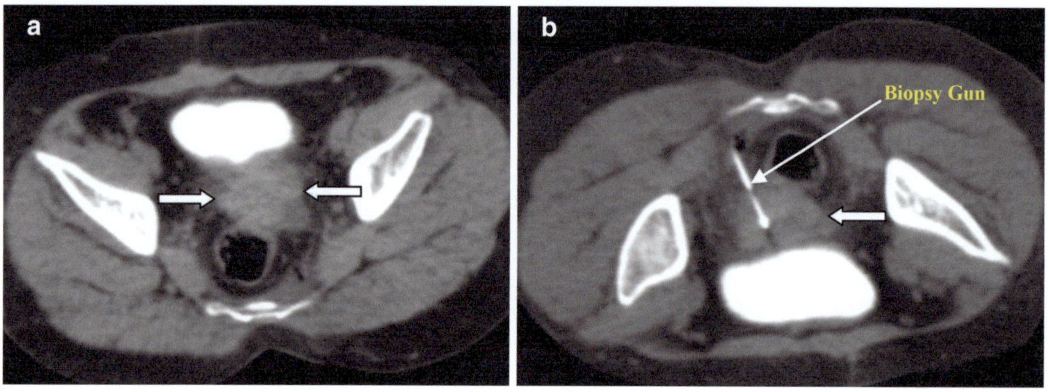

Fig. 25 Post-operative (total hysterectomy and bilateral salpingo-oophorectomy) case of cervical cancer on follow-up. (**a**) Follow-up CT showing pelvic mass (thick horizontal arrows) posterior to the bladder and anterior to rectum (suspicious recurrent tumour). (**b**) Percutaneous transgluteal CT guided core biopsy was done from the mass in prone position from posterior aspect. Biopsy gun (thin long arrow) is clearly seen with its cutting portion inside the mass. Biopsy confirmed recurrent tumour

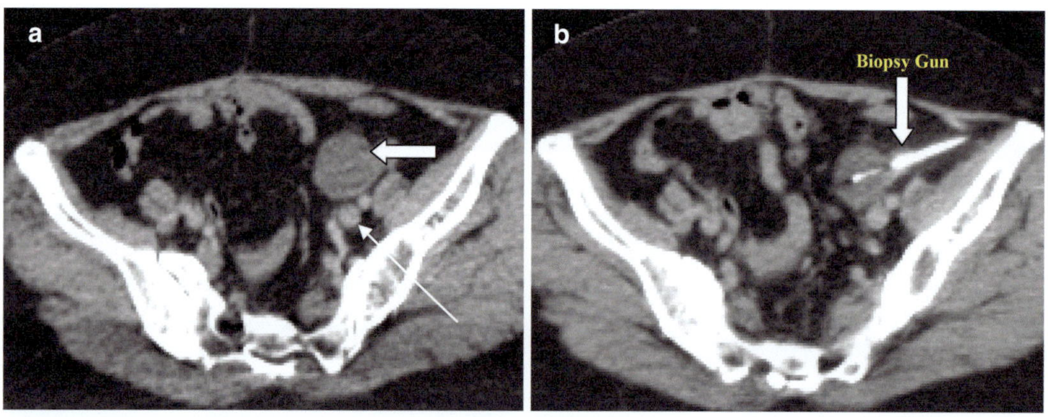

Fig. 26 Post-operative case of ovarian cancer on follow-up. (**a**) Follow-up CT showing an enlarged left iliac node (thick white arrow) abutting left iliac vessels (thin long arrow). (**b**) CT guided core biopsy was done from the nodal mass from left lateral aspect avoiding bowels and iliac vessels. Biopsy gun (thick white vertical arrow) is clearly seen with its cutting portion inside the nodal mass. Histopathology confirmed nodal metastasis

15 Conclusions

Common gynaecological malignancies include cervix, endometrium, vagina, vulva and adnexal masses. Imaging plays an essential role in management of malignant gynaecological diseases. Multiple modalities are utilized to investigate suspected gynaecological malignancy and these include ultrasound, CT, MRI and PET-CT. Each imaging modality has a different role in diagnosis, staging, management and follow-up. Ultrasound is the initial modality commonly used for endometrium and ovary. MRI is the cornerstone investigation for staging common gynaecological malignancies except ovary where contrast enhanced CT is the primary imaging modality. PET-CT is the most sensitive imaging modality for nodal involvement and distant metastases.

References

1. Laifer-Narin SL, Genestine WF, Okechukwu NC, Hecht EM, Newhouse JH. The role of computed tomography and magnetic resonance imaging in gynecologic oncology. PET Clin. 2018;13(2):127–41.
2. Sala E, Rockall A, Rangarajan D, Kubik-Huch RA. The role of dynamic contrast-enhanced and diffusion weighted magnetic resonance imaging in the female pelvis. Eur J Radiol. 2010;76(3):367–85.
3. Narayanan P, Sahdev A. The role of 18F-FDG PET CT in common gynaecological malignancies. Br J Radiol. 2017;90(1079):20170283.
4. Lakhani A, Khan SR, Bharwani N, Stewart V, Rockall AG, Khan S, Barwick TD. FDG PET/CT pitfalls in gynecologic and genitourinary oncologic imaging. Radiographics. 2017;37(2):577–94.
5. Bobdey S, Sathwara J, Jain A, Balasubramaniam G. Burden of cervical cancer and role of screening in India. Indian J Med Paediatr Oncol. 2016;37(04):278–85.
6. Weerakkody Y, Baba Y. Carcinoma of the cervix. 2021. https://radiopaedia.org/articles/carcinoma-of-the-cervix.
7. Prasad TV, Thulkar S, Hari S, Sharma DN, Kumar S. Role of computed tomography (CT) scan in staging of cervical carcinoma. Indian J Med Res. 2014;139(5):714.
8. Shaaban AM, Blodgett TM, Rezvani M, Heilbrun M, Salam ME, Roberts CC. Diagnostic imaging: oncology. Amirsys; 2011.
9. Silverman PM. Oncologic imaging: a multidisciplinary approach E-book: expert consult-online and print. Elsevier Health Sciences; 2012.
10. Creasman WT. Endometrial carcinoma guidelines. 2021. https://emedicine.medscape.com/article/254083-guidelines.
11. Balasubramaniam G, Sushama S, Rasika B, Mahantshetty U. Hospital-based study of endometrial cancer survival in Mumbai, India. Asian Pac J Cancer Prev. 2013;14(2):977–80.
12. Weerakkody Y, Vadera S. Endometrial carcinoma. 2021. https://radiopaedia.org/articles/endometrial-carcinoma.
13. Otero-García MM, Mesa-Álvarez A, Nikolic O, Blanco-Lobato P, Basta-Nikolic M, de Llano-Ortega RM, Paredes-Velázquez L, Nikolic N, Szewczyk-Bieda M. Role of MRI in staging and follow-up of endometrial and cervical cancer: pitfalls and mimickers. Insights Imaging. 2019;10(1):1–22.
14. Das SK, Niu XK, Wang JL, Zeng LC, Wang WX, Bhetuwal A, Yang HF. Usefulness of DWI in preoperative assessment of deep myometrial invasion in patients with endometrial carcinoma: a systematic review and meta-analysis. Cancer Imaging. 2014;14(1):1–1.
15. Gaillard F, Hacking C. Ovarian tumors. 2021. https://radiopaedia.org/articles/ovarian-tumours.
16. Knipe H, Vadera S. IOTA ultrasound rules for ovarian masses. radiopaedia.org. 2021. https://radiopaedia.org/articles/iota-ultrasound-rules-for-ovarian-masses.
17. Weerakkody Y, Saber M. Primary vaginal carcinoma. 2020. https://radiopaedia.org/articles/primary-vaginal-carcinoma.
18. Weerakkody Y, Bell D. Primary vulval cancer. 2018. https://radiopaedia.org/articles/primary-vulval-cancer.
19. Shaaban AM, Rezvani M, Haroun RR, Kennedy AM, Elsayes KM, Olpin JD, Salama ME, Foster BR, Menias CO. Gestational trophoblastic disease: clinical and imaging features. Radiographics. 2017;37(2):681–700.
20. Hameeduddin A, de Souza NM. Imaging of gynecological cancers. In: Pelvic cancer surgery. London: Springer; 2015. p. 235–54.

Principles and Practice of Surgery in Gynaecological Cancer

Gaurav Das, Shailesh V. Shrikhande, Vikram Chaudhari, and Amal Chandra Kataki

1 Introduction

Surgical oncology pertains to the application of oncological principles to surgically treat patients with cancer. A surgical oncologist is often the first specialist a patient with a possible diagnosis of cancer encounters and is responsible for a comprehensive clinical assessment. In that context, the clinical methods of a surgical oncologist assume paramount importance and a lot depends on the level of knowledge of the specialist regarding all existing therapies, whether surgical or non-surgical and standard or experimental. The term surgical oncology includes in its domain, by a broad definition, all the disciplines of surgery which are concerned with the treatment of cancer. This inclusive nature of the subject is owing to the fact that there are relatable surgical principles, regarded as oncologically sound, which are applicable to cancers arising from various organ systems of the body.

The importance of a cancer specialist with a working knowledge of all kinds of malignancies, together with a basic understanding of the surgical anatomy of the whole body cannot be undermined. A few examples can illustrate this subject matter. A patient with an undisclosed breast cancer or a patient with an unsuspected prostate cancer may often approach a clinician for back pain related to skeletal metastases. A patient with a testicular cancer may present to the doctor with only a neck or an abdominal swelling! A lady presenting with malignant ascites may have a multitude of possibilities as far as the organ of origin is concerned. A patient with a hypopharyngeal cancer may very well have a second primary in the esophagus! In an age when advanced imaging like whole body positron emission tomography (PET) scans are increasingly employed, detection of multiple sites of primary cancers in unrelated organ systems pose a problem to the clinician if the domain of understanding is restricted. The available literature is replete with such examples. A surgical oncologist has a detailed understanding of the core characteristics of cancer including its biology and natural history, the role of not only surgery, but also multidisciplinary treatment, including systemic therapies, radiation and palliative care.

G. Das (✉)
Department of Surgical Oncology, Dr. Bhubaneswar Borooah Cancer Institute (A Unit of Tata Memorial Centre, Mumbai), Guwahati, Assam, India

S. V. Shrikhande
GI and HPB Surgical Service, Tata Memorial Hospital, Mumbai, India

V. Chaudhari
GI and HPB, Department of Surgical Oncology, Advanced Centre for Treatment Research and Education in Cancer, Mumbai, India

A. C. Kataki
Department of Gynaecologic Oncology, Dr. Bhubaneswar Borooah Cancer Institute (A Unit of Tata Memorial Centre, Mumbai), Guwahati, Assam, India

A. C. Kataki, D. Barmon (eds.), *Fundamentals in Gynaecologic Malignancy*,
https://doi.org/10.1007/978-981-19-5860-1_6

On the other hand, it is only prudent that there have been organ-based divisions in the field of surgical oncology in the pursuit of surgical excellence. Such divisions that are prevalent include head and neck oncology, gynaecologic oncology, thoracic oncology, gastrointestinal oncology, musculoskeletal oncology, urological oncology, and neurosurgical oncology among others. There are also dedicated units super-specialized for the surgical treatment of cancers of only a limited surgical domain, like breast or colorectum or esophagus or stomach only.

The facts that stand out are that cancer incidence is increasing worldwide and the current goal is to achieve better patient outcomes in dedicated cancer care centers and surgeons specially trained in surgical management of cancer have a pivotal role to play in the multi-disciplinary scheme of things. A modern surgical oncologist should not only be adept in obtaining cancer-free surgical resection margins and adequate lymphadenectomy, where appropriate, but also apply concepts of integration of systemic treatment and radiation therapy in the pre- or post-surgery treatment plan.

2 History

We have come a long way since the period of 400 BC when Hippocrates propagated a negative view on the surgical treatment of cancer and stated that surgery would worsen survival. This was notwithstanding the fact that surgery was the oldest oncological discipline and surgical procedures for cancer were performed dating back to thousands of years [1]. However, the so-called foundation of the modern surgical oncology practice was developed over a period of about 100 years (1840–1940) and this is often referred to as the "century of the surgeon" [2]. The discovery of general anesthesia (1840s), antiseptic surgery (1860s) and progress in tissue microscopy with the publication of microscopic atlas of pathology and development of paraffin embedding technique (1840s) were positive strides that enabled the progress in the surgical field [3–5]. Several gifted surgeons have performed landmark complex oncological procedures in due course of time [6], a few of which have been listed in Table 1.

Table 1 A few important events in the history of surgical oncology

Timeline	Landmark
1600 BC	Egyptians used cautery to destroy breast cancer
First Century AD	Leonidas of Alexandria removed breast cancer with margins
1760s	John Hunter describes principles of surgical oncology including lymphatic spread
1809	E. MacDowell removed a large ovarian tumour
1846	JC Warren excised a vascular tumour from the neck: the first surgical procedure under modern anesthesia
1873	Theodore Billroth performed the first total laryngectomy for laryngeal cancer
1881	Theodore Billroth performed the first partial gastrectomy for cancer
1891	William Halsted did the first radical mastectomy for breast cancer
1906	Ernest Miles did the first abdominoperineal resection for rectal cancer
1927	First pulmonary metastasectomy by George Divis
1935	First pancreaticoduodenectomy for pancreatic cancer by A.O. Whipple
1960s	Walter Lawrence establishes a division of surgical oncology at the Medical College of Virginia
1975	The Society of Surgical Oncology (SSO) is established
1978	The term "surgical oncologist" is defined by SSO and NCI and SSO formulates guidelines for post-residency surgical oncology training

3 Roles of a Surgical Oncologist

The point where a surgeon transforms into a surgical oncologist is when he understands the biology and the natural history of cancer as well as the importance of other disciplines in the management plan, as part of a multi-disciplinary tumour board. The use of neoadjuvant or adjuvant treatment, before and after surgery respectively, requires collaboration with medical and radiation oncologists. Such neoadjuvant treatment may convert surgically inoperable tumours into operable ones. In other situations, intraoperative delivery of chemotherapy (as in hyperthermic intraperitoneal chemotherapy or HIPEC for peritoneal carcinomatosis and isolated limb perfusion for malignant melanoma) and intraoperative delivery of radiation (intraoperative radiation therapy or IORT) are practiced and need expertise and collaboration of the aforementioned specialists. A close collaboration with the radiology team is essential for a surgical oncologist to plan his surgeries and optimize resection margins. The pathology team is highly important for him in so much as to understand the disease subtype and biology and plan primary and adjuvant treatment as well as determine the adequacy and quality of surgery. The geneticist and team of genetic counselors aid the surgical oncologist with treatment, prevention and screening strategies of cancers with genetic origin, which do form a significant proportion of case load and such people require dedicated care. As part of the larger team of the surgical oncologist, the undeniable roles of the oncologic nursing team including stoma care nursing, the speech and swallowing therapist, the physiotherapist, the pain specialist and the palliative care team, among others, deserve special mention. The various roles of a surgical oncologist are discussed in the sections below.

4 Diagnosis and Staging

A surgical oncologist is primarily responsible for obtaining the final diagnosis and staging of solid cancers and aiding in the diagnosis of hematological cancers, where appropriate. Apart from his clinical methods, he has to choose the appropriate radiological investigations and provide the pathologist with cytological or histological specimens for detailed studies. He has to have a detailed knowledge about which one to choose and when and why and keep abreast with current recommendations. A surgical oncologist has at his disposal a wide array of tests to choose from but he should make the correct and rational choice. For example, a patient with rectal cancer will need magnetic resonance imaging (MRI) of the pelvis with a dedicated protocol for imaging of rectal cancer. Contrast-enhanced computed tomography (CECT) scan is not the option of choice in this case for the local imaging but is actually used simultaneously for metastatic work up in the same patient. Similarly, there are imaging modalities of choice for every such cancer in the body, whether it is for the local imaging or for the metastatic work up.

A surgical oncologist is also responsible for providing representative and adequate cytological or histological samples for the pathologist to study. Such techniques commonly include fine-needle aspiration cytology (FNAC), brush cytology, imprint cytology, fluid samples for cytology, core needle biopsy, incision biopsy or wedge biopsy, excision biopsy, punch biopsy, and node biopsy. He is expected to choose correctly for each cancer of a subsite. For example, for a gastric cancer, the usual practice is to obtain multiple endoscopic punch biopsies from the tumour. For a breast cancer, after an appropriate imaging which is in most instances a digital mammogram, the patient undergoes a core needle biopsy from the breast lump. For a musculoskeletal tumour, the patient undergoes a planned core needle biopsy from the tumour after review of the appropriate imaging, which is an MRI scan of the local part in case of extremity tumours. The performance of a good biopsy is a vital exercise in the management of cancer.

The appropriate staging of cancers is expected to be done in a structured and comprehensive manner and aids in their evidence-based management. Along with the clinical methods and radiological tests, the pathologist also plays a vital role towards this end. A surgical oncologist should have sufficient knowledge and collaborative mentality to strive towards excellence in this aspect.

There are cancers like ovarian cancer which require a surgical staging (staging laparotomy) and the surgical oncologist should know all the requisite steps and the reasoning behind each such step. The importance of non-spillage of tumour (and resultant tumour up-staging consequent to such spillage in various settings), mandatory peritoneal wash cytology, the performance of appropriate nodal dissection and getting the nodal yield and the resultant impact on staging, and peritoneal and omental biopsies together with removal of the primary ovarian tumour and gynaecological organs as appropriate, is a specialized surgical subject in itself. This is one of the umpteen examples in the purview of correct surgical oncologic practice.

The knowledge of specimen orientation and importance of transport of surgical specimen to the pathology laboratory in the correct manner is another essential practice. For example, it is absolutely necessary to orient the surgical specimen of a lumpectomy of breast on at least three sides before the specimen is detached from the body and then immediately upon removal, to immerse it completely in 10% neutral buffered formalin (NBF) within as minimum a time frame as possible, and then allow fixation time of not less than 6 h and not more than 72 h [7]. Such knowledge should not be a sole responsibility of the pathology team and the surgeon is also expected to have the know-how and the reasons behind it.

5 Curative Surgery

5.1 Surgery for Primary Cancer

A surgical oncologist is expected to know and have the technical skill to perform appropriate oncologically sound and evidence-based surgeries for any given primary cancer. For example, for a clinically staged cT3N any M0 (TNM staging) [8] distal gastric adenocarcinoma with tumour located in the antrum of the stomach, he would perform a standard distal gastrectomy which involves removal of the distal two-thirds of the stomach and do a D2 lymphadenectomy [8–15]. The D2 lymphadenectomy in this case [16] would entail complete removal of nodal stations 1, 3, 4d, 4sb, 5, 6, 7, 8a, 9, 11p, and 12a. In another example, surgery for a clinically staged cT3N1M0 adenocarcinoma of the right colon (ascending colon) would require a right hemicolectomy with a D3 lymphadenectomy [17, 18]. This would mean that the surgeon is expected to clear the lymph nodes at the root of the ileocolic and the middle colic vessels (apical nodes). The surgical oncologist is expected to keep abreast of all recent literature regarding the surgical management of such cancers, including the current developments about approaches, that is, in the context of the above mentioned cancers, the use of minimally invasive surgery, including laparoscopy or robotic approaches [19–40]. He or she also needs to continuously update his or her knowledge and be ready to adopt new development in science and technology related to surgery. Examples relevant to this statement have included, over the course of time, breast conservation therapy (BCT) in breast cancer, nephron sparing surgery (NSS) in renal cancer, complete mesocolic excision and central vascular ligation (CME + CVL) in colon cancer, total mesorectal excision (TME) in rectal cancer, minimally invasive surgery (MIS), and robotic surgery to name a few.

If we consider a different subsite, like breast cancer, the surgical oncologist should know the indications and contraindications (whether absolute or relative) of breast conservation surgery and be adept in counseling the patient about surgical treatment options. The judicious and evidence-based practice of neoadjuvant treatment [41–46] in the scenario of locally advanced breast cancer, large operable breast cancer and certain subsets of early stage breast cancer as well as the options of oncoplastic breast surgeries [47–49] and methods of reconstruction of the breast should all be known and understood by him. In the same vein, he must have stayed abreast of all the current developments of the management of axillary nodes in breast cancer [50–60].

5.2 Surgery for Metastatic Disease

The practice of metastasectomy with curative intent in evidence-based in certain subsites of cancer and such surgical exercise has often been rewarded with justifiable oncological outcomes [61, 62]. Examples include metastasectomy of hepatic and pulmonary metastases in colorectal cancers and pulmonary metastasectomy in musculoskeletal sarcomas (especially bone tumours). The practice of cytoreductive surgery (with hyperthermic intraperitoneal chemotherapy) for peritoneal carcinomatosis is another example where an extensive surgery is done in the scenario of metastatic disease but with the hope of achieving good tumour control. On another front, the curative potential of many metastatic cancers are being reconsidered and this has led to the emergence of the terminology like "oligometastatic" cancer which are increasingly being considered under the ambit of curative treatment. One such example would be "oligometastatic" lung cancer [63–65].

5.3 Palliative Surgery

In many instances the performance of a surgery would be required to alleviate the misery or in view of life threating complication like bleeding or hollow viscus perforation and not necessarily intended to improve survival owing to the metastatic stage of the disease. Examples include a palliative gastrectomy or a gastrojejunostomy done for metastatic gastric cancer to palliate bleeding or gastric outlet obstruction, a palliative mastectomy to improve the quality of life of a fungating tumour of the breast which is otherwise metastatic or a feeding jejunostomy to allow enteral feeding for a patient with esophageal cancer for whom even a self-expanding metallic stent could not be introduced due to complete occlusion of lumen.

5.4 Preventive or Prophylactic Surgery

This is considered in the setting of an elevated risk of cancer due to a proven genetic predisposition (Table 2). It is also known as risk-reduction surgery. The inputs of a geneticist and the irreplaceable role of a genetic counselor are vital in the conduct of such surgeries.

A surgical oncologist has to have the knowledge of the characteristic features of such genetic syndromes, the penetration levels as regards to

Table 2 List of genetic disorders [66] for which risk reducing surgeries are done

Disorder	Gene involved	Risk reducing surgery
Hereditary breast and ovarian cancer syndrome (HBOC)	BRCA1, BRCA2	Bilateral total mastectomy [67–69] Bilateral salpingo-oophorectomy [70]
Hereditary diffuse gastric cancer syndrome	CDH1	Total gastrectomy
Familial adenomatous polyposis (FAP)	APC	Total proctocolectomy and ileal pouch anal anastomosis [71] or Total colectomy with ileorectal anastomosis and endoscopic surveillance of the rectal segment
Hereditary non-polyposis colon cancer (HNPCC) syndrome	MMR genes (MSH1, MSH2, MSH3, MSH6, MLH1, PMS1, PMS2)	Total colectomy with ileorectal anastomosis [72, 73] Risk reducing hysterectomy and bilateral salpingo-oophorectomy
Multiple endocrine neoplasia (MEN) 2A, MEN 2B, and familial medullary thyroid cancer syndromes	RET oncogene	Total thyroidectomy [74]

the phenotypic expression of a particular malignancy and the appropriate timing of risk reduction surgery taking into account various considerations for every patient, namely, fertility issues and completion of family, long-term morbidities related to the procedure and the expected magnitude of risk reduction.

6 Conclusion

Whereas the domain of work of a surgical oncologist is a never-ending subject, it is the ability of the specialist to understand the same and dispense service and care in a highly judicious and responsible manner, with utmost precedence being given to evidence-based practice.

References

1. Faguet GB. A brief history of cancer: age-old milestones underlying our current knowledge database. Int J Cancer. 2015;136(9):2022–36. https://doi.org/10.1002/ijc.29134.
2. Bean WB. The century of the surgeon. AMA Arch Intern Med. 1959;103(3):506–7. https://doi.org/10.1001/archinte.1959.00270030162020.
3. Robinson DH, Toledo AH. Historical development of modern anesthesia. J Invest Surg. 2012;25(3):141–9. https://doi.org/10.3109/08941939.2012.690328. PMID: 22583009.
4. Worboys M. Joseph Lister and the performance of antiseptic surgery. Notes Rec R Soc Lond. 2013;67(3):199–209. https://doi.org/10.1098/rsnr.2013.0028.
5. Titford M. A short history of histopathology technique. J Histotechnol. 2006;29(2):99–110. https://doi.org/10.1179/his.2006.29.2.99.
6. Lawrence W. History of surgical oncology. In: Norton JA, et al., editors. Surgery. New York: Springer; 2008. https://doi.org/10.1007/978-0-387-68113-9_90.
7. Buesa RJ, Peshkov MV. How much formalin is enough to fix tissues? Ann Diagn Pathol. 2012;16(3):202–9. https://doi.org/10.1016/j.anndiagpath.2011.12.003. Epub 2012 Apr 5. PMID: 22483550.
8. Brierley J, Gospodarowicz MK, Wittekind C. TNM classification of malignant tumours. Chichester: Wiley; 2017.
9. Bonenkamp JJ, Songun I, Hermans J, et al. Randomised comparison of morbidity after D1 and D2 dissection for gastric cancer in 996 Dutch patients. Lancet. 1995;345:745–8.
10. Songun I, Putter H, Kranenbarg EM, Sasako M, van de Velde CJ. Surgical treatment of gastric cancer: 15-year follow-up results of the randomised nationwide Dutch D1D2 trial. Lancet Oncol. 2010;11(5):439–49. https://doi.org/10.1016/S1470-2045(10)70070-X. Epub 2010 Apr 19. PMID: 20409751.
11. Cuschieri A, Fayers P, Fielding J, et al. Postoperative morbidity and mortality after D1 and D2 resections for gastric cancer: preliminary results of the MRC randomised controlled surgical trial. The Surgical Cooperative Group. Lancet. 1996;347:995–9.
12. Kampschoer GH, Maruyama K, van de Velde CJ, et al. Computer analysis in making preoperative decisions: a rational approach to lymph node dissection in gastric cancer patients. Br J Surg. 1989;76:905–8.
13. Sano T, Sasako M, Yamamoto S, et al. Gastric cancer surgery: morbidity and mortality results from a prospective randomized controlled trial comparing D2 and extended para-aortic lymphadenectomy–Japan Clinical Oncology Group study 9501. J Clin Oncol. 2004;22:2767–73.
14. Smith DD, Schwarz RR, Schwarz RE. Impact of total lymph node count on staging and survival after gastrectomy for gastric cancer: data from a large US-population database. J Clin Oncol. 2005;23:7114–24.
15. Bouvier AM, Haas O, Piard F, et al. How many nodes must be examined to accurately stage gastric carcinomas? Results from a population based study. Cancer. 2002;94:2862–6.
16. Memon MA, Subramanya MS, Khan S, Hossain MB, Osland E, Memon B. Meta-analysis of D1 versus D2 gastrectomy for gastric adenocarcinoma. Ann Surg. 2011;253(5):900–11. https://doi.org/10.1097/SLA.0b013e318212bff6. PMID: 21394009.
17. Japanese Gastric Cancer Association. Japanese gastric cancer treatment guidelines 2018 (5th edition). Gastric Cancer. 2021;24(1):1–21. https://doi.org/10.1007/s10120-020-01042-y. Epub 2020 Feb 14. PMID: 32060757; PMCID: PMC7790804.
18. Emmanuel A, Haji A. Complete mesocolic excision and extended (D3) lymphadenectomy for colonic cancer: is it worth that extra effort? A review of the literature. Int J Colorectal Dis. 2016;31(4):797–804. https://doi.org/10.1007/s00384-016-2502-0. Epub 2016 Jan 30. PMID: 26833471.
19. Kanemitsu Y, Komori K, Kimura K, Kato T. D3 lymph node dissection in right hemicolectomy with a no-touch isolation technique in patients with colon cancer. Dis Colon Rectum. 2013;56(7):815–24. https://doi.org/10.1097/DCR.0b013e3182919093. PMID: 23739187.
20. Kitano S, Iso Y, Moriyama M, et al. Laparoscopy-assisted Billroth I gastrectomy. Surg Laparosc Endosc. 1994;4:146–8.
21. Cassidy MR, Gholami S, Strong VE. Minimally invasive surgery: the emerging role in gastric cancer. Surg Oncol Clin N Am. 2017;26:193–212.
22. Kitano S, Shiraishi N, Fujii K, et al. A randomized controlled trial comparing open vs laparoscopy-assisted distal gastrectomy for the treatment of early gastric cancer: an interim report. Surgery. 2002;131:S306–11.

23. Huang KH, Lan YT, Fang WL, et. al. Initial experience of robotic gastrectomy and comparison with open and laparoscopic gastrectomy for gastric cancer. J Gastrointest Surg. 2012;16:1303–10.
24. Hwang SI, Kim HO, Yoo CH, et al. Laparoscopic-assisted distal gastrectomy versus open distal gastrectomy for advanced gastric cancer. Surg Endosc. 2009;23:1252–8.
25. Kinoshita T, Uyama I, Terashima M, et al. Long-term outcomes of laparoscopic versus open surgery for clinical stage II/III gastric cancer: a multicenter cohort study in Japan (LOC-A study). Ann Surg. 2019;269(5):887–94.
26. Kim W, Kim HH, Han SU, et al. Decreased morbidity of laparoscopic distal gastrectomy compared with open distal gastrectomy for stage I gastric cancer: short-term outcomes from a multicenter randomized controlled trial (KLASS-01). Ann Surg. 2016;263:28–35.
27. Sakuramoto S, Yamashita K, Kikuchi S, et al. Laparoscopy versus open distal gastrectomy by expert surgeons for early gastric cancer in Japanese patients: short-term clinical outcomes of a randomized clinical trial. Surg Endosc. 2013;27:1695–705.
28. Yoo CH, Kim HO, Hwang SI, et al. Short-term outcomes of laparoscopic-assisted distal gastrectomy for gastric cancer during a surgeon's learning curve period. Surg Endosc. 2009;23:2250–7.
29. Huscher CG, Mingoli A, Sgarzini G, et al. Laparoscopic versus open subtotal gastrectomy for distal gastric cancer: five-year results of a randomized prospective trial. Ann Surg. 2005;241:232–7.
30. Vinuela EF, Gonen M, Brennan MF, et al. Laparoscopic versus open distal gastrectomy for gastric cancer: a meta-analysis of randomized controlled trials and high-quality nonrandomized studies. Ann Surg. 2012;255:446–56.
31. Chen K, Pan Y, Zhang B, et al. Robotic versus laparoscopic gastrectomy for gastric cancer: a systematic review and updated meta-analysis. BMC Surg. 2017;17:93.
32. Lacy AM, García-Valdecasas JC, Delgado S, Castells A, Taurá P, Piqué JM, et al. Laparoscopy-assisted colectomy versus open colectomy for treatment of non-metastatic colon cancer: a randomised trial. Lancet. 2002;359(9325):2224–9.
33. Liang J-T, Huang K-C, Lai H-S, Lee P-H, Jeng Y-M. Oncologic results of laparoscopic versus conventional open surgery for stage II or III leftsided colon cancers: a randomized controlled trial. Ann Surg Oncol. 2007;14(1):109–17.
34. Fleshman J, Sargent DJ, Green E, Anvari M, Stryker SJ, Beart RW, et al. Laparoscopic colectomy for cancer is not inferior to open surgery based on 5-year data from the COST Study Group trial. Ann Surg. 2007;246(4):655–62; discussion 662–4.
35. Kitano S, Inomata M, Mizusawa J, Katayama H, Watanabe M, Yamamoto S, et al. Survival outcomes following laparoscopic versus open D3 dissection for stage II or III colon cancer (JCOG0404): a phase 3, randomised controlled trial. Lancet Gastroenterol Hepatol. 2017;2(4):261–8.
36. Jeong S-Y, Park JW, Nam BH, Kim S, Kang S-B, Lim S-B, et al. Open versus laparoscopic surgery for mid-rectal or low-rectal cancer after neoadjuvant chemoradiotherapy (COREAN trial): survival outcomes of an open-label, non-inferiority, randomised controlled trial. Lancet Oncol. 2014;15(7):767–74.
37. Bonjer HJ, Deijen CL, Haglind E, COLOR II Study Group. A randomized trial of laparoscopic versus open surgery for rectal cancer. N Engl J Med. 2015;373(2):194.
38. Fleshman J, Branda M, Sargent DJ, Boller AM, George V, Abbas M, et al. Effect of laparoscopic-assisted resection vs open resection of stage II or III rectal cancer on pathologic outcomes: the ACOSOG Z6051 randomized clinical trial. JAMA. 2015;314(13):1346–55.
39. Stevenson ARL, Solomon MJ, Lumley JW, Hewett P, Clouston AD, Gebski VJ, et al. Effect of laparoscopic-assisted resection vs open resection on pathological outcomes in rectal cancer: the ALaCaRT randomized clinical trial. JAMA. 2015;314(13):1356–63.
40. Prete FP, Pezzolla A, Prete F, Testini M, Marzaioli R, Patriti A, et al. Robotic versus laparoscopic minimally invasive surgery for rectal cancer: a systematic review and meta-analysis of randomized controlled trials. Ann Surg. 2018;267(6):1034–46.
41. Fisher B, Brown A, Mamounas E, et al. Effect of preoperative chemotherapy on local-regional disease in women with operable breast cancer: findings from National Surgical Adjuvant Breast and Bowel Project B-18. J Clin Oncol. 1998;16:2672–85.
42. Bear HD, Anderson S, Smith RE, et al. Sequential preoperative or postoperative docetaxel added to preoperative doxorubicin plus cyclophosphamide for operable breast cancer: National Surgical Adjuvant Breast and Bowel Project Protocol B-27. J Clin Oncol. 2006;24:2019–27.
43. Gianni L, Eiermann W, Semiglazov V, et al. Neoadjuvant chemotherapy with trastuzumab followed by adjuvant trastuzumab versus neoadjuvant chemotherapy alone, in patients with HER2-positive locally advanced breast cancer (the NOAH trial): a randomised controlled superiority trial with a parallel HER2-negative cohort. Lancet. 2010;375:377–84.
44. Untch M, Loibl S, Bischoff J, et al. Lapatinib versus trastuzumab in combination with neoadjuvant anthracycline-taxane-based chemotherapy (GeparQuinto, GBG 44): a randomised phase 3 trial. Lancet Oncol. 2012;13:135–44.
45. De Azambuja E, Holmes AP, Piccart-Gebhart M, et al. Lapatinib with trastuzumab for HER2-positive early breast cancer (NeoALTTO): survival outcomes of a randomised, open-label, multicentre, phase 3 trial and their association with pathological complete response. Lancet Oncol. 2014;15:1137–46.
46. Schneeweiss A, Chia S, Hickish T, et al. Pertuzumab plus trastuzumab in combination with standard neoadjuvant anthracycline-containing and anthracycline-

free chemotherapy regimens in patients with HER2-positive early breast cancer: randomized phase II cardiac safety study (TRYPHAENA). Ann Oncol. 2013;24:2278–84.
47. Cochrane RA, Valasiadou P, Wilson ARM, Al-Ghazal SK, Macmillan RD. Cosmesis and satisfaction after breast-conserving surgery correlates with the percentage of breast volume excised. Br J Surg. 2003;90(12):1505–9.
48. Rainsbury RM. Surgery Insight: oncoplastic breast-conserving reconstruction—indications, benefits, choices and outcomes. Nat Clin Pract Oncol. 2007;4(11):657–64.
49. Masetti R, Pirulli PG, Magno S, Franceschini G, Chiesa F, Antinori A. Oncoplastic techniques in the conservative surgical treatment of breast cancer. Breast Cancer. 2000;7(4):276–80.
50. Donker M, van Tienhoven G, Straver ME, et al. Radiotherapy or surgery of the axilla after a positive sentinel node in breast cancer (EORTC 10981-22023 AMAROS): a randomised, multicentre, open-label, phase 3 non-inferiority trial. Lancet Oncol. 2014;15:1303–10.
51. Giuliano A, Hunt K. Axillary dissection vs. no axillary dissection in women with invasive breast cancer and sentinel node metastasis—Z11. JAMA. 2011;305:569–75.
52. Krag DN, Anderson SJ, Julian TB, et al. Sentinel lymph node resection compared with conventional axillary lymph node dissection in clinically node-negative patients with breast cancer: overall survival findings from the NSABP B-32 randomised phase 3 trial. Lancet Oncol. 2010;11:927–33.
53. Galimberti V, Cole BF, Zurrida S, et al. Axillary dissection versus no axillary dissection in patients with sentinel-node micrometastases (IBCSG 23-01): a phase 3 randomised controlled trial. Lancet Oncol. 2013;14:297–305.
54. Landin J, Weber WP. Lymph node surgery—stepwise retirement for the breast surgeon? Breast Care. 2016;11:282–6.
55. Kuehn T, Bauerfeind I, Fehm T, et al. Sentinel lymph node biopsy in patients with breast cancer before and after neoadjuvant chemotherapy (SENTINA): a prospective, multicentre cohort study. Lancet Oncol. 2013;14:609–18.
56. Boughey JC, Suman VJ, Mittendorf EA, et al. Sentinel lymph node surgery after neoadjuvant chemotherapy in patients with node-positive breast cancer: the ACOSOG Z1071 (Alliance) clinical trial. JAMA. 2013;310:1455–61.
57. Mamounas EP, Brown A, Anderson S, et al. Sentinel node biopsy after neoadjuvant chemotherapy in breast cancer: results from National Surgical Adjuvant Breast and Bowel Project protocol B-27. J Clin Oncol. 2005;23:2694–702.
58. Haffty BG, McCall LM, Ballman KV, et al. Patterns of local-regional management following neoadjuvant chemotherapy in breast cancer: results from ACOSOG Z1071. Int J Radiat Oncol Biol Phys. 2016;94:493–502.
59. Gentilini O, Veronesi U. Abandoning sentinel lymph node biopsy in early breast cancer? A new trial in progress at the European Institute of Oncology of Milan (SOUND: Sentinel node vs. Observation after axillary UltraSouND). Breast. 2012;21:678–81.
60. Jatoi I, Benson JR, Toi M. De-escalation of axillary surgery in early breast cancer. Lancet Oncol. 2016;17:e430–41.
61. Treasure T, Milošević M, Fiorentino F, et al. Pulmonary metastasectomy: what is the practice and where is the evidence for effectiveness? Thorax. 2014;69:946–9.
62. Morris EJ, Forman D, Thomas JD, et al. Surgical management and outcomes of colorectal cancer liver metastases. Br J Surg. 2010;97:1110.
63. Hellman S, Weichselbaum RR. Oligometastases. J Clin Oncol. 1995;13:8–10.
64. Niibe Y, Hayakawa K. Oligometastases and oligo-recurrence: the new era of cancer therapy. Jpn J Clin Oncol. 2010;40:107–11.
65. Ashworth A, Rodrigues G, Boldt G, Palma D. Is there an oligometastatic state in non-small cell lung cancer? A systematic review of the literature. Lung Cancer. 2013;82:197–203.
66. Garber JE, Offit K. Hereditary cancer predisposition syndromes. J Clin Oncol. 2005;23:276–92.
67. Eisen A, Rebbeck TR, Wood WC, et al. Prophylactic surgery in women with a hereditary predisposition to breast and ovarian cancer. J Clin Oncol. 2000;18:1980–95.
68. Meijers-Heijboer H, van Geel B, van Putten WL, et al. Breast cancer after prophylactic bilateral mastectomy in women with a BRCA1 or BRCA2 mutation. N Engl J Med. 2001;345:159–64.
69. Rebbeck TR, Friebel T, Lynch HT, et al. Bilateral prophylactic mastectomy reduces breast cancer risk in BRCA1 and BRCA2 mutation carriers: the PROSE Study Group. J Clin Oncol. 2004;22:1055–62.
70. Kauff ND, Satagopan JM, Robson ME, et al. Risk-reducing salpingo-oophorectomy in women with a BRCA1 or BRCA2 mutation. N Engl J Med. 2002;346:1609–15.
71. Nyam DC, Brillant PT, Dozois RR, et al. Ileal pouch-anal canal anastomosis for familial adenomatous polyposis: early and late results. Ann Surg. 1997;226:514–9.
72. Church JM. Prophylactic colectomy in patients with hereditary nonpolyposis colorectal cancer. Ann Med. 1996;28:479–82.
73. Syngal S, Weeks JC, Schrag D, et al. Benefits of colonoscopic surveillance and prophylactic colectomy in patients with hereditary nonpolyposis colorectal cancer mutations. Ann Intern Med. 1998;129:787–96.
74. Skinner MA, Moley JA, Dilley WG, et al. Prophylactic thyroidectomy in multiple endocrine neoplasia type 2A. N Engl J Med. 2005;353:1105–13.

Principles of Chemotherapy, Targeted Therapy, and Immunotherapy in Gynaecological Malignancies

Satya Sadhan Sarangi, Sudeep Gupta, and Amal Chandra Kataki

1 Introduction

In the management of cancer, both surgery and radiotherapy are essential local forms of treatments that are directed towards primary tumours and any loco-regional disease. Chemotherapy is a systemic modality and can treat distant metastases. Chemotherapy is used to improve the prognosis in majority of cancers, but is curative only in the minority of cancers. Chemotherapy is well known to cure lymphomas, leukemias, testicular cancers, and choriocarcinoma.

The main aim of delivering anti-neoplastic drugs is to eradicate cancer cells without causing excessive toxicity to normal cells. But anti-neoplastic drugs have considerable toxicity as it cannot easily differentiate between malignant cells from normal cells.

S. S. Sarangi (✉)
Department of Medical Oncology, Dr. Bhubaneswar Borooah Cancer Institute (A Unit of Tata Memorial Centre, Mumbai), Guwahati, Assam, India

S. Gupta
ACTREC (Advanced Centre for Treatment, Research and Education in Cancer), Navi Mumbai, Maharashtra, India
e-mail: sudeep.gupta@actrec.gov.in

A. C. Kataki
Department of Gynaecologic Oncology, Dr. Bhubaneswar Borooah Cancer Institute (A Unit of Tata Memorial Centre, Mumbai), Guwahati, Assam, India

2 Basic Principles

Chemotherapy agents are grouped into different categories based on the mechanism of action.

These categories include:

1. Alkylating agents
2. Topoisomerase inhibitors
3. Antimicrotubule agents
4. Antimetabolites
5. Plant alkaloids
6. Anthracyclines

In addition to the site of primary tumour and diagnosis, individual patient-related factors such as organ function, age, performance status, concurrent medical illness, and residual toxicities from the receipt of prior therapies also influence the selection of chemotherapy regimens. Depending on the goals of treatment and previous treatments the patient may require dose adjustments. Treating oncologist who is prescribing anticancer agents should understand the intent of care for the individual patient (curative vs. palliative) as well as the metabolism and toxicities of the chemotherapeutic agents prescribed. Patients and their families should be informed about the expected toxicities and aim of therapy.

A. C. Kataki, D. Barmon (eds.), *Fundamentals in Gynaecologic Malignancy*,
https://doi.org/10.1007/978-981-19-5860-1_7

3 Growth of Tumour Cell

Tumour growth is a complex and intricate process that is governed by genetic abnormalities within the cell and the interaction of tumour with its microenvironment. The understanding of cancer has accelerated significantly over the past decade, and Hanahan and Weinberg [1] have defined the distinguishing features of cancer detailing the following hallmarks in addition to genomic instability as an underlying premise of the make-up of cancer cells:

1. Promotion and sustaining proliferative signaling,
2. Activating invasion and metastasis,
3. Resisting cell death,
4. Allowing replicative immortality,
5. Induction of angiogenesis,
6. Evading growth suppressors,
7. Immune surveillance evasion,
8. Altered Energy reprogramming.

The proliferation and growth control of normal cells are not well understood, but the mitogenic signaling of cancer cells is increasingly better understood. Cancer cells acquire the ability to proliferate unchecked by several different mechanisms: self-production of growth factor ligands; control of the tumour microenvironment by signaling local stromal cells, which in turn produce factors leading to cancer growth; overexpression or enhanced signaling of transmembrane receptors; and growth factor independence via constitutive activation of tyrosine kinases within the receptor and/or downstream signaling molecules [2]. Enabling characteristics of cancer cells that allow the above changes to occur include overall genomic instability and the cancer cell's ability to avoid immune destruction [3].

4 Log Kill Hypothesis

Cell kinetics was originally described based on murine models, but later on it was seen that most human solid tumours do not grow exponentially. The log kill hypothesis was based on the L1210 murine leukemia model, which is fast-growing leukemia where 100% of the cells are actively progressing through the cell cycle [4]. Logarithmic kill hypothesis states that a given anticancer drug should kill a constant proportion or fraction of cells in contrast to a constant number of cells, and cell kill is proportional regardless of the bulk of tumour. For example, if a drug can lead to a 3 log kill of cancer cells and can reduce the cancer burden from 10^9 to 10^6, the same drug and dose can also reduce the tumour burden from 10^6 to 10^3. However, solid tumours tend to follow the Gompertzian model of tumour growth because most solid tumours do not grow and expand exponentially [5]. The Gompertzian model (Fig. 1) predicts that cell growth is faster at the start of the growth curve when a tumour is small compared to a larger tumour existing in the slower part of the growth curve, which thus has a lower growth fraction. The Gompertzian model also predicts that the sensitivity of cancer to chemotherapy depends on where the tumour is in its growth phase and that growth decreases exponentially over time. Similarly, the log kill produced by chemotherapy is higher in small-volume tumours than large-volume tumours because of the differences in growth kinetics.

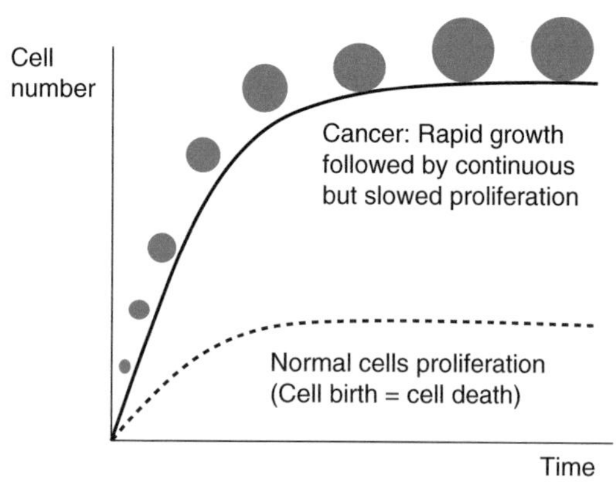

Fig. 1 Gompertzian growth curve. (Adapted with Permission from 2014 Pan Stanford Publishing Pte. Ltd through email communication)

5 Resistance to Chemotherapy

Resistance occurs with all cancers except for those that are curable. Multiple mechanisms are there, new mechanisms are also being discovered, and overlapping mechanisms can occur in tandem; tumour resistance to drug therapy results primarily from tumour growth and selection of existing resistant clones while sensitive cells are killed [6, 7]. One of the original hypotheses explaining drug resistance is the Goldie and Coldman hypothesis reported initially in 1979, which served as the basis for drug regimens used in hematologic malignancies and more recently in gynaecologic malignancies [8]. The tenets of the Goldie and Coldman hypothesis include the following:

1. Treatment should be started as soon as possible to treat the smallest amount and bulk of the tumour,
2. Multiple non-cross-resistant drugs should be used to avoid selection of resistant clones, and
3. Drugs should be used as frequently as possible and in doses that are higher than minimally cytotoxic doses.

In clinical trials that examine features of the Goldie and Coldman hypothesis, adjuvant breast cancer therapy has shown improvements in outcome by using this theory, but in the upfront treatment of ovarian cancer, the use of sequencing non-cross-resistant agents did not result in improved progression-free survival or overall survival [9]. Examples of mechanisms of drug resistance include alteration of drug movement across the cell membrane with respect to both influx and efflux, increased repair of DNA to offset damage done by certain agents, defective apoptosis so cancer cells are not receptive to drug effects, alteration of drug targets such as topoisomerase II alteration by point mutation, deletions or overexpression, and other mechanisms. The mechanisms of resistance associated with specific agents are discussed within the individual drug descriptions [6, 10]. Newly described drug resistance mechanisms include the identification of secondary mutations that restore the wildtype BRCA reading frame, which is likely a mediator of acquired resistance to platinum-based chemotherapy [11].

6 Dose Intensity

The therapeutic selectivity of chemotherapy is reliant on the outcome of dose-response between normal tissue and cancer tissue. Dose intensity is the amount of drug delivered per unit of time, and the dose intensity of each regimen is based on the time period during which the treatment is administered. Calculations can be made regarding the intended dose intensity as well as the actual dose intensity that the patient receives in total. By reducing the dose intensity to decrease toxicity, clinicians may compromise the predicted outcome of a patient, and therefore, clinicians must state the upfront intended outcome of administering chemotherapy (i.e., curative vs. palliative). The importance of maintaining dose intensity has been demonstrated in early-stage breast cancer patients using adjuvant cyclophosphamide, methotrexate, and 5-fluorouracil, as well as cyclophosphamide and doxorubicin. In gynaecologic cancers, the importance of dose intensity has been observed in older patients with ovarian cancer who may have worse outcomes compared to younger patients because of reduced dose intensity and less aggressive dosing of chemotherapy in older patients [12]. In another example, EMA-CO regimen is the most commonly used combination chemotherapy among other regimens that have been used in the management of high-risk GTN. Combination chemotherapy is often administered at 2- to 3-week intervals and timely administration is essential. Unnecessary treatment delays and dose reductions should be avoided as they may lead to tumour resistance and treatment failure. Several mechanisms to deliver chemotherapy in a dose-intense fashion are available to clinicians. First, doses of drugs can simply be escalated. Second, the same doses of drugs can be given in a reduced interval of time (i.e., "dose-dense administration"). For example, adjuvant cyclophosphamide and doxorubicin followed by paclitaxel in early breast cancer administered every 2 weeks rather than every 3 weeks demonstrated improvements in the dose-dense regimen [13]. The prophylactic use of growth factors has enabled chemotherapy to be delivered at higher doses safely without excess risk of neutropenic events and has enabled chemotherapy to be delivered in a dose-dense manner.

7 Single Versus Combination Therapy

Decisions regarding optimal choice of single agent versus combination therapy should be based on the objectives of therapy (curative vs. palliative treatment), published regimens for specific indications and dosing of agents, and predicted toxicities. Specific doses chosen should be based on published studies, but dose alterations can occur based on objectives of treatment; renal, hepatic, or bone marrow function; toxicities experienced by the patient during previous cycles; current performance status and comorbidities of the patient; direct measurement of drug levels in the individual patient when possible; and potential interactions with other concomitant medications. Although combination chemotherapy typically yields higher response rates overall compared to single agents, toxicities are usually higher; outcomes such as overall survival and progression-free survival may be better with combinations [14]. Scheduling of drugs is such that the most myelosuppressive agents are given on day 1 and scheduled every 2–4 weeks depending on the timing of the myelosuppression nadir. This allows for the recovery of bone marrow, gastrointestinal, dermatologic, and other organ toxicities without allowing significant tumour growth to occur. Mechanisms of action of the drugs and duration of infusion can also influence drug sequencing and toxicities.

8 Different Chemotherapy Types

Primary Therapy In which chemotherapy is the primary modality of treatment, e.g. Methotrexate in treatment of choriocarcinoma.

Adjuvant Therapy It is defined as the usage of systemic chemotherapy after surgery and/or radiotherapy with radical intent in patients who have subsequent high risk of recurrence.

Concurrent Chemoradiation Usage of chemotherapy in combination with radiation with curative intent to sensitize the tumour cell. Chemotherapy is used during radiation therapy to eradicate micrometastases within the radiation field and to increase the radio-responsiveness of tumour cells. Regimens using alternate radiation and chemotherapy aims to reduce toxicity to normal tissues and enhance tumour sensitivity by delivering each agent when the first agent has induced enhanced sensitivity to the other. The initial reduction of the tumour mass by chemotherapy results in improved tumour's blood supply, thus improving re-oxygenation, and improving radiation-induced tumour cell kill. Chemotherapy also plays an essential role in the segregation of the tumour cells in a favorable manner, permitting radiation to be more effective in a particular phase of the cell cycle. Conversely, radiation therapy may decrease the tumour mass, leading to improved blood supply [15] and optimal drug delivery. Few cancer chemotherapy agents function as radiation sensitizers, showing synergistic cancer cell kill when combined with radiation while having a lesser relative side effect on normal tissues.

Neoadjuvant Chemotherapy Defined as the use of chemotherapy in the treatment of the locally advanced disease that will assist in subsequent definitive treatment.

Induction Chemotherapy Initial systemic chemotherapy used in patients with the disseminated disease for which local modality (i.e., surgical resection or radiotherapy) is incomplete or not indicated.

Salvage Chemotherapy When chemotherapy is given for recurrence after initial treatment with chemotherapy or second-line chemotherapy if it does not respond to initial induction therapy. Generally, the intent is palliation.

Consolidation Chemotherapy Additional chemotherapy for more than the usual regimen.

Palliative Chemotherapy Chemotherapy when it is used for symptomatic relief in incurable cancer.

9 Routes of Administration

Intravenous Most chemotherapeutic agents are available only in an intravenous preparation, requiring venous access. Venous access can be temporary during chemotherapy administration or prolonged by surgically implanted intravascular devices, type of access must be chosen carefully for the anticipated duration, complexity, types of drugs (vesicants or non-vesicants), and anticipated need of fluid replacement, blood products, and antibiotics. Patient preference and quality of life issues also play a role.

Oral and Local Drug application intra-arterial (i.e., hepatic infusion, limb perfusion), intrathecal (meningeal metastasis), intraperitoneal (ovarian cancer, peritoneal carcinomatosis), intrapleural (pleurisy/pleural metastases), and intrapericardial (malignant pericardial effusion) are other routes of administration. Various agents are available in oral form, making intravenous access unnecessary. Besides their everyday use in various chemotherapy regimens, oral agents, have ease and convenience, also play a vital role in palliative therapy [16], where the quality of life issues are paramount. The use of oral agents is to be restricted in patients with functional or anatomical barriers for ingestion and absorption.

Intraperitoneal Therapy Direct intraperitoneal instillation of chemotherapy drugs provides a two- to five-fold and higher concentration advantage over systemic intravenous administration. It exposes tumour cells to both higher peak drug concentrations and area under the [17] concentration-time curve drug levels. Intraperitoneal therapy is typically accomplished through a surgically implanted intraperitoneal catheter, which may be either exteriorized or subcutaneous. Intraperitoneal therapy is best used to treat small-volume, diffuse intraperitoneal [18] disease, and has thus been used mainly in ovarian cancer, with less common application in intraperitoneal [19] gastrointestinal malignancies or mesothelioma. Drugs such as cisplatin, carboplatin, 5-fluorouracil (5-FU), and paclitaxel are used in intraperitoneal therapy.

10 Chemotherapeutic Drugs Used in the Treatment of Gynaecological Cancer

Majority of anticancer drugs cause damage to DNA with the help of various mechanisms, including disruption of cell cycle checkpoints, growth factors, growth factor receptors, and signal transduction.

10.1 Alkylating Agents

Alkylating agents are considered as one of the earliest chemotherapy agents that started to be used in the early 1940s. These agents block DNA replication by forming covalent bonds with DNA bases (cross-linking the DNA strands). Examples are cyclophosphamide, ifosfamide, melphalan, procarbazine, busulfan, etc. Chlorambucil can be given by mouth and is the least toxic. Cyclophosphamide and ifosfamide produces an acrolein metabolite that causes hemorrhagic cystitis. Use of mesna and hydration has largely overcome the hemorrhagic cystitis. Mesna inactivates the acrolein metabolites in the urine and is rapidly excreted in the urine. Cyclophosphamide can be used in patients with renal impairment. However, ifosfamide can cause cumulative renal tubular damage and resulting in Fanconi syndrome.

10.2 Platinum

The first platinum-based chemotherapy drug is cisplatin that was approved in 1978. Platinum can be considered as the most important chemotherapy drug used in gynaecological cancer. Platinum compounds form DNA cross-links by an action similar to the alkylating agents. Cisplatin, carboplatin, and recently oxaliplatin are platinum-based cytotoxic drugs. Cisplatin has more nephrotoxicity and ototoxicity than carboplatin. Carboplatin is a second generation and oxaliplatin is the third-generation platinum-based cytotoxic agent.

10.3 Anti-tumour Antibiotics and Anthracylines

Anti-tumour antibiotics have a variety of modes of action, including DNA cross-linking and topoisomerase inhibition. Some of these drugs intercalate between base pairs of DNA and RNA, inhibit RNA and DNA polymerase, generate oxygen-free radicals, and alter cell membrane function. The most important and commonly used members of this drug are doxorubicin and epirubicin. Doxorubicin is isolated from a mutated strain of streptomyces. Actinomycin D is also anti-tumour antibiotic (polypeptide antibiotic), which is isolated from the bacteria of the genus streptomyces. Doxorubicin, epirubicin, and idarubicin are also known as anthracycline drugs (anthracycline antibiotics). The short-term dose-limiting side effects of anthracycline drugs are myelosuppression and mucositis. Cardiomyopathy is also a dose-limiting side effect and can be prevented by controlling the total dose and the use of chemoprotection cardioxane (dexrazoxane) before treatment. Liposomal doxorubicin is the customized form of doxorubicin to enhance efficacy and reduce toxicity. The doxorubicin is encapsulated inside the liposome; liposome allows the doxorubicin to remain in the body for a longer duration. Encapsulated doxorubicin is also considered to reduce exposure of the active metabolite to myocardial tissue and therefore, decreasing myocardial toxicity. Currently, there are two types of liposomal doxorubicin available (differ in their lipid component), i.e. pegylated liposomal doxorubicin hydrochloride and Myocet. Myocet is indicated as a combination with cyclophosphamide in metastatic breast cancer. Bleomycin is also an anti-tumour antibiotic, discovered in the 1960s. Bleomycin acts by creating free oxygen radicals which break DNA strands, similar to anthracycline. These drugs are commonly used in the treatment of breast cancer, uterine sarcoma, and ovarian cancer.

10.4 Antimetabolites

Antimetabolites are cytotoxic agents which have structurally resemblance with naturally occurring purines, pyrimidines, and nucleic acids. They inhibit the key enzymes which are involved in DNA synthesis. They can add into the DNA or

RNA of the cancer cells and interfere with the cell division process. Examples are Methotrexate, 5-fluorouracil, 6-mercaptopurine, gemcitabine, etc. Methotrexate is an anti-folate drug, which is structurally similar to folic acid and inhibits the activity of DHFR enzyme leading to inhibition of DNA and RNA synthesis. Gemcitabine is a deoxycytidine analogue, a pyrimidine antimetabolite related to cytarabine. Gemcitabine is a pro-drug and metabolized intracellularly to the active forms known as dFdCDP and dFdCTP. Both active metabolites will incorporate into DNA and inhibit DNA synthesis resulting in apoptosis.

10.5 Vinca Alkaloids

Vinca alkaloids are plant derivatives (from the periwinkle plant), Vinca rosea (catharanthus roseus) that have been traditionally used by the natives of Madagascar to treat diabetes. Vinca alkaloids falls into the category of tubulin-binding drugs jointly with taxanes. Examples are vincristine, vinblastine, vinorelbine, and vindesine. Vinblastine and vincristine bind to tubulin dimers and prevent their assembly into microtubules. These are highly vesicant. This should be injected into a central venous line or cannula where there is no resistance to injection and where blood can be freely drawn back. Vinorelbine is a synthetic vinca alkaloid which is available both intravenously and orally.

10.6 Topoisomerase Inhibitors

Topoisomerase inhibitors (I and II) are a group of enzymes which allow unwinding and uncoiling of supercoiled DNA. Both Topoisomerase inhibitor I and II act by interfering with DNA transcription, replication, and function to prevent DNA supercoiling. Topoisomerase I inhibitors are extracted from the bark and wood of the Camptotheca accuminata, they form a complex with topoisomerase DNA. Topotecan and Irinotecan are topoisomerase inhibitor I. Topoisomerase II inhibitors are extracted from the alkaloids found in the roots of May Apple plants. Topoisomerase II enzyme binds covalently to complementary strands of double-strand DNA, cleaving both strands. The inhibitors of this enzyme will reseal these breaks. Examples are etoposide, teniposide, and amsacrine. They are also classified under epipodophyllotoxins chemotherapy agents. Hematological toxicity are the main side effects of topoisomerase inhibitors. These are excreted by the liver and renal tubules; hence, dose adjustment may be necessary with renal and hepatic impairment.

10.7 Taxanes

Taxanes are plant alkaloids which were initially developed for therapeutic use in 1963. These are extracted from the yew tree. Paclitaxel is the first taxane to be discovered in 1971 and was made available for clinical use in 1993. Paclitaxel is isolated from the bark of the Western Pacific yew tree. Docetaxel is the semi-synthetic second generation of taxanes derived from the needles of the European yew trees. Both drugs work in the M-phase of the cell cycle and stop the function of microtubules by binding with them resulting in a sustained block in mitosis. Summary of mecha-

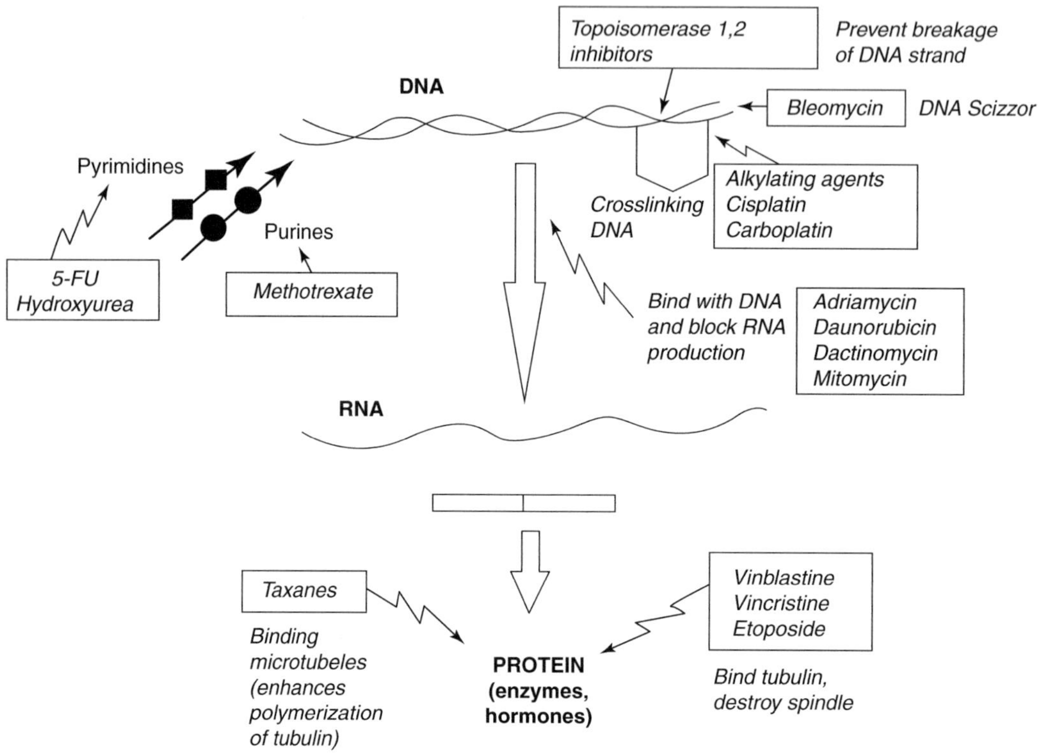

Fig. 2 Mode of action of chemotherapy agents used in Gynaecological Malignancies. (Adapted with Permission from 2014 Pan Stanford Publishing Pte. Ltd through email communication)

nism of action of different chemotherapeutic agents are shown in Fig. 2.

11 Targeted Therapies

The principal tenets of optimal disease management in women with gynaecologic malignancies have been the strategic utilization of surgery, cytotoxic chemotherapy, hormonal therapy, and radiotherapy. Although substantial progress has been realized from these practices, disease-specific mortality from gynaecologic malignancies still accounts for about 9% of all cancer-related deaths and underscores the need for the development of new therapeutic modalities. Investigation into the mechanisms governing cancer initiation, proliferation, metastases, autophagy, and apoptosis have uncovered a wealth of new opportunities, many of which harbor the potential of reversing the malignant phenotype, selectively inducing cancer cell death, overcoming primary and induced drug resistance, and optimistically improving overall outcomes for patients. The ability to pharmacologically and pharmacodynamically interact with these new "targets" has fostered rapid drug development, some of which is beginning to show merit in the treatment of women with gynaecologic malignancy. Because the biology of cancer growth often shares homology across different tumour types, targeted therapies are being investigated where the pathway of aberration is suspected to play an important or dominant role in disease pathogenesis. Although an "Achilles' heel," or a solitary activated pathway, is not present in most solid tumours, the opportunity to selectively target key regulatory and survival mechanisms in the tumour microenvironment holds great promise in expanding our therapeutic armamentarium for these women. We review some of these pathways and agents in this section.

11.1 Mechanisms of Action

One of the most common events defining the cancer process is the dysregulation of protein kinases that govern normal cellular function. In light of this observation, proteins are frequently the targets of anticancer agents. Although there are many ways to affect protein kinase function, including small molecules, monoclonal antibodies, antagomirs, antisense, RNA interference, immuno- and receptor drug conjugates, decoy receptors, allosteric inhibitors, and nanotubes, the intent is to target these aberrancies either restoring normal host function or inducing cell death. The principle challenge is to affect tumour cells without impacting the function of normal host cells. Three relevant mechanisms are important to review.

11.2 Interruption of Signal Transduction Pathways

Signal transduction is the process where a ligand, usually lipophobic (e.g., a growth factor), meets a receptor or channel on the cell surface and initiates a cascade of events such as kinase activity or dissociation of G-coupled proteins resulting in some cellular response. In contrast, lipophilic ligands (e.g., steroids) can penetrate the cell membrane and may affect cellular functions by direct binding to cytoplasmic or nuclear targets. Many of the "small molecules" being developed for cancer therapy involve blocking the tyrosine kinase activity of membrane-bound receptors that are usually influenced by a number of promoting ligands. The prototypical example of a relevant ligand-receptor signal transduction pathway in carcinogenesis is the epidermal growth factor receptor (EGFR). This receptor family is overexpressed and activated in many tumour types, including gynaecologic malignancies, and appears to play a key role in disease pathogenesis. Binding of the epidermal growth factor (EGF) ligand to the receptor induces tyrosine kinase activity, which leads to receptor dimerization and activation of the pathway driving multiple cellular functions such as cellular proliferation, enhanced cellular motility, resistance to apoptosis, and angiogenesis. Because of the broad spectra of activity, there has been intense interest in developing therapeutics against this pathway. Typically, these targeted agents are classified in two broad categories: competitive adenosine triphosphate (ATP)–pocket small-molecule inhibitors and monoclonal antibodies to the receptor's extracellular domain. The clinical experience of these molecules in gynaecologic cancer will be discussed later; however, the crafted directive of these targeted agents is to disrupt ligand/receptor activation in the hopes of blocking the signal transduction pathways leading to cancer cell survival. This receptor family is overexpressed and activated in many tumour types, including gynaecologic malignancies, and appears to play a key role in disease pathogenesis [20].

11.3 Induction of Apoptosis

Normal development and functional physiology are dependent on tight regulation of cellular growth and death. The representation of cancer as "uncontrolled cellular proliferation" attests to the importance dysregulated cellular programmed cell death, or apoptosis plays in human disease. Phenotypical transformation of a normal cell to a cancer cell is likely highly influenced by the loss of apoptotic function. In addition, resistance to chemotherapy-induced cytotoxicity is frequently the result of cellular escape from apoptotic inducement. Two dominant pathways govern cellular apoptosis: extrinsic, induced via a receptor–ligand interaction (death receptor), and intrinsic, induced via mitochondria-apoptosome signaling. The converging points for both pathways are the effector caspases, which are closely regulated by upstream signaling proteins either inducing apoptosis or preventing it. A caspase-independent pathway also exists and appears to be mediated through apoptosis-inducing factor (AIF), which is released from mitochondrial pores under control of Bcl-2 and induces nuclear chromatin clumping. The ultimate declaration of apoptosis is largely the balance of proapoptotic proteins (BAX, BID, BAK, and BAD) and anti-apoptotic proteins (Bcl-XI and Bcl-2). Numerous ligands have been identified as substrates for the death receptor including TNF, TNF-related apoptosis-inducing ligand (TRAIL), and Fas. Recently, novel targeted agents harboring agonist activation of this pathway at both the ligand and receptor levels have entered clinical trials [21]. p53, the most commonly mutated gene in human malignancy, functions as a transcription factor regulating downstream genes involved in DNA repair, cell cycle arrest, and both the intrinsic and extrinsic apoptotic pathways. p53, when activated, promotes the proapoptotic genes of the BCL-2 family, which inhibit Bcl-2 at the mitochondrial membrane, as well as activate expression of the death receptors, such as DR5 [21]. In this manner, cross-talk between the intrinsic and extrinsic pathways is extensive. When p53 is dysfunctional, one or both of these pathways may drive carcinogenesis; thus, this serves as a rationale to consider combinatorial treatment approaches, such as targeted therapy of the death receptor ligand in combination with cytotoxic chemotherapy.

11.4 Stimulation of the Immune Response

The immune system is a highly complex and interactive network of specialized cells and organs working in conjunction to maintain health. It is of no surprise that attempts at leveraging innate response or inducing a heightened response to cancer cells have been the subject of cancer therapeutic investigation for decades. The slow, albeit measured, clinical progress in this regard is a reflection of the complexity of the system, the evasiveness of cancer cells, and the imperfect models to preclinically study the system. However, the efficiency, selectivity, and sensitivity of the immune response make it one of the most promising avenues of targeted therapy and worthy of the effort. Key effectors of the immune response include cytokines, such as interferons and interleukins, and antibodies. Contemporary understanding of the interplay between cancer and the immune system suggests that although cancer cells are immunogenic, they do not always elicit a response. This “immunotolerance” is not well understood but may be mediated in part by local anti-inflammatory tumour cytokine production, which may prevent dendritic cells from properly processing tumour cell antigens for a robust immune, anticancer response. Nevertheless, several avenues of investigation have been pursued, the agents used in this regard are called biologic response modifiers (BRMs). The first BRMs to be created and used in cancer therapy were the interferons. As discussed earlier, this class of compounds has both direct and indirect activity on cancer cells. For example, the interferons can slow cancer cell growth or induce phenotypic transformation into normal cell behavior. Interferons also stimulate NK cells, T-cells, and macrophages, which may increase the efficiency of the immune response to effect better anticancer treatment. Several interferon compounds (α, β, and γ) have been US Food and Drug Administration (FDA) approved for cancer therapy, and many have entered mature clinical investigation, including for gynaecologic cancers, albeit with mixed results. For instance, an Austrian phase 3 study randomized 148 women with International Federation of Gynaecology and Obstetrics stage IC-IIIC disease to cisplatin/cyclophosphamide with or without subcutaneously administered interferon-γ. PFS at 3 years was significantly improved (17 vs. 48 months; Relative Risk (RR), 0.48; 95% CI, 0.28–0.82), and toxicity was considered comparable between the arms. However, a much larger phase 3 study conducted by the GRACES clinical trial consortium investigating combination paclitaxel/carboplatin with or without interferon-γ-1b in women with advanced-stage ovarian cancer was terminated early due to an interim futility analysis suggesting detrimental effects in the experimental cohort [22]. The second class of cytokines being investigated as cancer therapeutics is the interleukins (IL). These naturally occurring families of compounds have a vast cache of activities in multiple host systems, including lymphoproliferative organs and angiogenesis and immune system effectors, such as lymphocytes and platelets. Currently, IL-2 (aldesleukin), an IL that stimulates growth and differentiation of the T-cell response, is FDA approved for the treatment of metastatic renal cell carcinoma and melanoma. However, in light of the numerous functions ILs drive in the immune and host response to cancer cells, investigators continue to search for key treatment opportunities. For example, it has been known that IL-6, a proinflammatory cytokine that impacts hematopoietic stem cells, is a poor prognostic factor (associated with advanced disease, chemotherapy resistance, early recurrence, and short survival) of several solid tumours, including the gynaecologic cancers, and is closely linked to angiogenesis, particularly in ovarian cancer, where high levels are also identified in ascites [23]. It also may be an important mediator of the paraneoplastic thrombocytosis phenotype, which is commonly identified in patients with advanced-stage ovarian cancer.

Molecular pathways most commonly targeted in solid tumours are:-

(a) Epidermal growth factor receptors (EGFR),
(b) Vascular endothelial growth factors (VEGF),
(c) HER-2/neu.

The following pathways can be repressed at multi-levels: (a) binding and neutralizing ligands, (b) occupying receptor-binding sites, (c) blocking receptor signaling within the cancer cell, and (d) interfering with downstream intracellular molecules.

There are two types of targeted agents:

(a) Monoclonal antibody with larger molecules (large-molecule inhibitors): It targets extracellular component such as ligand and receptor. The route of administration of this group is intravenous. The examples of large-molecule inhibitors are bevacizumab, trastuzumab, alemtuzumab, cetuximab, gemtuzumab ozogamicin, panitumumab, and rituximab.
(b) Small-molecule inhibitors: They enter cells and inhibit receptor signaling (mainly tyrosine kinase) and interfering with downstream intracellular molecules. Tyrosine kinase signaling initiates a molecular cascade that leads to cell growth, proliferation, migration, and angiogenesis in normal and malignant tissues. As compared to large-molecule inhibitors, small-molecule inhibitors are commonly administered in oral form and are cheaper than large-molecule inhibitors. The examples of small-molecule inhibitors are bortezomib, dasatinib, erlotinib, gefitinib, and others such as imatinib, lapatinib, sorafenib, and sunitinib. Epidermal growth factor receptors are also present in normal cells; therefore, EGFR inhibitors can cause dermatologic complications such as skin rashes and gastrointestinal complications such as diarrhea and abdominal pain.

Anti-VEGF is also known as anti-angiogenesis; without new vessel formation, the tumour cannot grow. Due to better blood supply in the remaining tumour, the delivery of anticancer drugs will be more efficient. However, anti-VEGF will also affect normal blood vessels leading to bleeding, thrombosis, and proteinuria due to alteration in glomerular infiltration, bowel perforation, and hypertension. Bevacizumab is a humanized MoAb against VEGFA that is approved by the FDA for the treatment of metastatic colorectal, non-small-cell lung, renal cell, and breast cancers. Several phase 2 trials of this VEGFA antibody have been performed to assess its activity in gynaecologic cancers. Bevacizumab has been most extensively studied in recurrent ovarian cancer patients, where response rates have ranged from 16% to 24% and median overall survival is 10.7–17 months when administered either as a single agent or in combination with metronomic cyclophosphamide [24–26]. It has also been shown to have activity in the patient with recurrent or persistent endometrial cancer and patients with progressive or recurrent cervical cancer [27, 28]. Majority studies of bevacizumab in gynaecologic cancer have been performed in patients with recurrent or progressive disease. Following encouraging data in phase 2 studies compared with historical controls, two randomized phase 3 studies in untreated advanced ovarian cancer patients have been conducted: GOG 218 (NCT00262847) and ICON-7 (NCT00483782). Each of these trials included an experimental arm with a maintenance treatment phase, which was placebo-controlled in GOG 218 and open label in ICON7. Both trials showed enhanced clinical activity (hazard for progression) over control and, in the case of GOG 218, over combination of paclitaxel, carboplatin, and bevacizumab followed by placebo maintenance. Of interest, the PFS of these "winning" arms is substantively less than that reported by earlier phase 2 data despite a similar proportion of suboptimal stage IIIC patients.

11.5 PI3K/mTOR/Akt Pathway

PTEN (phosphate and tensin homolog detected on chromosome 10) is a tumour suppressor gene, which is important for normal cellular function. Mutations in PTEN can cause decreased apoptosis and these are seen in up to 83% of endometrioid carcinomas of the uterus. Due to mutation, there is decreased transcription which leads to less phosphatidylinositol 3-kinase (PI3K) inhibition, enhanced activity of Akt, and uncontrolled function of mammalian target of rapamycin (mTOR). Elevated activity of mTOR is seen in a vast majority of endometrial cancers as well as approximately 50% of cervical adenocarcinomas and 55% of ovarian carcinomas [29]. mTOR is a kinase that regulates cell growth and apoptosis [30]. Temsirolimus, ridaforolimus, and everolimus are mTOR inhibitors that have been tested as single agents in phase 2 studies and found to promote stable disease in 44% of patients with metastatic or recurrent cancer of the endometrium [31]. Myelosuppression, hyperlipidemia, hypercholesterolemia, and fatigue are most commonly seen side effects of these drugs. Because aberrations in the PI3K/Akt/mTOR pathway are prolific in gynaecologic cancers, drug discovery is keeping pace with several new agents entering the clinical domain. These drugs are being studied as single agents and in combination with chemotherapy and hormonal therapy [30].

11.6 Poly(ADP-Ribose) Pathway

There are a total of 17 members of the poly (ADP-ribose) polymerase (PARP) family, of which PARP-1 and PARP-2 orchestrate repair of single-stranded breaks in DNA [32]. These bind to DNA where there is damage and then start repair by ribosylation of nearby proteins, leading to base-excision repair at the site of damage and downstream effects on transcription and differentiation. Blocking of PARPs through competitive inhibition of the catalytic domain results in accumulation of DNA damage and cell death. BRCA1 and BRCA2 are tumour suppressor genes which plays important in DNA repair at sites of double-stranded breaks. Homologous recombination at DNA-damaged sites is an error free method of DNA repair mediated by Rad51 which is dependent on normal BRCA function. Mutations of BRCA genes drive the cellular machinery to rely on higher error prone methods of DNA repair and in turn promote genomic instability. The primitive studies of PARP inhibitors in BRCA-deficient tumours noted that, although mutations in BRCA increased tumour sensitivity to certain cytotoxic therapies, PARP inhibition causes cell death in this population which is approximately three-fold over conventional treatment. By letting single-stranded breaks unchecked by PARP inhibition, double-stranded DNA breaks are increased in cells that already lack DNA repair capability, a process which is known as synthetic lethality. Normal cells who have intact BRCA function will repair their double-stranded DNA breaks, making these tumour cells more prone to this treatment as compared to normal tissue.

PARP inhibitors are now being used in patients with BRCA-positive ovarian cancer. Among patients with BRCA mutations and ovarian carcinoma treated with olaparib, a response rate of 41–53% was noted [33]. Side effects of olaparib include secondary myeloid leukemias, GI complaints, fatigue, and myelosuppression. The activity of PARP inhibitors may not be limited to patients with germline BRCA mutations. Approximately 50% of undifferentiated and high-grade serous ovarian cancers have a loss of BRCA1 function [34]. Some tumours have BRCA-like functional losses by inactivation of BRCA genes or defects in other genes required for BRCA-associated DNA repair that give in a clinical outcome which is similar to cancers with BRCA mutations. Many evidences highlight that PARP inhibitors results in increased cytotoxic effects of chemotherapy and radiation without regard to BRCA function. These substitute mechanisms of propagating cytotoxic DNA damage has resulted in expansion of the usage of PARP inhibitors in substantial number of malignancies. PARP inhibitors are currently being tested alone and in combination with chemotherapeutic agents, which may induce a susceptible tumour homologous recombination phenotype, to evaluate the potential risks and benefits of these drugs among patients who have impaired and normal BRCA function.

11.7 Principles of Immunotherapy

11.7.1 Tumour Immunbiology and Immunotherapy

As stated by Rushdan Noor, Eng Hseon Tay, and Jeffrey Low in the handbook of gynaecologic oncology "it is an important aspect of cancer biology is the tumour microenvironment, which contributes to tumour initiation, tumour progression and responses to therapy. Cells and molecules of the immune system are basic parts of the tumour microenvironment. Tumour cells express majority of the same cell surface antigens (e.g. HLA antigen) as seen in normal cells. Many tumour cells express specific antigens that are not found in similar normal cells." These are termed as tumour-associated antigens (TAAs). See Fig. 3.

Recognition of antigen by T-cells involves binding of the T-cell receptor to specific major histocompatibility complex (MHC)-peptide combination. By studying the T-cells that identify tumours, many TAAs have now been discovered. Tumour-associated antigens can be classified into five broad groups: (1) mutated antigens (e.g. mutated beta-catenin, caspase, k-ras, in CML, (2) cancer-testis antigens (restricted to testis germ cells, ovary and trophoblast, e.g. MAGE, BAGE, etc.), (3) overexpressed antigen (can be found in normal cell, e.g. p53, Her2/neu), (4) differentiation antigens (only expressed on particular tissue types, e.g. prostate specific antigen, tyrosinase, etc.), (5) oncogenic viral products (in virally induced cancers, e.g. Epstein–Barr virus antigens in lymphomas, HPV virus antigens E6, E7 in anogenital cancers, etc.).

Arguable evidences which suggest humans have tumour limiting factors (immunosurveillance):

1. Spontaneous regression has been reported rarely in cancers such as melanoma, renal cancer, and neuroblastoma. Many have observed that this tumour regression was preceded by surgical intervention (e.g. biopsy, partial resection), infections, administration of bacterial vaccines, transfusion reaction, etc.).
2. Self-healing melanomas.
3. Regression of metastases after resection of primary neoplasms.
4. Regression of tumour after non-cytotoxic doses of chemotherapy.
5. Reappearance of metastases after a long latent period.
6. Frequent failure of circulating tumour cells to form metastases.
7. Infiltration of tumours by mononuclear cells.
8. Higher incidence of tumours after clinical immunosuppression.
9. High incidence of tumour in immune deficiency diseases.
10. Increased incidence of malignancy with aging.

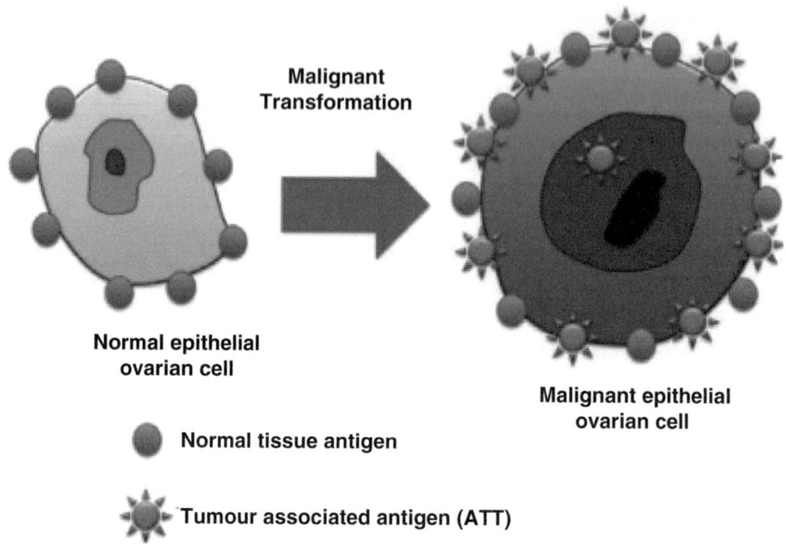

Fig. 3 Tumor-associated antigens are additionally expressed on the tumor cell surface. (Adapted with Permission from 2014 Pan Stanford Publishing Pte. Ltd through email communication)

The first report of successful immunotherapy was in 1881 by William Coley, who treat sarcomas by administrating bacterial toxins [35]. The ultimate goal of immunotherapy is the complete annihilation of all neoplastic cells. Effectiveness of immunotherapy is seen in neoplasms that are highly antigenic, such as Burkitt's lymphoma, malignant melanoma, and neuroblastoma. Tumour can change their antigenic profile and diminish the immune response. Some tumours can down-regulate many of the molecules that are involved in the processing and presentation of the peptide on MHC class I, and that changes occur in the antigenic profile of tumours as they progress and metastasize. The tumour microenvironment has also immunosuppressive properties because of hypoxia, induction, and recruitment of suppressor cells, oxidative stress, etc. This is why many immunotherapies have failed. They may be combined with radiotherapy or chemotherapy. Cancer vaccine has also shown quite a promise in immunotherapy. However, there are three main limitations: firstly, to identify the "correct antigen" that is dissimilar from a normal cell to minimize self-destruction, secondly to find the right adjuvant to enhance an immune response [at present only two adjuvants, aluminum-based salt and squalene oil-water–emulsion (MF56)]; other potential adjuvants are cytokines, bacterial products, heat shock protein, viral-like particles, etc., and finally to induce the right immune response, which is efficient in eradicating tumour cells, sustainable and excellent immune memory. The eventual goal of vaccine-based cancer immunotherapy is to obtain a robust immune response which will result in the eradication of the tumour as well as generate a long-term memory response in order to keep cancer in check.

12 Clinical Practice in Gynaecologic Oncology

12.1 Suitability for Immunotherapy

The outcome for patients can be improved by making primary therapy more effective or by exploring the application of "consolidation" or "maintenance" approaches to patients in a complete primary or subsequent remission. One important issue in evaluating immunotherapeutic approaches in ovarian cancer is to decide where the novel agent should be evaluated in the disease course. In general, the minimal disease state is sought, and the remission populations are best suited. The utility of additional treatment in patients who are in clinical complete remission was first recognized in acute leukemia, and additional "consolidation" or "maintenance" chemotherapy significantly enhanced the outcome for some of these patients. However, these concepts have not shown similar results in solid tumour therapy, and hence the nomenclature remains puzzling. Consolidation therapy is best applied to those strategies that are of limited duration, such as a fixed immunization course, and "maintenance" is best used to describe interventions that continue for years (or until progression) such as with trastuzumab. In ovarian cancer, there were no statistically significant improvement in overall survival, which was seen in randomized consolidation study. Negative randomized consolidation approaches include both subcutaneous and intraperitoneal interferon-α, high-dose chemotherapy, continued intravenous carboplatin versus whole abdominal radiotherapy (WART), chemotherapy versus observation versus WART, intraperitoneal radioactive phosphorus (phosphorus 32), "non-cross-resistant" chemotherapy in the form of cisplatin and 5-fluorouracil for three cycles or topotecan for four cycles, the monoclonal antibody oregovomab, which targets CA-125, and the SMART study [36–38]. Consolidation strategies have generally been used in the first remission population; investigational strategies in the second and third remission groups have been rare and all likewise negative to date [39]. Patients with ovarian cancer in remission are ideal candidates for an immunotherapeutic strategy. Recent data highlight the homogeneity of the second and third remission groups who have a progression-free survival (PFS) interval of fewer than 12 months so that hints of efficacy from a given immunotherapeutic approach could be recognized with a shorter follow-up interval than that required in the first remission. The number of therapeutic strategies under investigation for immunotherapy in patients with ovarian cancer is large. Most trials are pilot studies or phase 1 trials that has assessed safety and immunogenicity. Some of them have shown improved outcomes with surrogates such as an antibody or T-cell response, and most current trials aim to produce cellular responses. The number of adequately powered randomized trials is few, however, and none has shown definitive efficacy to date.

12.2 Antibodies Used as Immunogens

Although some antibodies are administered in the treatment of patients with cancer to convey passive immunity, they may also be used as immunogens and can elicit a complex immune response. Oregovomab (MAb B43.13), which is an IgG1k subclass murine monoclonal antibody that binds with high affinity (1.16×10^{10}/M) to circulating CA-125, has been evaluated. Both cellular and humoral immune responses have been seen with the production of anti-oregovomab antibodies (Ab2), T-helper cells, and cytotoxic T-cells in addition to the human anti-mouse antibody (HAMA) response. Nonrandomized studies have consistently shown longer overall survival with immune response. A randomized placebo-controlled trial in patients with stage III or IV epithelial ovarian cancer in first clinical remission receiving oregovomab or placebo showed no benefit using the intent-to-treat population. However, a favorable subgroup of patients showed a time to progression advantage favoring vaccination of 24 months versus 10.8 months (hazard ratio, 0.543; 95% CI, 0.287–1.025). This subgroup was appropriately considered to be hypothesis-generating, and a follow-up study enrolled 354 patients using the characteristics of this group as eligibility criteria. The median time to progression was 10.3 months (95% CI, 9.7–13.0 months) for the oregovomab group and 12.9 months (95% CI, 10.1–17.4 months) for the placebo group, showing no benefit to oregovomab immunotherapy [38]. Another antibody strategy is immunization with an anti-idiotype vaccine. The hypothesis is that the antigenicity of the immunogen can be increased by presenting the desired epitope to the now tolerant host in a different molecular environment. The "immune network hypothesis," which provided the foundation for this approach, was initially proposed in the early 1970s and explains an interconnected group of idiotypes that are expressed by antibodies. The proposed mechanism assumes that immunization with a given antigen will generate the production of antibodies against this antigen (termed Ab1). Ab1 can generate anti-idiotype antibodies against Ab1, classified as Ab2. Some of the anti-idiotypic antibodies (Ab2β) express the internal image of the antigen recognized by the Ab1 antibody and can be used as surrogate antigens. Immunization with Ab2β (the anti-idiotype antibody) can cause the production of anti-anti-idiotype antibodies (classified as Ab3) that recognize the corresponding original antigen identified by Ab1. Ab3 antibodies are also denoted Ab1′ to show that they may differ in their other epitopes compared with Ab1. A previous phase 1/2 study of abagovomab, the anti-idiotype monoclonal antibody whose epitope mirrors CA-125, suggested that Ab3 production was associated with overall survival. Other studies have shown an increase in interferon-γ expression of CA-125-specific CD8 + T-cells following immunization, but there has been no specific correlation between the induction of Ab3 and frequencies of CA-125-specific cytotoxic T-lymphocytes and T-helper cells. The efficacy of abagovomab in patients in the first remission was evaluated in an international phase 3, randomized, double-blind, placebo-controlled study ongoing in approximately 120 study locations (MIMOSA Trial). Outcomes were recurrence-free survival, overall survival, and safety. Preliminary blinded immunogenicity results were reported with 888 patients enrolled in the study and showed that 68% and 69% of all patients were positive for Ab3 (median values, 62,000 ng/mL and 337,000 ng/mL, respectively), whereas 53% and 63% of patients were positive for HAMA (median values, 510 ng/mL and 644 ng/mL, respectively).

12.3 Cancer-Testis Antigen Vaccines

Cancer-testis antigens represent a distinct class of differentiation antigens. The family has grown from the original melanoma-associated antigen 1 (MAGE-1) identified in a melanoma cell line to 100 cancer-testis genes or gene families identified in a recent database established by the Ludwig Institute for Cancer Research [40]. These antigens share several characteristics, including preferential expression in normal tissues on the testis and expression in tumours of varying histology (including ovarian cancer), and many are members of multigene families that are mostly encoded on chromosome X. Cancer-testis antigen expression has been correlated with clinical and pathologic parameters in a variety of tumours. MAGE-A4 expression shows an inverse correlation between expression and patient survival, for example, in ovarian cancer. The NY-ESO-1 antigen, initially defined by SEREX in esophageal cancer, is expressed in several tumours, including 40% of epithelial ovarian cancers. NY-ESO-1 MHC class I and II-restricted epitopes (recognized by CD8 + cytotoxic and CD4 + helper T-cells) have been characterized, including those recognized in conjunction with human leukocyte antigen (HLA)-A2 as well as with other haplotypes. Both NY-ESO-1 peptides and full recombinant protein have been administered to patients on protocols with immunogenicity as the primary endpoint with various adjuvants. Vaccination has been shown to induce both humoral and T-cell responses [41]. In a phase 1 trial in patients with epithelial ovarian cancer in the first remission immunized with HLA-A*0201–restricted NY-ESO-1b peptide with montanide ISA-51 as the adjuvant [42], treatment was well tolerated. Seven (77%) of nine patients showed T-cell immunity by tetramer and ELISPOT analyses. Multiple approaches have been used to try and enhance the inherently limited immunogenicity of these peptide vaccinations. Some have included amino acid substitution at different anchor positions of Melan-A/MART-126-352L; terminal alteration of MART-127-35; replacement of cysteine residues for NY-ESO-1; modification of T-cell receptor-interacting amino acid residues for carcinoembryonic antigen; and loading of peptides onto autologous dendritic cells. In addition, cytokines and costimulatory molecules have been administered.

12.4 Dendritic Cell-Based Vaccines

Dendritic cells act as antigen-presenting cells. They endocytose, process, and then present tumour antigens to T-cells. Many strategies are currently underway to manipulate the dendritic cell for use in immunotherapy. Dendritic cells have been pulsed with tumour-associated peptides or proteins and mRNA-encoded receptors such as folate receptor-α [43]. Other vaccines have been developed by the viral transduction of dendritic cells with tumour-specific genes or through transfection with liposomal DNA or RNA. Another strategy that has been tried to avoid the need to specifically define the effective tumour-associated antigens is to pulse them with tumour lysates or tumour protein extracts. In many cases, preclinical models have suggested protective immunity to subsequent tumour challenge, which supports further interest in investigating the approach. A specific example includes a study by Czerniecki et al. [44] in which advanced breast and ovarian cancer patients were treated with dendritic cells pulsed with HER-2/neu or MUC-1–derived peptides. In 50% of patients, peptide-specific cytotoxic T-cell lymphocytes were generated. Side effects were minimal. Gong and colleagues [45] fused human ovarian cells to human dendritic cells and likewise showed the proliferation of autologous T-cells, including cytotoxic T-cell activity with lysis of autologous tumour cells by an MHC class I restricted mechanism (i.e., demonstrating that the effector cells had the desired activity). Heat shock proteins, which are molecular chaperones that facilitate protein folding, have also been isolated, along with accompanying peptides and used as immunogens. Heat shock peptide complexes have been shown to interact with dendritic cells via the CD91 receptor. The heat shock proteins are taken up by endocytosis, are cross-presented by MHC-I molecules on the dendritic cells, and result in activation of naïve CD8 + cells along with upregulation of costimulatory molecules and the production of cytokines. Many reported studies have similar immunologic endpoints, but the clinical interpretation is often difficult from phase 1/2 trials without comparators.

12.5 Vaccines Designed to Generate Antibody Responses

Most current vaccines seek to generate cellular responses (often with an accompanying humoral response), but a vaccine is currently in phase 2 randomized trial in ovarian cancer (Gynaecology Oncology Group [GOG] Study 255) that evaluates a vaccine approach primarily designed to augment antibodies. Techniques for the chemical and enzymatic synthesis of carbohydrate and glycopeptide antigens have allowed the development of a range of synthetic vaccines that depend on antibody production and ADCC as the primary effectors. A variety of options such as different adjuvant therapies, schedules, and methods of conjugation have been tried to enhance immunogenicity. A proposed optimal construct has consisted of an antigen (single or multiple) with the carrier protein keyhole limpet hemocyanin (KLH) and the saponin adjuvant QS-21 (or OPT-821) [46].

12.6 Adoptive Cellular Therapy

Using the adoptive cellular therapy approach, one selects and activates many lymphocytes and introduces them into a modified host environment with a selected target. One way T-cells may be modified to recognize tumour-associated antigens is to introduce ex vivo a gene encoding artificial T-cell receptors termed chimeric antigen receptors (CARs) against a specific tumour-associated antigen. The first phase 1 study in patients with epithelial ovarian cancer using gene-modified autologous T-cells with reactivity against ovarian cancer-associated antigen α-folate receptor (FR) has been reported [47]. Cohort 1 received T-cells with IL-2 and cohort 2 received dual specific T-cells followed by allogeneic peripheral blood mononuclear cells. There was no reduction which was seen in tumour burden of any patient. Polymerase chain reaction examination showed that gene-modified T-cells were present in the circulation 2 days after transfer but thereafter declined. An inhibitory factor was developed in the serum of 3 out of 6 patients tested over the treatment period significantly reduced the ability of gene-modified T-cells to respond against FR-positive tumour cells. Further studies are needed to use strategies to increase T-cell persistence. The chimeric receptor approach continues to evolve in specificity against targets expressed in ovarian cancer such as the LeY carbohydrate antigen (expressed on 70% of ovarian cancer cells) or HER-2/neu. Most recently, receptors have been engineered to target the extracellular domain (termed MUC-CD) of MUC16 (CA125), which is expressed in most ovarian carcinoma [48]. In vitro, these CAR-modified, MUC-CD-targeted T-cells showed MUC-CD-specific cytolytic activity against ovarian cell lines, and infusion into severe combined immunodeficiency (SCID)-beige mice bearing orthotopic human MUC-CD–positive ovarian carcinoma tumours showed delayed disease progression or eradication. Clinical trials are planned. One necessary challenge to overcome is how to circumvent the multiple mechanisms in the tumour microenvironment that inhibit tumour-targeted T-cells. Options under investigation include administering T-cells after lymphodepleting chemotherapy, antibody-based blockade of inhibitory ligands, and infusion of proinflammatory cytokines such as IL-12.

12.7 Whole Tumour Antigen Vaccines

This strategy seeks to overcome some of the potential problems associated with trying to generate specific immune responses. In the latter case, the response may simply miss the target, it can be limited to only the epitopes provided on the stimulating antigen and drive variants of tumour cells that can evade the immune response (immunoediting), or it may be restricted to small numbers of patients of a certain HLA type, as in the case of using HLA-restricted peptides [42]. The reason for using whole tumour antigen vaccines is that it allows one to immunize without needing to define the tumour-associated antigens. They can be derived from autologous tumour cells or using an allogeneic strategy. One obvious challenge in using whole tumour antigen vaccines is that the tumour is currently residing in a host where tolerance to the tumour is already present. This tolerance is likely produced in multiple ways, including the production of IL-10 and transforming growth factor (TGF)-β to inhibit T-cell and dendritic cell functions, VEGF to inhibit dendritic cell maturation and differentiation, and soluble Fas ligand, which induces lymphocyte apoptosis. The whole tumour immunogen, therefore, is processed or modified in some way in an attempt to overcome this. Strategies have included using apoptotic whole tumour cells (developed with a lethal dose of irradiation), using necrotic tumour cell lysates (created with repetitive freezing and thawing and often administered as pulsed dendritic cells), and constructing dendritic cell/tumour fusion vaccines [49]. The issue of how to increase the immunogenicity of whole tumour vaccines remains a priority. One effective approach has been the use of a replication-deficient herpes simplex virus to infect tumour cells, which are subsequently engulfed and show enhanced ability to both activate NK cells and provide a costimulatory signal for T-cells.

12.8 Immune Checkpoint Inhibitors

Immune checkpoint synapses consist of several co-inhibitory molecules that are primarily responsible for limiting T-cell receptor signaling and abrogating immune responses. This strategic process set in place by the immune system is useful to halt immune responses in individuals after microbial infections are resolved, or in the development of self-tolerance to limit autoimmune disease. However, in cancer, high levels of immune checkpoint molecules on immune cells or on tumour cells are often associated with exhausted T-cells, which are incapable of developing aggressive anti-tumour responses, as well as with resistance to several classes of therapy [50–52]. .Immune checkpoints (IC) present potent immune-suppressive mechanisms in cancer, and blocking of two of these pathways in particular has provided useful therapeutic alternatives to improve survival in many cancer types. Briefly, the binding of CD28 on T-cells to B7-1/B7-2 (CD80/CD86) on antigen-presenting cells (APC) results in costimulatory anti-tumour responses. However, co-inhibitory molecule CTLA-4 on T-cells has a higher affinity for B7-1/B7-2 molecules than does CD28, and the preferential binding of CTLA-4 to B7-1/B7-2 blocks IL-2 release from T-cells and limits T-cell proliferation.

12.9 Immune Checkpoint Blockade Therapy in Endometrial Cancer

Immune checkpoint inhibitors have shown efficacy in multiple advanced solid tumours, predominantly among MMRd and MSI-H cancers and those with a high tumour mutational burden, such as endometrial cancer. The phase II KEYNOTE-158 study evaluated the anti-tumour activity and safety of pembrolizumab in previously treated, advanced non-colorectal MSI-H/MMRd cancers. Patients were treated with a fixed dose of pembrolizumab 200 mg IV once every 3 weeks for 2 years or until disease progression, unacceptable toxicity, or patient withdrawal. Among patients with a broad range of solid tumours including 27 tumour types, there were 49 patients with endometrial cancer (21% of the treatment population). In the cohort of patients with endometrial cancer, the ORR was 57.1%, with eight patients (16%) achieving a complete response and 20 patients (41%) achieving a partial response. The median PFS was 25.7 months. In the entire study cohort of 233 patients, 64.8% of patients had treatment-related adverse events and 14.6% had grade 3–5 treatment-related adverse events, with one grade 5 event related to pneumonia. The most common treatment-related adverse events were fatigue, pruritus, diarrhea, and asthenia. This study further indicated that MSI/MMRd status could be a predictor of the response to PD-1 blockade in endometrial cancer [53]. KEYNOTE-146/Study 111 was a single-arm, open label, phase Ib/II study to evaluate the safety and efficacy of lenvatinib plus pembrolizumab in advanced solid tumours, including endometrial carcinoma. Patients received lenvatinib 20 mg once daily orally plus pembrolizumab 200 mg IV once every 3 weeks, based on the recommended dosing from the phase Ib portion of the study. The final primary efficacy analysis was reported for the patient cohort with advanced endometrial carcinoma. The primary endpoint was ORR at 24 weeks (ORRWk24). The ORRWk24 was 38% in the cohort of 108 patients who were previously treated with conventional therapy. For 94 patients with MSS/MMRp tumours, ORR as measured by immune-related RECIST (irRECIST) was 37.2% versus 63.6% for 11 patients with MSI-H/MMRd tumours [54].

12.10 Immune Checkpoint Blockade Therapy in Cervical Cancer

Conventional treatment options for metastatic/recurrent cervical cancer additionally includes radiotherapy and chemotherapy, and this treatment is most often not sufficiently effective for disease management at this late stage. In a phase II KEYNOTE-158 trial, pembrolizumab was investigated in a single cohort trial of 98 patients with recurrent/metastatic cervical cancer. Of 77 patients, the ORR was 14.3% (95% CI: 7.4, 24.1), with 11.7% partial responses and 2.6% complete responses, whereas no responses were found in patients with tumours not expressing PD-L1 (NCT02628067). With this outcome, pembrolizumab was subsequently approved in 2018 for recurrent/metastatic cervical cancer patients with PD-L1 positive tumours [53].

References

1. Hanahan D, Weinberg RA. Hallmarks of cancer: the next generation. Cell. 2011;144:646–74.
2. Lemmon MA, Schlessinger J. Cell signaling by receptor tyrosine kinases. Cell. 2010;141:1117–34.
3. Negrini S, Gorgoulis VG, Halazonetis TD. Genomic instability: an evolving hallmark of cancer. Nat Rev Mol Cell Biol. 2010;11:220–8.
4. Skipper HE. Kinetics of mammary tumor cell growth and implications for therapy. Cancer. 1971;28:1479–99.
5. Norton LA. A Gompertzian model of human breast cancer growth. Cancer Res. 1988;48:7067–71.
6. Raguz S, Yague E. Resistance to chemotherapy: new treatments and novel insights into an old problem. Br J Cancer. 2008;99:387–91.
7. Gerlinger M, Swanton C. How Darwinian models inform therapeutic failure initiated by clonal heterogeneity in cancer medicine. Br J Cancer. 2010;103:1139–43.
8. Goldie JH, Coldman AJ. A mathematical model for relating the drug sensitivity of tumors to the spontaneous mutation rate. Cancer Treat Rep. 1979;63:1727–33.
9. Bookman MA, Brady MF, McGuire WP, et al. Evaluation of new platinum-based treatment regimens in advanced-stage ovarian cancer: a phase III trial of the Gynecologic Cancer InterGroup. J Clin Oncol. 2009;27:1419–25.
10. Tan DS-W, Gerlinger M, The B-T, et al. Anti-cancer drug resistance: understanding the mechanisms through the use of integrative genomics and functional RNA interference. Eur J Cancer. 2010;46:2166–77.
11. Sakai S, Swisher EM, Karlan BY, et al. Secondary mutations as a mechanism of cisplatin resistance in BRCA2-mutated cancers. Nature. 2008;451:1116–21.
12. Cress RD, O'Malley CD, Leiserowitz GS, et al. Patterns of chemotherapy use for women with ovarian cancer: a population based study. J Clin Oncol. 2003;21:1530–5.
13. Citron ML, Berry DA, Cirrincione C, et al. Randomized trial of dose-dense versus conventionally scheduled and sequential versus concurrent combination chemotherapy as postoperative adjuvant treatment of node-positive primary breast cancer: first report of Intergroup Trial C9741/Cancer and Leukemia Group B Trial 9741. J Clin Oncol. 2003;21:1431–9.
14. Pfisterer J, Plante M, Vergote I, et al. Gemcitabine plus carboplatin compared with carboplatin in patients with platinum-sensitive recurrent ovarian cancer: an intergroup trial of the AGO-OVAR, the NCIC CTG, and the EORTC GCG. J Clin Oncol. 2006;24:2699–707.
15. Siemann DW, Horsman MR. Modulation of the tumor vasculature and oxygenation to improve therapy. Pharmacol Ther. 2015;153:107–24.
16. Borner M, Scheithauer W, Twelves C, et al. Answering patients' needs: oral alternatives to intravenous therapy. Oncologist. 2001;4:12.
17. Dedrick RL, Myers CE, Bungay PM, et al. Pharmacokinetic rationale for peritoneal drug administration in the treatment of ovarian cancer. Cancer Treat Rep. 1978;62:1–9.
18. Markman M. Intraperitoneal therapy of ovarian cancer. Semin Oncol. 1998;25:356–60.
19. Markman M, Kelsen D. Efficacy of cisplatin-based intraperitoneal chemotherapy as treatment of malignant peritoneal mesothelioma. J Cancer Res ClinOncol. 1992;118:547–50.
20. Rocha-Lima CM, Soares HP, Raez LE, Singal R. EGFR targeting of solid tumors. Cancer Control. 2007;14(3):295–304.
21. Wiezorek J, Holland P, Graves J. Death receptor agonists as a targeted therapy for cancer. Clin Cancer Res. 2010;16(6):1701–8.
22. Alberts DS, Marth C, Alvarez RD, et al. Randomized phase 3 trial of interferon gamma-1b plus standard carboplatin/paclitaxel versus carboplatin/paclitaxel alone for first-line treatment of advanced ovarian and primary peritoneal carcinomas: results from a prospectively designed analysis of progression-free survival. Gynecol Oncol. 2008;109(2):174–81.
23. Giuntoli RL II, Webb TJ, Zoso A, et al. Ovarian cancer-associated ascites demonstrates altered immune environment: implications for antitumor immunity. Anticancer Res. 2009;29(8):2875–84.
24. Burger RA, Sill MW, Monk BJ, Greer BE, Sorosky JI. Phase II trial of bevacizumab in persistent or recurrent epithelial ovarian cancer or primary peritoneal cancer: a Gynecologic Oncology Group study. J Clin Oncol. 2007;25:5165–71.
25. Cannistra SA, Matulonis UA, Penson RT, et al. Phase II study of bevacizumab in patients with platinum-resistant ovarian cancer or peritoneal serous cancer. J Clin Oncol. 2007;25(33):5180–6.
26. Garcia AA, Hirte H, Fleming G, et al. Phase II clinical trial of bevacizumab and low-dose metronomic oral cyclophosphamide in recurrent ovarian cancer: a trial of the California, Chicago, and Princess Margaret Hospital phase II consortia. J Clin Oncol. 2008;26(1):76–82.
27. Aghajanian C, Sill MW, Darcy KM, et al. A phase II evaluation of bevacizumab in the treatment of recurrent or persistent endometrial cancer: a Gynecologic Oncology Group (GOG) study. J Clin Oncol. 2009;27(15_Suppl):5531.
28. Monk BJ, Sill MW, Burger RA, Gray HJ, Buekers TE, Roman LD. Phase II trial of bevacizumab in the treatment of persistent or recurrent squamous cell car-

cinoma of the cervix: a Gynecologic Oncology Group study. J Clin Oncol. 2009;27(7):1069–74.
29. Faried LS, Faried A, Kanuma T, et al. Expression of an activated mammalian target of rapamycin in adenocarcinoma of the cervix: a potential biomarker and molecular target therapy. Mol Carcinog. 2008;47(6):446–57.
30. Bansal N, Yendluri V, Wenham RM. The molecular biology of endometrial cancers and the implications for pathogenesis, classification, and targeted therapies. Cancer Control. 2009;16(1):8–13.
31. Slomovitz BM, Lu KH, Johnston T, et al. A phase 2 study of the oral mammalian target of rapamycin inhibitor, everolimus, in patients with recurrent endometrial carcinoma. Cancer. 2010;116(23):5415–9.
32. Miwa M, Masutani M. PolyADP-ribosylation and cancer. Cancer Sci. 2007;98(10):1528–35.
33. Fong PC, Boss DS, Yap TA, et al. Inhibition of poly(ADP-ribose) polymerase in tumors from BRCA mutation carriers. N Engl J Med. 2009;361(2):123–34.
34. Press JZ, De Luca A, Boyd N, et al. Ovarian carcinomas with genetic and epigenetic BRCA1 loss have distinct molecular abnormalities. BMC Cancer. 2008;8:17.
35. Coley WB. The treatment of malignant tumours by repeated inoculations of erysipelas: with a report of ten original cases. Am J Med Sci. 1893;105:487.
36. Alberts DS, Hannigan EV, Liu PY, et al. Randomized trial of adjuvant intraperitoneal alpha-interferon in stage III ovarian cancer patients who have no evidence of disease after primary surgery and chemotherapy: an intergroup study. Gynecol Oncol. 2006;100(1):133–8.
37. Verheijen RH, Massuger LF, Benigno BB, et al. Phase III trial of intraperitoneal therapy with yttrium90-labeled HMFG1 murine monoclonal antibody in patients with epithelial ovarian cancer after a surgically defined complete remission. J Clin Oncol. 2006;24(4):571–8.
38. Berek J, Taylor P, McGuire W, Smith LM, Schultes B, Nicodemus CF. Oregovomab maintenance monoimmunotherapy does not improve outcomes in advanced ovarian cancer. J Clin Oncol. 2009;27(3):418–25.
39. Sabbatini P. Consolidation therapy in ovarian cancer: a clinical update. Int J Gynecol Cancer. 2009;19(Suppl 2):S35–9.
40. van der Bruggen P, Traversari C, Chomez P, Lurquin C, De Plaen E, Van den Eynde B, Knuth A, Boon T. A gene encoding an antigen recognized by cytolytic T lymphocytes on a human melanoma. Science. 1991;254:1643–7.
41. Odunsi K, Qian F, Matsuzaki J, et al. Vaccination with an NY-ESO-1 peptide of HLA class I/II specificities induces integrated humoral and T cell responses in ovarian cancer. Proc Natl Acad Sci U S A. 2007;104(31):12837–42.
42. Diefenbach CS, Gnjatic S, Sabbatini P, et al. Safety and immunogenicity study of NY-ESO-1b peptide and montanide ISA-51 vaccination of patients with epithelial ovarian cancer in high-risk first remission. Clin Cancer Res. 2008;14(9):2740–8.
43. Hernando JJ, Park TW, Fischer HP, et al. Vaccination with dendritic cells transfected with mRNA encoded folate-receptor-alpha for relapsed metastatic ovarian cancer. Lancet Oncol. 2007;8(5):451–4.
44. Czerniecki BJ, Koski GK, Koldovsky U, et al. Targeting HER-2/neu in early breast cancer development using dendritic cells with staged interleukin-12 burst secretion. Cancer Res. 2007;67(4):1842–52.
45. Gong J, Apostolopoulos V, Chen D, et al. Selection and characterization of MUC1-specific $CD8^+$ T cells from MUC1 transgenic mice immunized with dendritic-carcinoma fusion cells. J Immunol. 2000;101(3):316–24.
46. Sabbatini PJ, Ragupathi G, Hood C, et al. Pilot study of a heptavalent vaccine-keyhole limpet hemocyanin conjugate plus QS21 in patients with epithelial ovarian, fallopian tube, or peritoneal cancer. Clin Cancer Res. 2007;13(14):4170–7.
47. Kershaw MH, Westwood JA, Parker LL, et al. A phase I study on adoptive immunotherapy using gene-modified T cells for ovarian cancer. Clin Cancer Res. 2006;12(20 Pt 1):6106–15.
48. Chekmasova AA, Brentjens RJ. Adoptive T cell immunotherapy strategies for the treatment of patients with ovarian cancer. Discov Med. 2010;9(44):62–70.
49. Hatfield P, Merrick AE, West E, et al. Optimization of dendritic cell loading with tumor cell lysates for cancer immunotherapy. J Immunother. 2008;31(7):620–32.
50. Sun C, Mezzadra R, Schumacher TN. Regulation and function of the PD-L1 checkpoint. Immunity. 2018;48:434–52.
51. Zhou G, Sprengers D, Boor PPC, Doukas M, Schutz H, Mancham S, Pedroza-Gonzalez A, Polak WG, de Jonge J, Gaspersz M, et al. Antibodies against immune checkpoint molecules restore functions of tumor-infiltrating T cells in hepatocellular carcinomas. Gastroenterology. 2017;153:1107–19.
52. Salmaninejad A, Valilou SF, Shabgah AG, Aslani S, Alimardani M, Pasdar A, Sahebkar A. PD-1/PD-L1 pathway: basic biology and role in cancer immunotherapy. J Cell Physiol. 2019;234:16824–37.
53. Marabelle A, Le DT, Ascierto PA, Di Giacomo AM, De Jesus-Acosta A, Delord JP, Geva R, Gottfried M, Penel N, Hansen AR, et al. Efficacy of pembrolizumab in patients with noncolorectal high microsatellite instability/mismatch repair-deficient cancer: results from the phase II KEYNOTE-158 study. J Clin Oncol. 2020;38:1–10.
54. Makker V, Taylor MH, Aghajanian C, Oaknin A, Mier J, Cohn AL, Romeo M, Bratos R, Brose MS, DiSimone C, et al. Lenvatinib plus pembrolizumab in patients with advanced endometrial cancer. J Clin Oncol. 2020;38:2981–92.

Principles and Practice of Radiation Oncology

Moirangthem Nara Singh, Rajesh Ashok Kinhikar, Jai Prakash Agarwal, and Sarbani Ghosh Laskar

1 Introduction

In radiation oncology, radiation is designated as a "2-Edges Swords" because it helps control and induces cancer [1]. Radiotherapy plays an essential part in dealing with more than 50% of all patients with cancer, among other modalities like surgery and chemotherapy [2]. In 1895, Wilhelm Conrad Roentgen discovered X-rays, one of the scientific community's milestones. In 1896, Henri Becquerel and Marie Curie discovered certain chemical elements that produced these energy rays and this phenomenon was coined as radioactivity, and they got a novel prize in 1905. The application of X-ray has been used in medical applications after 1 month of its discovery.

M. N. Singh (✉)
Department of Radiation Oncology, Dr. Bhubaneswar Booroah Cancer Institute, Guwahati, India

R. A. Kinhikar
Department of Medical Physics, Tata Memorial Centre, Mumbai, India

J. P. Agarwal · S. G. Laskar
Department of Radiation Oncology, Tata Memorial Centre, Mumbai, India
e-mail: agarwaljp@tmc.gov.in

2 Timeline of Radiation Therapy (RT)

The milestone timeline of discovery and development of radiation therapy practices and techniques are shown in Fig. 1 [3]. Nowadays, cancer treatment remains based on three primary treatment modalities: surgery, radiation therapy, and chemotherapy, along with other treatment tactics such as immunotherapy, targeted therapy, and gene therapy.

Radiation therapy (RT) has been an essential treatment for cancer patients for more than a century. Radiation therapy, also known as radiotherapy, is a treatment method that relies on radiation to damage tumour cells and eliminate them from growing and further dividing. About two-thirds of all cancer patients receive RT as a single treatment modality or as part of a more combined treatment modality. The new era of RT started in the 1970s with the introdcution of 3D based images systems, namely computed tomography (CT). The significant advantage of using ion beams is its controllability, which provides an excellent tool for cancer therapy and difficult-to-treat benign diseases [4, 5].

Primarily, radiation therapy used gamma-ray and X-ray radiations. Moreover, particle radiation such as electron, proton, carbo ions, and neutron are preferred due to their unique advantages over primary radiations. Conformal techniques also influence radiation, which has less toxicity than early treatment techniques able to treat in

A. C. Kataki, D. Barmon (eds.), *Fundamentals in Gynaecologic Malignancy*,
https://doi.org/10.1007/978-981-19-5860-1_8

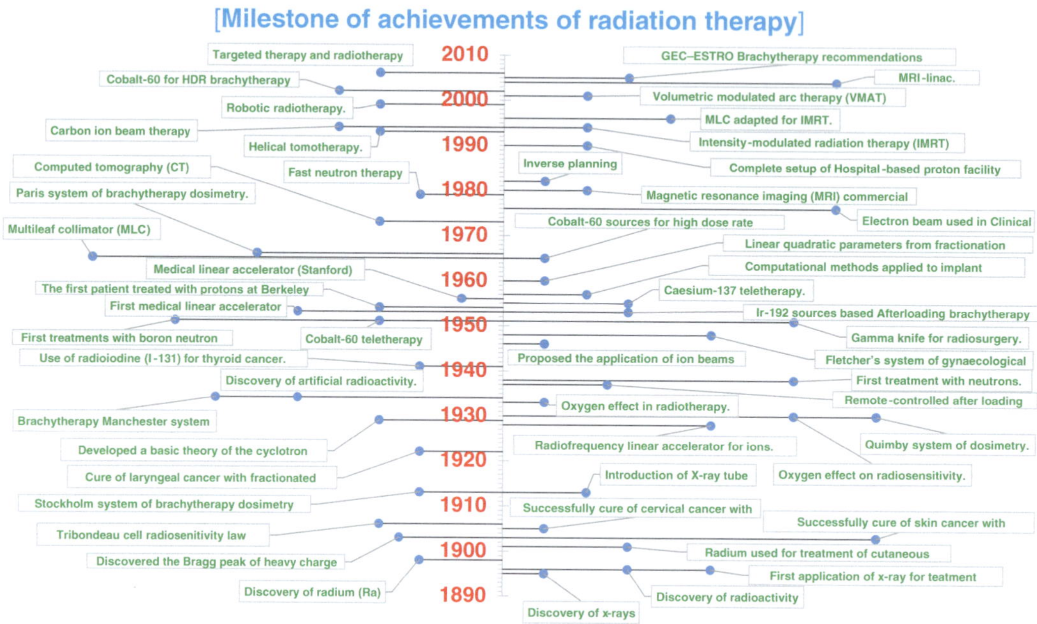

Fig. 1 Milestone achievements of radiation therapy

more efficacy and safer ways [6]. Image-guided radiotherapy (IGRT) enhanced the precision and accuracy of the advanced treatment techniques in radiation therapy [7].

3 Effects of Radiation Interaction

The main implications of the interaction of radiation with matter used in therapy physics or radio-diagnostic are radiation dosimetry, radiation detection, and radiation shielding [8].

(a) ***Radiation Shielding***

The nature of radiation intersection of shielding materials provides the situation shield for the particular type of radiation.

(b) ***Radiation Detection***

Radiation detection is a vital requirement to radiation workers for safety aspects. It detects/measures the number of secondary charges produced in the sensitive volume. The detector response depends on the charged or uncharged radiation type of interaction.

(c) ***Radiation Dosimetry***

Radiation dosimetry is the measurement of radiation quantities like absorbed dose, and it depends on the types of interaction of the incident radiation with the medium under consideration.

This section presents the interaction of different types of ionizing radiation mainly used in medical applications like the photons, particulate and uncharged with the matter, and physical aspects in radiation therapy. The main classification of ionizing radiation used in medical applications is shown in Fig. 2.

3.1 Interaction of Photons with Matter

When X-ray and γ-ray radiations incident on a medium, it may transfer part of its energy to the medium. Then, it produces some physical or chemical changes in the medium. The energy

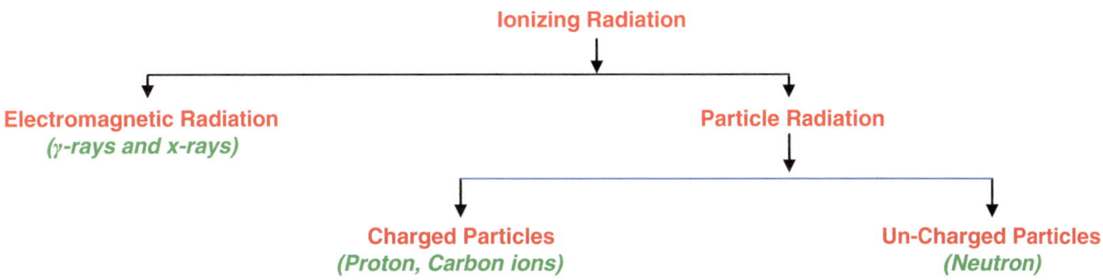

Fig. 2 Classification of type of radiation with examples

Table 1 Classification of photons interaction with matter

Type of interaction → / Interaction with ↓	Absorption	Scattering: Elastic (coherent)	Scattering: In-elastic (incoherent)
Atomic electrons	(a) Photoelectric effect	(b) Rayleigh scattering	(c) Compton scattering
Nucleons	(d) Photo-nuclear reaction	(e) Elastic nuclear scattering	(f) Nuclear resonance scattering
Electric field of nucleus/ electron	(g) Pair production (h) Triple production (i) Field of nucleus (j) Field of electron	(k) Delbruck scattering	–
Mesons	(l) Photo-meson production	–	–

transfer to the medium could be likely by 12 types of interactions as given in Table 1 with different interactions, such as interaction with the entire atom of the medium, the free electron of the atom, and the atomic nucleus or bound electron [9].

Photoelectric effects are predominant at low energy, but it reduces gradually with high energies of incident beams. The Compton process is predominant when the energy of incident radiation is from 200 keV to 5 MeV. Above 10 MeV, the total coefficient for air is constant because of the increase in pair productions. In pair production, the positron interacts with an electron and subsequently annihilate to produce two photons emitted 180° apart with energy 0.511 MeV. This principle is employed in the positron emission tomography (PET) [10].

In photodisintegration, photon energy (<10 MV) interacts with the atomic nucleus and produces radiation like neutron and alpha particles. Because of this effect, in medical linear accelerators with high energies photons need extra shielding in the room layout for neutron radiations [11].

3.2 Interaction of Charged Particles with Matter

Uncharged particle interactions, charge particles lose their energy entirely differently. Most of these interactions transfer some fractions of the incident particle's energy as if the particle is gradually losing its kinetic energy in a friction-like process, also known as continuous slowing down approximation (CSDA) [12]. The charged particle loses its kinetic energy or change from its path due to inelastic collision with atomic electron or soft collision, nucleus and elastic collision with a nucleus, an atomic electron [13].

3.2.1 Bragg Curve

The Bragg peak plots the energy loss of ionizing charged particle radiation such as protons, α-rays, and other ion rays, during its travel through matter [14]. When fast-moving charged particle passages through the medium, it starts to ionize and store a dose along its track. A peak is a presence in-depth dose profile due to the interaction cross-section increasing as the charged particle's energy decreases. The lost charged particles' energy is proportional to the inverse square of their velocity just before the particle comes to a complete stop [8].

3.2.2 Bremsstrahlung

The bremsstrahlung (continuous X-ray spectrum) is due to the Inelastic collision of electrons with the atomic nucleus. According to classical theory, it will radiate when a charged particle accelerates or decelerates. Therefore, an incident charged particle is deflected from its original path or changed of velocity, and it should emit radiation. The bremsstrahlung is dependent on the square of the atomic number of the absorbing material and is inversely proportional to the square of the mass of the incident particle. Hence, heavy particles like protons and α particle produce negligible bremsstrahlung X-rays. The shape of the spectral distribution of bremsstrahlung is independent of atomic number. At very low electron energies, X-ray intensity is predominant at right angles to the incident beam. When the electron energies increase, the maximum radiation intensity moves forward [8, 12].

3.3 Interaction of Neutron with Matter

Neutron interaction can broadly divide two types of neutron interaction: absorption (capture reaction) and scattering. It has lost some part of its energy during scattering. Because of the uncharged nature of the neutrons, their absorption in the matter cannot take place directly in the same manner as the charged particle. However, neutrons can experience a force when they come within highly close range of the nuclei. Hence their absorption in the matter is due to the exclusively short-range interaction with nuclei. Fast neutron loses their energies by colliding elastically with atoms and slowed down to thermal energies and then captured. Similarly to the gamma rays' effect, neutrons are removed exponentially from the beam. Hydrogenous compounds effectively slow down fast neutrons (paraffin, water). It should contain sufficient additives (boron, cadmium) to absorb slow neutrons, and borated polyethene is an excellent material for fast neutrons [15, 16]. K Okuno et al. developed effective neutron shielding concrete [17].

4 Biological Basis of Radiation Therapy

The effect of cell death due to radiation is an essential foundation of radiation therapy. Radiation interaction with living cells causes two levels of damage- molecular and cellular. In molecular damage due to radiation is double-stranded breaks of nuclear DNA [18]. Inhibition of division, chromosome aberrations (CA), gene mutation, and cell killing/cell death are observations of cellular damage. Normal cells have a better capability of repairing radiation damage than tumour cells. The cell death related to radiation is conceptually explained by survival fraction. It is a logarithmic curve of cell survival and radiation dose after exposure [19, 20].

Radiation therapy is based on the 5 *R*'s of radiobiology, such as repair, redistribution, repopulation, reoxygenation, and radiosensitivity [21]. RT significantly alters the immune landscape of cancer patients due to affecting immune activation and immunosuppressive pathways. The dose per fraction and successive fractions of radiation therapy have a tangible impact on this immune regulation. Because this activation of the immune response after radiation may rationalize adding the 6th R of Radiobiology, which represents "reactivation of the antitumor immune response" [21].

Different types of fractional schedules deliver radiation fractions in radiation therapy, but some are effectively used in a few cancer types or specific conditions. The most common types of fractionation [22]:

(a) ***Conventional fractionation***

Conventional fractionation is the most common tried fractionation schedule used in different types of cancer delivers daily doses of 1.8–2.0 Gy, 5 days a week, most often Monday to Friday.

(b) ***Hyper-fractionation***

Hyper-fractionation is doses per fraction less than conventional fraction per fraction (1.8–2.0 Gy) and the number of fractions increases.

(c) ***Hypofractionation***

Hypofractionation used a dose per fraction higher than conventional fractionation, i.e. more than 2.0 Gy per fraction and reduced the total number of fractions. Single-dose irradiation or hypofractionation with few fractions are widely used in palliative radiotherapy.

(d) ***Accelerated fractionation***

Accelerated fractionation treatment is used as the same total dose delivered in half the overall time by giving two or more fractions per day with an inter-fraction interval of 6 h.

(e) **Continuous Hyperfractionated Accelerated Radiation Therapy (CHART)**

Continuous hyperfractionated accelerated radiation therapy (CHART) protocol has 36 fractions, with three fractions delivered daily with an inter-fraction interval of 6 h over 12 consecutive days [23].

5 External Beam Therapy (EBRT)

External beam therapy (EBRT), also commonly known as teletherapy, and its literal meaning is *Tele* means far, or some distance and *therapy* mean treatment. It implies that the treatment target/tumour and radiation source have some distance apart between them. In the early radiation therapy, all therapy units were kilovoltage X-ray machines. These units have almost replaced megavolt therapy units in today's modern world, so this section discusses megavoltage units.

5.1 EBRT Treatment Machines

1. **Radiation isotope-based teletherapy unit**

In 1951, Dr Harold E. Johns discovered the Cobalt-60 isotope-based teletherapy unit to

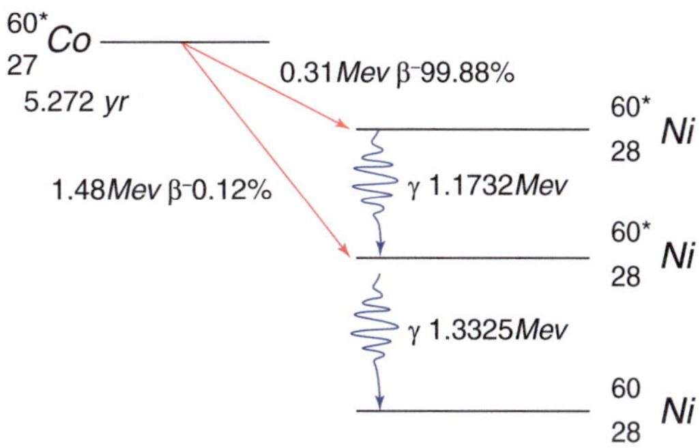

Fig. 3 Decay scheme of Cobalt-60 radioisotope

treat cancer patients. This Co-60 radioisotope source decays to Ni-60 by emitting two ß-particle and two γ-photons of energies, 1.17 and 1.33 MeV, with a half-life of 5.272 years shown in Fig. 3, and so this unit requires replacement of source every ~5 years. The Cobalt-60 sources are encapsulated in a stainless steel capsule which filters β-particles. The maximum source strength capacity of source housing of the teletherapy unit can hold up to 555 TBq [24]. The distance between the unit's isocentre and source position is 80 cm apart with the maximum field size of 35 × 35 cm^2.

The isotope-based teletherapy unit has two categories such as

(a) ***Standard telecobalt unit:*** It treated mainly conventional technique and 3DCRT, e.g., Theratron, Bhabhatron-II TAW.

(b) **Specialized telecobalt unit***:* This unit mainly treats stereotactic Radiosurgery (SRS) and stereotactic radiation therapy (SRT), e.g., Gamma-Knife.

The requirement properties of radionuclides for teletherapy are relatively long half-life, high energy and specific activity, simple means of production and no emission of toxic gaseous.

2. **Medical linear accelerator (Linac)**

Megavoltage linear accelerators are the most extensively used machines in radiation therapy. Initially, Van de Graaff accelerators were used for megavoltage medical applications but were discontinued. We use the linear accelerator (linac) for X-ray and electron beam radiations, and heavy particle units use cyclotron [12].

(a) Standard LINAC—It can treat conventional techniques and 3DCRT, IMRT, VMAT/Rapid Arc, and SRS/SRT, Stereotactic body radiotherapy (SBRT) as optional, such as Primus Trilogy, Synergy.
(b) Specialized LINAC—It is dedicated to SRS/SRT, SBRT, and spiral radiation delivered

- Helical beam delivery—Tomotherapy machine,
- Robotic beam delivery—Cyber-Knife,
- Medical Practice Accelerator: Medical Proton Cyclotron.

Comparative studies of Co-60, single and multiple energy linac are presented in Table 2.

5.2 Steps of Radiation Treatment Planning

The steps of radiation treatment of cancer patients have four subgroups: simulation, planning, radiation delivery, and quality assurance are shown in Fig. 4 [26]. The basic steps of radiation planning are as follows.

5.2.1 Patient Selection

For different sites of tumour positions, we need evaluations of the dosimetric benefits of treatment techniques in target and normal tissue doses.

5.2.2 Patient Simulation

1. ***Patient position and immobilization***

   The implication of patients' position is essential because of treatment accuracy and precision on treatment. A patient's comfortable position is a significant factor for reproducibility during treatment. Proper immobilization help reduce patient setup error and planning target volume (PTV) margins.
2. ***Imaging***

   After proper immobilization, patient images are taken for planning either in conventional or conformal techniques, and the mode of imaging like 2D or 3D depends on treatment techniques. Advanced treatments such as 3DCRT, IMRT, VMAT/Rapid Arc, SRS/SRT required 3D based images as computed tomography (CT) images, but the convention technique only required 2D X-ray orthogonal images. Moreover, other image modalities like Magnetic resonance imaging (MRI) and, PET-CT, Digital subtraction angiography (DSA) help delineate tumours, and soft tissue differentiation. Registration

Table 2 Comparison of the tele-isotope unit and linear accelerator unit [25]

Parameters	Cobalt-60 unit	Mono-energy linac	Variable-energy linac
The physical structure of the unit	Relatively very simple	Relatively complex in electrical and electronic equipment	Relatively very complex in electrical and electronic equipment and accessory
Radiation dosimetry	A cobalt-60 source with gamma-ray	6 MV X-ray energy	multiple X-ray and electron energies with variable dose rates plus FFF
Radiation room shielding	Concrete bunker and maze wall	Relatively thicker bunker with maze wall	Relatively more thicker bunker with maze wall and neutron shielding
Associated Staff	Basic requirement	Experience medical physicists, service and IT engineers	Advanced trained medical physicists, service and IT engineers
Cost involvement	Baseline	Slightly higher than baseline	Significantly higher than baseline
Source security	Require	NA	NA
Source replacement	Around 5 years	NA	NA
Clinical application	Basic treatment techniques	Advance treatment techniques	Advance treatment techniques with electrons
Patient load	Reduced due to source decay	Affected by poor maintenance	Affected by poor maintenance

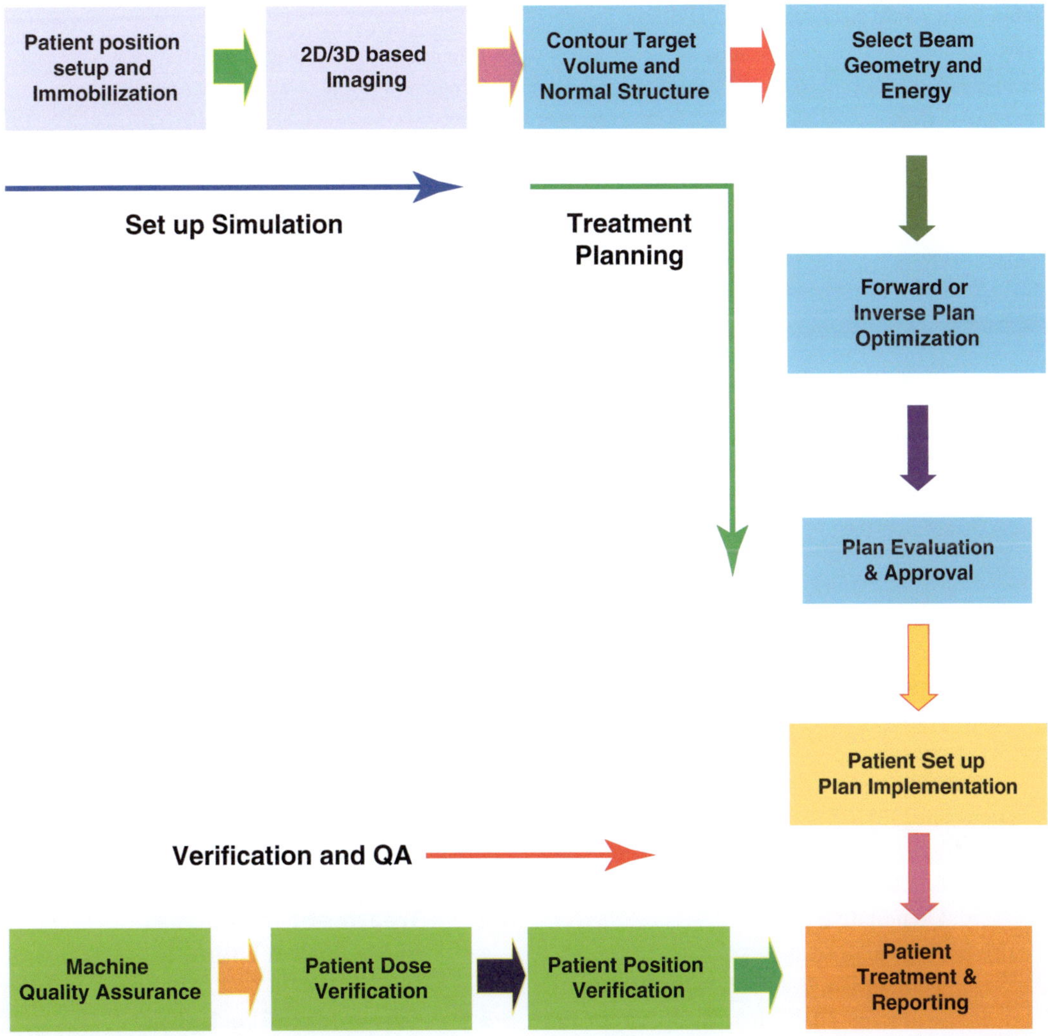

Fig. 4 Steps of the radiotherapy process

algorithms used in the fusion of planning CT and other images modalities should be accurate, precise, robust, flexible, automatic, and fast [27].

3. ***Contouring and planning***

The target and critical organs are contoured and relocated along with the images to the planning system using the CT and other image modalities, including magnetic resonance or positron emission tomography. ICRU 50 and 62 are essential documents for the delineation of targets [28, 29]. One of the challenges during treatment planning is the non-standardized nomenclatures of Target and OARs, which can cause systematic error. To minimize this problem, AAPM published task group (TG) 263 report regarding the uniform nomenclature of contours [30]. PTV margin depends on setup errors (systematic and random error), internal organ movement (varies from site to site) and needs to be individualized and carefully assessed. The optimum number of beams or arc and the direction of the beams are important parameters before planning. Routinely, the abdomen and pelvis site are treated with 15 or 18 MV, but head

Table 3 Treatment planning system (TPS) with the algorithm

TPS	Radiation	Company	Algorithm
Eclipse TPS	Photon Beam	Varian	Anisotropic Analytical Algorithm (AAA)
			Pencil Beam Convolution (PBC)
			Acuros XB
	Electron Beam		Electron Monte Carlo (eMC)
Monaco TPS	Photon Beam	Elekta	Photon Monte Carlo
CMS Xio TPS	Photon Beam		Multi grid superposition
			Fast Fourier Transform (FFT) Convolution
			Modified Clarkson sector integral
Oncentra Master Plan	Photon Beam	Nucletron[a]	3D pencil beam convolution
			Collapsed cone convolution
Pinnacle	Photon Beam	Phillips	Collapsed cone convolution

[a] Later change to Elekta

and neck, brain, and breast are using 6 MV photons [31, 32]. Treatment planning systems with various algorithms are presented in Table 3.

4. ***Plan evaluation***

   Plan evaluations of planning have two classes as [33]

   (a) Physical dose analysis
   - Qualitative (dose distribution)
   - Quantitative (DVH)

   (b) Biological dose analysis
   - Tumour Control Probability (TCP)
     – Increased by increasing target tissue dose
   - Normal Tissue Complication Probability (NTCP)
     – Decreased by reducing normal tissue dose

5. ***Patient-specific QA***

   Patient-specific dosimetric verification of advanced treatment techniques must be required to escape catastrophic accidents. It is the necessary procedure of IMRT/VMAT/SRS/SRT planning before radiation is delivered.

6. ***Patient setup/Plan implementation (PI)***

   After the plan is approved, planning parameters are transferred to the treatment room. Before radiation, delivery check patient setup verification with either CBCT or EPID. Once setup error is significantly less than the PTV margin, radiation is finally delivered [34].

7. ***Reporting***

   After treatment, dose per fraction and commutative doses are recorded. If any complications in the patient are observed, then further check-ups and evaluations are advised.

5.3 Treatment Techniques of Radiation Therapy

5.3.1 Conventional Technique

The conventional technique or two-dimensional (2D) radiation therapy has involved a single beam or up to four directions of beams. Usually, planning field setups were relatively simple and frequently consisted of opposed lateral fields or four fields, also known as boxes fields.

Limitation of Conventional Planning

One of the primary constraints of this technique has no information about 3D appreciations of tumour volume and its location concerning sensitive organs known as organ at risks (OARs). Conventional planning of a 3D tumour dose computation performs on a single transverse plane, and dose computation does not consider scattering contribution from adjacent body tissue.

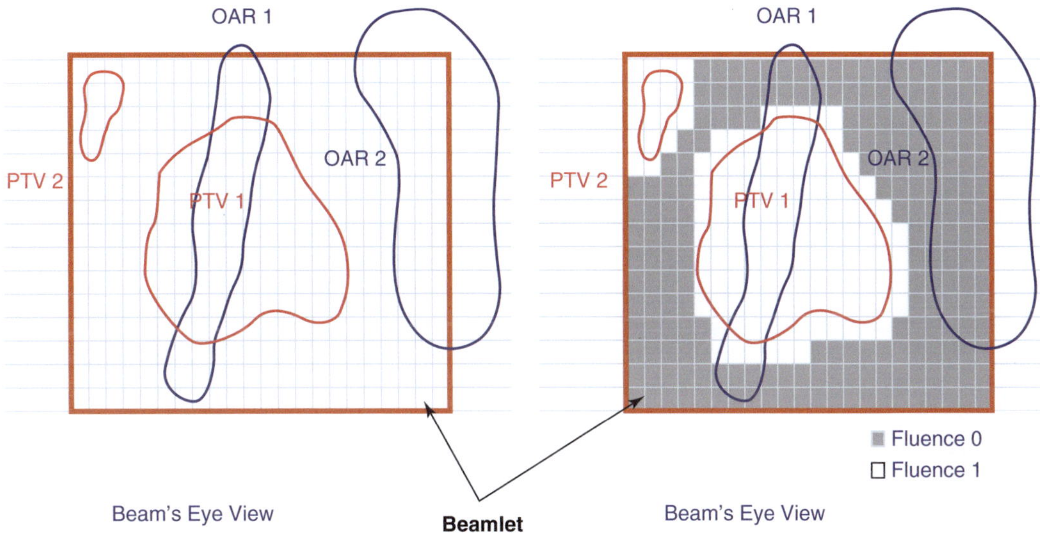

Fig. 5 Beamlet of intensity-modulated radiation therapy (IMRT)

5.3.2 Three-Dimensional Conformal Radiation Therapy (3DCRT)

Three-dimensional conformal radiation therapy (3DCRT) is CT-based planning, and it has overcome the limitation of the conventional technique. In 3DCRT, the radiation field is tightly conformed 3D shape of PTV by therapeutic dose-volume while minimizing surrounding normal tissue dose as low as possible.

Usually, a treatment session is of 3D-CRT comparatively similar to conventional technique around 10–20 min, except the first day of the session. To perform this technique in the teletherapy unit, it should have either multileaf collimator (MLC) or customized field-shaping blocks for the particular field of patients [35].

Conformal radiotherapy is planned using manual optimization techniques such as beam direction, number of fields, radiation energy, beam weights, beam modifier, shaping devices, and multiple iterative.

5.3.3 Intensity-Modulated Radiation Therapy (IMRT)

The intensity-modulated radiation treatment technique is quite similar to 3DCRT, but it has the non-uniform intensity of each field. Again, each field used in a divided small segment known as beamlet shown in Fig. 5 has a different radiation fluence. So it controls dose to normal tissues and better dose distribution with the target. Unlike 3DCRT, beam weighting is chosen by a computer algorithm, and it can determine the distribution of beam intensities throughout a target volume. IMRT is planned using inverse treatment planning techniques. The basic concept of IMRT is to modulate the intensity of the incident radiation. The flexibility of this technique achieved a higher degree of spatial arrangement resulting in dose distribution. IMRT effectively minimizes the intensity of rays to sensitive critical organs and increases the intensity of those rays that primarily see the target volume [36].

5.3.4 Arc Radiation Therapy

The limitations of fixed-field treatments, either radiation delivered by IMRT or 3DCRT, are image-guided radiotherapy and hypofractionation. Moreover, IMRT plans are more complex and take longer to treatment delivery [37]. Subsequently, it reduced patient throughput. IMRT can result in an increased integral dose which a larger volume of receives low doses of radiation to normal tissues. This effect is observed in the regions of the beams that enter and exit. Unlike fixed-field IMRT, the Arc therapy technique has better a conformal and same dose distribution of target and OAR sparing and higher dose falloff outside the target volume [38–40].

The significant theoretical advantage of arc therapy over standard fixed-field IMRT techniques is that

(a) The gantry is moved during the radiation is delivered around the patient,
(b) All angles (360°) are available to deliver radiation to the target,
(c) Better sparing critical structures,
(d) The choice of angles for fixed-field IMRT is pretty complex, but the arc technique simplifies with treated tumours from all angles with more degree of freedom [37].

VMAT, tomotherapy, fixed-field IMRT are advanced techniques and minor dosimetric differences. It depends on the user's expertise rather than the individual technology [26].

5.3.5 Stereotactic Techniques

Single fraction stereotactic radiosurgery (SRS) and fractionated stereotactic radiotherapy (SRT) are well-recognized treatment techniques for small lesions tumours. Nowadays, different technical methods are used with different radiation delivered systems. Hypofractionated or fractionated stereotactic radiotherapy is more efficient and effective than single fraction treatment SRS because of clinical outcome, post-treatment side effects, and the central field of development for radiosurgery. The next phase is completed in technological development, and proton or particle-based stereotactic radiosurgery will be used in the upcoming time [41].

W Jalbout et al. reported that 2.5 mm MLC has better clinically advantages for small target volume. 5.0 and 10.0 mm MLC could be applied in SRS/SRT for targets (PTV) diameter larger than 1 cm., but it is challenging to achieve PTV dose conformity for small target volume [42].

6 Image-Guided Radiation Therapy (IGRT)

Image-guided radiotherapy (IGRT) involves frequent imaging before radiation treatment and permits these images to make treatment decisions. The purpose of using IGRT is not only to decrease CTV-to-PTV margins but also to adequately define the tumour and normal tissue position, limiting the radiation dose exposed to an unwanted area. With the help of image-guided radiotherapy (IGRT), target volumes are fully optimized, and tumour doses can be delivered with proper control with slight complications [43]. IGRT is effectively achieved when proper devices help the patient position compensate for uncertainties in patient setup. Offline or online patient setup verifications are two methods in IGRT for patient setup verification. The changes of the patient's position during treatment and review setup margins are used in adaptive radiotherapy (ART) [44, 45]. The treatment plan is modified accordingly from offline or online imaging in adaptive planning, depending on the technique and tumour site. Offline adaptive planning is appropriate for systematic error or slow progressive changes, like weight loss and tumour regression. Online adaptive planning is preferred for significant potentially anatomical variations like bladder, cervix, or rectum [27].

The online setup of IGRT has reduced both systematic and random errors. Nowadays, many image-guidance technologies have been developed, including Exact Trac/Novalis Body system (BrainLAB AG), kV Cone-beam computed tomography (CBCT), and megavolt (MV) based Electronic portal imaging device (EPID) [43, 46, 47].

7 Advances 4D Radiation Therapy

Conventionally technology was not accessible to deal with patient-internal organ motion directly. However, extra margin as a safety margin to the target volume is provided to compensate for these uncontrolled internal organ movements. In the last two decades, the strategy of 4D based imaging, planning, and delivery technology has developed.

7.1 Imaging

The imaging principle is based on the consideration of the stationary position of the object during image acquisition. Thorax and upper abdomen imaging cause spatial image distortion and form reconstructed images during respiration. These artefacts reveal incorrect outlines in the image, misrepresentation of the object edge, reduced contrast resolution, and enlarged noise signal. Again, these artefacts are uncertainties in tumour identifying, delineating, and localisation. For acquiring image 4D imaging, time-resolved CT, MRI, PET/CT, SPECT, and US imaging with parallel multi-detector arrays have been used. During 4D delivery, CBCT imaging localization patient setup and fiducial markers for PTV motion tracking minimize the error in treatment delivery, providing better normal tissue control [36].

7.2 Radiation Therapy

Abdominal peristalsis and thoracic motion are challenging to perform the treatment, so we need to correct internal organ motion. The magnitude and shape of the motion, reproducibility during treatment, and closeness between moving targets and risk structures are factors that affect imaging and dose distribution. Management of the respiratory-induced motion of lung cancer is generally used 4D based imaging and therapy due to periodic motion and relative stability. It is performed using a gating and tracking system [48, 49].

7.3 Electron Beam Therapy

Electrons have been used in radiotherapy can treat superficial tumours. The energetic electron beam emerging from accelerators is a pencil beam which is not suitable for treatment. Hence the beam has to be spread to a larger area for treatment. Spread can be done by scattering foil. The scattering foils are composed of high *Z* material like gold interposed in an electron beam [50]. Different scattering foils are used for different electron energy. The characteristics of clinical electron beams such as depth dose, range parameters, energy specification, beam flatness, and symmetry and isodose distribution are required in clinical applications. Electron beams produced by medical linear accelerators for radiotherapy are nearly monoenergetic. Unlike photon beams, the depth dose of an electron beam is rapid dose fall beams after the depth of dose maximum (D_{max}) when the electron beams pass through a medium. It is due to the scattering and continuous energy loss. This depth dose profile reveals it is suitable for treating superficial tumours and tumours extending from the surface to a small depth. It is observed that the percentage surface dose of the electron beam increase with increasing energy in contrast to that of the photon beam.

Maximum range R_{max} (cm or g/cm^2) is the most significant infiltration depth of clinical electrons in the absorbing medium. The limitation of R_{max} is not giving a well-defined measurement depth. $E/4$ and $E/3$ approximately give a therapeutic range of R90 and R80 in cm of water, where E is the nominal kinetic energy in MeV of the electron beam. Several parameters are used to define the electron beam energy due to the complexity of its spectrum. The most commonly used parameters are most probable energy at the phantom surface ($E_{p,0}$), mean energy at the phantom surface (E_0) and R_{50} range [9].

For evaluating the flatness of electron beams, the beam profile should be measured at Z_{max} measured at a depth of maximum dose. Information of the beam flatness is essential from a clinical perspective in determining an acceptable field size to treat a particular area and an acceptable margin around the tumour.

The profile of individual electron isodose curves varies with electron beam energy, field size, collimation, source to surface distance (SSD), and the level of the isodose curve. Many factors can influence isodose curves' overall shape, including curvature of the patient body, inhomogeneous medium such as air, bone, lung, and high *Z* materials, and the effects of extended SSDs and field-shaping devices. When the electron beam passes through a medium, the beam enlarges rapidly below the surface because of scattering, and there is a spread of the isodose curve. The bulging of isodose curves increases the penumbra, while constriction of isodose curves indicates selecting a relatively larger field for treatment [26].

7.4 Heavy Particle Therapy

Heavy particle therapy uses proton beams, carbon ions, and pi Meson radiation. Proton therapy is an emerging treatment modality in the current scenario of cancer treatment due to its unique advantages over conventional radiotherapy. It effectively benefits the high-dose treatment area to the target and thus minimizes radiation dose surrounding normal tissue. Generally, particle radiation has high relative biologic effectiveness (RBE) and linear energy transfer (LET), advantages of particle radiation over photon radiation [51].

In particle therapy, the beam transverses and the dose deposited is constant until near the end of the range where the dose peaks out followed by raid falloff known as Bragg peak. Thus precisely confining the high-dose region to tumour volume and minimizing dose to surrounding normal tissue. Besides some limitations, it is not used on vast scales such as enormous cost required, complex and massive equipment required to accelerate particles, rigorous quality assurance needed, enough data not of side effects of treatment, and dose constraints [26].

8 Brachytherapy

The literal meaning of brachytherapy means brachy stands for short distance or nearby, and therapy stand for treatment. Simply, short distance therapy, where the source and target position are significantly less distant. Brachytherapy (also known as Curie therapy) is a short distance treatment with radiation produced from small sealed sources. The sources are kept directly or near the tumour volume. Brachytherapy has three main types: (1) Surface applicator or "Mould" Brachytherapy; (2) Interstitial Brachytherapy; (3) Intracavitary Brachytherapy (ICBT). Brachytherapy plays a crucial role in the management of invasive cervix cancer [52–54].

Most dose calculations in brachytherapy planning have been based on conventional TG-43 dose calculation formalism [55]. Recently, advanced TG-186 model-based dose calculation algorithms (MBDCAs) has been introduced [56].

8.1 Role Brachytherapy in Gynaecological Cancer

Intracavitary brachytherapy is primarily used to treat the cancer of the cervix, uterine, and vagina. Different applicators are employed to hold sources in a suitable configuration in the tumour, and its applicator has a central tube (tandem) and lateral capsules (ovoids).

8.2 2D Image-Based Intracavity Brachytherapy

2D image-based brachytherapy lacks target information, soft tissue, cervix, uterus, parametria, sigmoid colon, and small bowel. However, we can visualize the bladder, vaginal, rectum using radio-opaque gauze and markers. The orthogonal radiographs {Anteria Posteria (AP) and lateral images} are taken perpendicular, with the central axes of the X-ray beams lying nearly in the middle of the application. Dose specification in planning uses the oldest and the most extensively used Manchester system. Doses characterize defined points: Point A, Point B, Bladder point, and Rectum point.

In 2D intracavitary applicator planning system has significant uncertainties in the dose distribution from patient to patient. It was evident that the standard ICBT loading alone is not adequate due to a lack of information on source arrangement, tandem position relative to the ovoids, packing of the applicators, tumour size, and patient anatomy. Point A relates to the position of the sources and does not have a definite anatomic structure. Depending on the patient's cervix size, point A may lie inside the tumour or outside the tumour. Therefore, standard ICBT loading could risk under dosage of large or overdosage of small cervical.

The specification in planning uses the Manchester system, one of the primitive and the most widely used systems in the world. Doses characterize it to four points: Point A, Point B, Bladder point and Rectum point [57]. Point A is 2 cm superior to the external cervical (or cervical end of the tandem) and 2 cm lateral to the cervical canal. Point B is 3 cm lateral to point A. In the lateral radiograph, the AP line is drawn through the centre of the Foleys balloon, and the reference point is considered at its posterior surface. The rectal dose point falls at the maximum dose at the anterior rectal wall in the portions of the vaginal applicator. AP line is defined from the lower portion of intrauterine sources or middle of intravaginal sources in the lateral radiograph. The rectum reference point lies on this line 0.5 cm behind the posterior vaginal wall. In AP Radiograph, Reference Point is at the lower end of the intrauterine source.

8.3 3D Image-Based Intracavity Brachytherapy

To overcome the limitations of the standard ICBT Plan, a new advanced imaging and treatment planning system (TPS) has been introduced. Imaging techniques are computed tomography (CT) and magnetic resonance imaging (MRI), shown in Fig. 6. In MRI images, T1 images provide more applicators identification and reconstruction, and that of T2 series reveals recognizing and contouring the clinical target volume (CTV) and normal organs. If applicator reconstructions are not adequately performed, which can occur to geometrical uncertainties. These uncertainties affect the delivered dose's accuracy to CTV and normal organs. 100% isodose line of prescribed dose should cover HR-CTV (high risk-clinical target volume). We reported $D_{2\,cc}$, $D_{1\,cc}$, $D_{0.1\,cc}$ of the rectum, bladder, sigmoid, and small bowel that is dose to fixed volumes of 2 cc, 1 cc, and 0.1 cc of the rectum, bladder, sigmoid, and small bowel [58, 59].

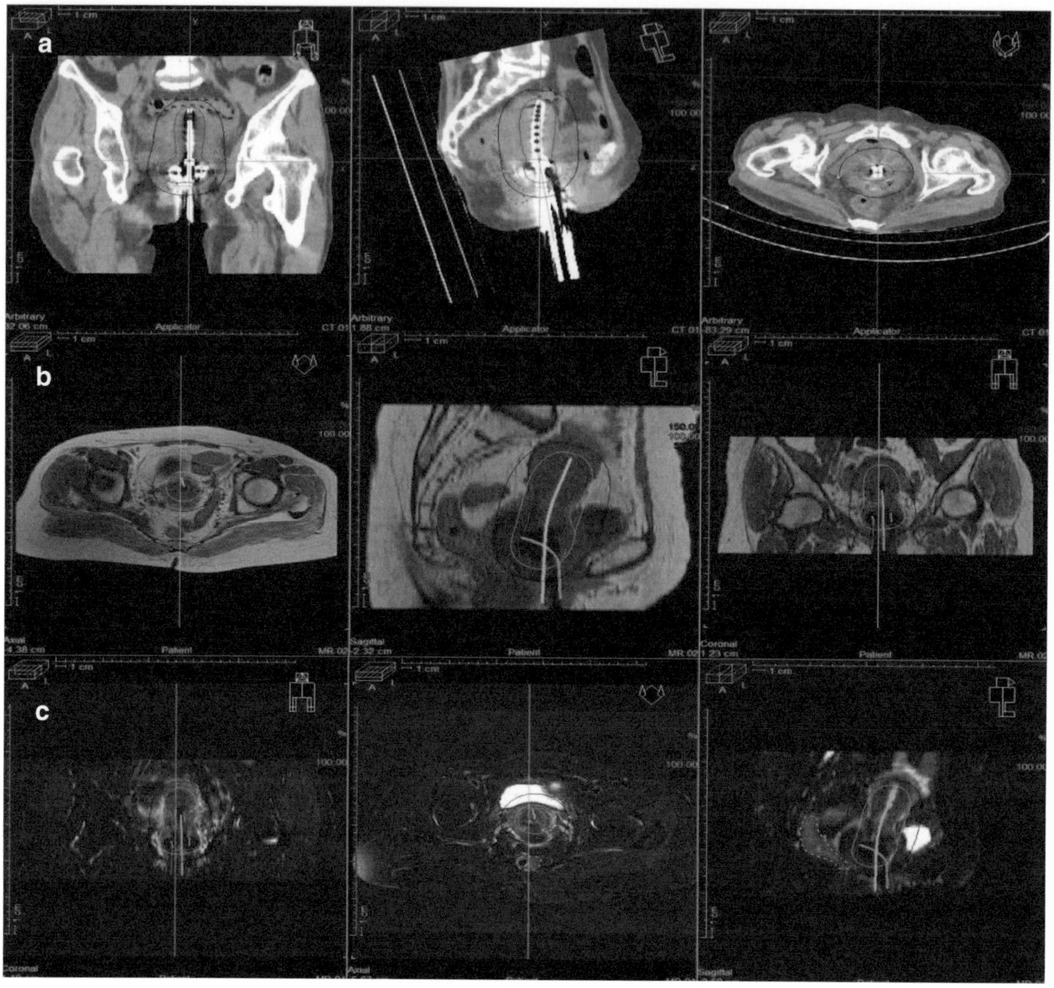

Fig. 6 Cather reconstruction in (**a**) CT image (**b**) T1 MRI image (**c**) T2 MRI image

9 Radiation Dosimetry in Radiation Therapy

Radiation dosimetry is a concern in the radiation therapy course for professional radiation workers and cancer patients. Therefore, radiation detectors play a critical role in radiation dosimetry, according to the purposed of detectors divided as personal monitoring and area survey detectors. The personal monitoring device is concerto radiation workers for estimation received during routine work. It is mainly a luminescent based dosimeter such as Thermolunescence dosimeter (TLD) and Optically stimulated luminescent dosimeter (OSLD). LiF: Mg, Ti (TLD-100) and $CaSO_4$:Dy (TLD-900) are the most commonly used TLD phosphors in personal and clinical applications. Aluminium oxide doped with carbon is the most sensitive OSL phosphor used in many developed countries for personal monitoring [60]. Moreover, pocket dosimeter as personal monitoring in an emergency during radiation process like telecobalt source struck and source replacement of telecobalt and brachytherapy unit.

Regarding patient safety and the achieved aim of radiation therapy, we need detectors that have good stability, independent of the energies of incident radiations, and low noise. Usually, output measurement of teletherapy units, ionization chamber is the proper choice among detectors. Ionization chambers have been used in the dosimetric QA of the therapy unit that calibrated against a national standard due to minor variation in response to energy, dose, dose rate, and reproducibility.

Ionization chambers have different shapes (cylindrical, spherical, and parallel plates) and sizes. There are different forms of ionization chambers for different uses in the QA of radiation units. For calibration of low energy radiation, we used a free ionization chamber. For output of megavoltages units, Farmer type ionization chambers are preferred. It has two electrodes, the inner and outer electrodes. It has an active volume of 0.6 cc filled with air and need temperature and pressure correction factors to apply before measurements. For relative dosimetry measured in radiation field analyser (RFA) equipment, the thimble chamber with 0.1 cc is used. Besides electron beam dosimetry, the parallel plate ionization chamber is recommended in TRS 398 IAEA [61]. Well type chambers (240 cc) are employed to calibrate brachytherapy sources.

Advance treatment techniques such as IMRT, VMAT/Rapid Arc, SRS/SRT, and SBRT required spatial dose distribution, revealing dose conformity, and homogeneity. Radiographic X-ray film provides an excellent 2D spatial resolution than other detectors because of some disadvantages of the radiographic film like non-reproducible, high cost, high maintenance, and darkroom management. Besides the above detectors, other detectors like diode detectors, Gel dosimeters, diamond detectors also play an essential role in dosimetry in radiation therapy. The peripheral dose measurement of patients is required to estimate the secondary cancer causes due to radiation therapy. In this process, TLD, OSL, diode detectors are used. Special treatments like total body irradiation (TBI), total skin electron therapy (TSET), dosimetry and commission required detectors to better results.

Semiconductor diode detectors are used extensively for beam data commissioning of therapy units. Diode detector has fast response, admirable spatial resolution, and high sensitivity. Besides, diode detector response depends on temperature, dose rate, and SSD, and some may also have angular dependence [62–64].

Diamond detectors are tissue equivalent and directional independent but have low dependence on dose rate and are expensive. It is ideal for small field dosimetry and profile measurements [65].

A film detector provides better spatial resolution with a permanent record, but it is not reproducible and expensive. Metal–oxide–silicon–semiconductor field-effect transistor (MOSFET) dosimeters are used in IMRT verification, small field dosimetry, brachytherapy, and in vivo dosimetry. The advantages of MOSFET dosimeters are reproducibility, linearity, energy, and angular responses [65].

Bang gel detectors are tissue equivalent and independent over a wide range of energies. In general, using gels is a lengthy process and has limited practicality in beam data commissioning except for SRS and IMRT [66, 67].

10 The Implication of Quality Assurance (QA) in RT

Several international and national organizations and other publications critically have discussions and recommendations on radiotherapy equipment quality assurance (QA). Quality assurance (QA) is performed in many radiation therapy fields, such as physical and technical features of treatment equipment, radiation dosimetry, and treatment delivery. The aim of QA in radiotherapy is the care and quality control of treatment equipment and delivery [68]. In radiation therapy, two types of errors, random and systematic errors, occur due to many uncertainties steps of radiation therapy processes. Therefore, QA takes a vital role to minimize errors in radiation therapy. Each of the steps of radiation therapy has many chances of errors are as follows [69].

(a) ***Diagnosis***

It is the initial stage of the whole process, but errors such as misdiagnosis, wrong histology, wrong staging can create catastrophic results after therapy.

(b) ***Imaging***

Images of patients like CT, MRI, PET-CT images reveal the confirmation of the disease at certain levels. Some errors during planning imaging, e.g. misconception, spatial distortions, density errors, provide wrong information to further process.

(c) ***Delineation of Volumes of Interest***

Contouring of target and OARs is necessary for planning and revealing received doses to particular countors. However, incorrect tumour identification incorrect normal tissue identification can cause misinterpretation of treatment and reporting.

(d) ***Prescription***

The prescribed doses to target are related to tumour control. If it is less or overestimated, it can cause underdose and overdose to target volume.

(e) ***Development of a plan of treatment***

The selection of beam direction and shapes of field, dose calculation algorithms, and treatment plan evaluation has the potential for error.

(f) ***Patient handling***

Improper patient immobilization, treatment positioning, and patient and organ movement responsibilities are challenging to control both errors.

(g) ***Treatment delivery***

In this last stage, improper treatment machine configuration and dose delivery have created severe patient problems.

11 Radiation Protection

Many international organizations provided dose limits of radiation workers on radiation exposure, which are given in Table 4. The motive of these recommendations is to prevent humans and the environment from the detrimental effects of ionizing radiation exposure.

In India, Atomic Energy Regulatory Board (AERB) provided dose limit of Radiation workers, Public and Trainee and Table 5 shows the limit equivalent dose of body parts.

Table 4 Comparison of the effective dose of radiation worker [26]

Dose limits	Occupational exposure	Public exposure
ICRP-26 1977	50 mSv/year	5 mSv/year
ICRP-60 1990	20 mSv per year over 5 years (100 mSv in 5 years) with no more than 50 mSv in a single year	1 mSv/year
ICRP-103 2007	20 mSv per year over 5 years (100 mSv in 5 years) with no more than 50 mSv in a single year	1 mSv/year
India AERB	20 mSv per year over 5 years (100 mSv in 5 years) with no more than 30 mSv in a single year	1 mSv/year
Europe 1996 BSS	20 mSv per year over 5 years (100 mSv in 5 years) with no more than 50 mSv in a single year	1 mSv/year

Table 5 the equivalent dose of radiation worker, public and trainee

Portion	Radiation worker	Public	Trainee
Lens of eyes	150 mSv in a year	15 mSv in a year	50 mSv in a year
Skin	500 mSv in a year	50 mSv in a year	150 mSv in a year
Extremities (hands and feet)	500 mSv in a year	–	150 mSv in a year

11.1 Classified Radiation Workers

Fewer radiation workers must be classified among them under existing regulations and codes. Those workers receive an effective dose that exceeds 6 mSv/year or 3/10ths of the average annual dose limits reported by the competent authority.

11.2 Pregnant Radiation Worker

Once a female radiation worker declares that pregnancy has been declared, she should inform the employer, licensee, and radiological safety officer (RSO) should modify the nature of work. The equivalent dose limit of the abdomen surface (lower trunk) and limiting intakes of radionuclide should be less than 2 mSv and by about 1/20 of the ALI.

11.3 Apprentices and Trainee

According to AERB, the occupational exposure of apprentices and trainees between 16 and 18 years shall maintain the dose limits should not exceed an effective dose of 6 mSv in a year.

References

1. Hall EJ, Wuu CS. Radiation-induced second cancers: the impact of 3D-CRT and IMRT. Int J Radiat Oncol Biol Phys. 2003;56(1):83–8. https://doi.org/10.1016/S0360-3016(03)00073-7.
2. Hall EJ, Henry S. Kaplan distinguished scientist award 2003: the crooked shall be made straight; dose-response relationships for carcinogenesis. Int J Radiat Biol. 2004;80(5):327–37. https://doi.org/10.1080/09553000410001695895.
3. Rosenblatt E, Zubizarreta E. Radiotherapy in cancer care: facing the global challenge. IAEA; 2017.
4. Gianfaldoni S, et al. An overview on radiotherapy: from its history to its current applications in dermatology. Open Access Maced J Med Sci. 2017;5(4):521–5. https://doi.org/10.3889/oamjms.2017.122.
5. Huh HD, Kim S. History of radiation therapy. Prog Radiat Ther. 2020;31:124–34. https://doi.org/10.3769/radioisotopes.60.385.
6. Mohan R. Field shaping for three-dimensional conformal radiation therapy and multileaf collimation. Semin Radiat Oncol. 1995;5:86–99. https://doi.org/10.1016/S1053-4296(95)80003-4.
7. Sterzing F, Engenhart-Cabillic R, Flentje M, Debus J. Image-guided radiotherapy. Dtsch Arztebl Int. 2011;108(16):274–81. https://doi.org/10.3238/arztebl.2011.0274.
8. Knoll FG. Radiation detection and measurement. Wiley; 2000.
9. Podgoršak EB. Radiation physics for medical physicists. Springer; 2010.
10. Ziegler SI. Positron emission tomography: principles, technology, and recent developments. Nucl Phys A. 2005;752:679–87. https://doi.org/10.1016/j.nuclphysa.2005.02.067.
11. Yücel H, et al. Measurement of photo-neutron dose from an 18-MV medical linac using a foil activation method in view of radiation protection of patients. Nucl Eng Technol. 2016;48(2):525–32. https://doi.org/10.1016/j.net.2015.11.003.
12. Podgorsak EB. Biological and medical physics, biomedical engineering: radiation physics for medical physicist. Springer; 2013.
13. Berger MJ, Inokuti M, Andersen HH, et al. ICRU report 49, stopping powers and ranges for protons and alpha particles. Rep Int Comm Radiat Units Meas. 1993;os-25(2):1–5. https://doi.org/10.1093/jicru_os25.2.1.
14. Brown A, Suit H. The centenary of the discovery of the Bragg peak. Radiother Oncol. 2004;73(3):265–8. https://doi.org/10.1016/j.radonc.2004.09.008.
15. IAEA. Safety Reports Series No. 47—radiation protection in the design of radiotherapy facilities. 2006:9.
16. Ahmed SN. Physics and engineering of radiation detection. Elsevier; 2007.
17. Okuno K, Kawai M, Yamada H. Development of novel neutron shielding concrete. Nucl Technol. 2009;168(2):545–52. https://doi.org/10.13182/NT09-A9241.
18. Little JB. Cellular, molecular, and carcinogenic effects of radiation. Hematol Oncol Clin North Am. 1993;7(2):337–52.
19. Supe SS, Naveen T, Ganesh KM, Samuel J. An overview of time dose fractionation models: NSD to BED. Pol J Med Phys Eng. 2006;12(4):165–201.
20. Hall EJ, Giaccia AJ. Radiobiology for the radiologist. Wolters Kluwer; 2012.
21. Steel GG, McMillan TJ, Peacock JH. The 5Rs of radiobiology. Int J Radiat Oncol Biol Phys. 1989;56:1045–8.
22. The Royal College of Radiologists. Radiotherapy dose fractionation, clinical oncology; 2019.
23. Saunders M, Dische S, Barrett A, Harvey A, Gibson D, Parmar M. Continuous hyperfractionated accelerated radiotherapy (CHART) versus conventional radiotherapy in non-small-cell lung cancer: a randomised multicentre trial. Lancet. 1997;350(9072):161–5. https://doi.org/10.1016/S0140-6736(97)06305-8.
24. Sahani G, Kumar M, Sharma DPK, et al. Compliance of Bhabhatron-II telecobalt unit with IEC standard—radiation safety. J Appl Clin Med Phys. 2009;10(2):120–30. https://doi.org/10.1120/jacmp.v10i2.2963.
25. Healy BJ, van der Merwe D, Christaki KE, Meghzifene A. Cobalt-60 machines and medical linear accelerators: competing technologies for external beam radiotherapy. Clin Oncol. 2017;29(2):110–5. https://doi.org/10.1016/j.clon.2016.11.002.
26. Levitt SH, Purdy JA, Perez CA, Vijayakumar S. Technical basis of radiation therapy. Springer; 2006.
27. Hutton BF, Braun M. Software for image registration: algorithms, accuracy, efficacy. Semin Nucl Med. 2003;33(3):180–92.
28. Landberg T, Chavaudra J, Dobbs J, et al. ICRU report 62: prescribing, recording and reporting photon beam therapy (supplement to ICRU report 50). Rep Int

Comm Radiat Units Meas. 1999;os-32(1):1–2. https://doi.org/10.1093/jicru_os32.1.1.
29. Landberg T, Chavaudra J, Dobbs J, et al. ICRU report 50: prescribing, recording and reporting photon beam therapy. Rep Int Comm Radiat Units Meas. 1993;os-26(1):67–70. https://doi.org/10.1093/jicru_os26.1.67.
30. Mayo CS, Moran JM, Bosch W, et al. AAPM TG 263: standardizing nomenclatures in radiation oncology. AAPM; 2018.
31. Bellon JR, Wong JS, Macdonald SM. Radiation therapy techniques and treatment planning for breast cancer. Springer; 2016.
32. Videtic GMM, Woody NM. Handbook of treatment planning in radiation oncology. Demos Medical; 2012.
33. Lee S, Cao YJ, Kim CY. Physical and radiobiological evaluation of radiotherapy treatment plan. Evol Ioniz Radiat Res. 2015; https://doi.org/10.5772/60846.
34. Agazaryan N. Patient specific quality assurance for the delivery of intensity modulated radiotherapy. J Appl Clin Med Phys. 2003;4(1):40. https://doi.org/10.1120/1.1525243.
35. Barrett A, Morris S, Dobbs J, Roques T. Practical radiotherapy planning. Hodder Arnold; 2009.
36. Bortfeld T. IMRT: a review and preview. Phys Med Biol. 2006;51:R363–79. https://doi.org/10.1088/0031-9155/51/13/R21.
37. Palma DA, Verbakel WFAR, Otto K, Senan S. New developments in arc radiation therapy: a review. Cancer Treat Rev. 2010;36(5):393–9. https://doi.org/10.1016/j.ctrv.2010.01.004.
38. Ślosarek K, Osewski W, Grzadziel A, et al. Integral dose: comparison between four techniques for prostate radiotherapy. Rep Pract Oncol Radiother. 2015;20(2):99–103. https://doi.org/10.1016/j.rpor.2014.10.010.
39. Lubbe WJ, Price R, Ruth K, et al. VMAT reduces moderate to high integral dose when compared to conventional IMRT for treatment of prostate cancer. Int J Radiat Oncol. 2011;81(2):S446. https://doi.org/10.1016/j.ijrobp.2011.06.742.
40. Kumar G, Bhushan M, Kumar L, et al. Dosimetric evaluation of low-dose spillage volumes for head and neck cancer using intensity-modulated radiation therapy and volumetric modulated arc therapy treatment techniques. Prog Med Phys. 2021;32(3):70–81. https://doi.org/10.14316/pmp.2021.32.3.70.
41. Münter MW, Welker H, Jensen AD, Wegner N. Stereotactic radiosurgery (SRS) and stereotactic radiation therapy (SRT) for neurooncological and neurological diseases: state of the art and future perspectives. Innov Neurosurg. 2013;1(3–4):157–64. https://doi.org/10.1515/ins-2013-0001.
42. Jalbout W, Zahr JA, Youssef B, Shahine B. On the feasibility of stereotactic radiosurgery with 5.0 and 10.0 mm mlc leaves as a function of target size and shape. Front. Oncol. 2019;9:3–10. https://doi.org/10.3389/fonc.2019.00741.
43. Verellen D, De Ridder M, Linthout N, Tournel K, Soete G, Storme G. Innovations in image-guided radiotherapy. Nat Rev Cancer. 2007;7(12):949–60. https://doi.org/10.1038/nrc2288.
44. Glide-Hurst CK, Lee P, Yock AD, et al. Adaptive radiation therapy (ART) strategies and technical considerations: a state of the ART review from NRG oncology. Int J Radiat Oncol Biol Phys. 2021;109(4):1054–75. https://doi.org/10.1016/j.ijrobp.2020.10.021.
45. Brock KK. Adaptive radiotherapy: moving into the future. Semin Radiat Oncol. 2019;29(3):181–4. https://doi.org/10.1016/j.semradonc.2019.02.011.
46. Chen GTY, Sharp GC, Mori S. A review of image-guided radiotherapy. Radiol Phys Technol. 2009;2(1):1–12. https://doi.org/10.1007/s12194-008-0045-y.
47. Jaffray D, Kupelian P, Djemil T, Macklis RM. Review of image-guided radiation therapy. Expert Rev Anticancer Ther. 2007;7(1):89–103. https://doi.org/10.1586/14737140.7.1.89.
48. Hugo GD, Rosu M. Advances in 4D radiation therapy for managing respiration: part I—4D imaging. Z Med Phys. 2012;22(4):258–71. https://doi.org/10.1016/j.zemedi.2012.06.009.
49. Keall PJ. Image-guided IMRT. Springer; 2006.
50. Patil B, Bhoraskar V, Dhole SC. Optimization of dual scattering foil for 6 to 20 MeV electron beam radiotheraphy. In: 2011 Part Accel Conf; 2011. p. 2157–9.
51. Murshed H. Proton radiation therapy. Fundam Radiat Oncol. 2019:161–71. https://doi.org/10.1016/b978-0-12-814128-1.00009-x.
52. Mayadev J, Benedict SH. Handbook of image-guided brachytherapy. Springer; 2017.
53. Eskander RN, Bristow RE. Gynecologic oncology: a pocketbook. Springer; 2015.
54. Banerjee R, Kamrava M. Brachytherapy in the treatment of cervical cancer: a review. Int J Women's Heal. 2014;6:555–64.
55. Rivard MJ, Coursey BM, DeWerd LA, et al. AAPM Task Group No. 43 Report: a revised AAPM protocol for brachytherapy dose calculations. Med Phys. 2004;31(3):633–74. https://doi.org/10.1118/1.1646040.
56. Beaulieu L, et al. Report of the Task Group 186 on model-based dose calculation methods in brachytherapy beyond the TG-43 formalism: current status and recommendations for clinical implementation. Med Phys. 2012;39(10):6208–36. https://doi.org/10.1118/1.4747264.
57. ICRU Report 38—Dose and volume specification for reporting intracavitary therapy in gynecology. 1985.
58. Pötter R, Haie-Meder C, Van Limbergen E, et al. Recommendations from Gynaecological (GYN) GEC ESTRO Working Group (II): concepts and terms in 3D image-based treatment planning in cervix cancer brachytherapy—3D dose volume parameters and aspects of 3D image-based anatomy, radiation physics, radiobiology. Radiother Oncol. 2006;78(1):67–77. https://doi.org/10.1016/j.radonc.2005.11.014.
59. Haie-Meder C, Pötter R, Van Limbergen E, et al. Recommendations from Gynaecological (GYN) GEC-ESTRO Working Group (I): concepts and terms in 3D

image based 3D treatment planning in cervix cancer brachytherapy with emphasis on MRI assessment of GTV and CTV. Radiother Oncol. 2005;74(3):235–45. https://doi.org/10.1016/j.radonc.2004.12.015.
60. Kry SF, Alvarez P, Cygler JE, et al. AAPM TG 191: clinical use of luminescent dosimeters: TLDs and OSLDs. Med Phys. 2020;47(2):e19–51. https://doi.org/10.1002/mp.13839.
61. IAEA. TRS 398 absorbed dose determination in external beam radiotherapy: an international code of practice for dosimetry based on standards of absorbed dose to water; 2006.
62. Saini AS, Zhu TC, Saini AS. Temperature dependence of commercially available diode detectors. Med Phys. 2002;2002(29):622–30. https://doi.org/10.1118/1.1461842.
63. Riknerf G, Grusellt E. General specifications for silicon semiconductors for use in radiation dosimetry. Phys Med Biol. 1987;32(9):1109–17.
64. Saini AS, Zhu TC, Saini AS. Dose rate and SDD dependence of commercially available diode detectors. Med Phys. 2004;31:914–24. https://doi.org/10.1118/1.1650563.
65. IAEA. TRS 483 dosimetry of small static fields used in external beam radiotherapy; 2017.
66. Das IJ, et al. Accelerator beam data commissioning equipment and procedures: report of the TG-106 of the Therapy Physics Committee of the AAPM. Med Phys. 2008;35(9):4186–215. https://doi.org/10.1118/1.2969070.
67. Ibbott GS, et al. Three-dimensional visualization and measurement of conformal dose distributions using magnetic resonance imaging of BANG polymer gel dosimeters. Int J Radiat Oncol Biol Phys. 1997;38(5):1097–103.
68. Ishikura S. Quality assurance of radiotherapy in cancer treatment: toward improvement of patient safety and quality of care. Jpn J Clin Oncol. 2008;38(11):723–9. https://doi.org/10.1093/jjco/hyn112.
69. Goitein M. Radiation oncology: a physicist's eye view. Springer; 2008.

Benign Breast Diseases

Gaurav Das, D. K. Vijayakumar,
Amal Chandra Kataki, and Lakshmi Malavika Nair

1 Introduction

In the present scenario where malignant diseases of the breast have been on the rise [1, 2], due to an increase in incidence as well as detection rates, the importance of understanding the entire subset of benign breast diseases cannot be overemphasized. A detailed history including presenting complaints, breast cancer risk factors including family history and menstrual and obstetric history are basic elements. A comprehensive examination of the breasts and draining nodal basins along with examination of other systems applying proper clinical methods is an indispensable component and should never be substituted for, but rather complemented by, relevant investigations.

2 Spectrum of Benign Breast Diseases

The symptoms that a patient may present with in case of benign breast diseases have significant overlap with those of malignant breast diseases (carcinomas, sarcomas including malignant phyllodes tumour and rarely, lymphoma). Table 1 illustrates a list of benign breast diseases that may be seen corresponding to a particular presenting symptom or clinical sign. It is important to know that each of the presenting complaints have malignant breast disease as one of the differential diagnoses, although the same has not been featured in the list, by virtue of the subject matter being discussed in this chapter. Only some benign breast diseases like ductal or lobular hyperplasia with atypia, confer an increased risk of development of breast cancer [3]. However, these are not to be regarded as premalignant lesions as the cancers do not necessarily develop in the areas of atypia [4–8].

G. Das (✉)
Department of Surgical Oncology, Dr. Bhubaneswar Borooah Cancer Institute (A Unit of Tata Memorial Centre, Mumbai), Guwahati, Assam, India

D. K. Vijayakumar
Surgical Oncology, Breast Diseases Division, AIMS, Kochi, India
e-mail: dkvijaykumar@aims.amrita.edu

A. C. Kataki
Department of Gynaecologic Oncology, Dr. Bhubaneswar Borooah Cancer Institute (A Unit of Tata Memorial Centre, Mumbai), Guwahati, Assam, India

L. M. Nair
Department of Surgical Oncology, Amrita Centre for Breast Diseases, Amrita Institute of Medical Sciences & Research Centre, Cochin, Kerala, India

A. C. Kataki, D. Barmon (eds.), *Fundamentals in Gynaecologic Malignancy*,
https://doi.org/10.1007/978-981-19-5860-1_9

Table 1 List of benign breast diseases according to presenting symptom/sign

Symptom/sign	Differential diagnoses
Breast lump/ swelling	Fibroadenoma Fibrocystic disease Fat necrosis Lactational adenoma Galactocele Lipoma Phyllodes tumour Simple and complex cysts Haematoma Hamartoma Haemangioma Lymphangioma Epidermal inclusion cyst Idiopathic granulomatous mastitis Tuberculosis Sarcoidosis Abscess Pseudoangiomatous stromal hyperplasia Seroma Amyloidosis Gynecomastia
Nipple discharge	Intraductal papilloma Multiple intraductal papillomas Juvenile papillomatosis Galactorrhoea Periductal mastitis and ductal ectasia
Pain, swelling, and redness	Lactational infection (mastitis/ abscess) Periareolar infection and mammary duct fistula Peripheral nonlactational breast abscess Cellulitis Eczema and secondary cellulitis Infected epidermoid cysts Hidradenitis suppurativa Intertrigo Pilonidal sinus Granulomatous lobular mastitis
Pain (mastalgia)	Cyclical mastalgia Noncyclical mastalgia • True noncyclic breast pain • Causes of chest wall pain

3 Approach to a Patient with Breast Disease

A thorough history is the first step in the proper evaluation of the disease. The components of such history include the details regarding the presenting complaint such as the duration, presence of any prior symptoms or any breast biopsies (needle or excisional), presence of any nipple discharge and its characteristics like colour, bilaterality or number of ducts involved, associated swellings in the axilla or neck or presence of systemic symptoms like fever, cough or dyspnoea, skin disease, bone pain, back pain, neurologic problems or blood disorders. Assessment of the risk factors for cancer is important including a detailed family history of cancer, menstrual history and history of previous breast biopsies and radiation to the chest. The history of breastfeeding is also documented. In postmenopausal women, the use of hormone replacement therapy is of importance as benign breast diseases are uncommon in such patients without exogenous hormones. In men, gynecomastia may be caused by hepatic dysfunction and drugs like H2 blockers and phenytoin, besides marijuana abuse.

Triple assessment includes physical examination, radiologic tests, and pathological assessment on needle biopsy (fine needle aspiration cytology or core needle biopsy, as indicated). The point to bear in mind is that patients who are clinically suspected to have a malignant tumour are subjected to core needle biopsy instead of fine needle aspiration cytology.

On physical examination, proper documentation of the clinical findings is of paramount importance (Table 2)

Table 2 List of essential clinical information in examination of the breast

Headings	Characteristics
Breast	Size, shape, symmetry
Nipple areola complex (NAC)	Position, symmetry, inversion, retraction, oedema, ulceration, discharge
Lump	
Number	Single/multiple
Location	Quadrant, O'clock positions, distance from NAC
Margins/borders	Ill-defined/well-defined
Shape	Spherical/oval/irregular
Consistency	Soft/firm/hard/cystic/variable
Surface	Smooth/irregular
Fixity	Skin/pectoralis muscle/chest wall
Skin over the breast	Dimpling, tethering, oedema including peau d'orange appearance, scar, ulcer
Nodal basins	
Axillary and supraclavicular	Palpable node(s), number, size, shape, consistency, discrete/matted, tenderness
Internal mammary	Visible swelling in parasternal regions, dull note on percussion in parasternal regions
General examination	
Systemic examination	Per abdomen, pelvic examination Respiratory system Cardiovascular system Nervous system Musculoskeletal system

4 Investigations

4.1 Ultrasound (US)

It can characterize whether a lump in the breast is solid or cystic (simple or complex). Simple cysts have a smooth and thin wall, are well-circumscribed, with few internal echoes, whereas complex cysts have a significant solid component, have septations and walls of thickness more than 0.5 mm, scalloped or irregular borders and internal echoes or fluid-debris level and absence of posterior wall enhancement. Simple cysts have negligible risk of cancer and do not usually require aspiration unless they cause symptoms like discomfort or pain. Complex cysts require aspiration to note the fluid content, and if it is sanguineous, the risk of malignancy is high. Benign cyst fluid is usually green, yellow or brown in colour and contains dead epithelial cells. In a cyst that recurs, repeat aspiration is done. However, multiple recurrences should be adequately evaluated with the addition of a mammogram and surgical excision is offered to a patient who does not desire repeated aspirations. Although the overall malignancy risk of a complex cyst is only 0.3%, one that contains a significant solid component carries a high risk. In case of solid breast lump in young women (less than 35 years), ultrasound can usually reliably differentiate a benign lesion from a malignant one [9, 10]. Malignant US features include spiculation, taller-than-wide orientation, angular margins, microcalcifications, and posterior acoustic shadowing. With these sonographic features, a negative predictive value of 99.5% and a sensitivity of 98.4% for the diagnosis of malignancy were achieved. These results have subsequently been validated by others and remain the cornerstone of US characterization of breast lesions today [11–16].

4.2 Mammography

A diagnostic mammogram is the standard of care for evaluation of abnormalities of the breast. The findings are reported according to the Breast Imaging-Reporting and Data System (BI-RADS system) (Table 3). The exception is in young women who have dense breasts in whom there can be some difficulty in identification of abnormalities and multicentric disease. In addition, it is a screening tool for breast cancer in people with average risk after 45 years of age. A mammogram cannot however differentiate a solid from cystic lesion.

4.3 Magnetic Resonance Imaging (MRI)

This is used when mammography and ultrasound have ambiguous findings and in patients who have dense breasts such as young ladies where mammography would not be properly interpreted

Table 3 BI-RADS categories [17]

Category	Malignancy risk	Management
0 Inconclusive	NA	Additional imaging
1 Negative	0%	Routine screening
2 Benign	0%	Routine screening
3 Probably benign	≤2%	Short-interval follow up (6 monthly)
4 Suspicious	4a Low suspicion of malignancy (2–10%) 4b Moderate suspicion of malignancy (10–50%) 4c High suspicion of malignancy (50–95%)	Tissue diagnosis
5 Highly suggestive of malignancy	≥95%	Tissue diagnosis
6 Biopsy-proven	100%	Treatment of malignancy

or would likely miss lesions. In the context of malignancy, MRI does carry a concern of detection of false-positive lesions, although there are definite indications for ordering the scan [18–20].

4.4 Fine-Needle Aspiration Cytology (FNAC)

Multiple passes are made percutaneously through the breast lump using a syringe and a fine needle of size ≥22G to aspirate cells for evaluation.

4.5 Core Needle Biopsy

An 18G or larger needle is used to do the biopsy and it yields tissue for characterization of histologic features. It is the current standard of care for evaluation of breast lumps.

4.6 Incision Biopsy

The only indication for this could be in an ulcerated or fungating breast mass and even then, a core biopsy can substitute this procedure as it may cause bleeding which can be avoided.

4.7 Excision Biopsy

This may be used for a high risk lesion like one with atypia, or in situations where needle biopsies are inconclusive or ambiguous or incongruous with imaging findings. The excision biopsy specimen should always be oriented properly in at least three sides. It is not a standard of care for the initial diagnosis of palpable breast lumps, in which case a core needle biopsy is the recommended option.

5 Classification of Benign Breast Lesions

A wide variety of lesions come under the spectrum of benign breast disease and these can be broadly divided into proliferative and non-proliferative ones [21, 22] (Table 4).

5.1 Breast Cysts

These are fluid-filled round or ovoid lumps that arise from the terminal duct lobular unit (TDLU) due to obstruction of the efferent ductule. In a prospective study of 2809 women at increased risk of breast cancer development, the American College of Radiology Imaging Network (ACRIN) 6666 protocol found that cysts were identified in 37.5% of all women screened, with the peak incidence between 35 and 50 years of age [23]. The ultrasound characteristics of breast cysts have been described in the previous section. A simple cyst and clustered simple microcysts usually do not need intervention. Fine needle aspiration of a simple cyst is only done

Table 4 Classification of benign breast lesions

Non-proliferative lesions	Proliferative lesions		Miscellaneous
Simple breast cysts	Without atypia	With atypia	Lipoma
Galactocele	Usual ductal hyperplasia	Atypical ductal hyperplasia	Fat necrosis
Papillary apocrine change	Intraductal papilloma(s)	Atypical lobular hyperplasia	Hamartoma
Mild hyperplasia of usual type	Sclerosing adenosis	Lobular carcinoma in situ (LCIS)	Sarcoidosis
	Radial scars		Idiopathic granulomatous mastitis
	Fibroadenomas		Diabetic mastopathy
	Adenomas		
	Pseudoangiomatous stromal hyperplasia		

when there are signs of infection and then the fluid is sent for culture and sensitivity testing. The fluid is usually not sent for cytology testing because such fluid invariably contains dead atypical cells. However, if the aspirate is sanguineous, then it is sent for both cytology and culture examinations. For complex cysts, an ultrasound guided core needle biopsy is essential. If this is technically not feasible, the ultrasound localization of the cyst followed by surgical excision is the treatment. However, if the imaging and core needle biopsy findings both indicate benign pathology, such cysts can be closely followed up every 6 months to document clinical stability, in the absence of which, a re-evaluation becomes necessary [24, 25].

5.2 Galactocele

The diagnosis of this clinical entity, also known as milk retention cysts, is made by a clinical history and milky aspirate. Mammogram may show a classic fat-fluid level or an indeterminate mass and ultrasound will show a well-defined lesion with thin echogenic walls and in long standing cases, there may be an appearance of a complex mass. Galactoceles can be followed up without the need for excision, unless it is bothersome for the patient [26–28].

5.3 Usual Ductal Hyperplasia

This is usually an incidental finding on the pathologic examination of biopsies done for mammographic abnormalities or breast lumps. No treatment is needed per se.

5.4 Intraductal Papillomas

A solitary ductal papilloma usually presents with nipple discharge, mostly bloody in nature or as a lump or a radiological finding (mammogram, ultrasound, MRI or a ductogram). Excision is recommended in cases of atypia, a palpable mass lesion, bloody nipple discharge (primarily for symptomatic relief), and/or pathology-imaging discordance, whereas small incidental benign solitary papillomas with imaging concordance may be offered close clinical and radiological follow-up [29].

5.5 Diffuse Papillomatosis (Multiple Papillomas)

Diffuse papillomatosis is defined as a minimum of five papillomas within a localized segment of breast tissue and is managed with surgical excision [30].

5.6 Juvenile Papillomatosis

This is a rare condition seen in girls and young women and the presentation may be with nipple discharge or as a breast lump with nipple discharge. This condition carries a slight increased risk of subsequent breast cancer and treatment is by surgical excision followed by surveillance [31–33].

5.7 Sclerosing Adenosis

It is a lobular lesion with increased fibrous tissue and interspersed glandular cells. This kind of proliferative lesion is commonly found in benign breast biopsies. There is prominence of stromal fibrosis and myoepithelium with enlarged and distorted lobules and crowded acini. In one study, sclerosing adenosis was present in 62.4% of biopsies with proliferative disease without atypia and 55.1% of biopsies with atypia [34]. The mere presence of sclerosing adenosis does not need surgical excision.

5.8 Radial Scars (Complex Sclerosing Lesions)

Histologically, these lesions have a fibroelastic core with radiating spokes of ducts and lobules and the latter are drawn into that radial configuration due to the contraction of the core. The ducts and lobules mentioned may contain a variety of proliferative changes and these include ductal hyperplasia, sclerosing adenosis, and cysts [35–37]. Radial scars are benign lesions but they present diagnostic dilemma at times due to the fact that it may be sometimes difficult to differentiate these lesions from malignant lesions like lobular carcinoma radiologically and pathologically these lesions may co-exist with high-risk lesions or frank malignancy. These are the reasons due to which the management to radial scar deserves special attention. When there is a pathological report of radial scar on a core needle biopsy, the lesion can either be excised surgically or closely followed up. The risk of subsequent breast cancer [38] being detected varies from 1.1% to 6.7%.

5.9 Galactorrhoea

When it is not associated with pregnancy or breast-feeding, the copious milky discharge from both breasts is related to hyperprolactinemia due to the use of psychotropic agents (drug-related) or hypothyroidism or a pituitary adenoma (prolactinoma). Hyperprolactinemia is usually associated with galactorrhoea, amenorrhea and relative infertility. Galactorrhoea disappears after appropriate drug therapy or cessation of offending drug or surgical removal of the pituitary adenoma. Drugs against hyperprolactinemia include cabergoline and bromocriptine [39–42].

5.10 Periductal Mastitis and Ductal Ectasia

Periductal mastitis is characterized clinically by periareolar inflammation and at times may be associated with a periareolar abscess or a lump or a mammary duct fistula. There is often nipple discharge with the content being a viscous, toothpaste like material or a greenish fluid. When dilated ducts are present, the condition is known as ductal ectasia. Ageing in itself is one of the predisposing factors to development of this condition and presence of bacterial infection, mostly anaerobic is probably one more inciting factor. Many women do have a history of smoking and the association has been reported. Microdochectomy is the surgery done for persistent single duct nipple discharge and it is done by either a radial or a circumareolar incision. The discharging duct is cannulated and methylene blue dye may be used to delineate the duct. Excision of that ductal system for about 5 cm is made. In case of complications associated with periductal mastitis with persistent nipple discharge from multiple ducts and in older women, complete duct excision can be performed [43–46].

5.11 Infective Conditions of the Breast

These include mastitis and cellulitis related to various microbial infections. The usual culprit is *Staphylococcal species,* apart from anaerobic streptococci and bacteroides and these usually respond to appropriate antibiotic course. The breast may be affected by tuberculosis, actinomycosis, syphilis, and mycosis and need cause-appropriate treatment. Hidradenitis suppurativa is a condition where there is infection of the apocrine sweat glands with abscess formation in the lower part of the breast and the axilla and it can be a recurrent condition. The condition requires good nursing care which includes keeping the area clean and dry and draining of all abscesses and culture sensitive antibiotic coverage. At times, debridement with skin grafting may become necessary. Granulomatous lobular mastitis is characterized by non-caseating granulomas and microabscesses in the breast and in some of the cases, may be associated with hyperprolactinemia or alpha-1 antitrypsin deficiency or Wegener's granulomatosis. The disease may be self-limiting within a year but any abscess that form need drainage or aspiration [47, 48].

5.12 Mastalgia

Breast pain may be cyclical, probably caused by hormonal stimulation of the normal breast lobules before menstruation, or it may be noncyclical related to several conditions. A few of such conditions include breast cysts, periductal mastitis, fat necrosis, focal mastitis, Mondor's disease, pressure from tight brassiere or nonbreast conditions like Tietze's syndrome (costochondritis) or radiculopathies. Pain relief is related to the control of the underlying cause.

5.13 Mondor's Disease [49]

This is a rare cause of breast pain (mastalgia) associated with multiple, tender subcutaneous cord like swellings related to superficial thrombophlebitis of the lateral thoracic vein and its tributaries. The condition is self-resolving but it is of clinical significance because it mimics malignancy.

5.14 Traumatic Fat Necrosis [50]

Fat necrosis is a benign non-suppurative inflammatory process of adipose tissue. They usually present as a palpable lump, typically periareolar, which can clinically mimic malignancy. A history of accidental trauma can be elicited from some patients, however, the absence of history of trauma does not exclude fat necrosis. The other common predisposing causes include surgery and radiation.

5.15 Gynecomastia

It is the benign proliferation of the glandular tissue of the male breast which presents with noticeable enlargement of the breast or a palpable swelling. The etiological factors related to gynecomastia is a vast subject [51–60] (Table 5).

It is important to differentiate two important conditions from gynecomastia and these are pseudogynecomastia which occurs due to excessive fat deposition rather than glandular proliferation and the other one is male breast cancer. The treatment of gynecomastia, if needed, depends on the underlying cause [61].

Table 5 Etiological factors of gynecomastia

Physiologic causes	Pathologic conditions
Neonatal	Idiopathic
Pubertal	Drug-induced • Hormones like androgens and anabolic steroids, oestrogens and its agonists, growth hormone • Anti-androgens like bicalutamide, cyproterone acetate, dutasteride • Antibiotics like isoniazid, metronidazole, ketoconazole • Cimetidine, rabeprazole, omeprazole • Amiodarone, digoxin, diltiazem, nifedipine, verapamil, amlodipine, captopril, spironolactone • Diazepam, haloperidol, olanzapine, venlafaxine • Alcohol, marijuana, amphetamine • Domperidone, pregabalin, phenytoin, gabapentin • Methotrexate, cyclosporine, alkylating agents
Ageing	Testicular tumours • Sertoli cell tumours • Leydig cell tumours • Germ cell tumours • Choriocarcinoma
	Adrenocortical carcinoma
	Liver disease
	Chronic renal failure
	Obesity
	Hyperthyroidism
	Testicular feminization
	Ectopic hCG production • Lung carcinoma • Liver carcinoma • Renal cell carcinoma • Gastric carcinoma
	Primary gonadal failure • Anorchia • Klinefelter's syndrome • Hermaphroditism • Viral orchitis • Castration • Granulomatous disease (e.g., leprosy)
	Testicular failure due to hypothalamic or pituitary disease

6 Benign Proliferative Stromal Lesions

6.1 Diabetic Fibrous Mastopathy

There is lymphocytic mastitis and stromal fibrosis seen in premenopausal women and rarely, men with long-standing type 1 insulin dependent diabetes mellitus with severe diabetic microvascular complications. It can present with breast lump(s) and mimic cancer. Core needle biopsy shows dense keloid-like fibrosis and classical B cell lymphocytic infiltration in periductal, lobular and perivascular locations along with presence of fibroblasts in the stroma. These patients need routine follow-up [62, 63].

6.2 Pseudoangiomatous Stromal Hyperplasia of the Breast

It comprises of myofibroblastic proliferation of the stroma of the breast and is mostly seen in premenopausal women or postmenopausal women taking hormone-replacement treatment. It presents as a well-circumscribed and rubbery mass, thus mimicking a fibroadenoma. Histologically, there is a complex network of anastomosing slit-like spaces with a densely collagenous stroma and hence it may cause some diagnostic confusion with angiosarcoma. The treatment of the condition is surgical excision [64, 65].

7 Benign Neoplasms

7.1 Fibroadenoma

A fibroadenoma is a solid, usually painless, benign breast tumour, with firm and rubbery consistency. Fibroadenomas are mostly seen in girls and young women and these often involute in the postmenopausal period. The purported aetiology is that the formation of fibroadenomas is oestrogen-driven [66]. Fibroadenomas are well-circumscribed but non-encapsulated lesions with pushing borders with no infiltration of the surrounding breast parenchyma due to which they have a characteristic 'free' mobility within the breast, leading to the terminology 'breast mouse'. Histologically, there is cellular proliferation of both glands and stromal cells with a uniform ratio throughout the lesion. Two growth patterns are noted in fibroadenomas. The intracanalicular pattern is characterized by the stroma compressing and distorting the glands into cleft-like spaces, whereas in the pericanalicular pattern the stroma does not distort the glands. There are some histologic variants of fibroadenomas. These include myxoid fibroadenomas [67] which have myxoid degeneration in the stroma, cellular fibroadenomas which have more cellularity than usual, juvenile fibroadenomas which have increased stromal cellularity and epithelial hyperplasia and commonly seen in young girls and complex fibroadenomas which have co-existent sclerosing adenosis, cysts, epithelial calcifications or papillary apocrine changes. Fibroadenomas larger than 5 cm in dimension are known as giant fibroadenomas. Most fibroadenomas do not require any treatment and are observed over time. Intervention is indicated only when there is rapid growth or when the lesion is causing symptoms or the patient desires removal. Surgical excision is the treatment of choice in such cases [68]. The alternatives to surgical excision includes ablative techniques like cryoablation or radiofrequency ablation or high-frequency focussed ultrasound (HIFU) or LASER ablation after histological confirmation. A mammotome is a vacuum-assisted breast biopsy device which can be used to remove a fibroadenoma.

7.2 Lipoma

A lipoma of the breast is a benign lesion which contains mature fat and is well-encapsulated. They do not have any malignant potential. There have been reports of giant lipomas of the breast which have been described to be more than 10 cm in dimension [69, 70]. The treatment is surgical excision.

7.3 Tubular Adenoma

It is a rare benign tumour seen in young women, with a characteristic histologic description of packed tubular structures within a small amount of fibrous tissue with the tubules being lined by normal epithelial and myoepithelial cells. The treatment is surgical excision [71].

7.4 Hamartoma

It is also known as a fibroadenolipoma or a 'breast within a breast' [72, 73]. A hamartoma is a rare tumour and is characterized by benign proliferation of fibrous, glandular and fatty tissues, surrounded by a thin pseudocapsule of connective tissue. Hamartomas have an association with Cowden syndrome [74]. Surgical excision is the definitive treatment.

7.5 Granular Cell Tumour

It is a rare benign tumour arising from Schwann cells [75]. The cells that compose this tumour have a characteristic granular, eosinophilic cytoplasm with typical nuclei and abundant lysosomes. Immunohistochemical staining shows positive results for neuron-specific enolase (NSE), S100 and CD68. Although it is essentially a benign tumour which is treated by surgical excision, in rare instances, a malignant variant has been described [76].

7.6 Phyllodes Tumour

It is an uncommon fibroepithelial breast tumour which can be histologically categorized into benign, borderline or malignant subtype based on features like cellular atypia, number of mitoses per high power field, stromal overgrowth and necrosis and type of margins [77–79]. There may be characteristic clinical presentation like rapid growth and presence of dilated veins in the overlying skin and at times, large tumours may cause pressure necrosis of the skin with ulceration. The treatment is by surgical excision with wide (≥1 cm) margins [80].

8 Conclusion

The spectrum of benign breast diseases is very vast and the knowledge of these conditions is important for any clinician involved in any oncological or non-oncological discipline related to the breast. Several benign breast diseases can closely mimic breast cancer, which can create a diagnostic challenge. Therefore, careful evaluation to differentiate the two become vital when treating a patient with a breast lump.

References

1. Schneider AP II, Zainer CM, Kubat CK, Mullen NK, Windisch AK. The breast cancer epidemic: 10 facts. Linacre Q. 2014;81(3):244–77. https://doi.org/10.1179/2050854914Y.0000000027. PMID: 25249706; PMCID: PMC4135458.
2. Ferlay J, Colombet M, Soerjomataram I, Mathers C, Parkin DM, Piñeros M, Znaor A, Bray F. Estimating the global cancer incidence and mortality in 2018: GLOBOCAN sources and methods. Int J Cancer. 2019;144(8):1941–53. https://doi.org/10.1002/ijc.31937. Epub 2018 Dec 6. PMID: 30350310.
3. Marshall LM, Hunter DJ, Connolly JL, Schnitt SJ, Byrne C, London SJ, Colditz GA. Risk of breast cancer associated with atypical hyperplasia of lobular and ductal types. Cancer Epidemiol Biomarkers Prev. 1997;6(5):297–301. PMID: 9149887.
4. Said SM, Visscher DW, Nassar A, Frank RD, Vierkant RA, Frost MH, Ghosh K, Radisky DC, Hartmann LC, Degnim AC. Flat epithelial atypia and risk of breast cancer: a Mayo cohort study. Cancer. 2015;121(10):1548–55. https://doi.org/10.1002/cncr.29243. Epub 2015 Jan 13. PMID: 25639678; PMCID: PMC4424157.
5. Hartmann LC, Sellers TA, Frost MH, Lingle WL, Degnim AC, Ghosh K, Vierkant RA, Maloney SD, Pankratz VS, Hillman DW, Suman VJ, Johnson J, Blake C, Tlsty T, Vachon CM, Melton LJ III, Visscher DW. Benign breast disease and the risk of breast cancer. N Engl J Med. 2005;353(3):229–37. https://doi.org/10.1056/NEJMoa044383. PMID: 16034008.
6. Dupont WD, Page DL. Risk factors for breast cancer in women with proliferative breast disease. N Engl J Med. 1985;312(3):146–51. https://doi.org/10.1056/NEJM198501173120303. PMID: 3965932.
7. Degnim AC, Visscher DW, Berman HK, Frost MH, Sellers TA, Vierkant RA, Maloney SD, Pankratz VS, de Groen PC, Lingle WL, Ghosh K, Penheiter L, Tlsty T, Melton LJ III, Reynolds CA, Hartmann LC. Stratification of breast cancer risk in women with atypia: a Mayo cohort study. J Clin Oncol. 2007;25(19):2671–7. https://doi.org/10.1200/JCO.2006.09.0217. Epub 2007 Jun 11. PMID: 17563394.
8. Hartmann LC, Radisky DC, Frost MH, Santen RJ, Vierkant RA, Benetti LL, Tarabishy Y, Ghosh K, Visscher DW, Degnim AC. Understanding the premalignant potential of atypical hyperplasia through its natural history: a longitudinal cohort study. Cancer Prev Res (Phila). 2014;7(2):211–7. https://doi.org/10.1158/1940-6207.CAPR-13-0222. Epub 2014 Jan 30. PMID: 24480577; PMCID: PMC4167687.
9. Houssami N, Irwig L, Ung O. Review of complex breast cysts: implications for cancer detection and clinical practice. ANZ J Surg. 2005;75(12):1080–5. https://doi.org/10.1111/j.1445-2197.2005.03608.x. PMID: 16398815.
10. Gerets JCWL, Kool M, Simons PCG, Aarts F, Vogelaar FJ. Prevalence of underlying malignancies in complex cysts of the breast. Breast Dis. 2022;41(1):89–95. https://doi.org/10.3233/BD-201057. PMID: 34542054.
11. Yao JP, Hao YZ, Chang Q, Geng CY, Chen Y, Zhao WP, Song Y, Zhou X. Value of ultrasonographic features for assessing malignant potential of complex cystic breast lesions. J Ultrasound Med. 2017;36(4):699–704. https://doi.org/10.7863/ultra.16.05012. Epub 2017 Jan 21. PMID: 28109002.
12. Masciadri N, Ferranti C. Benign breast lesions: ultrasound. J Ultrasound. 2011;14(2):55–65. https://doi.org/10.1016/j.jus.2011.03.002. Epub 2011 Apr 20. PMID: 23396888; PMCID: PMC3558101.
13. Tea MK, Grimm C, Heinz-Peer G, Delancey J, Singer C. The predictive value of suspicious sonographic characteristics in atypical cyst-like breast lesions. Breast. 2011;20(2):165–9. https://doi.org/10.1016/j.breast.2010.10.003. Epub 2010 Oct 28. PMID: 21035340.
14. Usami Y, Tsunoda H, Kajiura Y, Kawauchi N, Kikuchi M, Honda S, Saida Y, Suzuki K. Ultrasonographic evaluation of multiple cystic lesions in breast sonography. Choonpa Igaku. 2011;38(4):455–60. https://doi.org/10.3179/jjmu.38.455.
15. Apple SK, Doepke L, Bassett LW. Benign cystic lesions of the breast. In: Breast imaging; 2011. p. 239–54. https://doi.org/10.1016/B978-1-4160-5199-2.00015-1.
16. Rinaldi P, Ierardi C, Costantini M, Magno S, Giuliani M, Belli P, Bonomo L. Cystic breast lesions: sonographic findings and clinical management. J

Ultrasound Med. 2010;29(11):1617–26. https://doi.org/10.7863/jum.2010.29.11.1617. PMID: 20966473.
17. American College of Radiology. BI-RADS®—mammography. In: Breast imaging reporting and data system (BI-RADS) atlas. 4th ed. Reston, VA: American College of Radiology; 2003.
18. Saslow D, Boetes C, Burke W, Harms S, Leach MO, Lehman CD, Morris E, Pisano E, Schnall M, Sener S, Smith RA, Warner E, Yaffe M, Andrews KS, Russell CA, American Cancer Society Breast Cancer Advisory Group. American Cancer Society guidelines for breast screening with MRI as an adjunct to mammography. CA Cancer J Clin. 2007;57(2):75–89. https://doi.org/10.3322/canjclin.57.2.75. Erratum in: CA Cancer J Clin. 2007 May-Jun;57(3):185. PMID: 17392385.
19. Schelfout K, Van Goethem M, Kersschot E, Colpaert C, Schelfhout AM, Leyman P, Verslegers I, Biltjes I, Van Den Haute J, Gillardin JP, Tjalma W, Van Der Auwera JC, Buytaert P, De Schepper A. Contrast-enhanced MR imaging of breast lesions and effect on treatment. Eur J Surg Oncol. 2004;30(5):501–7. https://doi.org/10.1016/j.ejso.2004.02.003. PMID: 15135477.
20. Bluemke DA, Gatsonis CA, Chen MH, DeAngelis GA, DeBruhl N, Harms S, Heywang-Köbrunner SH, Hylton N, Kuhl CK, Lehman C, Pisano ED, Causer P, Schnitt SJ, Smazal SF, Stelling CB, Weatherall PT, Schnall MD. Magnetic resonance imaging of the breast prior to biopsy. JAMA. 2004;292(22):2735–42. https://doi.org/10.1001/jama.292.22.2735. PMID: 15585733.
21. Johansson A, Christakou AE, Iftimi A, Eriksson M, Tapia J, Skoog L, Benz CC, Rodriguez-Wallberg KA, Hall P, Czene K, Lindström LS. Characterization of benign breast diseases and association with age, hormonal factors, and family history of breast cancer among women in Sweden. JAMA Netw Open. 2021;4(6):e2114716. https://doi.org/10.1001/jamanetworkopen.2021.14716. PMID: 34170304; PMCID: PMC8233703.
22. Guray M, Sahin AA. Benign breast diseases: classification, diagnosis, and management. Oncologist. 2006;11(5):435–49. https://doi.org/10.1634/theoncologist.11-5-435. PMID: 16720843.
23. Berg WA, Sechtin AG, Marques H, Zhang Z. Cystic breast masses and the ACRIN 6666 experience. Radiol Clin North Am. 2010;48(5):931–87. https://doi.org/10.1016/j.rcl.2010.06.007. PMID: 20868895; PMCID: PMC3020576.
24. Hughes LE, Mansel RE, Webster DJ. Aberrations of normal development and involution (ANDI): a new perspective on pathogenesis and nomenclature of benign breast disorders. Lancet. 1987;2(8571):1316–9. https://doi.org/10.1016/s0140-6736(87)91204-9. PMID: 2890912.
25. Berg WA, Campassi CI, Ioffe OB. Cystic lesions of the breast: sonographic-pathologic correlation. Radiology. 2003;227(1):183–91. https://doi.org/10.1148/radiol.2272020660. PMID: 12668745.
26. Gómez A, Mata JM, Donoso L, Rams A. Galactocele: three distinctive radiographic appearances. Radiology. 1986;158(1):43–4. https://doi.org/10.1148/radiology.158.1.3940395. PMID: 3940395.
27. Sawhney S, Petkovska L, Ramadan S, Al-Muhtaseb S, Jain R, Sheikh M. Sonographic appearances of galactoceles. J Clin Ultrasound. 2002;30(1):18–22. https://doi.org/10.1002/jcu.10038. PMID: 11807850.
28. Stevens K, Burrell HC, Evans AJ, Sibbering DM. The ultrasound appearances of galactocoeles. Br J Radiol. 1997;70:239–41. https://doi.org/10.1259/bjr.70.831.9166046. PMID: 9166046.
29. Kiran S, Jeong YJ, Nelson ME, Ring A, Johnson MB, Sheth PA, Ma Y, Sener SF, Lang JE. Are we overtreating intraductal papillomas? J Surg Res. 2018;231:387–94. https://doi.org/10.1016/j.jss.2018.06.008. Epub 2018 Jun 29. PMID: 30278958; PMCID: PMC6173197.
30. Al Sarakbi W, Worku D, Escobar PF, Mokbel K. Breast papillomas: current management with a focus on a new diagnostic and therapeutic modality. Int Semin Surg Oncol. 2006;3:1. https://doi.org/10.1186/1477-7800-3-1. PMID: 16417642; PMCID: PMC1395317.
31. Rosen PP, Holmes G, Lesser ML, Kinne DW, Beattie EJ. Juvenile papillomatosis and breast carcinoma. Cancer. 1985;55(6):1345–52. https://doi.org/10.1002/1097-0142(19850315)55:6<1345::aid-cncr2820550631>3.0.co;2-b. PMID: 3971303.
32. Bazzocchi F, Santini D, Martinelli G, Piccaluga A, Taffurelli M, Grassigli A, Marrano D. Juvenile papillomatosis (epitheliosis) of the breast. A clinical and pathologic study of 13 cases. Am J Clin Pathol. 1986;86(6):745–8. https://doi.org/10.1093/ajcp/86.6.745. PMID: 3788861.
33. Rosen PP, Kimmel M. Juvenile papillomatosis of the breast. A follow-up study of 41 patients having biopsies before 1979. Am J Clin Pathol. 1990;93(5):599–603. https://doi.org/10.1093/ajcp/93.5.599. PMID: 2158224.
34. Visscher DW, Nassar A, Degnim AC, et al. Sclerosing adenosis and risk of breast cancer. Breast Cancer Res Treat. 2014;144(1):205–12. https://doi.org/10.1007/s10549-014-2862-5.
35. Wellings SR, Alpers CE. Subgross pathologic features and incidence of radial scars in the breast. Hum Pathol. 1984;15:475–9.
36. Kim EM, Hankins A, Cassity J, et al. Isolated radial scar diagnosis by core needle biopsy: is surgical excision necessary? Springerplus. 2016;5:398.
37. Ciatto S, Morrone D, Catarzi S, et al. Radial scars of the breast: review of 38 consecutive mammographic diagnoses. Radiology. 1993;187:757–60.
38. Lv M, Zhu X, Zhong S, Chen W, Hu Q, Ma T, Zhang J, Zhang X, Tang J, Zhao J. Radial scars and subsequent breast cancer risk: a meta-analysis. PLoS One. 2014;9(7):e102503. https://doi.org/10.1371/journal.pone.0102503. PMID: 25019286; PMCID: PMC4097058.
39. Huang W, Molitch ME. Evaluation and management of galactorrhea. Am Fam Physician. 2012;85(11):1073–80. PMID: 22962879.

40. Molitch ME. Drugs and prolactin. Pituitary. 2008;11(2):209–18. https://doi.org/10.1007/s11102-008-0106-6. PMID: 18404390.
41. Vroonen L, Daly AF, Beckers A. Epidemiology and management challenges in prolactinomas. Neuroendocrinology. 2019;109(1):20–7. https://doi.org/10.1159/000497746. Epub 2019 Feb 7. PMID: 30731464.
42. Christin-Maître S, Delemer B, Touraine P, Young J. Prolactinoma and estrogens: pregnancy, contraception and hormonal replacement therapy. Ann Endocrinol (Paris). 2007;68(2–3):106–12. https://doi.org/10.1016/j.ando.2007.03.008. Epub 2007 May 30. PMID: 17540335.
43. Dixon JM. Periductal mastitis and duct ectasia: an update. Breast. 1998;7(3):128–30. https://doi.org/10.1016/S0960-9776(98)90021-2.
44. Dixon JM, Anderson TJ, Lumsden AB, Elton RA, Roberts MM, Forrest AP. Mammary duct ectasia. Br J Surg. 1983;70(10):601–3. https://doi.org/10.1002/bjs.1800701011. PMID: 6684964.
45. Walker JC, Sandison AT. Mammary-duct ectasia. A clinical study. Br J Surg. 1964;51(5):350–5. https://doi.org/10.1002/bjs.1800510513.
46. Diaconu C, Socolov D, Dragomir C, Costachescu G, Florea N. 91 P—Periductal mastitis and mammary duct ectasia—two stages of the same disease? Eur J Cancer. 1996;32(Supplement 1):S19. https://doi.org/10.1016/0959-8049(96)84846-5.
47. Zhou F, Yu LX, Ma ZB, Yu ZG. Granulomatous lobular mastitis. Chronic Dis Transl Med. 2016;2(1):17–21. https://doi.org/10.1016/j.cdtm.2016.02.004. PMID: 29063020; PMCID: PMC5643750.
48. Going JJ, Anderson TJ, Wilkinson S, Chetty U. Granulomatous lobular mastitis. J Clin Pathol. 1987;40(5):535–40. https://doi.org/10.1136/jcp.40.5.535. PMID: 3584506; PMCID: PMC1141020.
49. Mondor H. Tronculite sous-cutané subaigue de laparoi thoracique antero-laterale. Mem Acad Chir (Paris). 1939;65:1271–8.
50. Taboada JL, Stephens TW, Krishnamurthy S, Brandt KR, Whitman GJ. The many faces of fat necrosis in the breast. AJR Am J Roentgenol. 2009;192(3):815–25. https://doi.org/10.2214/AJR.08.1250. PMID: 19234281.
51. Glass AR. Gynecomastia. Endocrinol Metab Clin North Am. 1994;23(4):825–37. PMID: 7705322.
52. Moore DC, Schlaepfer LV, Paunier L, Sizonenko PC. Hormonal changes during puberty: V. Transient pubertal gynecomastia: abnormal androgen-estrogen ratios. J Clin Endocrinol Metab. 1984;58(3):492–9. https://doi.org/10.1210/jcem-58-3-492. PMID: 6693546.
53. Mahoney CP. Adolescent gynecomastia. Differential diagnosis and management. Pediatr Clin North Am. 1990;37(6):1389–404. https://doi.org/10.1016/s0031-3955(16)37016-x. PMID: 2259545.
54. Mathur R, Braunstein GD. Gynecomastia: pathomechanisms and treatment strategies. Horm Res. 1997;48(3):95–102. https://doi.org/10.1159/000185497. PMID: 11546925.
55. Coen P, Kulin H, Ballantine T, Zaino R, Frauenhoffer E, Boal D, Inkster S, Brodie A, Santen R. An aromatase-producing sex-cord tumor resulting in prepubertal gynecomastia. N Engl J Med. 1991;324(5):317–22. https://doi.org/10.1056/NEJM199101313240507. PMID: 1986290.
56. Hertl MC, Wiebel J, Schäfer H, Willig HP, Lambrecht W. Feminizing Sertoli cell tumors associated with Peutz-Jeghers syndrome: an increasingly recognized cause of prepubertal gynecomastia. Plast Reconstr Surg. 1998;102(4):1151–7. https://doi.org/10.1097/00006534-199809040-00036. PMID: 9734436.
57. Agarwal VR, Takayama K, Van Wyk JJ, Sasano H, Simpson ER, Bulun SE. Molecular basis of severe gynecomastia associated with aromatase expression in a fibrolamellar hepatocellular carcinoma. J Clin Endocrinol Metab. 1998;83(5):1797–800. https://doi.org/10.1210/jcem.83.5.4773. PMID: 9589695.
58. Bowman JD, Kim H, Bustamante JJ. Drug-induced gynecomastia. Pharmacotherapy. 2012;32(12):1123–40. https://doi.org/10.1002/phar.1138. Epub 2012 Nov 16. PMID: 23165798.
59. Thompson DF, Carter JR. Drug-induced gynecomastia. Pharmacotherapy. 1993;13(1):37–45. PMID: 8094898.
60. Johnson RE, Murad MH. Gynecomastia: pathophysiology, evaluation, and management. Mayo Clin Proc. 2009;84(11):1010–5. https://doi.org/10.1016/S0025-6196(11)60671-X. PMID: 19880691; PMCID: PMC2770912.
61. Carlson HE. Approach to the patient with gynecomastia. J Clin Endocrinol Metab. 2011;96(1):15–21. https://doi.org/10.1210/jcem.96.9.zeg15a. PMID: 21209041.
62. Chan CL, Ho RS, Shek TW, Kwong A. Diabetic mastopathy. Breast J. 2013;19(5):533–8. https://doi.org/10.1111/tbj.12158. Epub 2013 Jul 29. PMID: 23895671.
63. Thorncroft K, Forsyth L, Desmond S, Audisio RA. The diagnosis and management of diabetic mastopathy. Breast J. 2007;13(6):607–13. https://doi.org/10.1111/j.1524-4741.2007.00489.x. PMID: 17983405.
64. Powell CM, Cranor ML, Rosen PP. Pseudoangiomatous stromal hyperplasia (PASH). A mammary stromal tumor with myofibroblastic differentiation. Am J Surg Pathol. 1995;19(3):270–7. https://doi.org/10.1097/00000478-199503000-00004. PMID: 7872425.
65. Virk RK, Khan A. Pseudoangiomatous stromal hyperplasia: an overview. Arch Pathol Lab Med.

2010;134(7):1070–4. https://doi.org/10.5858/2008-0686-RS.1. PMID: 20586640.
66. Krings G, Bean GR, Chen YY. Fibroepithelial lesions; The WHO spectrum. Semin Diagn Pathol. 2017;34(5):438–52. https://doi.org/10.1053/j.semdp.2017.05.006. Epub 2017 May 28. PMID: 28688536.
67. Lozada JR, Burke KA, Maguire A, Pareja F, Lim RS, Kim J, Gularte-Merida R, Murray MP, Brogi E, Weigelt B, Reis-Filho JS, Geyer FC. Myxoid fibroadenomas differ from conventional fibroadenomas: a hypothesis-generating study. Histopathology. 2017;71(4):626–34. https://doi.org/10.1111/his.13258. Epub 2017 Jul 5. PMID: 28513873; PMCID: PMC5597459.
68. Cowan ML, Argani P, Cimino-Mathews A. Benign and low-grade fibroepithelial neoplasms of the breast have low recurrence rate after positive surgical margins. Mod Pathol. 2016;29(3):259–65. https://doi.org/10.1038/modpathol.2015.157. Epub 2016 Jan 8. PMID: 26743469.
69. Ramírez-Montaño L, Vargas-Tellez E, Dajer-Fadel WL, Espinosa Maceda S. Giant lipoma of the breast. Arch Plast Surg. 2013;40(3):244–6. https://doi.org/10.5999/aps.2013.40.3.244. Epub 2013 May 16. PMID: 23730601; PMCID: PMC3665869.
70. delli Santi G, Bellioni M, Loreti A, Stagnitto D, La Pinta M, Dell'Osso A. Giant breast lipoma: a rare cause of breast asymmetry. Plast Reconstr Surg. 2006;117(3):1068–9. https://doi.org/10.1097/01.prs.0000201322.91566.42. PMID: 16525337.
71. Efared B, Sidibé IS, Abdoulaziz S, Hammas N, Chbani L, El Fatemi H. Tubular adenoma of the breast: a clinicopathologic study of a series of 9 cases. Clin Med Insights Pathol. 2018;11:1179555718757499. https://doi.org/10.1177/1179555718757499. PMID: 29449780; PMCID: PMC5808954.
72. Lee WF, Sheen-Chen SM, Chi SY, Huang HY, Ko SF. Hamartoma of the breast: an underrecognized disease? Tumori. 2008;94(1):114–5. PMID: 18468345.
73. Georgian-Smith D, Kricun B, McKee G, Yeh E, Rafferty EA, D'Alessandro HA, Kopans DB. The mammary hamartoma: appreciation of additional imaging characteristics. J Ultrasound Med. 2004;23(10):1267–73. https://doi.org/10.7863/jum.2004.23.10.1267. PMID: 15448315.
74. Seo M, Cho N, Ahn HS, Moon HG. Cowden syndrome presenting as breast cancer: imaging and clinical features. Korean J Radiol. 2014;15(5):586–90. https://doi.org/10.3348/kjr.2014.15.5.586. Epub 2014 Sep 12. PMID: 25246819; PMCID: PMC4170159.
75. Brown AC, Audisio RA, Regitnig P. Granular cell tumour of the breast. Surg Oncol. 2011;20(2):97–105. https://doi.org/10.1016/j.suronc.2009.12.001. Epub 2010 Jan 13. PMID: 20074934.
76. Akahane K, Kato K, Ogiso S, Sakaguchi K, Hashimoto M, Ishikawa A, Kato T, Fuwa Y, Takahashi A, Kobayashi K. Malignant granular cell tumor of the breast: case report and literature review. Breast Cancer. 2015;22(3):317–23. https://doi.org/10.1007/s12282-012-0362-1. Epub 2012 Mar 31. PMID: 22467405.
77. Rowell MD, Perry RR, Hsiu JG, Barranco SC. Phyllodes tumors. Am J Surg. 1993;165(3):376–9. https://doi.org/10.1016/s0002-9610(05)80849-9. PMID: 8383473.
78. World Health Organization. Histologic typing of breast tumors, vol. 2. 2nd ed. Geneva: WHO; 1981.
79. Rosen PP. Rosen's breast pathology. 2nd ed. New York: Lippincott William Wilkins; 2001.
80. Salvadori B, Cusumano F, Del Bo R, Delledonne V, Grassi M, Rovini D, Saccozzi R, Andreola S, Clemente C. Surgical treatment of phyllodes tumors of the breast. Cancer. 1989;63(12):2532–6. https://doi.org/10.1002/1097-0142(19890615)63:12<2532::aid-cncr2820631229>3.0.co;2-q. PMID: 2541890.

Breast Cancer

Duncan Khanikar, Kiran Kamalasanan, Arvind Krishnamurthy, Munlima Hazarika, and Amal Chandra Kataki

1 Incidence and Etiology

Breast cancer has been a major scourge for suffering and death in women throughout the world. As per GLOBOCAN 2020 [1], female breast cancer has now surpassed lung cancer as the leading cause of global cancer incidence in 2020, with an estimated 2.3 million new cases, representing 11.7% of all cancer cases. It is the fifth leading cause of cancer mortality worldwide, with 685,000 deaths. Among women, breast cancer accounts for 1 in 4 cancer cases and 1 in 6 cancer deaths, ranking first for incidence in the vast majority of countries (159 of 185 countries and for mortality in 110 countries).

Breast cancer accounts for nearly 25% of cancer cases and 15% of cancer-related deaths. However, there is a wide variation in incidence and mortality according to economic and geographic differences among countries. Breast cancer was more common in the richer and more industrialized nations, but recent trends suggest an equally alarming rise in the developing countries as well. Based on ICMR-National Centre for Disease Informatics and Research, in the North-Eastern region of India, the probability of developing Breast cancer (1 in 76 females) is the highest followed by that of cervix uteri (1 in every 86 females) and that of lung cancer (1 in every 109 females). This chapter attempts to highlight the salient features in the management of breast cancer.

D. Khanikar (✉) · M. Hazarika
Department of Medical Oncology, Dr. B Borooah Cancer Institute (A Unit of Tata Memorial Centre, Mumbai), Guwahati, Assam, India

K. Kamalasanan
Department of Surgical Oncology, Dr. B Borooah Cancer Institute (A Unit of Tata Memorial Centre, Mumbai), Guwahati, Assam, India

A. Krishnamurthy
Department of Surgical Oncology, Adyar Cancer Institute, Chennai, Tamilnadu, India

A. C. Kataki
Department of Gynaecologic Oncology, Dr. Bhubaneswar Borooah Cancer Institute (A Unit of Tata Memorial Centre, Mumbai), Guwahati, Assam, India

2 Risk Factors for Breast Cancer

It is to be noted that more than half of the breast cancer patients have no identifiable risk factors apart from increasing age and female gender. The risk factors that have been implicated can be gauged by the relative risk for breast cancer development. Most of these factors have a very high risk (RR > 2) and are mostly non-modifiable. They include increased breast density, precancerous breast lesions, and previous chest wall irradiation. Age, genetics, and an afflicted family tree do carry a stronger risk and demand better screening methods for the at-risk group.

A. C. Kataki, D. Barmon (eds.), *Fundamentals in Gynaecologic Malignancy*,
https://doi.org/10.1007/978-981-19-5860-1_10

The modifiable risk factors are mostly hormone-driven and based on poor lifestyle choices. They carry a low to minimal risk (RR < 2) and include early age at menarche, late menopause, nulliparity, exogenous estrogen exposure, and age at childbirth beyond 30 years of age. Increasing alcohol consumption, smoking, and less physical inactivity worsen any existing risk factor and predisposes to Breast cancer [2].

Increasing age—Age is a non-modifiable but important risk factor. According to SEER data [3], the probability of a woman developing breast cancer in the USA between 2013 and 2015 was:

- Birth to age 49—2.0 (1 in 49 women).
- Age 50 to 59—2.3 (1 in 42 women).
- Age 60 to 69—3.5 (1 in 28 women).
- Age 70 and older—6.7 (1 in 14 women).
- Birth to death—12.4 (1 in 8 women).

Women with breast cancer in India are found to be a decade younger in comparison to western women suggesting that breast cancer occurs at a younger premenopausal age in India. Cancers in the young, however, tend to be more aggressive [4].

Female gender—The incidence of breast cancer is 100 times more frequent in women than in men. As per United States data, more than 270,000 women suffer from Breast cancer annually, whereas less than 3000 cases are detected in men.

Weight and body fat—Obesity (defined as BMI ≥30 kg/m^2), per se worsens morbidity and mortality in women of all age groups.

Postmenopausal women—A higher BMI and/or perimenopausal weight gain have been consistently associated with a higher risk of breast cancer among postmenopausal women.

In a meta-analysis of more than 1000 epidemiologic studies of cancer risk, women with a higher BMI experienced an increased risk of postmenopausal breast cancer (relative risk [RR] 1.1 per 5 BMI units, 95% CI 1.1–1.2), particularly estrogen receptor (ER)-positive breast cancer [5].

The association between a higher BMI and postmenopausal breast cancer risk may be explained by higher estrogen levels resulting from the peripheral conversion of estrogen precursors (from adipose tissue) to estrogen. Arguing for this mechanism are data suggesting that, even among women with normal BMI, a higher body-fat percentage is associated with an elevated risk of breast cancer, particularly hormone receptor-positive breast cancer. In a secondary analysis of the Women's Health Initiative trial, among 3460 postmenopausal women with normal BMI, the multivariable-adjusted hazard ratios (HRs) for breast cancer risk among those with the highest quartile of body fat versus the lowest was 1.89 (95% CI 1.21–2.95) and 2.21 for ER-positive breast cancer (95% CI 1.23–3.67) [6].

In addition, hyperinsulinemia may also explain the obesity-breast cancer relationship because a high BMI is associated with higher insulin levels.

Premenopausal women—Unlike postmenopausal women, an increased BMI is associated with a lower risk of breast cancer in premenopausal women. In a multicenter analysis using pooled individual-level data from approximately 760,000 premenopausal women from 19 prospective cohorts, there was a 4.2-fold increased risk between the highest and lowest BMI categories (BMI ≥35 versus <17) [6].

The explanation of this finding remains unclear.

Tall stature—Increased height is an interesting risk factor for Breast cancer irrespective of menopausal status. The mechanism is not properly known but may be due to differential nutritional exposures during childhood and puberty [7].

Estrogen levels—Endogenous Estrogen, as well as Progesterone levels, carry an important risk in Breast cancer (more in Hormone receptor-positive) irrespective of menopausal status. The effect is more marked in postmenopausal women and this had led to therapies targeting the estrogen receptors and/or reducing estrogen levels.

Estrogen levels also play a role in the development of breast cancer among premenopausal women but, due to variations across the menstrual cycle, can be hard to measure. In a pooled analysis of data from seven studies, including 767 premenopausal women with breast cancer and 1699 matched controls, concentrations of estradiol, calculated free estradiol, estrone, androstenedione, dehydroepiandrosterone sulfate, and testosterone were positively associated with breast cancer risk [8]. For example, every twofold increase in estradiol concentration was associated with an odds ratio (OR) for breast cancer of 1.19 (95% CI 1.06–1.35). Concentrations of luteal-phase progesterone and calculated free testosterone were not significantly associated with such risk.

2.1 Breast Pathology

Benign breast disease—It includes a variety of common breast lesions, but only the proliferative types have a predisposition for developing Breast cancer.

Dense breast tissue—Breast tissue composition varies based on the relative amounts of adipose tissue and fibroglandular tissue. Fibroglandular tissue is radiodense and the major contributor to breast density. This component is also the harbinger of premalignant and malignant lesions. Mammographically, dense breast tissue is defined as fibroglandular tissue comprising more than 75% of the breast shadow [9]. Higher the breast density, the greater the risk of developing Breast cancer [10].

Although breast density is a largely inherited trait, exogenous hormones can influence density. For example, postmenopausal estrogen and progesterone hormone therapy increased breast density, while ER antagonists (i.e., tamoxifen) decrease breast density. In a prospective trial that included women randomly assigned to daily combined equine estrogens plus medroxyprogesterone acetate or placebo, women taking hormonal therapy had a 6% increase in the mean mammographic density at 1 year compared with women taking the placebo who had a mean 0.9% decrease in mean mammographic density [11]. Despite this association, breast density is not strongly correlated with endogenous hormone levels.

Bone mineral density—Bone homeostasis is intrinsically dependent on estrogen exposure and estrogen receptors play an important role in modulating the response. Bone Mineral Density (BMD) is considered a surrogate marker for estrogen exposure (both endogenous and exogenous). It has been observed in many studies that high BMD carries a greater Breast cancer risk. In a meta-analysis of eight prospective cohorts and two nested-control studies that included 70,878 postmenopausal women, of whom 1889 developed breast cancer, women in the highest hip BMD category were 62% more likely to develop breast cancer compared with women in the lowest BMD category (RR 1.62, 95% CI 1.17–2.06, $p < 0.001$) [12].

2.2 Other Hormonal Factors

Androgens—Androgens viz. Testosterone has also been implicated in Breast cancer risk. Studies suggest that elevated androgen levels increase the risk specifically for hormone receptor-positive breast cancers, and one study suggests they are associated with a lower risk of hormone receptor-negative breast cancers.

Insulin pathway and related hormones—A pooled analysis of 17 prospective studies have indicated that Insulin Growth Factor 1 is associated with Breast cancer risk in both premenopausal as well as postmenopausal women [13].

In addition, the Women's Health Initiative reported that higher endogenous insulin levels increased the risk of breast cancer among nondiabetic, postmenopausal women who did not take menopausal hormone therapy (HR for highest versus lowest quartile of insulin level 2.40, 95% CI 1.30–4.41) [14].

Diethylstilbestrol—Before 1971, in utero exposure to diethylstilbestrol that was given to mothers to prevent pregnancy complications has been linked to vaginal clear cell adenocarcinoma, and some studies have suggested an association with breast cancer.

Exogenous hormones—The impact of exogenous hormone use seems to depend as much on the agent used (estrogen-only versus estrogen plus progesterone preparations) and whether a woman is menopausal. For women undergoing in vitro fertilization, there does not appear to be an increased long-term risk of breast cancer.

Menopausal hormone therapy—Evidence supports cautious use of Hormone Replacement Therapy in Menopausal women. While the highest risk is with long-term use, short-term use of combined estrogen-progestin therapy (less than 3 years in previous users of estrogen) does not appear to significantly increase the risk of breast cancer.

Additional data on the risks of hormone therapy in young women, particularly centered on estrogen-progestin contraceptives, are discussed separately.

2.3 Reproductive Factors

Menarche at a younger age or later menopause—Menarche at a younger age is linked to a higher risk of breast cancer [15]. Compared to women who had menarche before the age of 13, women who had menarche at or after the age of 15 were less likely to develop ER−/progesterone receptor (PR)-positive breast cancer (HR 0.76, 95% CI 0.68–0.85). Women who reached menarche at or after the age of 15 had a 16% lower risk of developing ER-/PR-negative breast cancer. According to one study, every year that menarche was delayed resulted in a 5% reduction in the incidence of breast cancer [16].

Furthermore, the risk of breast cancer rises as women approach menopause and thereafter. After menopause, the Relative Risk rises by 1.03% each year, which is similar to the rise seen with menopausal hormone therapy.

Nulliparity and multiparity—Nulliparous women have an increased risk for breast cancer when compared with parous women (RR from 1.2 to 1.7). Although parous women have an increased risk for developing breast cancer within the first few years of delivery relative to nulliparous women, parity confers a protective effect decades after delivery. The effect of parity also differs depending upon the age of first birth.

Nulliparity and being overweight may have a synergistic effect on breast cancer risk for women >70 years of age.

Although studies have suggested that increasing the number of pregnancies might reduce breast cancer risk, it will be premature to conclude that multiparity has a protective effect on Breast cancer.

Infertility—There is some debate over the link between infertility and the risk of breast cancer. Infertility caused by anovulatory disorders has been linked to a lower risk of breast cancer in several epidemiological studies. After accounting for prior pregnancy history and age at first delivery, additional studies have found either no link or a minor increase in the increase of Breast cancer with infertility.

Increasing age at first pregnancy—Women who have their first child later in life are more likely to get breast cancer [17]. The cumulative incidence of breast cancer (up to age 70) was 20% lower, 10% lower, and 5% higher among women who delivered their first child at age 20, 25, or 35 years, respectively, according to the Nurses' Health Study as compared to nulliparous women at or near menopause [18]. A nulliparous woman's risk was similar to that of a woman who had her first full-term child at the age of 35.

Full cellular differentiation, which happens in the gland before and after pregnancy, is thought to protect the breast from developing breast cancer [19]. Because of the additional proliferative stimulation exerted on breast cells that are more likely to be fully grown and thus more susceptible to cell damage, later age at first birth may confer a greater risk than nulliparity.

2.4 History of Breast Cancer

A personal history of ductal carcinoma in situ (DCIS) or invasive breast cancer raises the risk of acquiring invasive breast cancer in the contralateral breast. During an average follow-up of 7.5 years in a 2010 study utilizing SEER data that included over 340,000 women with initial breast cancer, the incidence of invasive contralateral breast cancer (CBC) was 4% [20].

The risk of a CBC varied by age at the time of the index breast cancer diagnosis and the hormone receptor status of primary cancer:

- For women with prior ER-negative breast cancer—The rate was highest among women <30 years at diagnosis compared with those diagnosed at an older age (1.26 versus 0.85 at age 30–35 years and 0.45–0.64 for diagnoses ≥40 years).
- For women with prior ER-positive breast cancer—The rate (per 100 woman years) was slightly higher for women diagnosed under 30 years compared with those diagnosed at an older age (0.45 versus 0.25–0.37, respectively). Notably, these rates have been decreasing over time, most likely due to the wider use of hormonal therapy.

In a separate study, risks of CBC among those with hormone receptor-positive breast cancer were approximately 0.2% per year for the first 5 years after diagnosis (during adjuvant endocrine therapy), 0.5% for the subsequent 5 years (after endocrine treatment), and somewhere between these estimates for the following 5–10 years [21]. These rates were not altered with the inclusion of DCIS.

For women with a history of breast cancer, the risks of a CBC are even higher if there is a family history of breast cancer. For example, in a case-control study of women with CBC matched with women with unilateral breast cancer as controls, having a first-degree relative with breast cancer increased the risk of CBC by almost twofold [22]. Risks were further increased if the relative was diagnosed at age <40 years.

Family history of breast cancer—A positive family history of breast cancer in first-degree relatives (women) carries a higher risk of acquiring Breast cancer.

In a pooled analysis of >50,000 women with breast cancer and 100,000 controls, the risk of breast cancer was [23]:

- Increased almost two-fold if a woman had one affected first-degree relative.
- Increased three-fold if she had two affected first-degree relatives.

Breast cancer risk is also influenced by the age of the affected first-degree relative at diagnosis [23]. If a first-degree relative was diagnosed before the age of 30 (RR 3.0, 95% CI 1.8–4.9), women had a threefold increased risk, while the risk is only 1.5-fold increased if the affected relative was diagnosed after the age of 60.

However, family history is still an important risk factor even with relatives with a later age at diagnosis. In a prospective cohort study of over 400,000 women, a family history of breast cancer in a first-degree relative was associated with an increased risk of breast cancer, regardless of whether the relative was diagnosed before or after 50 years of age [24].

Breast cancer susceptibility genes (BRCA), such as BRCA1, BRCA2, p53, STK11, CDH1, PALB2, PTEN, and the mismatch repair genes, are inherited genetic mutations that predispose to breast cancer. Only 5 to 6% of all breast cancers are directly attributable to the inheritance of these high penetrance genes. These are discussed in more detail elsewhere.

2.5 Lifestyle Factors

Alcohol—Alcohol consumption increases the risk of breast cancer development.

Smoking—Multiple studies highlight a modestly increased risk of breast cancer in smokers [25]. Increased risks are most consistent in studies that evaluated early initiation, longer duration, and/or higher pack-years of smoking. For example, in a meta-analysis of 27 prospective observational studies, the risk of breast cancer was increased among patients with any history of smoking (summary RR [SRR] 1.10, 95% CI 1.02–1.14) [26]. Similar results were seen for passive smoking. However, 50% of women who smoke also consume alcohol, a known risk factor for breast cancer [27]. However, in studies among women who smoked but did not drink alcohol, there was still an increased risk of breast cancer associated with smoking [27].

Studies also suggest a possible association between breast cancer risk and exposure to passive smoking, but data are inconsistent. For example, in a meta-analysis of 11 prospective studies, the SRR for breast cancer was 1.07 (95% CI 1.02–1.13), with no heterogeneity [28]. Among 20 retrospective studies, the SRR was 1.30 but with high heterogeneity. Similarly, in an observational study including approximately 323,000 women, passive smoking exposure was associated with an increased risk of breast cancer (HR 1.10, 95% CI 1.01–1.20) [29]. However, a previous report from the Nurses' Health Study found no association between passive smoking and breast cancer risk among a cohort of over 1800 women (920 with a diagnosis of breast cancer) [30].

Night-shift employment is classified as a possible carcinogen by the International Agency for Research on Cancer and the World Health Organization, despite conflicting data. For example:

- In the Million Women Study, the RR for breast cancer among those with 20 or more years of night-shift work versus no night-shift work was 1.00 (95% CI 0.81–1.23) [31].
- However, in a prior systematic review including 10 studies, a pooled adjusted RR for the association between "ever exposed to night-shift work" and breast cancer was 1.19 (95% CI 1.05–1.35) [32].
- A 2012 study on nurses reported that working shifts after midnight was associated with an elevated risk of breast cancer (OR 1.8, 95% CI 1.2–2.8), with the highest risk noted in nurses working long-term day-to-night rotating shifts (OR 2.6, 95% CI 1.8–3.8) [33].

Therapeutic ionizing radiation exposure—Early exposure to ionizing radiation of the chest has been linked to an increased risk of breast cancer [24]. The risk appears to be greatest between the ages of 10 and 14 (prepuberty), while extra risk has been observed in women as old as 45. There does not appear to be any increased danger after the age of 45.

3 Protective Factors That May Reduce Breast Cancer Risk

Breastfeeding—Multiple case control and cohort studies and meta-analyses have revealed that nursing has a protective effect, the degree of which varies depending on the duration of breastfeeding and the confounding factor of parity.

A large pooled analysis from 47 epidemiologic studies (50,302 women with invasive breast cancer and 96,973 controls) stated that for every 12 months of breastfeeding, there was a 4.3% reduction in the relative risk (RR) of breast cancer. Another meta-analysis suggested that this association was stronger for hormone receptor-negative breast cancers. The protective effect of breastfeeding may stem from the fact that it may delay the re-establishment of ovulatory cycles.

Physical activity—While there is no direct evidence that inactivity is linked to an increased risk of breast cancer, regular physical exercise appears to provide modest protection against breast cancer, particularly in postmenopausal women. A 2016 review of epidemiologic studies estimated those at the risk of breast cancer were reduced among the most physically active women compared with women who were the least active (RR 0.88, 95% CI 0.85–0.90).

Given the paradoxical effect of weight in premenopausal and postmenopausal women, the reduction in breast cancer risk seen with exercise is likely not mediated through weight control alone. Increased physical activity may reduce breast cancer risk through hormonal influences such as reducing serum estrogens, insulin, and insulin growth factor-1 levels.

4 Epidemiology

Over the last decade, the incidence of breast cancer has been rising steadily and in India, 1 in every 29 women will develop Breast cancer during their lifetime [34].

In rural India, one out of every 64 women is thought to be at risk. This is in stark contrast to western research, which shows that one in every eight women is in danger of breast cancer. Breast cancer is the leading cancer among women in the subcontinent with age-adjusted incidence reported as high as 25.8 per 100,000 women and mortality 12.7 per 100,000 women. According to data from various national registries, the age-adjusted incidence rate of breast cancer was found to be as high as 41 per 100,000 women in Delhi, followed by Chennai (37.9), Bangalore (34.4), and Thiruvananthapuram District (33.7). A statistically significant increase in age-adjusted rate over time (1982–2014) in all the population-based cancer registries (PBCRs) namely Bangalore (annual percentage change: 2.84%), Barshi (1.87%), Bhopal (2.00%), Chennai (2.44%), Delhi (1.44%), and Mumbai (1.42%) was observed. Breast cancer projection for India predicts numbers to cross 170,000.

5 Role of Breast Imaging to Diagnose Breast Cancer

Mammography's present purpose is diagnostic, evaluating the ipsilateral breast for macrocalcification or multicentricity (if the woman wants to have her breasts conserved), or screening the opposite breast at the time of operation. (Less than 4% of women may have a contralateral lesion).

A combination of MG and USG can detect additional lesions than either of them alone but USG has a high false-positive rate, hence it is not routinely recommended in all patients. It can be used in cases when there the breasts are dense and the mass is occult or when there is clinical suspicion of multiple tumours. USG also serves as an adjunct for characterization of the mass, especially to differentiate a cystic lesion from solid.

Even when breast conservation surgery is planned, MRI is not suggested as a preoperative test for ipsilateral breast evaluation in all patients diagnosed with breast cancer. The COMICE trial is a randomized controlled trial (RCT) that found that using MRI in addition to triple assessment does not minimize the rate of reoperation in Breast conservation therapy patients [35].

The MONET study is another RCT that indicates an unfavorable effect of MRI in the form of higher re-excision rates in MRI patients. The ACRIN trial found that magnetic resonance imaging (MRI) can detect clinically and mammographically hidden breast cancer. However, according to the findings of this study, 12.5% of women required additional biopsies as a result of a positive MRI finding, of which less than 25% (24.8%) were positive for cancer, and only a little over half were positive for invasive cancer, with the rest being in situ. A comprehensive review and meta-analysis of incremental cancer detection and influence on surgical management of MRI breast results found that while MRI detects more tumours than traditional imaging, it is not always able to discriminate between benign and malignant findings.

Housammi et al. recently released an individual patient data meta-analysis examining the link between preoperative breast MRI and local and distant recurrence in breast cancer patients. There is no link between preoperative MRI and a lower risk of local or distant recurrence. Also, preoperative MRI is associated with increased odds of receiving ipsilateral mastectomy and contralateral prophylactic mastectomy as surgical treatment in newly diagnosed Breast cancer patients [36].

However, an MRI breast may be considered when the diagnosis of lobular carcinoma is made as there is an increased incidence of multifocal/bilateral tumours. It can also be used in cases of Paget's disease; with dense breasts on mammograms and no identifiable cause, as well as in situations of metastatic axillary adenopathy with negative dense mammograms.

6 Staging and Restaging

Conventional metastatic workup of a patient with advanced breast cancer includes a radionuclide bone scan to evaluate the skeletal system which is one of the commonest sites of disease spread (40). The commonly used tracer for this is 99mTc-methylene diphosphonate or hydroxy methylene diphosphonate. The skeletal lesions in breast cancer could be either osteoblastic, osteolytic, or mixed lesions. The sensitivity of planar bone scan for identifying bone metastases ranges from 62%·to 100%. The lower sensitivity is due to the inability to identify lytic lesions which do not incite high bone turnover as compared to the osteoblastic lesions having a high uptake due to the increased cell turnover. The specificity of these scans is between 78 and 100%; lower specificity is attributed to the traumatic, degenerative changes showing a false positive uptake. The specificity can be improved by doing a tomography of the suspicious area which is a 3-dimensional imaging of the region of interest called SPECT· Single Photon Emission Tomography. Additional anatomic imaging of the abnormality detected on scintigraphy could improve the specificity and this led to the advent of newer machines like positron emission tomography associated with computed tomography (PET/CT). PET /CT bone scan has higher sensitivity due to improved resolution of PET /CT scanner and a higher target to non-target delineation of fluoride which has 2–3 times higher uptake as compared to phosphates. The NCCN guidelines recommend an MDP bone scan for staging breast cancer and suggest an 18 Fluoride PET /CT bone scan if available.

A whole-body fluorodeoxyglucose (18F - FDG) PET /CT study works on the principle of the Warburg effect in cancer and its role in breast cancer has also been evaluated. FDG PET/CT is not sensitive in identifying small lesions (especially less than a centimeter); hence cannot be utilized to characterize small equivocal lesions located by other imaging modalities. Similarly, certain low-grade tumours may be falsely negative due to the absence of FDG uptake. Thus, it is not a suitable modality for screening or detection of primary breast cancer.

Extra axillary nodal disease FDG PET/CT has a better detection rate with higher sensitivity. The sensitivity for detection of internal mammary nodes using the FDG PET/CT method is high as shown in a preliminary study.

Few other larger studies evaluating the role of FDG PET/CT in Locally advanced breast cancer (LABC) have also confirmed better sensitivity in identifying both internal mammary and mediastinal nodes.

For bone metastases, FDG PET/CT is useful in identifying medullary lesions or lytic lesions, however, studies have shown a lower sensitivity for osteoblastic /sclerotic lesions. However, FDG PET /CT is used complementary with a bone scan to completely evaluate the skeletal system. NCCN guidelines suggest that if an FDG PET / CT scan is positive for a skeletal lesion an additional bone scan may not be performed.

Several studies have shown that FDG PET / CT has made a significant impact on the management of patients due to its high sensitivity; ranging from 84 to 93% to detect distant metastases.

6.1 TNM and Staging of Breast Cancer

Breast cancer staging follows the AJCC TNM staging (currently recommended, Eighth Edition) and incorporates T status, N status (clinical and pathologic), M status as per specific criteria.

The T stage includes the size of the tumour, its relation with the overlying skin and the chest wall (Table 1).

The N stage includes cN and pN which corresponds to clinical (physical examination and imaging) assessment and surgical assessment, respectively. Table 2 refers to cN and is determined by the levels of involved axillary lymph nodes. Table 3 indicates the Nodal staging based on the number of involved lymph nodes in the surgical specimen.

The M staging indicates the spread of disease to distant sites (Table 4).

Table 1 AJCC 8th edition TNM staging of breast cancer (definition of primary tumour (T)—clinical and pathological)

T Category	T Criteria
TX	Primary tumour cannot be assessed
T0	No evidence of primary tumour
Tis (DCIS)	Ductal carcinoma in situ
Tis (Paget)	Paget disease of the nipple NOT associated with invasive carcinoma and/or carcinoma in situ (DCIS) in the underlying breast parenchyma. Carcinomas in the breast parenchyma associated with Paget disease are categorized based on the size and characteristics of the parenchymal disease, although the presence of Paget disease should still be noted
T1	Tumour ≤20 mm in greatest dimension
T1mi	Tumour ≤1 mm in greatest dimension
T1a	Tumour >1 mm but ≤5 mm in greatest dimension (round any measurement 1.0–1.9 mm to 2 mm)
T1b	Tumour >5 mm but ≤10 mm in greatest dimension
T1c	Tumour >10 mm but ≤20 mm in greatest dimension
T2	Tumour >20 mm but ≤50 mm in greatest dimension
T3	Tumour >50 mm in greatest dimension
T4	Tumour of any size with direct extension to the chest wall and/or to the skin (ulceration or macroscopic nodules); invasion of the dermis alone does not qualify as T4
T4a	Extension to the chest wall; invasion or adherence to pectoralis muscle in the absence of invasion of chest wall structures does not qualify as T4
T4b	Ulceration and/or ipsilateral macroscopic satellite nodules and/or edema (including peau d'orange) of the skin that does not meet the criteria for inflammatory carcinoma
T4c	Both T4a and T4b are present
T4d	Inflammatory carcinoma

(***Source:*** *Reprinted with Permission from Wiley Global Permissions: Wiley Publication, ACS JOURNALS, Breast Cancer—Major changes in the American Joint Committee on Cancer eighth edition cancer staging manual by Armando E. Giuliano* et al, *Vol. 67, Issue4, p. 290-303, 2017,* https://doi.org/10.3322/caac.21393; Copyright *2017 by American cancer Society*)

Table 2 Definition of regional lymph nodes—clinical

cN Category	cN Criteria
cNX	Regional lymph nodes cannot be assessed (e.g., previously removed)
cN0	No regional lymph node metastases (by imaging or clinical examination)
cN1	Metastases to movable ipsilateral level I, II axillary lymph node(s)
cN1mi	Micrometastases (approximately 200 cells, larger than 0.2 mm, but none larger than 2.0 mm)
cN2	Metastases in ipsilateral level I, II axillary lymph nodes that are clinically fixed or matted
	Or in ipsilateral internal mammary nodes in the absence of axillary lymph node metastases
cN2a	Metastases in ipsilateral level I, II axillary lymph nodes fixed to one another (matted) or to other structures
cN2b	Metastases only in ipsilateral internal mammary nodes in the absence of axillary lymph node metastases
cN3	Metastases in ipsilateral infraclavicular (level III axillary) lymph node(s) with or without level I, II axillary lymph node involvement
	Or in ipsilateral internal mammary lymph node(s) with level I, II axillary lymph node metastases;
	Or metastases in ipsilateral supraclavicular lymph node(s) with or without axillary or internal mammary lymph node involvement
cN3a	Metastases in ipsilateral infraclavicular lymph node(s)
cN3b	Metastases in ipsilateral internal mammary lymph node(s) and axillary lymph node(s)
cN3c	Metastases in ipsilateral supraclavicular lymph node(s)

(***Source:*** *Reprinted with Permission from Wiley Global Permissions: Wiley Publication, ACS JOURNALS, Breast Cancer—Major changes in the American Joint Committee on Cancer eighth edition cancer staging manual by Armando E. Giuliano* et al, *Vol. 67, Issue 4, p. 290-303, 2017,* https://doi.org/10.3322/caac.21393; Copyright *2017 by American cancer Society*)

Table 3 Definition of regional nodes—pathological pN0

pN Category	pN Criteria
pNX	Regional lymph nodes cannot be assessed (e.g., not removed for pathological study or previously removed)
pN0	No regional lymph node metastasis identified or ITCs only
pN0(i+)	ITCs only (malignant cell clusters no larger than 0.2 mm) in regional lymph node(s)
pN0(mol+)	Positive molecular findings by reverse transcriptase polymerase chain reaction (RT-PCR); no ITCs detected
pN1	Micrometastases; or metastases in 1–3 axillary lymph nodes; and/or clinically negative internal mammary nodes with micrometastases or macrometastases by sentinel lymph node biopsy
pN1mi	Micrometastases (approximately 200 cells, larger than 0.2 mm, but none larger than 2.0 mm)
pN1a	Metastases in 1–3 axillary lymph nodes, at least one metastasis larger than 2.0 mm
pN1b	Metastases in ipsilateral internal mammary sentinel nodes, excluding ITCs
pN1c	pN1a and pN1b combined
pN2	Metastases in 4–9 axillary lymph nodes; or positive ipsilateral internal mammary lymph nodes by imaging in the absence of axillary lymph node metastases
pN2a	Metastases in 4–9 axillary lymph nodes (at least one tumour deposit larger than 2.0 mm)
pN2b	Metastases in clinically detected internal mammary lymph nodes with or without microscopic confirmation; with pathologically negative axillary nodes
pN3	Metastases in 10 or more axillary lymph nodes
	Or in infraclavicular (level III axillary) lymph nodes
	Or positive ipsilateral internal mammary lymph nodes by imaging in the presence of one or more positive level I, II axillary lymph nodes
	Or in more than three axillary lymph nodes and micrometastases or macrometastases by sentinel lymph node biopsy in clinically negative ipsilateral internal mammary lymph nodes
	Or in ipsilateral supraclavicular lymph nodes
pN3a	Metastases in 10 or more axillary lymph nodes (at least one tumour deposit larger than 2.0 mm);
	Or metastases to the infraclavicular (level III axillary lymph) nodes
pN3b	pN1a or pN2a in the presence of cN2b (positive internal mammary nodes by imaging);
	Or pN2a in the presence of pN1b
pN3c	Metastases in ipsilateral supraclavicular lymph nodes

(***Source:*** *Reprinted with Permission from Wiley Global Permissions: Wiley Publication, ACS JOURNALS, Breast Cancer—Major changes in the American Joint Committee on Cancer eighth edition cancer staging manual by Armando E. Giuliano* et al, *Vol. 67, Issue 4, p. 290-303, 2017,* https://doi.org/10.3322/caac.21393; Copyright *2017 by American cancer Society*)

Table 4 Definition of distant metastasis (M)

M Category	M Criteria
M0	No clinical or radiographic evidence of distant metastases
cM0(i+)	No clinical or radiographic evidence of distant metastases in the presence of tumour cells or deposits no larger than 0.2 mm detected microscopically or by molecular techniques in circulating blood, bone marrow, or other nonregional nodal tissue in a patient without symptoms or signs of metastases
M1	Distant metastases detected by clinical and radiographic means (cM) and/or histologically proven metastases larger than 0.2 mm (pM)

(***Source:*** *Reprinted with Permission from Wiley Global Permissions: Wiley Publication, ACS JOURNALS, Breast Cancer—Major changes in the American Joint Committee on Cancer eighth edition cancer staging manual by Armando E. Giuliano* et al, *Vol. 67, Issue 4, p. 290-303, 2017,* https://doi.org/10.3322/caac.21393; Copyright *2017 by American cancer Society*)

6.2 Changes in T Classification Between 7th and 8th Edition

- Lobular carcinoma in situ (LCIS) is now considered a benign entity and is no longer classified as Tis.
- Tumours >1 mm and <2 mm should now be rounded to 2 mm, so as not to classify tumours between 1 and 1.5 mm as microinvasive (T1mi) carcinomas.
- The eighth edition confirmed that small, microscopic, satellite tumour foci around a primary should not be added to the maximum tumour size.
- It also clarified that the T size for multiple synchronous tumours is that of the largest tumour, but the suffix “m” should be appended to the *T* score.
- It defined T4b lesions as macroscopic satellite tumour nodules to the skin that are separate from the primary tumour. Microscopic skin and dermal tumour satellite nodules do not qualify and should be classified based on tumour size.

6.3 Changes in N Classification from 7th to 8th Edition

The eighth edition clarified that the largest contiguous tumour deposit should define pN. Dimensions of satellite deposits are not added.

Furthermore, clarification was added that cNX should only be used when a nodal basin has been removed and cannot be examined by imaging or clinical exam. cN0 is assigned to tumours in which nodal exam and imaging if obtained, are negative.

6.4 Changes in Metastases (M) Classification

In the eighth edition, clarification was added that pM0 should not be used. Cases are either cM0 or cM1, and if cM1 disease is confirmed by biopsy, then pM1 should be used.

The clinical prognostic stage is the primary prognostic staging system for patients who receive neoadjuvant treatment or for those who do not receive upfront surgery. It is based on clinical T, N, and M; grade; and does not include genomic profile information (Table 5).

For patients who receive surgical resection as initial treatment, a pathologic prognostic stage is assigned, which is based on pathologic T, N, and M; grade; HER2 and hormone receptor status; and for T1 to T2 N0, ER-positive, HER2-negative disease, the result of genomic testing (Table 6).

Table 5 AJCC Anatomic Stage Groups

When T is…	And N is…	And M is…	Then the stage group is…
Tis	N0	M0	0
T1	N0	M0	IA
T0	N1mi	M0	IB
T1	N1mi	M0	IB
T0	N1	M0	IIA
T1	N1	M0	IIA
T2	N0	M0	IIA
T2	N1	M0	IIB
T3	N0	M0	IIB
T0	N2	M0	IIIA
T1	N2	M0	IIIA
T2	N2	M0	IIIA
T3	N1	M0	IIIA
T3	N2	M0	IIIA
T4	N0	M0	IIIB
T4	N1	M0	IIIB
T4	N2	M0	IIIB
Any T	N3	M0	IIIC
Any T	Any N	M1	IV

(***Source:*** *Reprinted with Permission from Wiley Global Permissions: Wiley Publication, ACS JOURNALS, Breast Cancer—Major changes in the American Joint Committee on Cancer eighth edition cancer staging manual by Armando E. Giuliano* et al, *Vol. 67, Issue 4, p. 290-303, 2017,* https://doi.org/10.3322/caac.21393; Copyright *2017 by American cancer Society*)

Table 6 Clinical Prognostic Stage (AJCC Cancer staging Manual, Eighth Edition)

When TNM is…	And grade is…	And HER2 status is…	And ER status is…	And PR status is…	Then the pathologic prognostic stage group is…
Tis(c or p)N0M0	Any	Any	Any	Any	0
T1[a]N0M0, T0N1miM0, T1[a]N1miM0	1	Positive	Positive	Positive	IA
				Negative	IA
			Negative	Positive	IA
				Negative	IA
		Negative	Positive	Positive	IA
				Negative	IA
			Negative	Positive	IA
				Negative	IA
	2	Positive	Positive	Positive	IA
				Negative	IA
			Negative	Positive	IA
				Negative	IA
		Negative	Positive	Positive	IA
				Negative	IA
			Negative	Positive	IA
				Negative	IB
	3	Positive	Positive	Positive	IA
				Negative	IA
			Negative	Positive	IA
				Negative	IA
		Negative	Positive	Positive	IA
				Negative	IA
			Negative	Positive	IA
				Negative	IB
T0N1[b]M0, T1N1[b]M0, T2N0M0	1	Positive	Positive	Positive	IA
				Negative	IB
			Negative	Positive	IB
				Negative	IIA
		Negative	Positive	Positive	IA
				Negative	IB
			Negative	Positive	IB
				Negative	IIA
	2	Positive	Positive	Positive	IA
				Negative	IB
			Negative	Positive	IB
				Negative	IIA
		Negative	Positive	Positive	IA
				Negative	IIA
			Negative	Positive	IIA
				Negative	IIA

(continued)

Table 6 (continued)

When TNM is…	And grade is…	And HER2 status is…	And ER status is…	And PR status is…	Then the pathologic prognostic stage group is…
	3	Positive	Positive	Positive	IA
				Negative	IIA
			Negative	Positive	IIA
				Negative	IIA
		Negative	Positive	Positive	IB
				Negative	IIA
			Negative	Positive	IIA
				Negative	IIA
T2N1M0, T3N0M0	1	Positive	Positive	Positive	IA
				Negative	IIB
			Negative	Positive	IIB
				Negative	IIB
		Negative	Positive	Positive	IA
				Negative	IIB
			Negative	Positive	IIB
				Negative	IIB
	2	Positive	Positive	Positive	IB
				Negative	IIB
			Negative	Positive	IIB
				Negative	IIB
		Negative	Positive	Positive	IB
				Negative	IIB
			Negative	Positive	IIB
				Negative	IIB
	3	Positive	Positive	Positive	IB
				Negative	IIB
			Negative	Positive	IIB
				Negative	IIB
		Negative	Positive	Positive	IIA
				Negative	IIB
			Negative	Positive	IIB
				Negative	IIIA
T0N2M0, T1N2M0, T2N2M0, T3N1M0, T3N2M0	1	Positive	Positive	Positive	IB
				Negative	IIIA
			Negative	Positive	IIIA
				Negative	IIIA
		Negative	Positive	Positive	IB
				Negative	IIIA
			Negative	Positive	IIIA
				Negative	IIIA
	2	Positive	Positive	Positive	IB
				Negative	IIIA
			Negative	Positive	IIIA
				Negative	IIIA
		Negative	Positive	Positive	IB
				Negative	IIIA
			Negative	Positive	IIIA
				Negative	IIIB

Table 6 (continued)

When TNM is…	And grade is…	And HER2 status is…	And ER status is…	And PR status is…	Then the pathologic prognostic stage group is…
	3	Positive	Positive	Positive	IIA
				Negative	IIIA
			Negative	Positive	IIIA
				Negative	IIIA
		Negative	Positive	Positive	IIB
				Negative	IIIA
			Negative	Positive	IIIA
				Negative	IIIC
T4N0M0, T4N1M0, T4N2M0, T(any)N3M0	1	Positive	Positive	Positive	IIIA
				Negative	IIIB
			Negative	Positive	IIIB
				Negative	IIIB
		Negative	Positive	Positive	IIIA
				Negative	IIIB
			Negative	Positive	IIIB
				Negative	IIIB
	2	Positive	Positive	Positive	IIIA
				Negative	IIIB
			Negative	Positive	IIIB
				Negative	IIIB
		Negative	Positive	Positive	IIIA
				Negative	IIIB
			Negative	Positive	IIIB
				Negative	IIIC
	3	Positive	Positive	Positive	IIIB
				Negative	IIIB
			Negative	Positive	IIIB
				Negative	IIIB
		Negative	Positive	Positive	IIIB
				Negative	IIIC
			Negative	Positive	IIIC
				Negative	IIIC
T(any)N(any)M1	Any	Any	Any	Any	IV

For cases in which HER2 is determined to be equivocal by in situ hybridization (ISH; fluorescence ISH or chromogenic ISH) testing under the 2013 ASCO/College of American Pathologists HER2 testing guidelines, the HER2-negative category should be used for staging in the pathologic prognostic stage group table. The prognostic value of these prognostic stage groups is based on populations of persons with breast cancer who have been offered and mostly treated with appropriate endocrine and/or systemic chemotherapy (including anti-HER2 therapy)

(**Source**: *Reprinted with permission from ASCO Educational Book "American Society of Clinical Oncology Educational Book: List of issues: volume 38: New and Important Changes in the TNM Staging System for Breast Cancer" by Gabriel N. Hortobagyi, MD, Stephen B. Edge, MD, and Armando Giuliano, MD, 2018, 10.1200/EDBK_201313; Copyright 2018 American Society of Clinical Oncology)*

[a] Includes T1mi

[b] Does not include N1mi

7 Approach to a Patient with a Suspected Breast Cancer

Breast cancer diagnosis involves the triple test, first described in 1975, which includes clinical examination, radiological investigations (mammography), and histopathological confirmation [3].

An abnormal mammography, ultrasound (US), or MRI may not always mean malignancy, and in the presence of an abnormal physical exam finding, normal imaging does not reliably exclude carcinoma. Further, in the setting of an abnormal mammography or US, a normal MRI does not obviate the need for biopsy to rule out malignancy.

7.1 Biopsy Techniques in Nonpalpable or Palpable Breast Lesions

Fine needle aspiration (FNA), core needle biopsy, and excisional biopsy are all options for biopsy. Needle biopsy techniques (FNA or core biopsy) are chosen because they are less expensive than surgical excision and eliminate a surgical scar and potential cosmetic deformities because most breast lesions are benign.

FNA requires a trained cytopathologist for accurate specimen interpretation and, when targeting primary breast lesions, does not reliably distinguish invasive cancer from DCIS. FNA is commonly used to evaluate palpable abnormalities and asymmetric breast tissue in a perceived high-risk situation, to screen high-risk patients for biological markers indicative of current active proliferation to assess temporal breast cancer risk, or to monitor prevention drug trials. A 22–25 G needle and a 10 cc syringe are generally used for FNA. Local anesthesia is achieved by injecting a dermal anesthetic into the biopsy site. The best specimen is obtained by rigorously jiggling the biopsy needle in and out under a vacuum and then releasing the vacuum before extracting the needle. This can be quickly mastered by the operator's immediate evaluation of specimen cellularity. Initially, air-dried smears were used, but aspirate material is increasingly being injected into a liquid. Biomarker evaluation for ER, PR, HER2, and other markers can often be performed on fine needle aspirate by centrifuging the cellular material and performing immunohistochemical (IHC) staining on the resulting cell block.

In contrast, core needle biopsy provides a histologic specimen with maintained architecture; facilitates ER, PR, and HER2 testing, which have become a critical component of multidisciplinary treatment planning; and allows for placement of a clip to mark the area of interest if subsequent surgical excision or definitive breast cancer treatment is indicated.

Both core needle biopsy and FNA can produce false-negative results due to sampling errors. Additional tissue should be acquired, usually by excisional biopsy, if there is no concordance between the core biopsy or FNA diagnosis and the clinical and imaging findings. The availability of large, vacuum-assisted biopsy machines that expand the area of lesion sample, together with the establishment of clearly defined reasons for follow-up surgical biopsy, has alleviated concerns about the false-negative rate of image-guided core biopsy. Core biopsy false-negative rates are now consistently around 1%. Surgical excision of all lesions displaying ALH or LCIS is no longer routinely suggested, despite the detection of atypical ductal hyperplasia on a core biopsy being universally acknowledged as a justification for open surgical biopsy. On a core biopsy, papillary carcinoma in situ can be difficult to identify from benign papillary lesions, and the radial scar can be difficult to separate from tubular carcinoma without removing the tumour completely.

Core biopsy for the identification of mammographic abnormalities is cost-effective and enhances the possibility that the patient will only need one surgical surgery for conclusive cancer treatment. Excisional biopsy should be used only in patients who have imaging abnormalities that cannot be targeted with core biopsy. A small margin of the anatomically normal breast should be excised around the tumour during an excisional biopsy for diagnosis, orienting sutures should be applied, and the material should be inked to allow margin examination.

8 Breast Cancer Immunohistochemistry

8.1 Receptor Expression Scoring

There has never been a standard way of interpreting IHC results. Others employ a continuous reporting system, while some pathologists use a binary approach (totally negative or unambiguously positive). There has yet to be established a universally agreed cut-off point for optimism.

8.2 *H*-Score

McCarty introduced the *H*-score, a semiquantitative grading system, in 1985. The *H*-score is calculated by multiplying the percent of tumour cells that stain the reagent by an ordinal value that corresponds to the intensity level (0 = none, 1 = weak, 2 = moderate, and 3 = high), with a maximum score of 300. A score of 1 is deemed negative, a score of 100 is weakly positive (1+), a score of 101–200 is moderately positive (2+), and a score of 201–300 is very positive (3+) according to the modified *H*-score [37].

8.3 Allred/Quick Score

The Allred score is the sum of the proportion and the intensity scores.

On a scale of 0 to 5, the proportion of positive staining cells is scored (0 = no staining; 1 = less than 1%; 2 = 1%–10%; 3 = 11%–33%; 4 = 34%–66%; 5 = 67%–100%), while the intensity of tumour cell staining is scored (0 = none; 1 = weak; 2 = moderate; 3 = strong). The total of these ratings provides a final score ranging from 0 to 8. A score of 0 to 2 is regarded as negative, while a score of 3 to 8 is considered positive. It has been demonstrated that malignancies with an Allred score of 2 have similar outcomes to tumours that are fully ER-negative. The majority of breast cancers have an Allred score of 7 or 8, indicating a favorable response to treatment. Tumours with scores of 3 or 4 are not well studied. Any score above 2 is considered positive [38].

8.4 *J*-Score

The *J*-score was developed by Japanese researchers to evaluate the number of positive cells without taking the staining intensity into account. The requirements for the *J*-score are as follows, with cut-off thresholds of 1% and 10%.

J-score 0: no staining.
J-score 1: less than 1% stained cells.
J-score 2: stained cells more than 1% but less than 10%, and.
J-score 3: more than 10% stained cells.

The conclusion on hormone receptor status was divided into three categories: negative (*J*-score 0), ambiguous (*J*-score 1 and 2), and positive (*J*-score 1 and 2). (*J*-score 3). In the Western world, this scoring system has not found favor.

9 American Society of Clinical Oncology/College of American Pathologists Recommendations

As per the 2010 American Society of Clinical Oncology (ASCO) and College of American Pathologists (CAP) Guidelines, the test is considered positive when 1% or more of the tumour cell nuclei are immunoreactive to ER or PR. Higher ER levels indicate a better chance of responding to treatment. Although controversial, clinical response has been linked to ER expression as little as 1% positive staining. As a result, clinicians can weigh the benefits of hormone therapy vs. hazards on a case-by-case basis by reporting low or weak ER expressions in the range of 1% to 10% [47, 49]. The choice of a 1% cut-off was based on this. Less than 1% of immunoreactive tumour cells (in the presence of positive internal controls) are classified receptor-negative, according to ASCO/CAP standards. For receptor quantification, Allred scores, *H*-scores, or simply reporting the percentage of positive cells are utilized [39].

10 Surgical Anatomy of the Breast

Traditionally the anatomy of the breast is taught thus: between the second and sixth ribs, and between the sternal border and the mid-axillary line, the breast is anatomically surface marked [40]. Skin, subcutaneous tissue, epithelial and stromal parts of breast parenchyma make up the breast. The ligaments of Cooper support the breast. They run from the skin through the breast and attach to muscles on the chest. Perforating branches of the internal mammary and lateral thoracic arteries deliver blood to the breast. Breast lymphatic drainage is carried out by a superficial and deep lymphatic plexus, with >95% of lymphatic breast drainage passing through the axillary lymph nodes and the remainder passing through the internal mammary nodes. Berg classified the axillary nodes into three categories based on their proximity to the pectoralis minor muscle [41].

Fifty years ago, a basic knowledge of classical anatomy stood any surgeon in good stead. Today's complex oncoplastic surgeries do not afford that luxury. They stress both form and function and frequently incorporate locoregional flaps or may involve a microvascular transfer. This requires an intimate knowledge of functional anatomy.

Every surgical oncologist during his/her training undergoes an initiation into surgical oncology with the modified radical mastectomy, very much as the general surgeon is initiated into practice with an appendicectomy. Some extra attention during this procedure will result in a knowledge of the onco-vascular anatomy of the important breast subunits.

A careful observation of the large constant perforators when lifting the breast of the chest wall should draw the surgeon's attention toward the blood supply to the nipple which arises from the fifth rib region, and sometimes even a few of the intercostal perforators.

10.1 Surgical Anatomy Pertinent to the Oncoplastic Breast Surgeon

The breast is held in place by attachments to the skin around the nipple-areola complex and the medial and inframammary zones of adherence.

The breast is enveloped within the superficial and deep fascia. The superficial fascia lies under the dermis and the deep fascia lies over the chest wall. The chest wall is very loosely attached to the breast.

The breast has both a deep and a superficial blood supply. The deep vessels penetrate the breast from its under surface (contained within Würinger's septum) and spread out through the breast. The superficial vessels are pushed upward as the breast develops; they travel over the top of the breast in the subcutaneous tissue and supply the breast from the periphery.

If the surgeon understands the deep and superficial vascular supply, the design of pedicles and locoregional flaps becomes more predictable in both primary and secondary breast surgery.

The breast has four main arterial blood supply patterns:

1. Deep perforator at the fourth interspace from the internal mammary system.
2. Superficial descending branch from the second interspace from the internal mammary system.
3. Superficial branch from the third interspace from the internal mammary system.
4. Lateral thoracic system.

11 Surgery for Breast Cancer

Hippocrates proposed in 400 A.D. that breast cancer is a systemic disease from the start, and that local treatment had no effect on long-term cure and survival. Over the years the original Halstedian theory has given way to Fisher's theory that breast cancer is a systemic disease at inception. This has led to a paradigm shift toward conservation in locoregional treatment with the advances in systemic therapy. However, the foundation of locoregional therapy still stands on the complete eradication of all malignant cells from the breast and the draining nodal basin.

Radical mastectomy: In 1882 William Halstead first described radical mastectomy, an en bloc resection of the breast, pectoral muscles, and lymphatics thus acting upon the hypothesis that breast cancer was a local disease. He reported 3-year local and loco-regional recurrence rates of 3% and 22%, respectively. In the 1920s, Handley et al. hypothesized that internal mammary nodes (IMLN) could be a pathway for metastatic spread of breast cancer, with 33% of IMLN being positive for metastasis, 54% in cases of medially located tumours, and 69% IMLN positive in cases of existing metastases to ipsilateral axillary nodes (111). However, radical mastectomy fell out of favor with surgeons given poor cosmetic results, excessive blood loss, and low survival rates despite extensive surgery.

Modified radical mastectomy: It was during this period that Patey DH and Dyson WH described the procedure of modified radical mastectomy. Patey in 1932 performed the first documented modified radical mastectomy and reported equivalent local recurrence and survival rates between radical and modified radical surgery in 146 breast cancer patients. The landmark NSABP B-04 trial by Bernard Fisher, aimed to answer the question of equivalence between radical mastectomy and total mastectomy with or without radiation. The results of this trial transformed the understanding of the biology of breast cancer a 25 years follow-up of NSABP B-04 also failed to show any survival difference (both OS and DFS) between the treatment groups [42].

Indications of MRM today include diffuse malignant appearing microcalcifications, inflammatory breast cancer, persistently positive margins despite repeated attempts at margin revision, and patients' choice.

Breast Conservation Therapy: In 1922 Geoffrey Keynes pioneered the idea of breast conservation. The safety of breast conservation therapy, with the benefit of radiation, was established by six randomized trials initiated in the 1970s: NSABP B-06 [42], Milan [43], EORTC 10801 [44], DBCG-82TM [45], Poggi [46], and Arriagada [47].

The greatest predictive predictor for local recurrence after conservative surgery is adequate surgical excision and clear margins. Revision of margins on a regular basis might lead to a bad cosmetic result, negative psychological reactions, a delay in initiating oncological treatments, and increased costs. Thus, emphasizing the importance of careful patient selection for breast conservation surgery, adequate surgical excision, and obtaining tight margins during primary surgery.

There has been a paradigm shift in the way clinically node-negative breast cancer has been managed in the last 15 years with the introduction of sentinel lymph node biopsy, which has circumvented the morbidity of the traditional axillary lymph node dissection.

11.1 What Constitutes a Clear Margin?

A 2-mm margin reduces the risk of IBTR compared to smaller negative margins, according to the Society of Surgical Oncology-American Society for Radiation Oncology-American Society of Clinical Oncology Consensus Guideline on Margins for Breast-Conserving Surgery with Whole-Breast Irradiation in Ductal Carcinoma in Situ. When compared to 2-mm margins, wider clear margins have no significant effect on IBTR [48].

The SSO-ASTRO-ASCO guideline for Invasive cancers undergoing BCT recommends the use of no ink on tumours as the standard for an adequate margin as it is linked to a lower risk of IBTR and has the potential to lower re-excision rates, improve cosmetic outcomes, and save money on health care [49].

11.2 Oncoplastic Breast Surgery

Oncoplastic interventions essentially refer to a set of surgical innovations to solve malignant and concomitantly esthetic problems according to the individual anatomy and available expertise.

Oncoplastic surgery has been defined in several ways. However, the American Society of Breast Surgeons (ASBS) has sought to unify the definition and classification of Oncoplastic surgery in a recently published consensus.

ASBS Definition of Breast Cancer—Oncoplastic surgery is a type of breast-conservation surgery that entails oncologic removal: with a partial mastectomy, ipsilateral reconstruction with volume displacement or volume replacement procedures, and contralateral symmetry surgery if necessary.

The choice of oncoplastic surgical technique is based upon multiple factors, including the location of cancer in the breast, the degree of anatomic ptosis, the desires of the patient, the patient's overall health, and the skill set of the surgeon or team of surgeons (Table 7).

A detailed discussion of surgical techniques for Oncoplastic Breast surgeries is beyond the scope of this chapter. A few examples are shown below. Figures 1 and 2 portrays Lateral intercostal artery Flap. Figures 3 and 4 picturizes the Bellini's Round Block Technique.

Despite these extreme oncoplastic options, there are several conditions that preclude breast conservation [50].

- Locally widespread disease;
- Multicentricity;
- Diffuse (malignant) microcalcifications;
- I or II trimester;
- Patients with mutations on BR-CA1 and 2 genes;
- Already irradiated thoracic wall.
- Persistently positive margins despite attempts at re-excision.

In addition to the above situations, low socio-economic economic considerations must be included in the decision-making process as has been discussed by Krishnamurthy et al. [51].

Table 7 Classification of oncoplastic breast surgeries

Volume displacement	Examples
Level 1: \20% breast tissue removed	Local tissue rearrangement Crescent mastopexy Doughnut mastopexy
Level 2: 20–50% of breast tissue removed	Circumvertical mastopexy design Reduction of mammaplasty designs (including free nipple graft)
Volume replacement	Examples:
>50% of breast tissue removed	Implant-based reconstruction Local/regional flap reconstruction: Thoracodorsal artery perforator, etc.

(**Source**: *Reprinted by permission from Springer Nature Customer Service Centre GmbH: SPRINGER NATURE, An Oncoplastic Surgery Primer: Common Indications, Techniques, and Complications in Level 1 and 2Volume Displacement Oncoplastic Surgery by Krishnabhai Patel MD* et al, *July 24,2019; DOI: 10.1245/s10434-019-07592-5; Copyright 2019, Society of Surgical Oncology*)

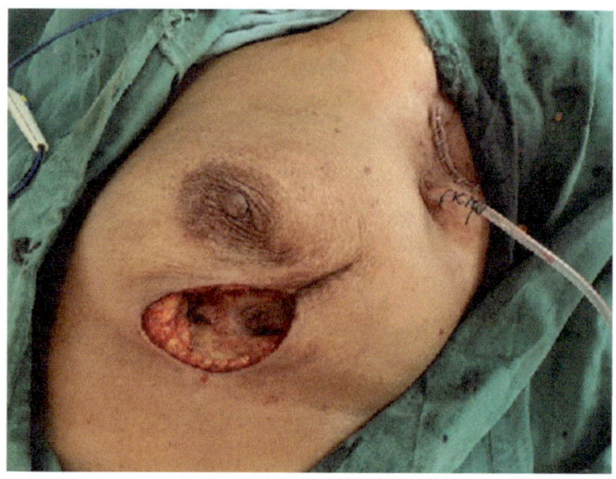

Fig. 1 Lateral Intercostal artery Flap. (Courtesy Dr. Kiran Kamalasanan, n.d.)

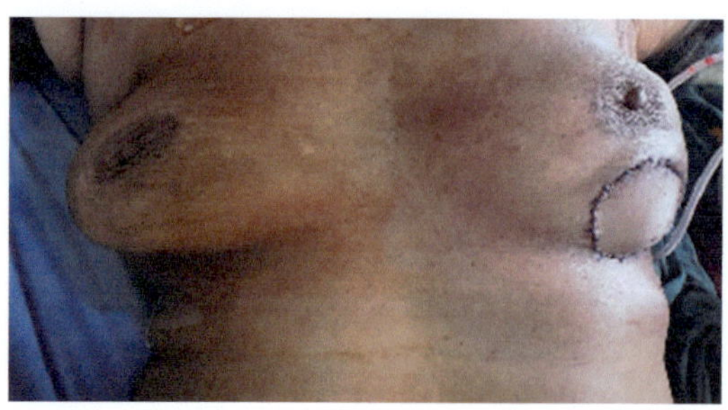

Fig. 2 Lateral Intercostal artery Flap. (Courtesy Dr. Kiran Kamalasanan, n.d.)

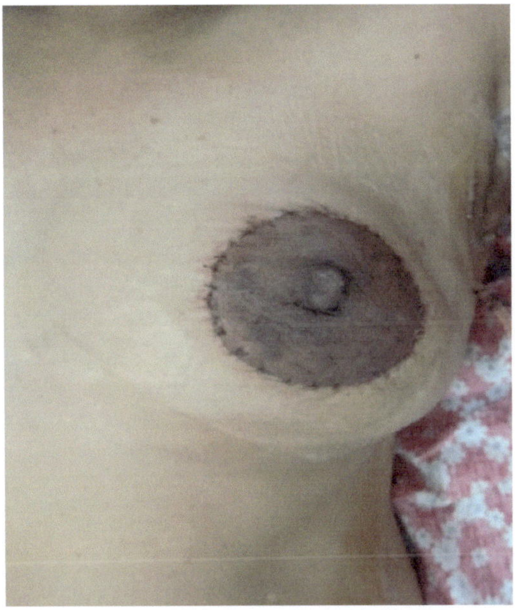

Fig. 3 Bellini's Round Block Technique. (Courtesy Dr. Kiran Kamalasanan, n.d.)

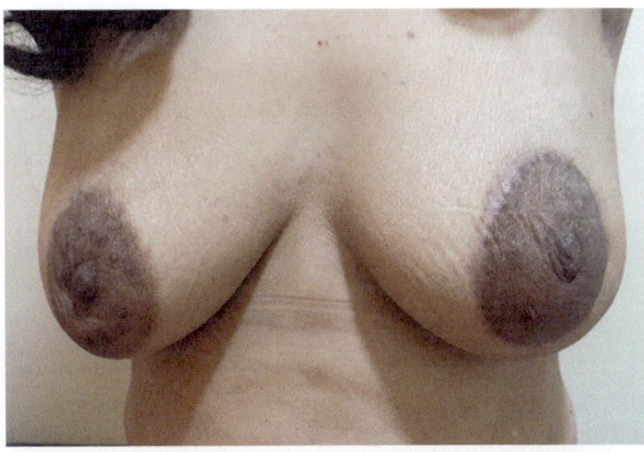

Fig. 4 Bellini's Round Block Technique. (Courtesy Dr. Kiran Kamalasanan, n.d.)

11.3 Sentinel Lymph Node Biopsy

The first use of the term sentinel lymph node can be traced back to Leonard R. Braithwaite, who used the term to describe the node draining lymphatics from the omentum in cats [52]. This was followed by the detection of the sentinel lymph node in parotid gland by Gould in 1960 [53]. The concept was then extended to Carcinoma Penis by Cabanas et al. [54] and in Melanoma by Morton [55]. The use of Sentinel lymph node biopsy in Breast cancer began in the early 1990s with studies on the blue dye technique was by Armando Guiliano in 1994 [56], which followed the description of the radiolabeled dye technique by Krag et al. [57] in 1993.

The use of sentinel lymph nodes has been validated by several large studies. The largest of these in the NSABP B-32 Trial which established the noninferiority of Sentinel lymph node biopsy vs. Axillary lymph node dissection [58]. The sentinel lymph node detection rate was 97% while the false-negative rate was less than 10%.

11.3.1 Technique of Sentinel Lymph Node Biopsy

SLNB can be performed with the blue dye, the radioactive colloid, or both tracers; the choice is determined by the surgeon and institutional preference. Although excellent results are reported in single-institution series using either radioactive colloid or blue dye combined use of both tracers appears to be complementary, minimizing the false-negative rate in most of the studies.

At Dr. B. Borooah Cancer institute, the technique of sentinel lymph node biopsy uses Blue dye in the form of methylene blue diluted in a 1:1 ratio with normal saline. 3–4 mL of the diluted dye is injected in a peri-areolar fashion at 12,3,6, and 9'o clock positions subdermally. This is followed by a systematic massage of the breast in a clockwise and counterclockwise fashion for around 5 min (note bene-slightly longer in women >60 years of age. Next, an axillary incision is made centered around a point at the intersection between the left mid-axillary line and a line tangential to and 1 cm below the lower hairline. The incision is deepened to identify the anterior lamina of the axillary fascia. Next, the anterior lamina is incised the open the axillary lympho-adipose tissue. The identification of the sentinel lymph node is usually preceded by the detection of the blue lymph lymphatic duct. Careful and precise dissection proximal to the duct usually identifies the sentinel lymph node. In the event, the node is not detected identification of constant landmarks assists in their localization. The Clough's cross is formed by the lateral thoracic vein and the second intercostobrachial nerve divides the axilla into four zones. Most nodes are found in zone a, followed by zone c and d, and a search for the nodes in that particular order usually leads to the identification of the sentinel lymph node(s) [59].

11.3.2 Management of Positive Sentinel Lymph Nodes

- The management of positive sentinel lymph nodes has undergone a philosophical change ever since the publication of several landmark trials. Earlier, all patients with a pathologically node-positive lymph node were subjected to a completion axillary lymph node dissection.
- ACOSOG Z0011 was a large trial where the noninferiority of observation for up to two positive lymph nodes was demonstrated in patients with primary tumours <5 cm and those who would undergo whole breast radiotherapy [60]. The so-called ZOO11 Criteria has significantly impacted practice all over the world.

11.3.3 Sentinel Lymph Node Biopsy in the Setting of Neoadjuvant Chemotherapy

The approach to the axilla depends on the presence of suspicious nodes prior to neoadjuvant therapy (either on an exam or the axillary US), the results of a fine needle aspiration (FNA) or core needle biopsy (CNB) of suspicious nodes prior to treatment, and clinical node status following neoadjuvant therapy.

Patients with no evidence of lymph node involvement prior to or during neoadjuvant therapy, or those who had negative needle biopsies of any suspicious nodes at diagnosis, should undergo post-neoadjuvant therapy sentinel lymph node biopsy (SLNB).

Data in support of performing an SLNB after neoadjuvant therapy include a meta-analysis of 16 studies encompassing 1456 women with clinically node-negative breast cancer who underwent SLNB and axillary lymph node dissection (ALND) after neoadjuvant chemotherapy (NACT). In this population, the sentinel node identification rate was 96% and the false-negative rate (FNR) was 6%.

For patients undergoing a post-treatment SLNB, the procedure is performed concurrently with breast surgery. Patients are advised that an ALND may be performed at the same time if intraoperative analysis, usually by frozen section, demonstrates persistent disease in the sampled nodes, and if results of the final SLNB pathology differ from the intraoperative findings, subsequent axillary surgery may be recommended.

- If the SLNB post-treatment is negative (ypN0), no further axillary treatment is required.
- If the SLNB post-treatment is positive (ypN+), we proceed with ALND There is interest in assessing whether axillary radiation is as effective as ALND in this setting, and ongoing trials address this question; however, data comparing these two in the post-neoadjuvant therapy setting are not yet available. For patients keen to avoid ALND, axillary radiation may be considered as an alternative, with appropriate counseling that the equivalence of this approach in terms of locoregional disease control has not been demonstrated.
- Patients in whom sentinel node mapping is not technically successful require an ALND.

12 Postmastectomy Radiation Therapy

For a significant subset of the patient population, postmastectomy RT (PMRT) offers two advantages: it reduces the rate of locoregional recurrence while also improving long-term breast cancer-specific and overall survival.

12.1 Indications for PMRT

- T4 disease.
- Select cases of positive margins at mastectomy with other poor prognostic features (e.g., age ≤ 50 years, T2 or higher primary lesions, triple-negative histology, high grade, or lymphovascular invasion.
- Select cases of T2 and T3 disease with other poor prognostic features (e.g., age ≤ 50 years, triple-negative histology, high grade, or lymphovascular invasion).
- Node-positive disease.

The 2005 Early Breast Cancer Trialists' Collaborative Group (EBCTCG) meta-analysis, which had 8500 patients with mastectomy, axillary dissection, and node-positive disease enrolled in trials of radiotherapy (radiotherapy to the chest wall and regional lymph nodes) versus no radiotherapy. For women with node-positive disease, PMRT resulted in improved breast cancer-specific survival (54.7% versus 60.1% with no RT) and reduced local recurrence at 15 years (7.8% versus 29% with no RT) [61].

12.2 For 1–3 Nodes

In the 2005 Metanalysis, detailed results for women with one to three involved nodes were not provided. Data in support of PMRT for these patients come from a 2014 EBCTCG meta-analysis of trials between 1964 and 1986 [62]. This analysis included approximately 1300 women with one to three involved lymph nodes receiving mastectomy and axillary dissection, and demonstrated that radiotherapy to the chest wall and regional nodes reduced locoregional recurrence (3.8% versus 20.3%), overall recurrence (34% versus 45.7%; rate ratio [RR] 0.68, 95% CI 0.57–0.82), and breast cancer mortality (42% versus 50%; RR 0.80, 95% CI 0.67–0.95). However, these data must be cautiously interpreted, as they were taken from trials where either no systemic therapy was given or less than contemporary systemic regimens were used. Therefore, the outcomes were worse in the control groups compared with what is currently observed. Additional data come from the European Organization for Research and Treatment of Cancer (EORTC) 22,922/10925 trial, which included almost 1000 patients who had undergone a mastectomy, the majority of whom had fewer than four involved lymph nodes, as well as the British Columbia series, in which PMRT improved breast cancer-free survival among premenopausal women with node-positive disease, regardless of whether they had four (RR 0.59, 95% CI 0.38–0.91) or one to three involved nodes (RR 0.64, 0.42–0.97) [63].

BIG 2-04 P88 MRC/EORTC SUPREMO is a randomized controlled trial that is examining the role of postmastectomy radiation therapy in intermediate-risk patients. Patients are randomly assigned to undergo postmastectomy radiation therapy [64].

12.3 T3N0

Among node-negative patients with a tumour size >5 cm, patients treated with mastectomy alone with adjuvant systemic therapy had a locoregional failure rate as low as 5% on five of the NSABP chemotherapy trials. A SEER analysis of 1865 patients showed no increase in cancer-specific survival with PMRT for women with T3N0 breast cancer [65]. This lends further support to the hypothesis that T3N0 disease post-mastectomy represents a favorable subset of locally advanced breast cancer.

12.4 Complete Nodal Response After Neoadjuvant Chemotherapy

The current PMRT recommendations are based on the clinical stage designated prior to the start of any treatment. However, in these individuals, a good response to neoadjuvant chemotherapy lowers the chance of locoregional recurrence. Many contend that because these patients have been effectively down-staged to a lower risk category, PMRT may no longer be of value to them.

Patients with pathologically affected lymph nodes who have a complete pathologic response to neoadjuvant chemotherapy are randomized to either comprehensive regional nodal RT or chest wall radiation exclusively in the NSABP B-51 (NCT01872975) randomized controlled study. However, the NCCN and professional organizations presently oppose skipping postmastectomy radiation therapy in these patients [66].

12.5 Internal Mammary Node Coverage

Studies have shown the incidence of metastatic involvement of the internal mammary nodes to vary between 4% and 9% in patients with axillary node-negative breast cancer and between 16% and 65% in patients with axillary node-positive breast cancer. Patients with the following conditions have a high risk of IMNS metastasis: (1) patients with 4 or more positive ALNs. (2) patients with medial tumour and positive ALNs. (3) patients with T3 tumour and younger than 35 years. (4) patients with T2 tumour and positive ALNs. (5) patients with T2 tumour and medial tumour. The incidences of IMNS metastasis for these patients exceed 20%.

Internal mammary nodes should be included in the radiation field if they are pathologically enlarged on CT and/or metabolically active on PET, or positive in the rare IMN Sentinel biopsies. IMN coverage by choice is divisive. The radiation fields in the PMRT trials included all of the breast's draining lymphatics, including the axillary, supraclavicular, and internal mammary nodal (IMN) chains. However, investigations have revealed a low prevalence of IMN nodal positive and clinical IMN recurrence, at the cost of a higher risk of long-term heart and lung damage.

Several big trials have looked at the volume of elective nodal irradiation (ENI) in patients with central/medial tumours, positive lymph nodes, or node-negative individuals with high-risk disease following mastectomy [63]. The outcomes of patients treated with entire breast, chest wall radiation, supraclavicular, and axillary apex radiation with or without internal mammary node irradiation were compared in the French and Danish investigations. While the French study was randomized, the Dutch study irradiated the internal mammary nodes of patients with right-sided disease while skipping IMNI in patients with the left-sided disease to reduce heart dose. Patients with right-sided breast cancer who were assigned to IMNI [67] had a substantial 2.5% improvement in breast cancer-specific survival, according to the Dutch study. The French trial, on the other hand, failed to show a survival benefit. Another large randomized trial, EORTC 22922, compared comprehensive nodal irradiation with IMN to standard breast radiation alone in patients with high-risk node-negative, central/medially located tumours, and/or positive showed a 3% improvement in disease-free survival and a 2% reduction in breast cancer mortality in patients with high-risk node-negative, central/medially located tumours and/or positive. Only about a quarter of these patients, however, had had mastectomy [63].

The recent EBCTCG metanalysis on regional nodal irradiation, presented at the San Antonio Breast Conference in 2018 concluded that RT to regional lymph nodes in older (1961–78) studies increased the overall risk of death, probably explained by radiation exposure to the lungs and heart. Nodal RT in more recent (1989–2003) studies reduced breast cancer recurrence, breast cancer mortality, and overall mortality without increasing non-breast cancer mortality. Details of the meta-analysis are yet to be published [18].

In conclusion, comprehensive lymph node coverage may offer a small improvement in disease-free survival and possibly even breast cancer-specific survival in a small subset of patients, but given the lack of evidence, a multidisciplinary expert panel on postmastectomy management recommends that if comprehensive nodal radiation is recommended, the radiation treatment field should include the IMN, supraclavicular, and apical axillary regions, as well as the chest wall [68].

12.6 Postmastectomy Radiation Therapy After Implant/Tissue Expander

High rates of capsular contracture, revision procedures, reconstructive failures, and overall inferior cosmetic outcomes have been linked to postmastectomy radiation therapy after breast reconstruction [69]. The type of breast reconstruction (i.e., autologous versus implant-based) and the time of the breast reconstruction (i.e., immediate versus delayed) are crucial issues that require an informed discussion by the patient in collaboration with the multidisciplinary team prior to surgery.

Implant reconstruction is usually done in two stages, with a tissue expander placed first and then a permanent implant. When radiation was given to the tissue expander rather than the permanent implant, studies examining the best sequence reconstruction with irradiation revealed increased rates of reconstructive failures ranging from 32% to 40% [70]. Patients who choose immediate expander/implant reconstruction should be well informed about the hazards of postmastectomy radiation in the context of breast reconstruction.

Additional data from two ongoing North American studies will be used to answer these questions. Patients are randomized to 50 Gy in 2-Gy fractions or 42.56 Gy in 2.66-Gy fractions to the rebuilt breast and Regional Nodal Irradiation (RNI), including IMNs, in the Alliance for Clinical Trials in Oncology Phase III study (Alliance A221505/ RT CHARM; ClinicalTrials.gov identifier: NCT03414970). Patients with tissue expander/implant-based immediate reconstruction are randomly assigned to 50 Gy to the chest wall and 46 to 50 Gy to supraclavicular nodes in 2-Gy fractions or 42.56 Gy to the chest wall and 39.9 Gy to supraclavicular nodes in 2.66-Gy fractions in the FABREC trial (ClinicalTrials.gov identifier: NCT03422003) (with or without other regional nodes).

12.7 Whole Breast Radiation After Breast Conservation Therapy

Following breast-conserving therapy, WBRT lowers the chance of locoregional recurrence and death from breast cancer. The Early Breast Cancer Trialists' Collaborative Group (EBCTCG) completed a meta-analysis in 2011 that included approximately 10,000 women (pathologically node-negative or positive) in 17 trials [71], demonstrating the benefits of WBRT. WBRT resulted in a roughly 50% reduction in the 10-year chance of any first recurrence compared to breast-conserving surgery alone, according to the meta-analysis (19% versus 35%, respectively; relative risk [RR] 0.52, 95% CI 0.48–0.56). The decrease in recurrence rate linked with RT was attributed to a reduction in locoregional recurrences rather than distant recurrences. This has resulted in a 15-year reduction in the chance of dying from breast cancer (21% versus 25%; RR 0.82, 95% CI 0.75–0.90).

Conventional versus hypofractionated schedules—Historically, most women have received conventionally dosed WBRT, which is delivered to the entire breast in 1.8–2 Gy daily fractions over 4.5–5 weeks to a total dose of 45–50 Gy. However, another option is a shorter fractionation ("hypofractionated") schedule, which has been associated with equivalent tumour control and fewer toxicities, and is now preferred for many patients. In general, a hypofractionated regimen delivers more radiation per dose, but the overall treatment duration is shorter (typically 40 to 42.5 Gy in approximately 3–5 weeks without or with a boost). The American Society for Radiation Oncology (ASTRO) favored hypofractionated RT in all women with invasive breast cancer or ductal carcinoma in situ (DCIS) for whom the intent is to treat only the whole breast without an additional field to cover the regional lymph nodes, provided that dose homogeneity goals can be achieved (dose homogeneity of >7% and the volume of breast tissue receiving >105% of the prescription dose should be minimized)

[72]. This is independent of any age, stage, or use of systemic therapy. Importantly, however, there is insufficient evidence to support hypofractionation when regional RT is indicated.

Cosmetic and disease outcomes have been equivalent between hypofractionated and conventional schedules. The efficacy of a hypofractionated schedule was shown in a 2016 meta-analysis of nine randomized trials ($n = 8228$ women) that compared it with conventionally scheduled WBRT [10]. Shorter fractionation resulted in:

- No difference in breast cancer-specific survival (RR 0.91, 95% CI 0.78–1.06).
- No difference in 10-year mortality (RR for mortality 0.91, 95% CI 0.80–1.03).
- No difference in breast appearance (RR 0.90, 95% CI 0.81–1.01).
- No difference in late RT subcutaneous toxicity (RR 0.93, 95% CI 0.83–1.05).
- A decrease in acute RT toxicity (RR 0.32, 95% CI 0.22–0.45).

A further meta-analysis of the 10-year follow-up of two of the trials included (START-A and START-B) found no significant difference between the shorter fractionation and normally dosed RT schedules [73]. This was true regardless of age, main surgery type, axillary node status, tumour grade, adjuvant chemotherapy administration, or the use of a tumour-bed boost RT [73].

Schedules as short as 1 week have also been explored for WBRT, with similar results. In a subsequent randomized trial of over 4000 breast cancer patients, the 5-year incidence of ipsilateral breast tumour relapse was 2.1% with the standard 40 Gy in 15 fractions over 3 weeks versus 1.4% with 26 Gy in five fractions over 1 week (5.2 Gy per fraction; hazard ratio [HR] 0.67, 95% CI 0.38–1.16) and 1.7% with 27 Gy in five fractions over 1 week (5.4 Gy per fraction; HR 0.86, 95% CI 0.51–1.44) [74] .

In regard to toxicities, cosmesis results have been somewhat mixed with hypofractionated versus standard schedules and likely depend at least in part on the specific schedule used. Other long-term toxicities appear to be similar:

- In the 10-year follow-up of the FAST trial, there were no significant differences in normal tissue effects for the standard 50 Gy in 25 fractions schedule versus a once-weekly schedule for 5 weeks totaling 28.5 Gy, but normal tissue effects were higher with a weekly schedule for 5 weeks totaling 30 Gy (odds ratio relative to standard radiation 2.12, 95% CI 0.55–2.89) [75]. Similarly, in the FAST-FORWARD trial discussed above evaluating five fractions over 1 week, moderate or marked tissue effects in the breast or chest wall were more common among patients receiving 27 Gy (15%) than either 40 Gy (10%) or 26 Gy (12%), but differences between the 40-Gy and 26-Gy groups were not statistically different [74].
- By contrast, a separate randomized trial showed similar or better cosmetic outcomes among patients receiving a hypofractionated schedule (40 Gy in 15 fractions) compared with standard fractionation (50 Gy in 25 fractions), among over 1800 patients with node-negative breast cancer or DCIS (246 patients) [76]. Radiation-associated cardiac and lung diseases were comparable between the groups.
- Additional research is needed to better understand both efficacy and toxicity in specific subgroups, such as those with more advanced tumours (T-size >5 cm), those who have had a mastectomy with or without reconstruction, and those who have positive nodes.
- More studies are needed before hypofractionation can be recommended for those in whom regional RT is indicated.
- More research is needed to assess the efficacy and safety of hypofractionated irradiation in the treatment of primary breast tumours with unusual histologies, in patients who have had breast augmentation, and in patients who have collagen vascular disease.
- There is not enough information to assess the acceptability of shorter fractionation when combined with other treatments (i.e., chemotherapy or monoclonal antibodies).

RT boost to the tumour bed—RT boost to the tumour bed is intended to decrease locoregional recurrence rates. While RT to the tumour bed following breast-conserving surgery and WBRT is recommended in younger women, its routine use in older women is less clear. A common practice, which we support, is that all patients receive an RT boost after WBRT, except for selected women aged 60 and older with stage 0 to I luminal phenotypes resected with negative margins, for whom it is optional. The degree of benefit and the associated potential skin toxicities following a boost in patients who had received hypofractionated RT is unclear. The decision to give a boost to these patients should be made after a discussion between the patient and the treating radiation oncologist.

If an RT boost is given, the dose is usually 10–14 Gy in 2 Gy or 2.5 Gy fractions, with the boost dose being somewhat determined by the dose and fractionation given to the full breast. The technical aspects of delivering an RT boost are discussed in detail elsewhere.

Two trials that looked at the efficacy of an RT boost found that it reduced the number of recurrences and, as a result, the number of future mastectomies; however, there was no discernible benefit in overall survival (OS) [77, 78]. Women with stage I or II breast cancer who were having WBRT were randomly randomized to receive an RT increase or no additional treatment [79] in one of the largest trials. Of note, the majority of patients (95.5%) in this trial had negative resection margins. With a 17.2-year median follow-up, among women with a negative resection margin ($n = 5318$), an RT boost resulted in [79]:

- A significant reduction in the local recurrence rate (9% versus 13% in those who did not receive a boost; HR 0.65, 95% CI 0.52–81). In all age categories, the relative reduction in the risk of local recurrence was comparable. However, the absolute amount of the reduction was largest among younger women (50 years) with DCIS (15% versus 31% in those who did not receive a boost; HR 0.37, 95% CI 0.22–0.62).
- A lower rate of mastectomy as first salvage for those with in-breast tumour recurrence (75% versus 79%).
- No difference in OS, breast cancer mortality, or disease-free survival (DFS) at 20 years.
- A higher rate of severe fibrosis (5.2% versus 1.8%).

A gene expression-based classifier assay has been shown to identify patients at particularly high risk of locoregional recurrence, who are thus more likely to benefit from a tumour-bed boost, and possibly regional nodal RT. However, we await prospective validation prior to routine clinical use.

13 Chemotherapy in Breast Cancer

There have been considerable advancements in the diagnosis and treatment of breast cancer in the recent few decades, with significant survival implications. The use of adjuvant therapies in a standardized manner has reduced mortality by 23% across all stages and considering all major variables.

Traditional adjuvant therapy indications were based on anatomic and pathologic variables such as tumour size, tumour grade, LN status hormone, and HER 2-receptor status. However, genomic profiling approaches and the identification of tumour subtypes based on molecular expression patterns have advanced significantly during the last decade. All of these advancements have sparked interest in tailoring therapy for those who are most likely to respond while avoiding negative effects in "non-responders." The most difficult task is determining which patients require adjuvant treatment and which do not. The purpose of adjuvant chemotherapy is to eliminate local or distant microscopic illness, hence improving DFS and OS.

Breast cancers are classified into four subgroups based on gene expression patterns: luminal A and B (estrogen-sensitive BC), HER2-enriched, and basal-like tumours (negative ER/PR and negative HER2). The use of hormone therapy for luminal A tumours, HER2-targeting therapy for HER2-enriched tumours, and chemotherapy for luminal B and basal tumours have resulted from the molecular classification, which has led to a focused approach for breast cancer medicines.

The first clinical trials in the field of adjuvant chemotherapy for breast cancer began in the late 1960s to establish its role in node-positive breast cancer and compare the effects of different chemotherapy regimens to observation after surgery alone to remove the primary tumour [80]. These studies convincingly demonstrated that adjuvant chemotherapy improves survival in patients who are at high risk of recurrence.

Anthracyclines In breast cancer: The efficacy of cyclophosphamide, methotrexate, and 5-fluorouracil (CMF) as adjuvant treatment for patients with nodal positive breast cancer was reported by Bonadonna et al. in 1976 [81]. Inoperable breast cancer patients, CMF-decreased the annual probabilities of recurrence and mortality by 24% and 14%, respectively. Anthracycline-containing adjuvant combinations were explored in prospective randomized trials in the late 1970s and early 1980s. In comparison to CMF, the Anthracycline regimens (5-fluorouracil, doxorubicin, and cyclophosphamide (FAC); doxorubicin and cyclophosphamide (AC); and 5-fluorouracil, epirubicin, and cyclophosphamide (FEC) were associated with 2% reductions in the risk of recurrence and 16% reduction in mortality. After 5 years, the advantage is roughly 3%, and at 10 years, it is about 4%. In NSABP B-15 and B-23, the NSABP group investigated the differences between anthracycline and CMF regimens, finding that four cycles of AC were comparable to six cycles of conventional CMF in terms of disease-free survival (DFS) and overall survival (OS). Other randomized investigations, as well as a meta-analysis, convincingly showed the same [82].

The FASG- 01 trial looked at the best duration of adjuvant chemotherapy, and found that six cycles of adjuvant FEC were preferable to three cycles of the same regimen in patients with operable breast cancer [83]. As a result, during the 1990s, it was widely agreed that six cycles of an anthracycline-based combination were the best adjuvant treatment for node-positive operable breast cancer.

13.1 Role of Taxanes

Taxanes were added to the chemotherapeutic agents for breast cancer in the 1990s. The taxanes were developed as part of the conventional treatment for metastatic breast cancer because they have a partial lack of cross-resistance with anthracyclines. Taxanes have been studied in the adjuvant context in several phase I clinical trials. Several pooled analyses or meta-analyses found that taxanes-based adjuvant chemotherapy improves DFS and OS (by 5% and 3%, respectively) when compared to standard anthracycline-based therapy, regardless of the type of taxanes used, the schedule of administration, the extent of nodal involvement, or hormone-receptor expression status. They also proposed that taxanes and anthracyclines can be given together or separately.

13.2 Trials Evaluating Sequential Administration of Taxanes to Anthracyclines

In the PACS 01 trial, 1999 women with operable node-positive breast cancer were randomly assigned to either six cycles of FEC or three cycles of FEC followed by three cycles of Docetaxel, both administered every 21 days. Five-year DFS rates were 73.2% with FEC and 78.4% with FEC-D after a median follow-up of 60 months, indicating an 18% reduction in the relative risk of relapse with FEC-D. Overall survival rates were 86.7% with FEC and 90% with FEC-D after 5 years, resulting in a 27% lower relative risk of death [84].

A total of 1246 women with lymph node-positive disease were properly randomized to therapy with FEC or FEC followed by weekly paclitaxel in the GEICAM 9906 study (FEC-P). DFS episodes were reduced by 26% in the taxane arm (FEC90 ->P) at a median follow-up of 66 months, with a nonsignificant increase in overall survival ($p = 0.11$) [85].

In the UK TACT trial, 41 62 women with node-positive or high-risk node-negative operable early breast cancer were randomized to FEC (fluorouracil 600 mg/m(2), epirubicin 60 mg/m(2), cyclophosphamide 600 mg/m^2 at 3-weekly intervals) for four cycles, followed by docetaxel (100 mg/m^2 at 3-weekly intervals) for four cycles, and compared with control arm FEC for 8 cycles. The primary goal was to assess recurrence. The FEC-D regimen had no advantage in terms of DFS or overall survival. The use of a low dose of epirubicin (60 mg/m^2 instead of I 00 mg/m^2) [86] was the cause for no benefit for taxanes in this experiment.

The WGO/ AGO trial randomized 2011 patients with primary breast cancer and 1–3 positive lymph nodes to four cycles EC 90 followed by four cycles of docetaxel 100 or six cycles of CEF 100 or six cycles of CMF. There was a statistically significant benefit in DFS with the use of Docetaxel [87].

13.3 Trials Evaluating Concurrent Administration of Taxanes with Anthracyclines

BCIRG 001 trial randomized 1491 women with axillary node-positive breast cancer to six cycles of either TAC or FAC after surgery. Adjuvant chemotherapy with TAC, as compared with FAC, significantly improves the rates of di ease-free and overall survival in women with operable node-positive breast cancer. However, the TAC regimen is associated with significant toxicities. The rate of febrile neutropenia was 24.7% with TAC compared to 2.5% with FAC [88].

The GEICAM 9805 trial had similar design and treatment arms as in BCIRG001 except that GEICAM included only node-negative breast cancer patients. The study demonstrated that node-negative patients benefited significantly from the addition of a taxane to an anthracycline-containing regimen [88].

13.4 Trial Replacing Anthracyclines with Taxanes

The US Oncology trial USO 9375 randomized 2016 patients either lymph node-negative or positive to 4 standard doses of AC vs. TC. At 7 years follow-up, TC was superior to AC in both DFS and OS.

This trial supports the selection of a non-anthracycline-containing regimen for women with node-negative, and lower risk node-positive breast cancer, especially in patients who have cardiac dysfunction or are at risk for cardiac morbidity [89].

13.5 Optimal Taxane Dose and Schedule

The CALGB 9342 trial found that increasing the dose of paclitaxel from 175 mg/m^2 to 250 mg/m^2 every 3 weeks did not affect response rate, time to progression, or overall survival. However, increasing the dose of docetaxel from 60 mg/m^2 to 100 mg/m^2 every 3 weeks was linked to a better response rate and time to progression [90, 91].

The optimum taxane administration regimens were studied in the ECOG 1199 experiment. After four cycles of AC, 5000 patients with node-positive or high-risk node-negative were randomized to one of four taxane regimens: paclitaxel 175 mg/m^2 every 3 weeks for four cycles (control), paclitaxel 80 mg/m^2 every 3 weeks for four cycles, docetaxel 100 mg/m^2 every 3 weeks for four cycles, or docetaxel 35 mg/m^2 every 3 weeks for four cycles. When compared to the usual every 3-week paclitaxel group [92], 5-year DFS was significantly better in the group getting weekly paclitaxel (HR 1.27, 95% CI 1.03-1.57) and in the group receiving docetaxel every 3 weeks (HR 1.23, 95% Cl 1.00–1.52).

13.6 Dose-Dense Chemotherapy

The CALBG 9741 experiment was the first of these dose-dense trials, and it was designed to see if dose-dense chemotherapy (every 2 weeks) was better than conventional chemotherapy (every 3 weeks); and if sequential Adriamycin and cyclophosphamide (A—>C) was better than concurrent (AC) [93]. In a 2 × 2 factorial design, node-positive breast cancer patients were randomly assigned to one of four treatment arms: sequential chemotherapy with doxorubicin, cyclophosphamide, and paclitaxel, or concurrent chemotherapy with doxorubicin and cyclophosphamide followed by paclitaxel at 14-day (with growth factor support) versus 21-day intervals. Dose-dense regimens outperformed traditional timed regimens in terms of DFS (HR 50.74, *P* 0.0072) and OS (RR 50.69, P.0014). The DFS for the 4-year period was 82%.

In the AGO research, 1284 patients with four or more affected axillary lymph nodes were randomly assigned to receive IDD-ETC (intense dose-dense sequential epirubicin, paclitaxel, and cyclophosphamide) every 2 weeks or epirubicin/cyclophosphamide followed by paclitaxel every 3 weeks. The conventional arm had a 5-year EFS of 62%, while the IDD-ETC arm had a 5-year EFS of 70%, representing a 28% reduction in the relative risk of relapse (P.001). Menopausal status, hormone receptor, and human epidermal growth factor receptor 2 status did not affect this benefit [94]. The OS benefit of IDD-EPC in comparison to conventionally dosed EC P has been enhanced to an absolute difference of 10% [95] after 10 years.

13.7 Timing of Chemotherapy

The importance of timely initiation of systemic therapy was reconfirmed in a retrospective analysis of 2594 patients who had early-stage breast cancer. The investigators demonstrated that delays in initiating chemotherapy were associated with significant increases in relapse risk and adverse survival, particularly if the delay from definitive surgery exceeded 12 weeks.

14 Targeted Therapy in HER 2 Neu Positive Breast Cancer

The HER2 receptor belongs to the epidermal growth factor receptor (EGFR) family, and it is overexpressed in about 20% to 25% of human breast tumours. Overexpression of the HER2 gene is a strong predictor of poor prognosis [96]. This worsening prognosis can be addressed by combining anti-HER2 therapy with Trastuzumab (a monoclonal antibody that targets the extracellular region of the HER2 protein), which has been shown to enhance DFS and OS when combined with chemotherapy in the adjuvant setting. Various trials that looked at the benefits of adding trastuzumab to chemotherapy, either sequentially or concurrently, have been successfully performed to date.

In the Herceptin Adjuvant (HERA) trial, 5102 patients were randomly assigned to one of three arms: chemotherapy followed by observation, or trastuzumab after chemotherapy (sequential administration) for 1 or 2 years. The trastuzumab group had significantly better DFS and OS [97].

In the North Central Cancer Treatment Group study, simultaneous trastuzumab and paclitaxel were compared to sequential trastuzumab administered after anthracycline-based therapy. At a median follow-up of 6 years, the data showed that concurrent administration of trastuzumab and paclitaxel was preferable to sequential administration.

In the NSABP B-31 study, patients were randomly assigned to receive either chemotherapy (AC followed by paclitaxel) or concurrent trastuzumab and paclitaxel. The combined analysis of N9831 and the NSABP trial B-31 revealed that combining trastuzumab with paclitaxel after doxorubicin/cyclophosphamide (AC) significantly improved DFS (HR 0.49, 95% Cl 0.41–0.58, P.0001) and OS (HR 0.63, 95% Cl 0.49–0.81, PS.0004) when compared to chemotherapy alone [98]. In patients with HER2-positive breast cancer larger than 1 cm, these trials have led to the recommendation of using trastuzumab in conjunction with chemotherapy.

The Breast Cancer International Research Group 006 (BCIRG 006) trial looked at trastuzumab in combination with either docetaxel after AC (AC-TH) or carboplatin plus docetaxel (TCarboH), using doxorubicin/cyclophosphamide as a control. The trastuzumab-containing arms (TCH and AC-TH) showed statistically significant improvements in both DFS (AC-TH 84 percent, TCH 81 percent versus AC-T 75 percent, P0.001) and OS (AC-TH 92 percent, TCH 91 percent versus AC-T 87%, p 0.001) compared to the non-trastuzumab-containing arm (ACT) [99] after a median follow-up of 65 months. The results for the two trastuzumab-containing arms were not statistically different, although the trial was not powered to detect differences between these two regimens.

14.1 Duration of HER 2 Targeted Therapy

Because the decision to treat with trastuzumab for a year in the previous studies was arbitrary, it was investigated whether a shorter duration of trastuzumab could be similarly beneficial while lowering costs and reducing cardiac toxicity.

The FinHer trial used trastuzumab for 9 weeks and found that it offered a similar benefit to 1 year of trastuzumab; however, it was a small trial (n = 232), and the SOLD trial followed, which found that the 9-week regimen was not noninferior to regular Trastuzumab [100] treatment.

The SOLD trial 2176 patients were randomized to either docetaxel plus trastuzumab for 9 weeks, followed by three cycles of fluorouracil, epirubicin, and cyclophosphamide in both groups, with the control arm continuing Trastuzumab for 1 year. Nine weeks of trastuzumab was not noninferior to 1 year of trastuzumab when given with similar chemotherapy. Cardiac safety was better in the 9-week group. The docetaxel dosing with trastuzumab requires further study [101].

In the PHARE trial, 3480 patients were randomly assigned to receive trastuzumab for 6 or 12 months, either concurrently or sequentially with chemotherapy. It was a noninferiority trial, with a 1.15 noninferiority margin. The 4-year DFS rates for 6 months versus 12 months of trastuzumab were 84.9% and 87.8%, respectively, according to the intent-to-treat analysis, with an HR of 1.28 and a confidence interval (Cl) of l.05–1.56. The HR of 1.28 implies that trastuzumab [102] for 12 months has a benefit.

Longer-term trastuzumab therapy was the focus of the HERA trial. One year of trastuzumab was compared against 2 years of trastuzumab in this study. The 8-year analysis revealed that disease-free survival (DFS) rates for the 1- and 2-year treatment groups were identical, at 76% and 75.8%, respectively, with a hazard ratio (HR) of 0.99, implying that 1 year of Trastuzumab is the standard of care [97].

The SHORT HER study and the HORG trial failed to show the noninferiority of a shorter trastuzumab administration. One-year trastuzumab remains the standard. However, a 9-week administration decreases the risk of severe cardiac toxicity and can be an option for patients with cardiac events during treatment and those with a low risk of relapse [103, 104].

Meanwhile, the multicenter PERSEPHONE trial in 4088 women has shown that disease-free survival was comparable whether patients were treated with 6 or 12 months of adjuvant trastuzumab [105].

However, in a recent Metanalysis, a shorter duration of adjuvant trastuzumab was noninferior to its 1-year administration and resulted in lower rates of cardiac toxic effects [106]. These results suggest that a shorter duration may be the preferred option for patients with the low-risk disease or a predisposition to cardiac toxic effects.

In clinical practice, 1 year of HER 2 targeted therapy is advised and is the standard of care if the drug is easily accessible. Trastuzumab for a shorter period may be an alternative for persons with restricted finances.

15 Role of Neo-Adjuvant Chemotherapy (NACT) in Breast Cancer

Neo-adjuvant or preoperative chemotherapy in breast cancer is a treatment option in locally advanced breast cancer, inflammatory breast cancer patients, and operable breast cancer where breast conservation is desired but not technically feasible upfront. The intention of induction chemotherapy is to enhance the likelihood of attaining negative margins and to improve breast conservation rates. Compared to adjuvant chemotherapy, NACT is associated with high rates of clinical response, including complete pathological responses (path CR) and a higher likelihood of permitting cosmetically acceptable surgery. However, it has no effect on disease-free survival (DFS) or overall survival (OS).

Chemotherapy regimens based on anthracyclines and taxanes are the most commonly utilized as neoadjuvant therapy. A total of 2411 patients in the NSABP B27 study were given four cycles of neoadjuvant AC before being randomly assigned to no additional chemotherapy [107], four cycles of neoadjuvant docetaxel (100 mg/m^2) every 3 weeks, or surgery followed by four cycles of adjuvant docetaxel. Docetaxel pre-surgery resulted in a better overall clinical response rate and a higher pathologically complete response rate than AC alone, but no difference in overall survival.

Patients with HER2-positive cancers have a relatively high rate of pathologic complete response to NACT, particularly if treatment includes a HER2-directed agent [108].The benefit of adding trastuzumab to chemotherapy was shown in a pooled analysis of two randomized studies that evaluated NACT with or without trastuzumab with an improvement in the rate of pCR, a reduction in the relapse rate, and a trend toward a lower mortality rate though it was not statistically significant [108].

The Indian experience on NACT in locally Advanced breast cancer has been favorable as shown in a cohort study of 664 patients at Tata Memorial Hospital Mumbai, in whom the 3-year local DFS was better post-conservation than after mastectomy (87% vs. 78%, $P = 0.02$). The disease-free survival (DFS) was also superior after BCT, 72% vs. 52% ($P < 0.001$) at 3 years and 62% vs. 37% ($P < 0.001$) at 5 years, respectively [109].

16 Evolving Role of Chemoimmunotherapy for Triple-Negative Breast Cancer

Several studies have looked into the impact of the addition of immunotherapy agents to NACT on pathologic complete response (pCR) rates in HER2-negative breast cancer, especially triple-negative breast cancer [108, 110–112].

While results from some of these studies are encouraging regarding the impact of adding an Immune checkpoint inhibitor to NACT on pCR rates in TNBC, many questions remain. These include the choice of agent, timing and duration of treatment, selection of the accompanying NACT regimen, the appropriate target population (PD-L1-negative cancers vs. only PD L1 positive), as well as the impact of immunotherapy on long-term outcomes such as EFS and overall survival. Until then use of these agents in neoadjuvant regimens remains investigational.

17 Endocrine Therapy in Breast Cancer

The two primary steroid receptors tested for in breast cancer are the estrogen receptors (ERs) and the progesterone receptors (PgRs) which are primarily nuclear hormonal receptors that function as transcription factors.

The use of the selective estrogen receptor modulator Tamoxifen, in breast cancer, was started in the 1970s and the review of various RCTs suggested that it was as effective as high dose estrogens and Megestrol acetate (which were initially used as first-line hormonal agents in advanced breast cancer) but had a much safer side effect profile and tolerability. Since then, tamoxifen has been used as a first-line hormonal agent and the Oxford review established its role in breast cancer in pre as well as postmenopausal women with equal efficacy in all stages, of the disease. In estrogen receptor (ER)-positive disease, (N = I0,645), 5 years of Tamoxifen substantially reduced recurrence rates throughout the first 10 (RR 0.53 [SE 0.03] during years 0–4 and RR 0.68 [0.06] during years 5–9 [both $p < 0.00001$] but RR 0.97 [0.10] during years 10–14, suggesting no further gain or loss after year 10). Breast cancer mortality was reduced by a third throughout the first 15 years (RR 0.71 during years 0–4, 066 during years 5–9, and 068 during years

10–14; $p < 00001$ for extra mortality reduction during each separate time period), Tamoxifen also reduces the incidence of contralateral breast cancer by almost 50%. The carry-over effect of Tamoxifen for 5 years beyond completion of 5 years of treatment gave rise to the idea that extended treatment would give more benefit, especially in premenopausal women in whom a longer duration of treatment is desired [113].

Hence, extending the treatment for 5 more years with Tamoxifen itself was tested in two trials, aTToM [Adjuvant Tamoxifen Treatment offer more?] and ATLAS [Adjuvant Tamoxifen: Longer Against Shorter).

The aTTom trial comprised 6953 women with breast cancer [ER + −2755, ER unknown- 4198-80% estimated to be positive] who were randomized to receive 5 years of Tamoxifen versus 10 years of Tamoxifen, and the results showed that continuing Tamoxifen for 10 years produces a further reduction in breast cancer recurrence from seventh year and breast cancer mortality after tenth year: However, the relative risk of developing endometrial carcinoma was higher in the group which received Tamoxifen for 10 years(RR 2.20}, not reaching significant difference [114].

The ATLAS trial reported similar results on 6846 women with ER + early breast cancers. Ten years of Tamoxifen was seen to reduce both breast cancer recurrence rates as well as mortality as compared to 5 years of Tamoxifen. Additionally, breast cancer mortality is almost halved in the second decade with 10 years of Tamoxifen [115].

Aromatase inhibitors (Als) were introduced in the treatment of breast cancer in the 1990s. Sequential use of Tamoxifen with an Al was first examined in the Italian Co-operative Study in 2001 [116]. This study randomized 380 postmenopausal women, who had already received 3 years of Tamoxifen to receive 2 years of aminoglutethimide or continue the standard 5 years of Tamoxifen. Although the study used a low dose of oral aminoglutethimide (250 mg daily), many women discontinued the drug because of its side effects. The study failed to recruit the desired number of participants and was stopped in 1998 after the availability of Anastrozole.

The ATAC (Arimidex, Tamoxifen, Alone or in Combination) trial was the first large randomized trial that showed a disease-free survival (DFS) benefit for 5 years of Anastrozole over 5 years of Tamoxifen. In this trial, in ER+ early breast cancers, there was a significant improvement in DFS (HR 0.85), time to recurrence (HR 0.76), time to distant recurrence (HR 0.84) and also, the Anastrozole arm showed significantly lower ipsilateral and contralateral breast cancer rates (HR 0.60, absolute benefit in ER + arm 2.8%). The combination arm was discontinued after following up for 33 months since it was seen to be inferior to the Anastrozole arm and equivalent to the Tamoxifen arm [117].

The Breast international group (BIG 1·98) study randomized over 8000 women with ER+ early breast cancer and randomized them to four arms (Letrozole 5 years, Tamoxifen 5 years, Tamoxifen for 2 years, Letrozole for 3 years, Letrozole 2 years, Tamoxifen for 3 years). It included DFS as the primary endpoint which apart from local invasive recurrence and distant recurrence from primary breast cancer, included any other non-breast cancer and not DCIS (as against the ATAC trial) and showed that Letrozole monotherapy was significantly better than Tamoxifen (DFS HR 0.86, OS HR 0.87) and that addition of an Al at any point of time in the treatment was better than Tamoxifen alone [118].

Another large trial, Tamoxifen Exemestane Adjuvant Multinational (TEAM) study randomized close to 10,000 patients, but when the IES study results were declared, the study protocol was amended and the Tamoxifen arm was changed to a sequential cross over the arm to Exemestane after 2–3 years of Tamoxifen. The initial part of the study (before witching) showed better DFS in the Exemestane arm (HR 0.85, p-0.12) not reaching significance, but after the switch over, both arms showed similar DFS [119].

Several trials evaluated the role of extending treatment with Als after 5 years of Tamoxifen and the largest of these is the MA 17 trial, which was terminated after the first interim analysis which demonstrated significantly better DFS in the Letrozole group (HR 0.58) [120].

The Suppression of ovarian function (SOFT) and Tamoxifen and Exemestane (TEXT) trials randomized about 5000 premenopausal (age < 50 years) women with early hormone receptor-positive breast cancer to ovarian ablation + tamoxifen /Exemestane or Tamoxifen alone. They concluded that Exemestane + LHRH agonists as compared to Tamoxifen + LHRH agonists significantly improved DFS (4% absolute benefit] but not OS and this benefit was seen maximum in women with age < 40 yrs., tumour size >2 cm, and axillary lymph node-positive for metastasis [121].

17.1 Neoadjuvant Hormone Therapy

Neoadjuvant hormonal therapy is restricted to patients unfit for receiving any form of chemotherapy. However, now this option is being explored for women with strong hormone receptor-positive breast cancers. The pathological complete response (pCR) rates with NAHT are reported around 5–10% · The greater the duration of NAHT, the more the rates of pCR. The optimal duration varies for individual patients depending on the response to NAHT but relapses within less than 12 months appear rare.

A response to endocrine therapy is usually seen after 3–4 months or more, and maximal response may not be achieved until much later. Thus, the duration of endocrine treatment prior to surgery must be individualized based on the patient's clinical status and the clinical response.

18 Metastatic Breast Cancer

Around 10% of women have metastatic disease at the time of presentation and up to 30% of women with localized disease at diagnosis will develop distant metastatic disease. While metastatic breast cancer is not curable, improvements in survival have been seen, with the Introduction of newer systemic therapies. The goals of the treatment of metastatic breast cancer are to improve quality of life by reducing cancer-related symptoms and prolonging survival.

Depending upon the type of breast cancer, a therapy used to achieve this goal can be chemotherapy, hormonal therapy, or Her 2-directed therapy.

Cytotoxic chemotherapy may be used in the following situations:

1. Hormone receptor-negative breast cancer.
2. Hormone receptor-positive breast cancer in whom disease has progressed following more than one endocrine therapy (le. endocrine-resistant disease) or large tumour burden involving visceral organs.

Choice of chemotherapy: For patients in whom chemotherapy is recommended, the choice of regimen (i.e., single-agent or a combination) and selection of a specific therapy depend on multiple factors, like tumour burden, ECOG performance status of the patient, prior treatments, and toxicities, and patient preference. For patients with a limited tumour burden, single-agent chemotherapy is preferred. Sequential single-agent treatment is less toxic and results in similar overall survival compared with combination chemotherapy. For a select group of patients with a large tumour burden (extensive liver metastases, or dyspnea related to diffuse lung metastases) a combination regimen rather than a single-agent is preferred.

Duration of treatment—Unlike in the adjuvant setting, there is no predetermined duration of treatment in metastatic disease. The duration of chemotherapy should be individualized based on the patient's performance status, the presence of treatment toxicities, and alternative options that might be available. In general, patients should continue chemotherapy for the best response, disease progression, or till unacceptable toxicities. There is some data to suggest that there are benefits to continuing treatment beyond their best response. A meta-analysis of randomized trials compared maintenance treatment with treatment over a prespecified duration (range, 3–8 cycles) [122]. Longer duration chemotherapy was associated with improvement in progression-free survival (IHR 0.64, 95% Cl 0.55–0.76) and overall survival HR 0.91, 95% Cl 0.84–0.99). A randomized trial was recently published in which 324 patients with metastatic (breast cancer were treated with paclitaxel and gemcitabine [123]. Patients who had established disease control were randomly allocated to either observation or maintenance treatment with the same drugs until the disease progressed. Maintenance chemotherapy resulted in a greater 6-month PFS rate (60% versus 36%, respectively; HR-0.73) and improved OS when compared to observation (median, 32 versus 24 months; HR 0.65).

Common single-agent protocols used in metastatic breast cancer:

1. Paclitaxel (80 mg/m^2 weekly), docetaxel (75 mg/m^2 3 weekly),
2. Anthracyclines—Doxorubicin 60 mg/m^2 3 weekly, Epirubicin 90 mg/m^2 3 weekly,
3. Capecitabine—1000 mg/m^2 (Day 1 to Day 14, then 7 days off),
4. Platinum agents are rarely used as single agents in metastatic breast cancer, however, in combination regimens, these drugs are preferred especially in patients with BRCA 1 mutation or in triple-negative breast cancer.

Common combination regimens used are.

1. AC—(Doxorubicin and cyclophosphamide, ORR—47–54%),
2. AP—(Doxorubicin and paclitaxel, ORR—40%).
3. Capecitabine plus docetaxel—(ORR—45%).
4. CMF (Cyclophosphamide, methotrexate, and fluorouracil, ORR-30%).

18.1 Her 2 Positive Metastatic Breast Cancer

18.1.1 First-Line Therapy

I. Trastuzumab: Slamon et al. [124] provided the first definitive evidence of the efficacy of anti-HER2 medicines in a critical clinical trial. Chemotherapy with or without trastuzumab was given to patients with HER2-positive metastatic breast cancer who had not previously undergone systemic therapy for metastatic illness.

Chemotherapy plus trastuzumab resulted in a significantly higher rate of objective response. When compared to chemotherapy alone, there was a longer time to progression (TTP; 7.4 vs. 4.6 months; *P* 0.001) and better overall survival (OS; 25 vs. 20 months; *P* = 0.01). There have been several phase III trials that have established the efficacy of trastuzumab and the possibility of combining chemotherapy with HER 2-focused therapy.

II. Lapatinib: Chemotherapy with or without lapatinib was tested in a randomized experiment. The lapatinib group had a median OS of 20.7 months against 20.5 months in the chemotherapy-only arm [125]. The MA 31 study evaluated lapatinib with trastuzumab, both of which were used in combination with taxane treatment. PFS was shown to be inferior with lapatinib (8.8 months vs. 11.4 months with trastuzumab) [126] at the interim analysis. Trastuzumab-based regimens should be regarded as the best option based on the information presented above. Although lapatinib has activity against HER 2 positive breast cancer, it is not recommended in first-line settings.

Ill. Trastuzumab Plus Pertuzumab: The Cleopatra trial [127] examined whether pertuzumab could be added to regular taxane and trastuzumab therapy. A statistically significant improvement in OS in favor of pertuzumab was reported after a median follow-up of 60 months (56.5 months in the pertuzumab arm compared with 40.8 months with placebo).

18.1.2 Second-Line Therapy

Several phase III clinical trials have demonstrated that continuing anti-HER2 therapy in the second-line scenario is related to improved outcomes, including improved survival, in patients whose illness has progressed on first-line trastuzumab-based therapy. Currently, available treatment options include combining trastuzumab with another chemotherapy regimen, adding the mTOR pathway inhibitor Everolimus, switching to a Capecitabine plus lapatinib combination, or switching to the new T-DM 1.

18.1.3 Third Line Therapy and Beyond

THERESA [128] is the only phase 3 trial looking at the efficacy of anti-her2 treatment in the third-line scenario. Patients who had had both trastuzumab and lapatinib for advanced illness were randomized 2:1 to T-DM1 or physician's choice of therapy in this study. Treatment with T-DM 1 was linked to an increase in PFS (6.2 months vs. 3.3 months), as well as a tendency toward improved OS.

In the HER2CLIMB study, adding tucatinib to capecitabine and trastuzumab to patients with progressive metastatic breast cancer who had been treated with trastuzumab, pertuzumab, and trastuzumab emtansine resulted in improved progression-free survival (33.1% at 1 year vs. 10% for the placebo combination arm) and overall survival at 2 years (44.9% in the tucatinib. On December 20, 2019, the US Food and Medication Administration (FDA) granted fast approval to trastuzumab deruxtecan, a drug that targets Her2neu-positive breast tumours [129].

Hormone receptor-positive metastatic breast cancer. ET is the recommended approach for pre- and perimenopausal women with OFS/OFA, men (ideally with an LHRH agonist), and postmenopausal women with HR-positive disease, even in the context of visceral disease, unless there is a visceral crisis. Menopausal state, comorbidities, and adjuvant medications are all factors in deciding which endocrine agent to use. Endocrine therapies should be used with anti-HER-2 medicines (trastuzumab, lapatinib) in cases of ER-positive/HER-2 positive breast cancer with no indication for chemotherapy since they lead to a considerable improvement in progression-free survival compared to endocrine therapy alone.

18.1.4 Premenopausal Patients

Young women with ER-positive ABC should have appropriate OFS/OFA and then be treated with endocrine medications, with or without targeted therapy, in the same way, that postmenopausal women are managed.

18.1.5 Postmenopausal Patients

Given the OS benefit seen in several trials, both in the first- and second-line settings, substantial PFS benefit, and good toxicity profile, cyclin-dependent kinase (CDK)4/6 inhibitors combined with endocrine therapy (ET) have become the standard of care for ER-positive/HER2-negative metastatic breast cancer in the last 2 years [130–133].

The SOLAR-1 phase III, randomized, placebo-controlled trial evaluated the role of alpelisib, an oral inhibitor of the phosphoinositide 3-kinase alpha (PI3Kα) isoform, in combination with fulvestrant, for postmenopausal women and men who had previously been treated with an AI.59 In the PIK3CA-mutated cohort, alpelisib provided a PFS benefit of 11.0 months versus 5.7 months [hazard ratio (HR) for progression or death: 0.65; 95% confidence interval (CI) 0.50–0.85, $P < 0.001$). OS data are not yet available [134].

There is no data to determine the best therapy sequence for this ABC subtype, but the authors believe that using a CDK4/6 inhibitor plus ET as the first line, followed by alpelisib plus ET in patients with PIK3CA-mutated tumours or everolimus plus ET in patients with PIK3CA-wild type or unknown tumours, is the most appropriate sequence in settings where all drugs are accessible.

AIs are the preferable alternative in resource-constrained environments, such as in India, because they are superior to tamoxifen in terms of overall response and time to progression. Tamoxifen, fulvestrant, and everolimus are all alternatives after AI therapy.

Chemotherapy should be provided to patients who have clear signs of endocrine resistance. There is no consensus on how many lines of endocrine therapy should be used before transitioning to chemotherapy. Chemotherapy is chosen based on the patient's response to earlier endocrine therapies, the presence of symptoms and/or quickly progressing or life-threatening disease, patient preference and performance level, and chemotherapy's expected tolerability.

18.2 Triple-Negative Metastatic Breast Cancer

Sacituzumab govitecan induced clinical benefit over physician's choice of therapy (PCT) in patients with metastatic triple-negative breast cancer (TNBC), irrespective of Trop-2 expression; however, greater efficacy was observed in those who had a medium or high Trop-2 score, according to data from an exploratory biomarker analysis of the phase 3 ASCENT trial (NCT02574455) that was presented during the 2020 San Antonio Breast Cancer Symposium [135].

Male Breast Cancer: Male breast cancer accounts for less than 1% of all breast cancers and 0.5% of all malignancies in men. As a result, the most available evidence is from large retrospective series and treatment guidelines are extrapolated from the results of studies on women with breast cancer. Predisposing factors for MBC include family history (in the first-degree relative). Hormones (high estrogen and prolactin levels), radiation exposure, diseases associated with hyperestrogenemia like cirrhosis of the liver, and genetic syndromes. 90% of the tumours in men are hormone receptor-positive and 2–15% are Her2neu positive. The treatment protocols are the same as that for women with breast cancer, except that loco-regional surgery entails a radical mastectomy and adjuvant treatment is based on the stage of presentation.

Cancer Institute (WIA), Adyar, have published their experience with neoadjuvant chemoradiation in male breast cancers. The median age of the patients in the study was 53 years. Stage IIB disease was observed in 8/31 (26%) patients, stage III in 20/31 (64%), and stage IV in 3/31 (10%) patients [136]. The standard of care for treating breast cancer is not neoadjuvant concomitant chemoradiation (CTRT). It has, however, been frequently utilized at the Cancer Institute (WIA) in patients with locally advanced breast cancer to shrink the tumour and make it amenable to surgery.

19 Management of Breast Cancer in the Elderly

Breast cancer is a major concern in the older population, with 1 in 15 women >70 years likely to develop breast cancer. Older women often are treated less aggressively than younger women, owing to co-existing comorbidities, which may contribute to inferior outcomes seen in this population. However, overtreatment should be avoided if a patient is more likely to die from causes unrelated to breast cancer.

Treatment considerations should be individualized based on general prognostic tumour-related markers (biology and extent of disease), global health status (providing information on life expectancy and treatment tolerance), and patient preference, but not on chronological age per se.

For patients with estrogen receptor-positive disease who are not initially candidates for surgery based on the extent of their disease, neoadjuvant endocrine therapy may allow for less aggressive surgery to be performed at a later date.

For patients with hormone receptor-positive, small (<2 cm) tumours and clinically negative axilla who will receive adjuvant endocrine therapy, both axillary surgery and breast radiation may be able to be avoided, without an adverse effect on survival. Decision-making should occur in a multidisciplinary setting.

Adjuvant chemotherapy may be needed in some patients, with the choice of regimen influenced by tumour biology, tumour extent, and patient preference, as in the general population. However, general health status also affects treatment decisions. If chemotherapy is deemed appropriate, for most patients ≥65 years treated for early, HER2-negative breast cancer, four cycles of cyclophosphamide and docetaxel are better tolerated compared to other chemotherapy regimens. However, for fit patients with the higher-risk disease (e.g., node-positive disease, T3 tumours), an anthracycline- and taxane-based regimen may be preferred.

For the patient who is unlikely to tolerate concurrent multiagent chemotherapy, it is reasonable to offer a "deconstructed regimen" (i.e., sequential single-agent treatment; e.g., doxorubicin, followed by paclitaxel, followed by cyclophosphamide, each for four cycles).

Over the past two decades, three prospective randomized trials demonstrated that elderly women with early-stage hormone-positive breast cancer had equivalent disease-specific mortality regardless of axillary surgery. In 2016, the Choosing Wisely campaign encouraged patients and providers to reconsider the role of axillary surgery in this population.

Despite evidence supporting the safety of axillary observation in this patient population, the use of axillary surgery remains high. Surgeons must balance patient-specific comorbidities and life expectancy with surgical risks when making decisions about patient treatment. Surgeons continue to play an important role in guiding shared decision-making in axillary surgery.

20 Current Status of Screening for Breast Cancer

The United States Preventive Services Task Force (USPSTF) recommends biennial screening mammography for women aged 50–74 years [137]. Breast cancer screening is not available to women under the age of 5O or above the age of 75. Only women under the age of 50 who have a high risk of developing breast cancer may be offered screening and genetic testing. Women aged 50–74 should have a mammogram every 2 years, according to current worldwide guidelines.

Level I evidence from NBSS from Canada has shown no benefit of adding mammography to clinical breast examination [138]. Screening for breast cancer for women under the age of 50 years-. The US preventive task force recommends that the decision to start regular, biennial screening mammography before the age of 50 years should be an individual one and taken with the patient's context into account, including the patient's values regarding specific benefits and harms [137]. Randomized clinical trials have shown no benefit of mammography over CBE in women under 50 years of age [139, 140]. There is, however, a significant risk of over-diagnosis (25%) and harms related to it. Table 8 summarizes the approved screening recommendations by various Oncology Societies and Screening Guidelines that are followed throughout the World.

There is no nationalized screening program for breast cancer in India. In fact, any form of screening that may occur is at the very least opportunistic. Mammographic screening for early detection of breast cancer, being a resource-intensive proposition is not a viable option for most developing nations.

Until recently there was no evidence for an overall mortality reduction for breast self-exams or clinical breast exams, but in developing countries such as India, the lower incidence rates, limited access to healthcare, fewer treatment facilities, and advanced stage distribution of disease may yield different optimal screening strategies, such as clinical breast examination (CBE) and ultrasound. In a prospective cluster, randomized clinical trial of 538 women aged 35–64 with no history of breast cancer, conducted in Mumbai Mitra et al. concluded that clinical breast examination conducted every 2 years by primary health workers significantly downstage breast cancer at diagnosis and led to a nonsignificant 15% reduction in breast cancer mortality overall (but a significant reduction of nearly 30% in mortality in women aged ≥50). No significant reduction in mortality was seen in women younger than 50 years. Hence, clinical breast examination should be considered for breast cancer screening in low- and middle-income countries.

Table 8 Summary of screening recommendations as per different standard guidelines

	U.S. Preventive Services Task Force	American Cancer Society	American College of Obstetricians and Gynecologists	International Agency for Research on Cancer	American College of Radiology	American College of Physicians	American Academy of Family Physicians
Women aged 40 to 49 years with an average risk	The decision to start screening with mammography in women before age 50 years should be an individual one. Women who place a higher value on the potential benefit than the potential harms may choose to begin screening once every 2 years between the ages of 40 and 49 years	Women aged 40–44 years should have the choice to start breast cancer screening once a year with mammography if they wish to do so. The risks of screening as well as the potential benefits should be considered. Women aged 45–49 years should be screened with mammography annually	After counseling and if an individual desires screening, mammography may be offered once a year or once every 2 years and clinical breast exams may be offered once a year. Decisions between screening with mammography once a year or once every 2 years should be made through shared decision-making after appropriate	There is limited evidence that screening with mammography reduces breast cancer mortality in women 40–49 years of age	Screening with mammography is recommended once a year	Clinicians should discuss whether to screen for breast cancer with mammography before age 50 years. Discussion should include the potential benefits and harms and a woman's preferences. The potential harms outweigh the benefits in most women aged 40–49 years	The decision to start screening with mammography should be an individual one. Women who place a higher value on the potential benefit than the potential harms may choose to begin screening

(continued)

Table 8 (continued)

	U.S. Preventive Services Task Force	American Cancer Society	American College of Obstetricians and Gynecologists	International Agency for Research on Cancer	American College of Radiology	American College of Physicians	American Academy of Family Physicians
Women aged 50 to 74 years with average risk	Screening with mammography once every 2 years is recommended The evidence is insufficient to assess the additional benefits and harms of clinical breast examination	Women aged 50 to 54 years should be screened with mammography annually. For women aged 55 years and older, screening with mammography is recommended once every 2 years or once a year. Women aged 55 years and older should transition to biennial screening or have the opportunity to continue screening annually. Among average-risk women, clinical breast examination to screen for breast cancer	Screening with mammography is recommended once a year or once every 2 years. Decisions between screening with mammography once a year or once every 2 years should be made through shared decision-making after appropriate counseling Clinical breast exams may be offered annually Clinical breast exams should be offered in the context of a shared, informed decision-making approach that recognizes the uncertainty of additional benefits and harms of clinical breast examination beyond screening mammography	There is sufficient evidence that screening with mammography reduces breast cancer mortality to an extent that its benefits substantially outweigh the risk of radiation-induced cancer from mammography There is inadequate evidence that clinical breast examination reduces breast cancer mortality. There is sufficient evidence that clinical breast examination shifts the stage distribution of tumours detected toward a lower stage	Screening with mammography is recommended once a year	Clinicians should offer screening with mammography once every 2 years. In average-risk women of all ages, clinicians should not use clinical breast examination to screen for breast cancer	Screening with mammography is recommended once every 2 years Current evidence is insufficient to assess the benefits and harms of clinical breast exams

Women aged 75 years or older with average risk	Current evidence is insufficient to assess the balance of benefits and harms of adjunctive screening for breast cancer using breast ultrasonography, magnetic resonance imaging (MRI), digital breast tomosynthesis (DBT), or other methods in women identified to have dense breasts on an otherwise negative screening mammogram	Women should continue screening with mammography as long as their overall health is good and they have a life expectancy of 10 years or more	The decision to stop screening should be based on a shared decision-making process. The decision-making process should include a discussion of the woman's health status and longevity	Not addressed	The age to stop screening with mammography should be based on each woman's health status rather than an age-based determination	In average-risk women aged 75 years or older or in women with a life expectancy of 10 years or less, clinicians should discontinue screening for breast cancer	Current evidence is insufficient to assess the balance of benefits and harms of screening with mammography

(continued)

Table 8 (continued)

	U.S. Preventive Services Task Force	American Cancer Society	American College of Obstetricians and Gynecologists	International Agency for Research on Cancer	American College of Radiology	American College of Physicians	American Academy of Family Physicians
Women with dense breasts	Current evidence is insufficient to assess the balance of benefits and harms of adjunctive screening for breast cancer using breast ultrasonography, magnetic resonance imaging (MRI), digital breast tomosynthesis (DBT), or other methods in women identified to have dense breasts on an otherwise negative screening mammogram	Evidence is insufficient to recommend for or against yearly MRI screening	Other than screening with mammography, the organization does not recommend routine use of alternative or additional tests. Health care providers should comply with state laws that may require disclosure to women of their breast density as recorded in a mammogram report	There is inadequate evidence that ultrasonography as an adjunct to mammography reduces breast cancer mortality. There is limited evidence that ultrasonography as an adjunct to mammography increases the breast cancer detection rate. There is sufficient evidence that ultrasonography as an adjunct to mammography increases the proportion of false-positive screening outcomes	In addition to mammography, contrast-enhanced breast MRI is also recommended. After weighing the benefits and risks, ultrasound can be considered for those who cannot undergo MRI	There is insufficient evidence on the benefits and harms of screening strategies in women who have dense breasts	Current evidence is insufficient to assess the balance of benefits and harms of adjunctive screening for breast cancer using breast ultrasonography, MRI, DBT, or other methods

(**Source**: *Compiled from Recommendations of Standard Oncology Societies and Oncology Groups*)

References

1. Sung H, Ferlay J, Siegel RL, Laversanne M, Soerjomataram I, Jemal A, et al. Global cancer Statistics 2020: GLOBOCAN estimates of incidence and mortality worldwide for 36 cancers in 185 countries. CA Cancer J Clin. 2021;71(3):209–49.
2. Krishnamurthy A, Soundara V, Ramshankar V. Preventive and risk reduction strategies for women at high risk of developing breast cancer: a review. Asian Pac J Cancer Prev. 2016;17(3):895–904.
3. Siegel RL, Miller KD, Jemal A. Cancer statistics, 2020. CA Cancer J Clin. 2020;70(1):7–30.
4. Chopra B, Kaur V, Singh K, Verma M, Singh S, Singh A. Age shift: breast cancer is occurring in younger age groups—is it true? Clin Cancer Investig J. 2014;3:526.
5. Lauby-Secretan B, Scoccianti C, Loomis D, Grosse Y, Bianchini F, Straif K. Body fatness and cancer—viewpoint of the IARC Working Group. N Engl J Med. 2016;375(8):794–8.
6. Iyengar NM, Arthur R, Manson JE, Chlebowski RT, Kroenke CH, Peterson L, et al. Association of body fat and risk of breast cancer in postmenopausal women with normal body mass index: a secondary analysis of a randomized clinical trial and observational study. JAMA Oncol. 2019;5(2):155–63.
7. Pooled Analysis of Prospective Cohort Studies on Height, Weight, and Breast Cancer Risk | American Journal of Epidemiology | Oxford Academic [Internet]. https://academic.oup.com/aje/article/152/6/514/75807. Accessed 20 Jul 2021.
8. Sex hormones and breast cancer risk in premenopausal women: collaborative reanalysis of seven prospective studies. Lancet Oncol. 2013;14(10):1009–19.
9. McCormack VA, dos Santos Silva I. Breast density and parenchymal patterns as markers of breast cancer risk: a meta-analysis. Cancer Epidemiol Prev Biomark. 2006;15(6):1159–69.
10. Kerlikowske K, Ichikawa L, Miglioretti DL, Buist DSM, Vacek PM, Smith-Bindman R, et al. Longitudinal measurement of clinical mammographic breast density to improve the estimation of breast cancer risk. J Natl Cancer Inst. 2007;99(5):386–95.
11. McTiernan A, Investigators for the WHIMDS, Martin CF, Investigators for the WHIMDS, Peck JD, Investigators for the WHIMDS, et al. Estrogen-plus-progestin use and mammographic density in postmenopausal women: Women's health initiative randomized trial. JNCI. J Natl Cancer Inst. 2005;97(18):1366–76.
12. Buist DS, LaCroix AZ, Barlow WE, White E, Weiss NS. Bone mineral density and breast cancer risk in postmenopausal women. J Clin Epidemiol. 2001;54(4):417–22.
13. Endogenous Hormones and Breast Cancer Collaborative Group. Insulin-like growth factor 1 (IGF1), IGF binding protein 3 (IGFBP3), and breast cancer risk: pooled individual data analysis of 17 prospective studies. Lancet Oncol. 2010;11(6):530–42.
14. Gunter MJ, Hoover DR, Yu H, Wassertheil-Smoller S, Rohan TE, Manson JE, et al. Insulin, insulin-like growth factor-I, and risk of breast cancer in postmenopausal women. J Natl Cancer Inst. 2009;101(1):48–60.
15. Height, weight, weight change and risk of breast cancer in Rio de Janeiro, Brazil [Internet]. https://www.scielo.br/scielo.php?pid=S1516--31802001000200005&script=sci_arttext&tlng=en. Accessed 12 Nov 2020.
16. Menarche, menopause, and breast cancer risk: individual participant meta-analysis, including 118 964 women with breast cancer from 117 epidemiological studies. Lancet Oncol. https://www.thelancet.com/journals/lanonc/article/PIIS1470-2045(12)70425-4/fulltext. Accessed 12 Nov 2020.
17. Rosner B, Colditz GA, Willett WC. Reproductive risk factors in a prospective study of breast cancer: the nurses' health study. Am J Epidemiol. 1994;139(8):819–35.
18. Colditz GA, Rosner B. Cumulative risk of breast cancer to age 70 years according to risk factor status: data from the nurses' health study. Am J Epidemiol. 2000;152(10):950–64.
19. Colditz GA, Frazier AL. Models of breast cancer show that risk is set by events of early life: prevention efforts must shift focus. Cancer Epidemiol Biomarkers Prev. 1995;4(5):567–71.
20. Declining Incidence of Contralateral Breast Cancer in the United States From 1975 to 2006 [Internet]. https://www.ncbi.nlm.nih.gov/pmc/articles/PMC3082975/. Accessed 12 Nov 2020.
21. Pan H, Gray R, Braybrooke J, Davies C, Taylor C, et al. 20-year risks of breast-cancer recurrence after stopping endocrine therapy at 5 years. N Engl J Med. 2017;377:1836.
22. Breast cancer family history and contralateral breast cancer risk in young women: an update from the women's environmental cancer and radiation epidemiology study—PubMed [Internet]. https://pubmed.ncbi.nlm.nih.gov/29620998/. Accessed 12 Nov 2020.
23. Collaborative Group on Hormonal Factors in Breast Cancer. Familial breast cancer: collaborative reanalysis of individual data from 52 epidemiological studies including 58,209 women with breast cancer and 101,986 women without the disease. Lancet. 2001;358(9291):1389–99.
24. Braithwaite D, Miglioretti DL, Zhu W, Demb J, Trentham-Dietz A, Sprague B, et al. Family history and breast cancer risk among older women in the breast cancer surveillance consortium cohort. JAMA Intern Med. 2018;178(4):494–501.
25. Gaudet MM, Carter BD, Brinton LA, Falk RT, Gram IT, Luo J, et al. Pooled analysis of active cigarette smoking and invasive breast cancer risk in 14 cohort studies. Int J Epidemiol. 2017;46(3):881–93.

26. Wang K, Li F, Zhang X, Li Z, Li H. Smoking increases risks of all-cause and breast cancer specific mortality in breast cancer individuals: a dose-response meta-analysis of prospective cohort studies involving 39725 breast cancer cases. Oncotarget. 2016;7(50):83134–47.
27. Gram IT, Park S-Y, Kolonel LN, Maskarinec G, Wilkens LR, Henderson BE, et al. Smoking and risk of breast cancer in a racially/ethnically diverse population of mainly women who do not drink alcohol: the MEC study. Am J Epidemiol. 2015;182(11):917–25.
28. Macacu A, Autier P, Boniol M, Boyle P. Active and passive smoking and risk of breast cancer: a meta-analysis. Breast Cancer Res Treat. 2015;154(2):213–24.
29. Dossus L, Boutron-Ruault M-C, Kaaks R, Gram IT, Vilier A, Fervers B, et al. Active and passive cigarette smoking and breast cancer risk: results from the EPIC cohort. Int J Cancer. 2014;134(8):1871–88.
30. Passive cigarette smoke exposure during various periods of life, genetic variants, and breast cancer risk among never smokers | American Journal of Epidemiology | Oxford Academic [Internet]. https://academic.oup.com/aje/article/175/4/289/117058. Accessed 12 Nov 2020.
31. Night shift work and breast cancer incidence: three prospective studies and meta-analysis of published studies | JNCI: Journal of the National Cancer Institute | Oxford Academic [Internet]. https://academic.oup.com/jnci/article/108/12/djw169/2706931. Accessed 12 Nov 2020.
32. Wang F, Yeung KL, Chan WC, Kwok CCH, Leung SL, Wu C, et al. A meta-analysis on dose-response relationship between night shift work and the risk of breast cancer. Ann Oncol. 2013;24(11):2724–32.
33. Hansen J, Stevens RG. Case-control study of shift-work and breast cancer risk in Danish nurses: impact of shift systems. Eur J Cancer. 2012;48(11):1722–9.
34. Mathur P, Sathishkumar K, Chaturvedi M, Das P, Sudarshan KL, Santhappan S, et al. Cancer Statistics, 2020: Report from National Cancer Registry Programme, India. JCO Glob Oncol [Internet]. https://ascopubs.org/doi/pdf/10.1200/GO.20.00122. Accessed 16 Jul 2020.
35. Peters NHGM, van Esser S, van den Bosch MAAJ, Storm RK, Plaisier PW, van Dalen T, et al. Preoperative MRI and surgical management in patients with nonpalpable breast cancer: the MONET—randomised controlled trial. Eur J Cancer. 2011;47(6):879–86.
36. Houssami N, Turner RM, Morrow M. Meta-analysis of pre-operative magnetic resonance imaging (MRI) and surgical treatment for breast cancer. Breast Cancer Res Treat. 2017;165(2):273–83.
37. Estrogen receptor analyses. Correlation of biochemical and immunohistochemical methods using monoclonal antireceptor antibodies—PubMed [Internet]. https://pubmed.ncbi.nlm.nih.gov/3893381/. Accessed 10 Nov 2020.
38. Allred DC, Harvey JM, Berardo M, Clark GM. Prognostic and predictive factors in breast cancer by immunohistochemical analysis. Mod Pathol. 1998;11(2):155–68.
39. Hammond MEH, Hayes DF, Wolff AC, Mangu PB, Temin S. American Society of Clinical Oncology/College of American Pathologists Guideline Recommendations for immunohistochemical testing of Estrogen and progesterone receptors in breast cancer. J Oncol Pract. 2010;6(4):195–7.
40. Westreich M. Anthropomorphic breast measurement: protocol and results in 50 women with aesthetically perfect breasts and clinical application. Plast Reconstr Surg. 1997;100(2):468–79.
41. Berg JW. The significance of axillary node levels in the study of breast carcinoma. Cancer. 1955;8(4):776–8.
42. Fisher B, Jeong J-H, Anderson S, Bryant J, Fisher ER, Wolmark N. Twenty-five-year follow-up of a randomized trial comparing radical mastectomy, total mastectomy, and total mastectomy followed by irradiation. N Engl J Med. 2002;347(8):567–75.
43. Veronesi U, Cascinelli N, Mariani L, Greco M, Saccozzi R, Luini A, et al. Twenty-year follow-up of a randomized study comparing breast-conserving surgery with radical mastectomy for early breast cancer. N Engl J Med. 2002;347(16):1227–32.
44. Litière S, Werutsky G, Fentiman IS, Rutgers E, Christiaens M-R, Van Limbergen E, et al. Breast conserving therapy versus mastectomy for stage I-II breast cancer: 20 year follow-up of the EORTC 10801 phase 3 randomised trial. Lancet Oncol. 2012;13(4):412–9.
45. Blichert-Toft M, Nielsen M, Düring M, Møller S, Rank F, Overgaard M, et al. Long-term results of breast conserving surgery vs. mastectomy for early stage invasive breast cancer: 20-year follow-up of the Danish randomized DBCG-82TM protocol. Acta Oncol. 2008;47(4):672–81.
46. Poggi MM, Danforth DN, Sciuto LC, Smith SL, Steinberg SM, Liewehr DJ, et al. Eighteen-year results in the treatment of early breast carcinoma with mastectomy versus breast conservation therapy: the National Cancer Institute randomized trial. Cancer. 2003;98(4):697–702.
47. Arriagada R, Lê MG, Rochard F, Contesso G. Conservative treatment versus mastectomy in early breast cancer: patterns of failure with 15 years of follow-up data. Institut Gustave-Roussy breast cancer group. J Clin Oncol. 1996;14(5):1558–64.
48. Morrow M, Van Zee KJ, Solin LJ, Houssami N, Chavez-MacGregor M, Harris JR, et al. Society of Surgical Oncology-American Society for Radiation Oncology-American Society of Clinical Oncology consensus guideline on margins for breast-conserving surgery with whole-breast irradiation in ductal carcinoma in situ. Pract Radiat Oncol. 2016;6(5):287–95.
49. Moran MS, Schnitt SJ, Giuliano AE, Harris JR, Khan SA, Horton J, et al. Society of Surgical Oncology-

American Society for Radiation Oncology consensus guideline on margins for breast-conserving surgery with whole-breast irradiation in stages I and II invasive breast cancer. J Clin Oncol. 2014;32(14):1507–15.
50. Morrow M. Limiting breast surgery to the proper minimum. Breast. 2005;14(6):523–6.
51. Tewari M, Krishnamurthy A, Shukla HS. Breast conservation in locally advanced breast cancer in developing countries: wise or waste. Surg Oncol. 2009;18(1):3–13.
52. Braithwite LR. The flow of lymph from the ileocaecal angle, and its possible bearing on the cause of duodenal and gastric ulcer. Br J Surg. 1923;11:7–26.
53. Gould EA, Winship T, Philbin PH, Kerr HH. Observations on a "sentinel node" in cancer of the parotid. Cancer. 1960;13:77–8.
54. Cabanas RM. An approach for the treatment of penile carcinoma. Cancer. 1977;39(2):456–66.
55. Morton DL, Wen DR, Wong JH, et al. Technical details of intraoperative lymphaticmapping for early stagemelanoma. Arch Surg. 1992;127:392–9. Google Search [Internet]. https://www.google.com/search?q=Morton+DL%2C+Wen+DR%2C+Wong+JH%2C+et+al.+Technical+details+of+intraoperative+lymphaticmapping+for+early+stagemelanoma.+Arch+Surg.+1992%3B127%3A392%E2%80%93399.&oq=Morton+DL%2C+Wen+DR%2C+Wong+JH%2C+et+al.+Technical+details+of+intraoperative+lymphaticmapping+for+early+stagemelanoma.+Arch+Surg.+1992%3B127%3A392%E2%80%93399.&aqs=chrome..69i57.178j0j4&sourceid=chrome&ie=UTF-8. Accessed 16 Nov 2020.
56. Giuliano AE, Kirgan DM, Guenther JM, Morton DL. Lymphatic mapping and sentinel lymphadenectomy for breast cancer. Ann Surg. 1994;220(3):391–401.
57. Krag DN, Weaver DL, Alex JC, Fairbank JT. Surgical resection and radiolocalization of the sentinel lymph node in breast cancer using a gamma probe. Surg Oncol. 1993;2(6):335–9; discussion 340.
58. Krag DN, Anderson SJ, Julian TB, Brown AM, Harlow SP, Costantino JP, et al. Sentinel-lymph-node resection compared with conventional axillary-lymph-node dissection in clinically node-negative patients with breast cancer: overall survival findings from the NSABP B-32 randomised phase 3 trial. Lancet Oncol. 2010;11(10):927–33.
59. Clough KB, Nasr R, Nos C, Vieira M, Inguenault C, Poulet B. New anatomical classification of the axilla with implications for sentinel node biopsy. Br J Surg. 2010;97(11):1659–65.
60. Giuliano AE, Ballman KV, McCall L, Beitsch PD, Brennan MB, Kelemen PR, et al. Effect of axillary dissection vs no axillary dissection on 10-year overall survival among women with invasive breast cancer and sentinel node metastasis: the ACOSOG Z0011 (Alliance) randomized clinical trial. JAMA. 2017;318(10):918–26.
61. Clarke M, Collins R, Darby S, Davies C, Elphinstone P, Evans V, et al. Effects of radiotherapy and of differences in the extent of surgery for early breast cancer on local recurrence and 15-year survival: an overview of the randomised trials. Lancet. 2005;366(9503):2087–106.
62. Group E Early BCTC. Effect of radiotherapy after mastectomy and axillary surgery on 10-year recurrence and 20-year breast cancer mortality: meta-analysis of individual patient data for 8135 women in 22 randomised trials. Lancet. 2014;383(9935):2127–35.
63. Internal mammary and medial supraclavicular irradiation in breast cancer | NEJM [Internet]. https://www.nejm.org/doi/full/10.1056/NEJMoa1415369. Accessed 9 Nov 2020.
64. Thomas JS, Hanby AM, Russell N, van Tienhoven G, Riddle K, Anderson N, et al. The BIG 2.04 MRC/EORTC SUPREMO trial: pathology quality assurance of a large phase 3 randomised international clinical trial of postmastectomy radiotherapy in intermediate-risk breast cancer. Breast Cancer Res Treat. 2017;163(1):63–9.
65. McCammon R, Finlayson C, Schwer A, Rabinovitch R. Impact of postmastectomy radiotherapy in T3N0 invasive carcinoma of the breast: a surveillance, epidemiology, and end results database analysis. Cancer. 2008;113(4):683–9.
66. NCCN Guidelines Version 5.2020.
67. Hennequin C, Bossard N, Servagi-Vernat S, Maingon P, Dubois J-B, Datchary J, et al. Ten-year survival results of a randomized trial of irradiation of internal mammary nodes after mastectomy. Int J Radiat Oncol Biol Phys. 2013;86(5):860–6.
68. Recht A, Comen EA, Fine RE, Fleming GF, Hardenbergh PH, Ho AY, et al. Postmastectomy radiotherapy: an American Society of Clinical Oncology, American Society for Radiation Oncology, and Society of Surgical Oncology focused guideline update. Pract Radiat Oncol. 2016;6(6):e219–34.
69. Christante D, Pommier SJ, Diggs BS, Samuelson BT, Truong A, Marquez C, et al. Using complications associated with postmastectomy radiation and immediate breast reconstruction to improve surgical decision making. Arch Surg. 2010;145(9):873–8.
70. Nava MB, Pennati AE, Lozza L, Spano A, Zambetti M, Catanuto G. Outcome of different timings of radiotherapy in implant-based breast reconstructions. Plast Reconstr Surg. 2011;128(2):353–9.
71. Early Breast Cancer Trialists' Collaborative Group (EBCTCG), Darby S, McGale P, Correa C, Taylor C, Arriagada R, et al. Effect of radiotherapy after breast-conserving surgery on 10-year recurrence and 15-year breast cancer death: meta-analysis of individual patient data for 10,801 women in 17 randomised trials. Lancet. 2011;378(9804):1707–16.
72. Smith BD, Bellon JR, Blitzblau R, Freedman G, Haffty B, Hahn C, et al. Radiation therapy for the whole breast: executive summary of an American

Society for Radiation Oncology (ASTRO) evidence-based guideline. Pract Radiat Oncol. 2018;8(3):145–52.
73. Haviland JS, Owen JR, Dewar JA, Agrawal RK, Barrett J, Barrett-Lee PJ, et al. The UK standardisation of breast radiotherapy (START) trials of radiotherapy hypofractionation for treatment of early breast cancer: 10-year follow-up results of two randomised controlled trials. Lancet Oncol. 2013;14(11):1086–94.
74. Brunt AM, Haviland JS, Wheatley DA, Sydenham MA, Alhasso A, Bloomfield DJ, et al. Hypofractionated breast radiotherapy for 1 week versus 3 weeks (FAST-Forward): 5-year efficacy and late normal tissue effects results from a multicentre, non-inferiority, randomised, phase 3 trial. Lancet. 2020;395(10237):1613–26.
75. Brunt AM, Haviland JS, Sydenham M, Agrawal RK, Algurafi H, Alhasso A, et al. Ten-year results of FAST: a randomized controlled trial of 5-fraction whole-breast radiotherapy for early breast cancer. J Clin Oncol. 2020;38(28):3261–72.
76. Offersen BV, Alsner J, Nielsen HM, Jakobsen EH, Nielsen MH, Krause M, et al. Hypofractionated versus standard fractionated radiotherapy in patients with early breast cancer or ductal carcinoma in situ in a randomized phase III trial: the DBCG HYPO trial. J Clin Oncol. 2020;38:3615–25. https://ascopubs.org/doi/pdf/10.1200/JCO.20.01363. Accessed 12 Nov 2020.
77. Romestaing P, Lehingue Y, Carrie C, Coquard R, Montbarbon X, Ardiet JM, et al. Role of a 10-Gy boost in the conservative treatment of early breast cancer: results of a randomized clinical trial in Lyon, France. J Clin Oncol. 1997;15(3):963–8.
78. Bartelink H, Horiot JC, Poortmans P, Struikmans H, Van den Bogaert W, Barillot I, et al. Recurrence rates after treatment of breast cancer with standard radiotherapy with or without additional radiation. N Engl J Med. 2001;345(19):1378–87.
79. Bartelink H, Horiot J-C, Poortmans PM, Struikmans H, Van den Bogaert W, Fourquet A, et al. Impact of a higher radiation dose on local control and survival in breast-conserving therapy of early breast cancer: 10-year results of the randomized boost versus no boost EORTC 22881-10882 trial. J Clin Oncol. 2007;25(22):3259–65.
80. Surgical adjuvant chemotherapy in cancer of the breast: results of a decade of cooperative investigation. [Internet]. https://www.ncbi.nlm.nih.gov/pmc/articles/PMC1387335/. Accessed 16 Nov 2020.
81. Bonadonna G, Valagussa P, Moliterni A, Zambetti M, Brambilla C. Adjuvant cyclophosphamide, methotrexate, and fluorouracil in node-positive breast cancer: the results of 20 years of follow-up. N Engl J Med. 1995;332(14):901–6.
82. Martin M, Villar A, Sole-Calvo A, Gonzalez R, Massuti B, Lizon J, et al. Doxorubicin in combination with fluorouracil and cyclophosphamide (i.v. FAC regimen, day 1, 21) versus methotrexate in combination with fluorouracil and cyclophosphamide (i.v. CMF regimen, day 1, 21) as adjuvant chemotherapy for operable breast cancer: a study by the GEICAM group. Ann Oncol. 2003;14(6):833–42.
83. Randomized trial comparing six versus three cycles of Epirubicin-based adjuvant chemotherapy in premenopausal, node-positive breast cancer patients: 10-year follow-up results of the French Adjuvant Study Group 01 Trial | J Clin Oncol [Internet]. https://ascopubs.org/doi/pdf/10.1200/JCO.2003.04.148. Accessed 11 Nov 2020.
84. Roché H, Fumoleau P, Spielmann M, Canon J-L, Delozier T, Serin D, et al. Sequential adjuvant epirubicin-based and docetaxel chemotherapy for node-positive breast cancer patients: the FNCLCC PACS 01 trial. J Clin Oncol. 2006;24(36):5664–71.
85. Martín M, Rodríguez-Lescure A, Ruiz A, Alba E, Calvo L, Ruiz-Borrego M, et al. Randomized phase 3 trial of fluorouracil, epirubicin, and cyclophosphamide alone or followed by paclitaxel for early breast cancer. J Natl Cancer Inst. 2008;100(11):805–14.
86. Ellis P, Barrett-Lee P, Johnson L, Cameron D, Wardley A, O'Reilly S, et al. Sequential docetaxel as adjuvant chemotherapy for early breast cancer (TACT): an open-label, phase III, randomised controlled trial. Lancet. 2009;373(9676):1681–92.
87. Nitz U, Gluz O, Huober J, Kreipe HH, Kates RE, Hartmann A, et al. Final analysis of the prospective WSG-AGO EC-doc versus FEC phase III trial in intermediate-risk (pN1) early breast cancer: efficacy and predictive value of Ki67 expression. Ann Oncol. 2014;25(8):1551–7.
88. Martin M, Pienkowski T, Mackey J, Pawlicki M, Guastalla J-P, Weaver C, et al. Adjuvant docetaxel for node-positive breast cancer. N Engl J Med. 2005;352(22):2302–13.
89. Jones S, Holmes FA, O'Shaughnessy J, Blum JL, Vukelja SJ, McIntyre KJ, et al. Docetaxel with cyclophosphamide is associated with an overall survival benefit compared with doxorubicin and cyclophosphamide: 7-year follow-up of US oncology research trial 9735. J Clin Oncol. 2009;27(8):1177–83.
90. Winer EP, Berry DA, Woolf S, Duggan D, Kornblith A, Harris LN, et al. Failure of higher-dose paclitaxel to improve outcome in patients with metastatic breast cancer: cancer and Leukemia group B trial 9342. J Clin Oncol. 2016;22:2061. Accessed 6 Nov 2020.
91. Harvey V, Mouridsen H, Semiglazov V, Jakobsen E, Voznyi E, Robinson BA, et al. Phase III trial comparing three doses of docetaxel for second-line treatment of advanced breast cancer. J Clin Oncol. 2006;24(31):4963–70.
92. Long-term follow-up of the E1199 Phase III Trial Evaluating the Role of Taxane and Schedule in Operable Breast Cancer [Internet]. https://www.ncbi.nlm.nih.gov/pmc/articles/PMC4500829/. Accessed 17 Nov 2020.
93. Citron ML, Berry DA, Cirrincione C, Hudis C, Winer EP, Gradishar WJ, et al. Randomized trial of dose-

dense versus conventionally scheduled and sequential versus concurrent combination chemotherapy as postoperative adjuvant treatment of node-positive primary breast cancer: first report of intergroup trial C9741/cancer and Leukemia group B trial 9741. J Clin Oncol. 2003;21(8):1431–9.
94. Moebus V, Jackisch C, Lueck H-J, du Bois A, Thomssen C, Kurbacher C, et al. Intense dose-dense sequential chemotherapy with epirubicin, paclitaxel, and cyclophosphamide compared with conventionally scheduled chemotherapy in high-risk primary breast cancer: mature results of an AGO phase III study. J Clin Oncol. 2010;28(17):2874–80.
95. Möbus V, Jackisch C, Lück HJ, du Bois A, Thomssen C, Kuhn W, et al. Ten-year results of intense dose-dense chemotherapy show superior survival compared with a conventional schedule in high-risk primary breast cancer: final results of AGO phase III iddEPC trial. Ann Oncol off J Eur soc. Med Oncol. 2018;29(1):178–85.
96. Thomas E, Berner G. Prognostic and predictive implications of HER2 status for breast cancer patients. Eur J Oncol Nurs. 2000;4(Sa):10–7.
97. Piccart-Gebhart MJ, Procter M, Leyland-Jones B, Goldhirsch A, Untch M, Smith I, et al. Trastuzumab after adjuvant chemotherapy in HER2-positive breast cancer. N Engl J Med. 2005;353(16):1659–72.
98. Romond EH, Perez EA, Bryant J, Suman VJ, Geyer CE, Davidson NE, et al. Trastuzumab plus adjuvant chemotherapy for operable HER2-positive breast cancer. N Engl J Med. 2005;353(16):1673–84.
99. Slamon D, Eiermann W, Robert N, Pienkowski T, Martin M, Press M, et al. Adjuvant trastuzumab in HER2-positive breast cancer. N Engl J Med. 2011;365(14):1273–83.
100. Joensuu H, Kellokumpu-Lehtinen P-L, Bono P, Alanko T, Kataja V, Asola R, et al. Adjuvant docetaxel or vinorelbine with or without trastuzumab for breast cancer. N Engl J Med. 2006;354(8):809–20.
101. Joensuu H, Fraser J, Wildiers H, Huovinen R, Auvinen P, Utriainen M, et al. Effect of adjuvant trastuzumab for a duration of 9 weeks vs 1 year with concomitant chemotherapy for early human epidermal growth factor receptor 2-positive breast cancer: the SOLD randomized clinical trial. JAMA Oncol. 2018;4(9):1199–206.
102. 6 months versus 12 months of adjuvant trastuzumab in early breast cancer (PHARE): final analysis of a multicentre, open-label, phase 3 randomised trial. Lancet [Internet]. https://www.thelancet.com/journals/lancet/article/PIIS0140-6736(19)30653-1/fulltext. Accessed 11 Nov 2020.
103. Conte P, Frassoldati A, Bisagni G, Brandes AA, Donadio M, Garrone O, et al. Nine weeks versus 1 year adjuvant trastuzumab in combination with chemotherapy: final results of the phase III randomized short-HER study. Ann Oncol. 2018;29(12):2328–33.
104. Mavroudis D, Saloustros E, Malamos N, Kakolyris S, Boukovinas I, Papakotoulas P, et al. Six versus 12 months of adjuvant trastuzumab in combination with dose-dense chemotherapy for women with HER2-positive breast cancer: a multicenter randomized study by the Hellenic oncology research group (HORG). Ann Oncol. 2015;26(7):1333–40.
105. Earl HM, Hiller L, Vallier A-L, Loi S, McAdam K, Hughes-Davies L, et al. 6 versus 12 months of adjuvant trastuzumab for HER2-positive early breast cancer (PERSEPHONE): 4-year disease-free survival results of a randomised phase 3 non-inferiority trial. Lancet. 2019;393(10191):2599–612.
106. Evaluation of 1-year vs shorter durations of adjuvant trastuzumab among patients with early breast cancer: an individual participant data and trial-level meta-analysis | Breast Cancer | JAMA Network Open | JAMA Network [Internet]. https://jamanetwork.com/journals/jamanetworkopen/fullarticle/2769686. Accessed 15 Jun 2021.
107. Bear HD, Anderson S, Smith RE, Geyer CE, Mamounas EP, Fisher B, et al. Sequential preoperative or postoperative docetaxel added to preoperative doxorubicin plus cyclophosphamide for operable breast cancer: National Surgical Adjuvant Breast and Bowel Project Protocol B-27. J Clin Oncol Off J Am Soc Clin Oncol. 2006;24(13):2019–27.
108. Cortazar P, Zhang L, Untch M, Mehta K, Costantino JP, Wolmark N, et al. Pathological complete response and long-term clinical benefit in breast cancer: the CTNeoBC pooled analysis. Lancet. 2014;384(9938):164–72.
109. Parmar V, Krishnamurthy A, Hawaldar R, Nadkarni MS, Sarin R, Chinoy R, et al. Breast conservation treatment in women with locally advanced breast cancer—experience from a single Centre. Int J Surg. 2006;4(2):106–14.
110. Pembrolizumab for Early Triple-Negative Breast Cancer | NEJM [Internet]. https://www.nejm.org/doi/full/10.1056/NEJMoa1910549. Accessed 17 Nov 2020.
111. Nanda R, Liu MC, Yau C, Shatsky R, Pusztai L, Wallace A, et al. Effect of pembrolizumab plus neoadjuvant chemotherapy on pathologic complete response in women with early-stage breast cancer: an analysis of the ongoing phase 2 adaptively randomized I-SPY2 trial. JAMA Oncol. 2020;6(5):676–84.
112. Mittendorf EA, Zhang H, Barrios CH, Saji S, Jung KH, Hegg R, et al. Neoadjuvant atezolizumab in combination with sequential nab-paclitaxel and anthracycline-based chemotherapy versus placebo and chemotherapy in patients with early-stage triple-negative breast cancer (IMpassion031): a randomised, double-blind, phase 3 trial. Lancet. 2020;396(10257):1090–100.
113. Group (EBCTCG) EBCTC. Relevance of breast cancer hormone receptors and other factors to the efficacy of adjuvant tamoxifen: patient-level meta-analysis of randomised trials. Lancet. 2011;378(9793):771–84.
114. Gray RG, Rea D, Handley K, Bowden SJ, Perry P, Earl HM, et al. aTTom: long-term effects of continu-

ing adjuvant tamoxifen to 10 years versus stopping at 5 years in 6,953 women with early breast cancer. J Clin Oncol. 2013;31(18_suppl):5.

115. Davies C, Pan H, Godwin J, Gray R, Arriagada R, Raina V, et al. Long-term effects of continuing adjuvant tamoxifen to 10 years versus stopping at 5 years after diagnosis of oestrogen receptor-positive breast cancer: ATLAS, a randomised trial. Lancet. 2013;381(9869):805–16.
116. Sequential Tamoxifen and Aminoglutethimide Versus Tamoxifen Alone in the Adjuvant Treatment of Postmenopausal Breast Cancer Patients: Results of an Italian Cooperative Study | J Clin Oncol [Internet]. https://ascopubs.org/doi/pdf/10.1200/JCO.2001.19.22.4209. Accessed 17 Nov 2020.
117. Howell A, Cuzick J, Baum M, Buzdar A, Dowsett M, Forbes JF, et al. Results of the ATAC (Arimidex, tamoxifen, alone or in combination) trial after completion of 5 years' adjuvant treatment for breast cancer. Lancet. 2005;365(9453):60–2.
118. Regan MM, Neven P, Giobbie-Hurder A, Goldhirsch A, Ejlertsen B, Mauriac L, et al. Assessment of letrozole and tamoxifen alone and in sequence for postmenopausal women with steroid hormone receptor-positive breast cancer: the BIG 1-98 randomised clinical trial at 8·1 years median follow-up. Lancet Oncol. 2011;12(12):1101–8.
119. van de Velde CJ, Rea D, Seynaeve C, Putter H, Hasenburg A, Vannetzel J-M, et al. Adjuvant tamoxifen and exemestane in early breast cancer (TEAM): a randomised phase 3 trial. Lancet. 2011;377(9762):321–31.
120. Goss PE, Ingle JN, Martino S, Robert NJ, Muss HB, Piccart MJ, et al. Randomized trial of letrozole following tamoxifen as extended adjuvant therapy in receptor-positive breast cancer: updated findings from NCIC CTG MA.17. J Natl Cancer Inst. 2005;97(17):1262–71.
121. Francis PA, Pagani O, Fleming GF, Walley BA, Colleoni M, Láng I, et al. Tailoring adjuvant endocrine therapy for premenopausal breast cancer. N Engl J Med. 2018;379(2):122–37.
122. Gennari A, Stockler M, Puntoni M, Sormani M, Nanni O, Amadori D, et al. Duration of chemotherapy for metastatic breast cancer: a systematic review and meta-analysis of randomized clinical trials. J Clin Oncol. 2011;29(16):2144–9.
123. Park YH, Jung KH, Im S-A, Sohn JH, Ro J, Ahn J-H, et al. Phase III, multicenter, randomized trial of maintenance chemotherapy versus observation in patients with metastatic breast cancer after achieving disease control with six cycles of gemcitabine plus paclitaxel as first-line chemotherapy: KCSG-BR07-02. J Clin Oncol. 2013;31(14):1732–9.
124. Use of chemotherapy plus a monoclonal antibody against HER2 for metastatic breast cancer that overexpresses HER2 | NEJM [Internet]. https://www.nejm.org/doi/full/10.1056/nejm200103153441101. Accessed 15 Nov 2020.
125. Guan Z, Xu B, DeSilvio ML, Shen Z, Arpornwirat W, Tong Z, et al. Randomized trial of lapatinib versus placebo added to paclitaxel in the treatment of human epidermal growth factor receptor 2-overexpressing metastatic breast cancer. J Clin Oncol. 2013;31(16):1947–53.
126. Gelmon KA, Boyle FM, Kaufman B, Huntsman DG, Manikhas A, Di Leo A, et al. Lapatinib or trastuzumab plus Taxane therapy for human epidermal growth factor receptor 2-positive advanced breast cancer: final results of NCIC CTG MA.31. J Clin Oncol. 2015;33(14):1574–83.
127. Swain SM, Baselga J, Kim S-B, Ro J, Semiglazov V, Campone M, et al. Pertuzumab, trastuzumab, and docetaxel in HER2-positive metastatic breast cancer. N Engl J Med. 2015;372(8):724–34.
128. Krop IE, Kim S-B, González-Martín A, LoRusso PM, Ferrero J-M, Smitt M, et al. Trastuzumab emtansine versus treatment of physician's choice for pretreated HER2-positive advanced breast cancer (TH3RESA): a randomised, open-label, phase 3 trial. Lancet Oncol. 2014;15(7):689–99.
129. Tucatinib, Trastuzumab, and Capecitabine for HER2-Positive Metastatic Breast Cancer | NEJM [Internet]. https://www.nejm.org/doi/full/10.1056/NEJMoa1914609. Accessed 15 Jun 2020.
130. Im S-A, Lu Y-S, Bardia A, Harbeck N, Colleoni M, Franke F, et al. Overall survival with Ribociclib plus endocrine therapy in breast cancer. N Engl J Med. 2019;381(4):307–16.
131. Slamon DJ, Neven P, Chia S, Fasching PA, De Laurentiis M, Im S-A, et al. Overall survival with Ribociclib plus Fulvestrant in advanced breast cancer. N Engl J Med. 2020;382(6):514–24.
132. Palbociclib and Letrozole in Advanced Breast Cancer | NEJM [Internet]. https://www.nejm.org/doi/full/10.1056/NEJMoa1607303. Accessed 16 Nov 2020.
133. Sledge GW Jr, Toi M, Neven P, et al. The effect of abemaciclib plus fulvestrant on overall survival in hormone receptor-positive, erbb2-negative breast cancer that progressed on endocrine therapy-MONARCH 2: a randomized clinical trial. JAMA Oncol. 2019;6(1):116–24. Google Search [Internet]. https://www.google.com/search?q=Sledge+GW%2C+Jr.%2C+Toi+M%2C+Neven+P%2C+et+al.+The+effect+of+abemaciclib+plus+fulvestrant+on+overall+survival+in+hormone+receptor-positive%2C+erbb2-negative+breast+cancer+that+progressed+on+endocrine+therapy-MONARCH+2%3A+a+randomized+clinical+trial.+JAMA+Oncol.+2019%3B6(1)%3A116-124.&oq=Sledge+GW%2C+Jr.%2C+Toi+M%2C+Neven+P%2C+et+al.+The+effect+of+abemaciclib+plus+fulvestrant+on+overall+survival+in+hormone+receptor-positive%2C+erbb2-negative+breast+cancer+that+progressed+on+endocrine+therapy-MONARCH+2%3A+a+randomized+clinical+trial.+JAMA+Oncol.+2019%3B6(1)%3A116-124.&aqs=chrome..69i57.301j0j4&sourceid=chrome&ie=UTF-8. Accessed 16 Nov 2020.

134. André F, Ciruelos E, Rubovszky G, Campone M, Loibl S, Rugo HS, et al. Alpelisib for PIK3CA-mutated, hormone receptor–positive advanced breast cancer. N Engl J Med. 2019;380(20):1929–40.
135. Bardia A, Hurvitz SA, Tolaney SM, Loirat D, Punie K, Oliveira M, et al. Sacituzumab Govitecan in metastatic triple-negative breast cancer. N Engl J Med. 2021;384(16):1529–41.
136. Iyer P, Balasubramanian A, Selvaluxmy G, Sridevi V, Krishnamurthy A, Radhakrishnan V. Neoadjuvant concurrent chemoradiation in male breast cancer: experience from a tertiary cancer center. Indian J Cancer. 2019;56(1):37–40. Google Search [Internet]. https://www.google.com/search?q=Iyer+P%2C+Balasubramanian+A%2C+Selvaluxmy+G%2C+Sridevi+V%2C+Krishnamurthy+A%2C+Radhakrishnan+V.+Neoadjuvant+concurrent+chemoradiation+in+male+breast+cancer%3A+Experience+from+a+tertiary+cancer+center.+Indian+J+Cancer.+2019+Jan-Mar%3B56(1)%3A37-40&oq=Iyer+P%2C+Balasubramanian+A%2C+Selvaluxmy+G%2C+Sridevi+V%2C+Krishnamurthy+A%2C+Radhakrishnan+V.+Neoadjuvant+concurrent+chemoradiation+in+male+breast+cancer%3A+Experience+from+a+tertiary+cancer+center.+Indian+J+Cancer.+2019+Jan-Mar%3B56(1)%3A37-40&aqs=chrome..69i57j69i59.1459j0j9&sourceid=chrome&ie=UTF-8. Accessed 16 Jun 2020.
137. Recommendation: Breast Cancer: Screening | United States Preventive Services Taskforce [Internet]. https://www.uspreventiveservicestaskforce.org/uspstf/recommendation/breast-cancer-screening. Accessed 17 Nov 2020.
138. Twenty five year follow-up for breast cancer incidence and mortality of the Canadian National Breast Screening Study: randomised screening trial | The BMJ [Internet]. https://www.bmj.com/content/348/bmj.g366. Accessed 17 Nov 2020.
139. Nelson HD, Fu R, Cantor A, Pappas M, Daeges M, Humphrey L. Effectiveness of breast cancer screening: systematic review and meta-analysis to update the 2009 U.S. preventive services task force recommendation. Ann Intern Med. 2016;164(4):244–55.
140. Oeffinger KC, Fontham ETH, Etzioni R, Herzig A, Michaelson JS, Shih Y-CT, et al. Breast cancer screening for women at average risk: 2015 guideline update from the American Cancer Society. JAMA. 2015;314(15):1599.

Cervical Cancer Screening

Roma Jethani, Debabrata Barmon,
and Amal Chandra Kataki

1 Introduction

Globally, cervical cancer is the fourth most common cancer in women, following breast, colorectal, and lung cancer, with estimated 604,127 new cases and 341,831 new deaths in 2020 [1]. There is substantial variation in the incidence of cervical cancer based on HDI (human development index) levels [2]. The highest age standardized incidence and mortality rate was reported in Eastern Africa which is approximately threefold higher than the global estimates. India contributes significantly to the incidence of cervical cancer as it accounts for 36% of the population among lower HDI (human development index) countries [3].

Cervical cancer is preventable due to availability of highly effective primary (HPV vaccination) and secondary (screening) prevention measures. The two most important factors which have paved the path to huge success of cervical cancer screening programs are definite precursor lesions and definitive treatment options available for such lesions. Incorporation of routine screening for cervical cancer along with introduction of HPV vaccination has drastically reduced the incidence and mortality in developed countries, such as Australia [4].

WHO announced **90-70-90** targets to achieve elimination of cervical cancer by 2030, i.e. to maintain incidence rate of below 4 per 1,00,000 women. The targets to be met are:

1. 90%—Girls fully vaccinated with the HPV vaccine by the age of 15.
2. 70%—Women screened using a high-performance test by the age of 35, and again by the age of 45.
3. 90%—Women with pre-cancer treated and 90% of women with invasive cancer managed [5].

2 Methods of Cervical Cancer Screening

Over the years, several methods have been described for screening of cervical cancer. The screening methods are based on direct identification of gross abnormalities with naked eye or with magnification using colposcope, cytological examination of cervical scrapings/smear, and identification of the culprit viral (human papilloma virus). The methods vary in their sensitivity and specificity in detecting pre-invasive lesions. The low-cost and low-technology cervical cancer screening modalities, such as VIA, are useful in low- and middle-income countries [6].

R. Jethani (✉) · D. Barmon · A. C. Kataki
Department of Gynaecologic Oncology,
Dr. Bhubaneswar Borooah Cancer Institute
(A Unit of Tata Memorial Centre, Mumbai),
Guwahati, Assam, India
e-mail: dydiracademic@bbci.tmc.gov.in

A. C. Kataki, D. Barmon (eds.), *Fundamentals in Gynaecologic Malignancy*,
https://doi.org/10.1007/978-981-19-5860-1_11

1. Visual screening	Visual inspection of cervix • VIA (Visual inspection with acetic acid) [6] • VILI (Visual Inspection with Lugol's Iodine) [6] • VIAM (Visual inspection with acetic acid under low magnification) [7]
	Colposcopy • Colposcope [8] • Video Colposcope [8] • POCket colposcope [9] • Gynocular [9] • EVA COLPO [9]
	Automated Visual Evaluation (AVE) [9]
	Smart Scope [10]
2. Physical	Polar probe (Truscreen) [9]
	Fluorescence Spectroscopy [11]
	Colpo-probe [12]
	Electrical impedance spectroscopy (ZedScan) [13]
3. Cytology	Conventional cytology (Pap test) [14]
	Liquid-based cytology [14]
4. HPV testing	Primary HPV testing [14]
	Co-testing (Pap test and HPV testing) [14]
5. Newer modalities	p16 and Ki67 [14]
	DNA methylation (QIAsure methylation test) [14]
	E6 and E7 mRNA [14]
	HPV self-sampling [14]
	HPV DNA in urinary sample [15]
	HPV DNA in menstrual blood [16]
	HPV DNA in blood—liquid biopsy [17]

SAVE-Cervix is an on-going project funded by IARC (International Agency for Research on Cancer) for development of an artificial intelligence (AI) image recognition device to improve screening and management of pre-invasive lesions in LMIC (low- and middle-income countries) [18].

2.1 HPV Testing

The causal association of cervical cancer with human papilloma virus is proven beyond doubts [19] thus, detection of HPV (DNA/RNA) has gained popularity as primary screening test. The screening intervals can be prolonged to 5 years owing to the high sensitivity and negative predictive value of HPV test [14]. Evidence suggests that as compared to screening with VIA or cytology, the cervical cancer incidence and deaths are reduced if HPV testing is used as primary screening test [20].

Indications of HPV testing:

1. Primary screening test.
2. In combination with cytology (Co-testing).
3. Triage tests for women with borderline cytology.

The 14 high-risk HPV genotypes identified are HPV16, 18, 31, 33, 35, 39, 45, 51, 52, 56, 58, 59, 66, and 68. HPV16 and 18 are the most common types associated with cervical cancers [21]. HPV DNA testing detects high-risk strains of HPV, which cause almost all cervical cancers. HPV mRNA detects HPV infections leading to cellular transformation [22].

The HPV tests can report either partial genotyping or extended genotyping:

1. Partial Genotyping- tests report HPV 16 and 18 (including HPV 45 in some cases) and other carcinogenic types separately.
2. Extended Genotyping- tests reporting additional types, such as HPV31, 33, 35, 45, 52 and 56 [20].

WHO 2021 recommendations allow inclusion of both self-sampling and provider sampling for HPV DNA testing (nucleic acid amplification test) [20]. The FDA approved HPV devices are Digene Hybrid Capture (HC2) HPV DNA test, Cervista HPV HR test, Cervista HPV 16/18, Cobas HPV test, Aptima HPV (FDA approved for ThinPrep), Aptima HPV 16, 18/45, BD Oncolarity HPV assay [23].

Self-sampling of HPV—Self-HPV testing makes HPV testing more efficient, painless, female friendly, and less costly. A meta-analysis of 33 studies with 369,000 total participants: 29

RCTs and 4 observational studies, concluded that the acceptance of self-sampling of HPV was high. There is strong evidence that HPV self-sampling can increase cervical cancer screening uptake compared with standard of care, with no negative effect on linkage to clinical assessment/treatment. This evidence is mainly from high income countries. Self-collection of samples for HPV testing is likely to increase equity by reducing cultural, socioeconomic, gender and logistic barriers to screening [24].

The self-collected sampling kit consists of:

1. Swab or cervical brush (single-use).
2. Tube (containing the collection/transport media) [20].

Examples of self-sampling kit available are Qvintip, Evalyn Brush, FLOQSwabsTM, SelfCerv [9].

2.2 Cytology

The Papanicolaou or PAP smear, conceptualized by Dr. George Papanicolaou and Dr. Herbert Traut, involves analysis of vaginal smears for screening of cervical and vaginal cancers [25].

Two types of cervical cytology preparation methods:

1. Conventional Pap smear (Pap test).
2. Liquid-based cytology (LBC) [14].

Currently, two commercially available liquid-based cytology systems are approved by the U.S. Food and Drug Administration

(a) ThinPrep (Hologic).
(b) SurePath (Becton Dickinson).

Liquid-based cytology improves specimen adequacy and reduces screening time as compared to Convention smears, however, prospective studies have failed to prove superiority of LBC over conventional smears in terms of sensitivity and specificity [6]. The National Cancer Institute developed a uniform system of diagnostic terminologies for PAP tests in Bethesda, Maryland, in 1988. It was revised in 2001 and again in 2014 which is in use till date [26]. The results of cytology guide further evaluation by colposcopy and/or biopsy.

2.3 Visual Inspection with Acetic Acid (VIA)

Visual assessment of cervix after application of 3–5% acetic acid, called a VIA, is the most feasible test in limited resource settings due to low cost, simple technique, and immediate results. The test, however, is not appropriate in post-menopausal women due to recession of transformation zone within the endocervix. The success of VIA led cervical screening programs are dependent on validated training and evaluation procedures [14]. Owing to the variable sensitivity and specificity of VIA, WHO has instructed countries to switch over from VIA test to HPV testing for cervical cancer screening [20]. Figure 1 shows quick clinical reference chart for VIA [27].

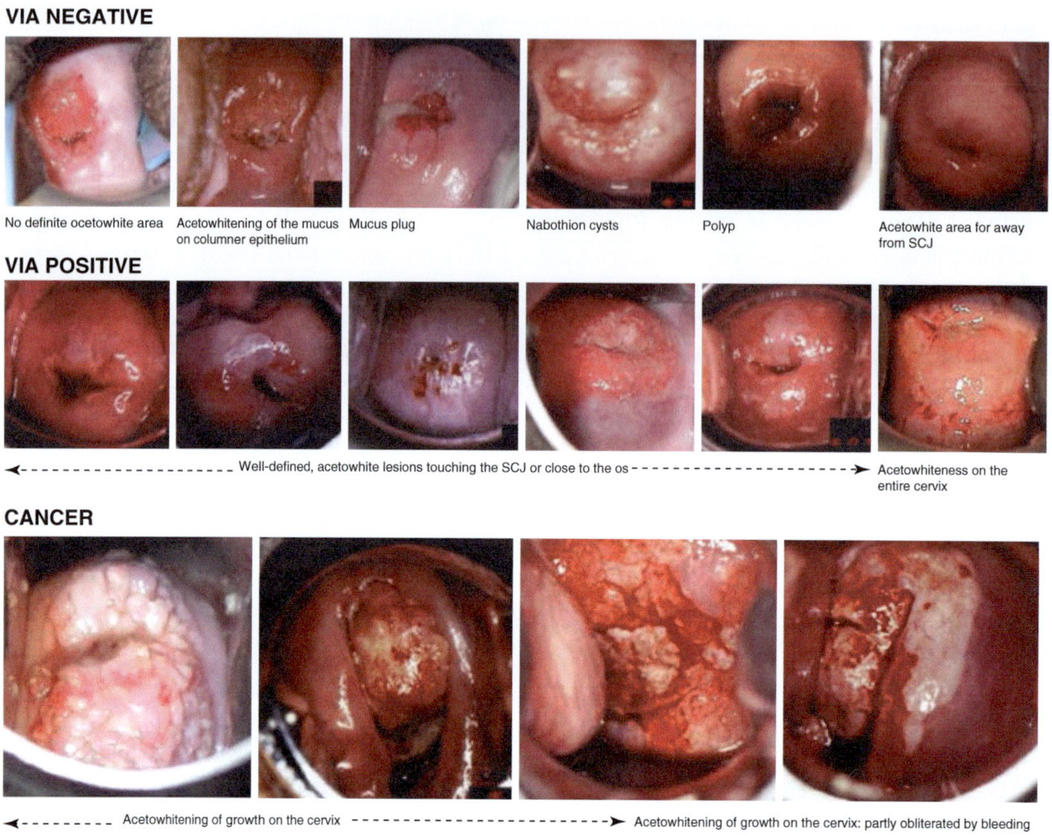

Fig. 1 Quick reference chart for Visual inspection with Acetic acid (VIA). (Reprinted with permission from International Agency for Research on Cancer/World Health Organization, Quick clinical reference chart for visual inspection with acetic acid (VIA), IARC Screening Group, Copyright (2005))

2.4 Colposcopy

Examination of lower genital tract under illumination and magnification using colposcope is used for screening, diagnosing, and managing cervical pre-invasive lesions. Examination of cervix under colposcope consists of four steps, examination after successive application of:

1. Normal saline followed by
2. 3–5% acetic acid and
3. Lugol's Iodine [28].

Figure 2 shows colposcopic pictures of a 35-years-old female.

Modified Reid's Colposcopy index (RCI) includes four parameters—color of aceto-white area, margin and surface configuration of aceto-white lesion, vessels, iodine staining. A score of 0–2 indicate likely Cervical Intraepithelial Neoplasia(CIN)-1; 3–4 indicates overlapping lesions, likely CIN1–2; 5–8 indicate CIN2–3 lesions [29]. Swede score includes size of lesion, along with above mentioned parameters, for predicting the severity of disease [30]. Apart from traditional video colposcope, newer portable devices such as smart colposcope are being increasingly used.

The International Federation of Cervical Pathology and Colposcopy developed nomenclature for clinical and colposcopic terminology of the cervix, vagina in 2011 [31]. IFCPC terminology of the vulva was published in 2012 [32].

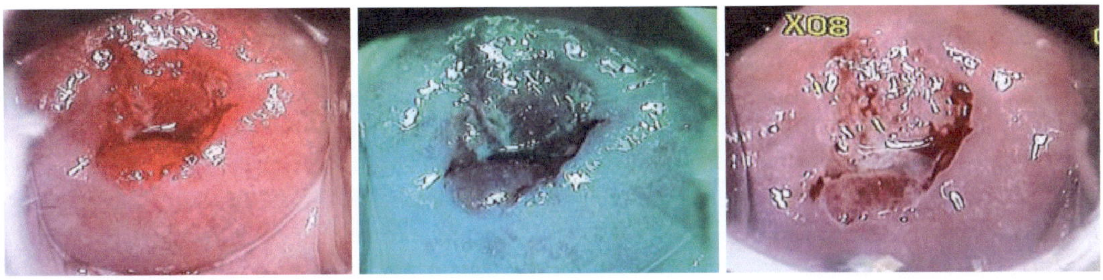

After application of Normal saline | With green filter | After application of acetic acid

Fig. 2 Colposcopic pictures showing Type 1 transformation zone, with no abnormal vessels. Aceto-whitening of Endocervical epithelium with no aceto-white areas on the Squamous epithelium is seen

3 Federation of Obstetrics and Gynaecological Societies of India Good Clinical Practice Recommendations (FOGSI GCPR) 2018

In 2018, the FOGSI GCPR formulated cervical cancer screening guidelines keeping in mind diversity in socio-cultural practices, poor accessibility to health care facilities, lack of trained staff, and infrastructure in India. There recommendations based on availability of healthcare facilities: good resource setting and limited resource setting. The three main screening methods are human papillomavirus (HPV) testing, cytology (Pap smear), and visual inspection by acetic acid (VIA).

In good resource setting- Screening is started at 25 years of age with either primary HPV testing (every 5 years), co-testing (every 5 years), cytology alone (every 3 years), or VIA till 65 years of age.

In limited resource setting- Screening is started at 30 years of age with either VIA (every 5 years, at least 1–3 times in a lifetime) or affordable HPV test till 65 years of age.

4 WHO Guidelines for Cervical Cancer Screening [20]

In order to meet the global target of elimination of cervical cancer by 2030, WHO updated the existing guidelines. There are 23 recommendations and 7 good practice statements with the objective of improving national strategies for screening and treatment to prevent cervical cancer in all women, including women living with HIV.

The two screening and treatment approaches described are:

Screen-and-treat approach—treatment based on finding on primary screening test only.

Screen, triage, and treat approach—treatment depends on positive primary screening test which is supplemented with positive triage test (with/without) histologically confirmed diagnosis.

4.1 IA. Recommendations for All Women (General Population and Women with HIV)

1. **Primary screening test**: HPV DNA detection rather than VIA or cytology in screening and treatment approaches among both the general population of women and women living with HIV. Remarks: Screening with quality-assured cytology as primary screening test can be continued in existing programs till HPV DNA testing becomes operational. Due to inherent challenges with quality assurance WHO strongly discourages the use of VIA as the primary screening test.
2. **Method of collection (HPV DNA test)**: WHO suggests using either samples taken by a healthcare provider or self-collected samples among both the general population of women and women living with HIV.

3. **When to stop screening**: After the age of 50 years, WHO suggests screening is stopped after two consecutive negative screening results consistent with the recommended regular screening intervals among both the general population of women and women living with HIV.
4. **Interval of screening**: Where HPV DNA testing is not yet operational, WHO suggests a regular screening interval of every 3 years when using VIA or cytology as the primary screening test among both the general population of women and women living with HIV.
5. **After triaging test**: WHO suggests that women from both the general population and women living with HIV who have screened positive on a cytology primary screening test and then have normal results on colposcopy are retested with HPV DNA testing at 12 months and, if negative, move to the recommended regular screening interval.
6. **Treatment**: WHO suggests large-loop excision of the transformation zone (LLETZ) or cold knife conization (CKC) for women from the general population or women living with HIV who have histologically confirmed adenocarcinoma in situ (AIS). Remarks: Loop excision may be preferred in women of reproductive age, in settings with greater availability of LLETZ and by providers with greater expertise performing LLETZ. CKC may be preferred when interpretation of the margins of the histological specimen is imperative.

4.2 IB. Recommendations Specific for General Population of Women

1. **Primary screening test**: WHO suggests using an HPV DNA primary screening test either with triage or without triage to prevent cervical cancer among the general population of women.
2. In a **screen-and-treat approach** using HPV DNA detection as the primary screening test among the general population of women, WHO suggests treating women who test positive for HPV DNA.

   In a **screen, triage, and treat approach** using HPV DNA detection as the primary screening test among the general population of women, WHO suggests using partial genotyping, colposcopy, VIA or cytology to triage women after a positive HPV DNA test.
3. **Age of starting screening**: WHO recommends starting regular cervical cancer screening at the age of 30 years among the general population of women.
4. **Interval of screening**: WHO suggests a regular screening interval of every 5–10 years when using HPV DNA detection as the primary screening test among the general population of women.
5. **After triaging test**: WHO suggests that women from general population who have screened positive on an HPV DNA primary screening test and then negative on a triage test are retested with HPV DNA testing at 24 months and, if negative, move to the recommended regular screening interval.

4.3 IC. Recommendations Specific for Women with HIV

1. **Primary screening test**: WHO suggests using an HPV DNA primary screening test with triage rather than without triage to prevent cervical cancer among women living with HIV.
2. In a **screen, triage and treat approach** using HPV DNA detection as the primary screening test among women living with HIV, WHO suggests using partial genotyping, colposcopy, VIA or cytology to triage women after a positive HPV DNA test.
3. **When to start screening**: WHO suggests starting regular cervical cancer screening at the age of 25 years among women living with HIV. Remarks: Low-certainty evidence found that there are likely to be small numbers of women living with HIV with cervical cancer who are below the age of 25. This recommendation applies to women living with HIV

regardless of when they first tested positive for HIV.

4. **Interval of screening**: WHO suggests a regular screening interval of every 3–5 years when using HPV DNA detection as the primary screening test among women living with HIV.
5. **After triaging test**: WHO suggests that women living with HIV who have screened positive on an HPV DNA primary screening test and then negative on a triage test are retested with HPV DNA testing at 12 months and, if negative, move to the recommended regular screening interval.
6. **Follow up**: WHO suggests that women living with HIV who have been treated for histologically confirmed CIN2/3 or adenocarcinoma in situ (AIS), or treated as a result of a positive screening test are retested at 12 months with HPV DNA testing when available, rather than with cytology or VIA or co-testing, and, if negative, are retested again at 12 months and, if negative again, move to the recommended regular screening interval.

4.4 IIA. Good Practice Guideline for All Women

1. While transitioning to a program with a recommended regular screening interval, screening even just twice in a lifetime is beneficial among both the general population of women and women living with HIV.
2. As programs introduce HPV DNA testing, use this test at the woman's next routine screening date regardless of the test that was used at prior screening. In existing programs with cytology or VIA as the primary screening test, rescreening with the same test should be continued until HPV DNA testing is operational among both the general population of women and women living with HIV.
3. Once a decision to treat a woman is made—whether from the general population of women or women living with HIV—it is good practice to treat as soon as possible within 6 months to reduce the risk of loss to follow-up. However, in women who are pregnant, good practice includes deferral until after pregnancy. In circumstances when treatment is not provided within this time frame, it is good practice to re-evaluate the woman before treatment.

4.5 IIB. Good Practice Guidelines for General Population of Women

1. Priority should be given to screening women aged 30–49 years in the general population of women. When tools are available to manage women aged 50–65 years, those in that age bracket who have never been screened should also be prioritized.

4.6 IIIC. Good Practice Guidelines for Women with HIV

1. Priority should be given to screening women living with HIV aged 25–49 years. When tools are available to manage women living with HIV aged 50–65 years, those in that age bracket who have never been screened should also be prioritized.

Annexure 1 [20]

Strength of Recommendations

Strong recommendations (worded as "WHO recommends") when all the desirable consequences of the intervention clearly outweighed the undesirable consequences in most settings.

Conditional recommendations (worded as "WHO suggests") were made when the desirable consequences of the intervention probably outweighed the undesirable consequences in most settings.

References

1. Sung H, Ferlay J, Siegel RL, Laversanne M, Soerjomataram I, Jemal A, Bray F. Global cancer statistics 2020: GLOBOCAN estimates of incidence and mortality worldwide for 36 cancers in 185 countries. CA Cancer J Clin. 2021;71(3):209–49.
2. Fidler MM, Soerjomataram I, Bray F. A global view on cancer incidence and national levels of the human development index. Int J Cancer. 2016;139(11):2436–46.
3. Bray F, Ferlay J, Soerjomataram I, Siegel RL, Torre LA, Jemal A. Global cancer statistics 2018: GLOBOCAN estimates of incidence and mortality worldwide for 36 cancers in 185 countries. CA Cancer J Clin. 2018;68(6):394–424.
4. Berek JS, Hacker NF, MD. Berek and Hacker's gynecologic oncology. 7th ed. Philadelphia: Wolter Kluwer Health; 2021. p. 634–5.
5. https://www.who.int/initiatives/cervical-cancer-elimination-initiative.
6. International Agency for Research on Cancer (IARC). IARC Handbooks of Cancer Prevention: Volume 10-Cervix Cancer Screening. Lyon: IARC Press; 2005. http://www.iarc.fr/en/publications/pdfs-online/prev/handbook10/HANDBOOK10.pdf. Accessed 18 Mar 2022.
7. Sankaranarayanan R, Shastri SS, Basu P, Mahé C, Mandal R, Amin G, Roy C, Muwonge R, Goswami S, Das P, Chinoy R. The role of low-level magnification in visual inspection with acetic acid for the early detection of cervical neoplasia. Cancer Detect Prev. 2004;28(5):345–51.
8. Basu P, Sankaranarayanan R. Atlas of colposcopy—principles and practice: IARC Cancer Base no. 13 [internet]. Lyon: International Agency for Research on Cancer; 2017. https://screening.iarc.fr/atlascolpo.php. Accessed 18 Mar 2022.
9. https://unitaid.org/assets/Cervical_Cancer_Technology-landscape-2019.pdf.
10. Rahatgaonkar V, Uchale P, Oka G. Comparative study of smart scope® visual screening test with naked eye visual screening and pap test. Asian Pac J Cancer Prev. 2020;21(12):3509.
11. Pandey K, Pradhan A, Agarwal A, Bhagoliwal A, Agarwal N. Fluorescence spectroscopy: a new approach in cervical cancer. J Obstetr Gynecol India. 2012;62(4):432–6.
12. Canfell K, Chow C. Real-time devices for the screening and diagnosis of cervical neoplasia. Cervix. 2006;3:387–98.
13. Tidy JA, Brown BH. Clinical utility of ZedScan when used as an adjunct to colposcopy. Indian J Gynecol Oncol. 2021;19(3):1–6.
14. https://www.fogsi.org/fogsi-gcpr-on-screening-hpv-vaccination/.
15. Piyathilake CJ, Badiga S, Chambers MM, Brill IK, Matthews R, Partridge EE. Accuracy of urinary human papillomavirus testing for the presence of cervical human papillomaviruses and higher grades of cervical intraepithelial neoplasia. Cancer. 2016;122(18):2836–44.
16. Budukh A, Palayekar V, Maheshwari A, Deodhar K, Purwar P, Bagal S, Vadigoppula A, Lokhande M, Panse N, Dikshit R, Badwe R. Menstrual pad, a cervical cancer screening tool, a population-based study in rural India. Eur J Cancer Prev. 2018;27(6):546–52.
17. Gu Y, Wan C, Qiu J, Cui Y, Jiang T, Zhuang Z. Circulating HPV cDNA in the blood as a reliable biomarker for cervical cancer: a meta-analysis. PLoS One. 2020;15(2):e0224001.
18. https://screening.iarc.fr/cervical_cancer.php.
19. Walboomers JMM, Jacobs MV, Manos MM, Bosch FX, Kummer JA, Shah KV, Snijders PJF, Peto J, Meijer CJLM, Munoz N. Human papillomavirus is a necessary cause of invasive cervical cancer worldwide. J Pathol. 1999;189:12–9.
20. WHO guideline for screening and treatment of cervical pre-cancer lesions for cervical cancer prevention, second edition. Geneva: World Health Organization; 2021. Reprinted with permission from World Health Organization, second edition, WHO guideline for screening and treatment of cervical pre-cancer lesions for cervical cancer prevention, Copyright (2021).
21. Berek JS, Hacker NF, MD. Berek and Hacker's gynecologic oncology. 7th ed. Philadelphia: Wolter Kluwer Health; 2021. p. 618.
22. https://www.who.int/news-room/fact-sheets/detail/cervical-cancer.
23. US Food and Drug Administration (FDA). FDA executive summary: new approaches in the evaluation for high-risk human papillomavirus nucleic acid detection devices. Prepared for the march 8, 2019 meeting of the microbiology devices panel of the medical devices advisory committee. FDA; 2019.
24. https://www.who.int/reproductivehealth/self-care-interventions/human-papillomavirus-testing/en/.
25. Shaw PA. The history of cervical screening I: the Pap test. J SOGC. 2000;22(2):110–4.
26. Nayar R, Wilbur DC. The pap test and Bethesda 2014. Cancer Cytopathol. 2015 May;123(5):271–81.
27. Sankaranarayanan R, Wesley RS. A practical manual on visual screening for cervical neoplasia. IARC technical report n°41. Lyon: IARC; 2005. https://publications.iarc.fr/Book-And-Report-Series/Iarc-Technical-Publications/A-Practical-Manual-On-Visual-Screening-For-Cervical-Neoplasia-2003 and https://screening.iarc.fr/quick_clinical_reference.php.
28. Prendiville W, Sankaranarayanan R. Colposcopy and treatment of cervical precancer. International Agency for Research on Cancer, World Health Organization; 2017.
29. Reid R, Scalzi P. Genital warts and cervical cancer. VII. An improved colposcopic index for differentiating benign papillomaviral infections from high-grade cervical intraepithelial neoplasia. Am J Obstet Gynecol. 1985;153:611–8.

30. Bowring J, Strander B, Young M, Evans H, Walker P. The swede score: evaluation of a scoring system designed to improve the predictive value of colposcopy. J Low Genit Tract Dis. 2010;14(4):301–5.
31. Bornstein J, Bentley J, Bösze P, Girardi F, Haefner H, Menton M, Perrotta M, Prendiville W, Russell P, Sideri M, Strander B. 2011 Colposcopic terminology of the International Federation for Cervical Pathology and Colposcopy. Obstet Gynecol. 2012;120(1):166–72.
32. Bornstein J, Sideri M, Tatti S, Walker P, Prendiville W, Haefner HK. 2011 terminology of the vulva of the International Federation for Cervical Pathology and Colposcopy. J Low Genit Tract Dis. 2012;16(3):290–5.

Management of Precancerous Lesions of Cervix

Ranajit Mandal, Helen Kamei, Puja Chatterjee, and Debabrata Barmon

1 Introduction

Cancer cervix accounted for 604,000 new cases and 342,000 deaths worldwide in 2020. It is the fourth leading cause of cancer deaths in women [1]. Since the last few decades, incidence of cervical cancer has declined, but the statistics in low- and middle-income countries reflect high disease burden. Cervical cancer in India is still a major health problem. Amongst the gynaecological malignancy in Indian women, it is the second most frequent cancer [2].

Human papilloma virus (HPV) infection a necessary event in the evolution of cervical cancer has helped in understanding the natural history of cervical cancer better. In May 2018, the WHO Director-General announced a global call for action to eliminate cervical cancer [3]. Each country should meet the 90-70-90 targets by 2030 to get on the path to eliminate cervical cancer within the next century. Achieving that goal rests on the following key points:

- **Vaccination:** 90% of girls fully vaccinated with the HPV vaccine by the age of 15.
- **Screening:** 70% of women screened using a high-performance test by the age of 35, and again by the age of 45.
- **Treatment:** 90% of women with pre-cancer treated and 90% of women with invasive cancer managed.

2 Anatomy

Cervix is a fibromuscular structure lined by single layered columnar epithelium in the endocervical canal and multi-layered squamous epithelium in the ectocervix (basal layer, parabasal layer, intermediate and superficial layer). Squamo-columnar junction, SCJ refers to a point where these lining epithelia meet. This junction in foetal life termed as original SCJ defines the extent of metaplastic process in the cervix. With the start of puberty, oestrogen production causes increase in volume of the cervix with eversion of the endocervical lining to the ectocervix. It also causes the vaginal epithelium to fill up with glycogen. The lactobacilli act on the glycogen reducing the vaginal pH [4–6], which in turn stimulates the subcolumnar reserve cells to undergo metaplasia. The columnar epithelium is

R. Mandal (✉) · P. Chatterjee
Department of Gynaecological Oncology, Chittaranjan National Cancer Institute, Kolkata, West Bengal, India

H. Kamei
Department of O&G, JNIMS, Imphal, Manipur, India

D. Barmon
Department of Gynaecologic Oncology, Dr. Bhubaneswar Borooah Cancer Institute (A Unit of Tata Memorial Centre, Mumbai), Guwahati, Assam, India
e-mail: dydiracademic@bbci.tmc.gov.in

A. C. Kataki, D. Barmon (eds.), *Fundamentals in Gynaecologic Malignancy*,
https://doi.org/10.1007/978-981-19-5860-1_12

replaced by immature, undifferentiated, stratified squamous metaplastic epithelium [2]. This metaplastic epithelium undergoes maturation producing a mature squamous epithelium thus forming a new site for SCJ; hence, called the new SCJ. Transformation zone, TZ refers to the area between the original and new SCJ [7, 8]. Once the TZ matures, the original SCJ limit is identified by identifying gland openings and nabothian follicles. TZ marks the site for origin of cervical neoplasia. On colposcopy three types of transformation zone may be identified: **Type 1 TZ** where TZ is completely ectocervical and is fully visible; **Type 2 TZ** where the TZ is endocervical but may is fully visible (Cogan's endocervical speculum or artery forceps may be used for visualization of TZ), and **Type 3 TZ** where the TZ is not visible completely.

3 Etiopathogenesis

HPV is double stranded DNA virus. There are over 100 documented genotypes; of these, 13 types (16, 18, 31, 33, 35, 39, 45, 51, 52, 56, 58, 59, 63) are categorized as high risk as they are known to cause cancer cervix with Type 16 and 18 accounting for majority of the cases [9–11]. Type 6 and 11 are examples of low risk types associated with condyloma accuminata, subclinical HPV infection, and low grade CIN lesions. Based on the nucleotide sequence of the open reading frames or ORF coding for the capsid protein L1, HPV viruses are divided into different genera of which alpha-papilloma virus group is particularly important in pathogenesis of cervical precancers and cancers. Alpha-HPVs infect mucosal tissue whereas beta-, gamma-, nu-, and mu-subtypes infect cutaneous sites. HPV 16 and 18 belongs to the Alpha-papillomavirus 9 and 7, respectively [12].

The genome is divided into three major functional regions:

(a) the E region codes- E 1,2,4,5,6,7,
(b) the L region codes- L1,2,
(c) the non coding region.

Majority of HPV infection clears off within 2 years in sexually active women [13]. However, if the infection is persistent, especially more with specific type HPV, the chance of spontaneous clearance is lowered and the risk for precancerous lesion of the cervix is increased [14, 15]. HPV infection targets the immature basal cells of the metaplastic epithelium through cracks or micro-abrasions within it [16]. In infected cells, stable viral genome is maintained. However, with persistent carcinogenic type, E1 and E2 genes help integration into host genome and E6 and E7 genes cause cellular transformation, immortalizing it [17, 18]. E6 and E7 bind with the tumour suppressor genes p53 and retinoblastoma gene, pRb, respectively, thus influencing the apoptosis of host cells [19, 20]. The average time from HPV infection to the development of precancerous lesion is short, 5 years, while the development of invasive cancer from precancerous lesion is variable [21, 22]. Factors such as smoking, contraceptive use, nutrition, multiparity, age at first pregnancy, and infection with other sexually transmitted disease influence persistence of infection and progression to precursor lesions and malignancy [23–25].

4 Terminology

Precancerous and cancerous lesion of cervix is screened by cytological assessment of the cervix and HPV testing. Other screening modalities include Co testing, Visual Inspection under Acetic Acid or VIA, Colposcopy, and other newer modalities.

Cytological assessment is reported using the Bethesda system (SIL), which was last revised in 2015 [26]. Histological assessment of precancerous lesion of ectocervix is reported as CIN, cervical intraepithelial neoplasia. The glandular or endocervical lesion is reported as glandular cervical neoplasia. Depending on the degree of atypical cellular changes, CIN is graded as CIN1, 2 or 3. CIN 1 has mild cellular changes in the lower third of epithelium. It is considered low grade lesion and Koilocytes are often seen. Koilocytes are cytopathic changes noted due to HPV infection. In CIN 2, moderately atypical cellular changes involve basal 2/third of the epithelium, while CIN 3 show severe atypical cellular changes involving greater than 2/third to full thickness of the epithelium. For CIN 2 to be graded as precancerous, p16 immunostaining can be done. CIN 1 is referred to as LSIL and CIN 3 as HSIL.

The lower anogenital squamous terminology (LAST Project) 2012 publication re-evaluated the terminology of HPV associated lesions of the lower genital tract. For non-invasive HPV associated lesion, a two-tiered nomenclature was recommended with appropriate –IN, intraepithelial neoplasia terminology. HPV associated lesions should be classified as low grade squamous intraepithelial lesion (LSIL) and high grade squamous intraepithelial lesion (HSIL); with use of p16 marker as arbitration [27].

5 Colposcopy

International Federation of Cervical Pathology and Colposcopy Nomenclature is preferably used for documentation of colposcopy findings [28]. In IFCPC nomenclature, the findings are described in the following broad headings:

1. **General Assessment**: Adequacy of assessment, Type of TZ, Visibility of Squamo-columnar junction.
2. **Normal Colposcopy Findings** like cervical Ectopy, Nabothian Follicles, Deciduosis of Pregnancy.
3. **Abnormal Colposcopy Findings**: Description of Acetowhite Epithelium including Size and Location. Grade 1 or minor lesions include thin acetowhite lesions with irregular margins and fine punctations. Grade 2 or major lesions include dense acetowhite lesion with sharp or raised border, cuffed crypt openings, and coarse punctations. Exophytic growth or ulcers are suggestive of invasive cancer. Ridge sign and Inner border sign indicate high grade lesions. *Ridge sign* is a thick opaque acetowhite epithelium with irregular raised margin and *Inner border sign* refers to a sharp acetowhite demarcation within a less opaque acetowhite area.
4. **Non-specific and miscellaneous findings** like Leucoplakia, cervical polyp, Congenital Transformation Zone.

Swede score may be used for description also along with a schematic diagram indicating the site of lesion. A score of 1–4 is regarded as low grade or normal; score 5–6 as high grade, not suspicious of cancer or CIN 2; and score 7–10 as high grade lesion suspicious of cancer or CIN 3. It is scored with respect to Acetowhite uptake, Margin, Vessels, Lesion Size, and Lugol's Iodine staining [29].

6 Management

Monitoring and timely treatment of patients with CIN helps prevention of progression of patients with CIN to cervical cancer. However, it is an established fact that some cases with HPV infection and/or precursor lesion of cancer cervix tends to regress in most cases. Persistent infections with HPV define the risk of progression from precancerous to cancerous lesion. Certain risk factors (HPV related and non-related) contribute to the causation of cancer cervix [30–32]. Treatment options include ablative or excisional procedures. The treatment modalities, available for the treatment of precancerous lesions, even though effective carry the chances of adverse effects. Therefore, it is essential to consider the risk of progression and morbidity related to treatment modality while considering treatment for CIN.

Age and grade of CIN are important predictors of progression to cervical cancer, aside from HPV subtype and cytology preceding the diagnosis of CIN [33–36]. Despite high rate of HPV infection in younger population, infection tends to regress spontaneously as do most of the associated CIN lesions [39]. Most CIN 1 lesion tends to regress, unlike CIN2 and CIN 3 lesions [37, 38]. With CIN3 the chances of progression to invasive lesion are higher and spontaneous regression tends to be lower compared to CIN 2. HPV 16 and 18 are highly oncogenic compared to other oncogenic subtypes and more commonly associated with CIN 3 [40].

6.1 CIN1, Women ≥25 Years

For CIN 1 lesion preceded by LSIL, ASCUS, NILM but positive for HPV, observation is recommended with HPV-based testing after 1 year. For CIN 1 lesion with negative HPV, routine screening for subsequent follow-up is done, as the chances for development of malignancy are low. Observation entails HPV testing and colposcopy at 1 year. For CIN 1 lesion with preceding ASC-H or HSIL cytology, intervention is required, as there is chance of development of high grade lesions, ≥CIN3 lesions [41, 42]. Intervention is absolute following HSIL but with ASC H lesion, observation is still an option. Observation entails colposcopy and HPV testing provided the entire SCJ is visible and endocervical curettage, ECC is negative for precursor lesions or malignancy. In resource rich settings, repeat negative HPV testing allows for long-term surveillance. Abnormal observation requires repeat colposcopy and management depends on biopsy. Intervention following HSIL will take into account patient's reproductive status and preferences along with compliance for follow-up. Excisional intervention might have repercussions on patient's future pregnancy [43]. CIN 1 preceded by atypical glandular cells (AGC) have increased risk for development of high grade lesions; hence should be evaluated by colposcopy and ECC. For women with AGC-endometrial, endometrial sampling and ECC should be done [41, 44]. AGC maybe NOS (not other specified) or favours neoplastic, adenocarcinoma in situ or adenocarcinoma. Invasive disease is more likely in later groups compared to NOS [44].With persistent CIN1, the risk of progression to high grade lesion is low, so observation with subsequent follow-up can be done. Intervention with ablative or excisional procedure is an option for women who do not require conservative approach.

6.2 CIN2 and CIN3, Women ≥25 Years

Both CIN 2 and 3 have high risk of progression to invasive lesion. Hence, prompt treatment is recommended. CIN3 requires definitive treatment and observation in such case though not common, if done, it entails cytology and colposcopy at 6 and 12 months [41]. Observation in CIN 2 can be considered for women with reproductive issues, if squamo-columnar junction and lesion are easily visualized and endocervical curettage show low grade lesion.

6.3 CIN in Special Populations

1. <25 years patients
2. Pregnant patients.
3. Immunocompromised patients.
4. Heterosexual partners and Sexual Minority Women(SMW).

6.3.1 CIN in <25 Years Women

CIN1 preceded by LSIL, ASCUS or NILM, should have repeat cytology in 1 year. Repeat cytology showing NILM can go for routine screening. Colposcopy should be considered for lesions showing ≥ ASCUS. If the preceding lesion is ASC H or HSIL, observation can be considered for cases with adequate colposcopy and ECC less than CIN 2. Persistent high grade cytology during observation calls for diagnostic excisional procedures. With preceding AGC, since the risk of underlying invasive disease is high, subsequent evaluation should be done. CIN 2 and 3 in young patients are more likely to regress [45]. Observation is usually not an option with CIN 3; if it is done cytology and colposcopy are performed at 6 and 12 months [41]. Treatment consists of excisional procedures with ablation as an alternative.

6.3.2 Pregnant Patients

With CIN1, patients should be reassessed postpartum and subsequent management depends on the outcome of the re-evaluation. With CIN 2 or 3, if invasive disease is not suspected then observation with colposcopy or cytology or HPV (age appropriate) every 12 to 24 weeks during pregnancy, with indication of repeat biopsy if there is worsening of lesion appearance or invasive cytology report [41]. Diagnostic excisional procedure is recommended only when invasive disease is suspected [46].

6.3.3 Adolescents

Management will follow the recommendations for women less than 25 years of age, in whom risk of infection is as high as the spontaneous clearance rate [47]. Screening in adolescents is not routine; the follow-up is for those cases where screening was done inadvertently.

6.3.4 Immunocompromised

HIV patients show higher incidence of cervical cancer precursor lesions than non-HIV patients [48]. If the viral load is low and CD4 count level is stable, low grade lesions show regression. For high grade lesion and persistent CIN 1, ablation or excisional treatment is acceptable. Effective antiretroviral therapy plays a very important role in the natural history of precursor lesions in HIV patients [49, 50]. While data is lacking regarding long-term follow-up results, it is a known fact that recurrences and progression to invasive lesion is more compared to general population [51]. Adjuvant use of topical Fluorouracil (FU) to ablative or excisional procedures is limited even though it does reduce recurrence [52].

6.3.5 Sexual Partners and Sexual Minority Women (SMW)

Data on screening strategies for SMW are scant, but screening and awareness should be offered as HPV infection is known to occur [53]. High risk HPV infection and penile intraepithelial neoplasia are known to occur in male partners of women with CIN. Condom use is recommended, as it promotes regression of lesions associated with HPV infection in both partners [54, 55].

6.3.6 HPV Vaccination

For pre-existing HPV infection or precancerous cervical lesion, vaccination does not have therapeutic role. There are data available for the role of vaccination in reducing recurrences. This concept also applies to health care workers, who bears the risk of developing HPV infection and HPV associated nasal and oropharyngeal disease [56, 57].

7 Treatment

Ablative or excisional therapy can be used effectively for the treatment of CIN. Cone knife conization (CKC), Loop electrosurgical excision procedure, LEEP/large loop excision of the transformation zone, LLETZ, and laser conization are the various options under excisional treatments, while ablative therapies include cryotherapy, CO_2 laser ablation, and thermal ablation (e.g., diathermy, cold coagulation). Excisional therapies have both therapeutic and diagnostic advantages, while ablative therapies have therapeutic effect only. The World Health Organization recommends use of LEEP, if easily accessed [54]. Hysterectomy is not a primary option in the treatment of CIN. Medical therapies have limited data as alternative in the treatment of cervical intraepithelial neoplasia.

Important factors that need considerations while choosing ablation or excision for the treatment of precursor lesions are the size of the lesions, extension into the endocervical canal and risk of invasive disease. Presence of glandular disease, ECC $\geq$ CIN2 or previous history of excision favours excisional therapy over ablation [41, 58]. For patients, planning pregnancy, ablation seems to be preferable to excision considering adverse outcomes in relation to excision. However, excision has been related to less chance of persistent disease and recurrence and some studies report no or little difference in adverse outcomes [59]. Cost and availability of infrastructure are important considerations as well.

7.1 Ablative Therapy

Pre-requisites for performing ablation include the following [58]:

1. Lesion should be entirely on ectocervix.
2. Lesion should not have endocervical and/or vaginal extension.
3. Lesion should occupy less than half of the cervical quadrants.
4. The largest cryoprobe tip should adequately cover the lesion.
5. No suspicion of malignancy or obvious cervical growth or irregular surface.
6. No post coital bleeding /postmenopausal bleeding.

7.1.1 Cryosurgery

It can be done as office procedures and is usually ideal for small low grade lesions and located entirely on the ectocervix. A cryoprobe gun with a metal cryoprobe tip ranges from 19 to 25 mm diameter and maybe shaped as cone or flat is used to carry out this procedure (Figs. 1, 2, and 3). The refrigerant gas (N2O or CO_2) at −20 degree Celsius is used to induce crystallization of intracellular water resulting in cell death. An ice ball in the cervical tissue is formed due to hypothermia induced through the probe by refrigerant gas, covering the entire TZ. This will ensure complete coverage of the lesion and a 5 mm depth. Under colposcopic guidance, the cervix is visualized and the area of lesion is mapped out and the cryoprobe tip is placed over the target after applying water soluble gel to the tip. *A Freeze Thaw Freeze* method (3 min freeze, 5 min slow thaw, and repeat 3 min freeze followed by 5 min slow thaw) is done after activating the cryotherapy unit [58].

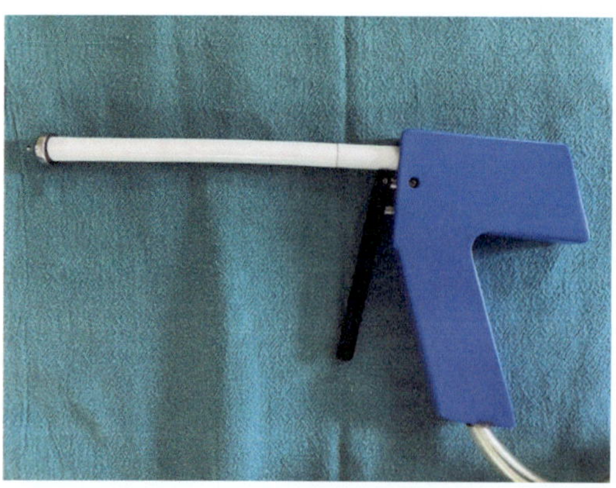

Fig. 1 A Cryogun with the cryoprobe attached to it

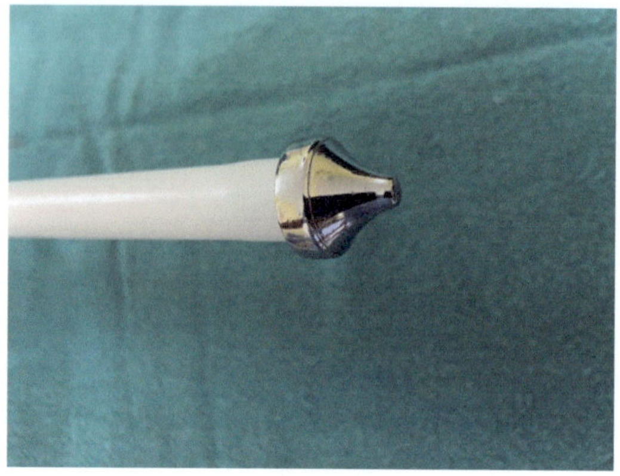

Fig. 2 A Cone shaped cryoprobe

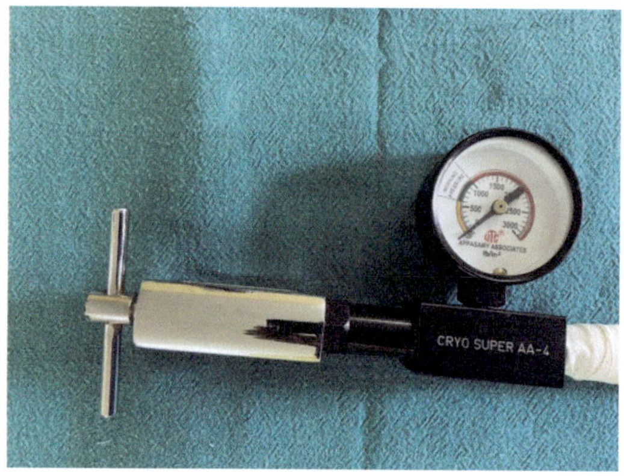

Fig. 3 Pressure gauge device

The probe should be allowed to fall off by itself and cervix defrosted till pink in colour.

7.1.2 Laser Ablation

It requires specialized training and is done using CO_2 with a high power laser setting. The cervical tissue absorbs laser beam, the water in the cells boil and subsequently explodes into vapour. The power density is kept within the range of 750–2000 W/cm^2 [60]. Under colposcopy, the cervix is visualized and area of lesion is mapped out. The micromanipulator attached to the colposcope carries out selective ablation of the lesion and controls tissue vaporization by delivering short bursts of laser energy. The control of depth and width of the tissue ablated during the procedure and rapid healing are advantages of laser ablation.

7.1.3 Thermocoagulation or Cold Coagulation

A portable device with a reusable metallic probe is used for thermocoagulation (Figs. 4 and 5). The cervical epithelial and stromal tissue destruction is achieved by electrically heating to approximately 100 °C. The metallic probe is applied over the area of interest and heated for 20–40 s. Multiple overlapping applications depending on the size of lesions can be done [61] and is a definite advantage over cryosurgery. See and treat approach is easier with the use of thermocoagulation.

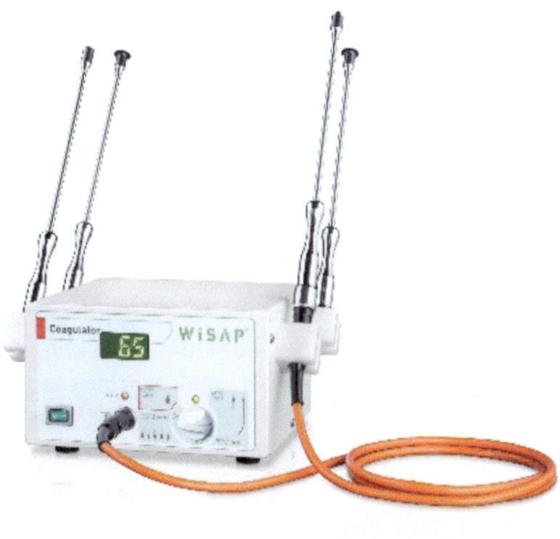

Fig. 4 Wisap Cold Coagulator (Mobile version)

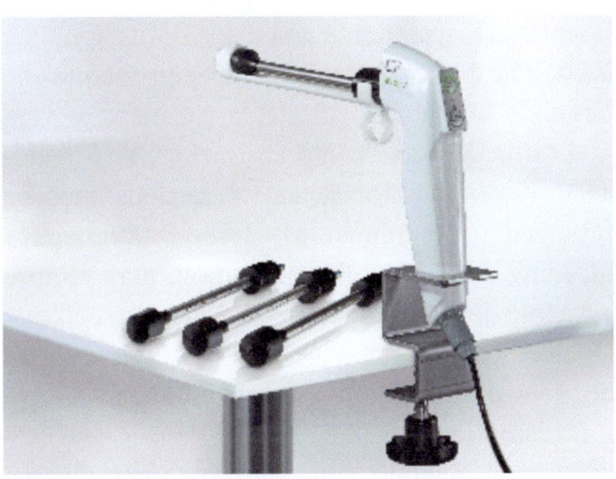

Fig. 5 Wisap Cold Coagulator (Desktop version)

7.1.4 Diathermy

Diathermy is done with cautery. The cautery is attached to the electrosurgical unit set to 30–35 Watts [62], and after visualizing, the cervical tissue is ablated. Multiple applications can be done depending on requirement.

Post-ablation, patient should be advised to abstain from sexual activity and not to use tampons for at least 4 weeks. For 2–3 weeks, watery, blood stained discharge is expected. About 1–2% complications follow ablation of cervical lesions [63]. Discharge is common post ablation. Bleeding can be treated with haemostatic agents or in rare cases, by suturing or packing even. Pelvic infection is not a frequent complication. Cervical stenosis is rare complication associated with ablation [64, 65].

7.2 Excisional Therapy

Excisional procedures have the advantage of being both diagnostic and therapeutic. It may be carried out under regional or general anaesthesia. The excision treatment may be categorized into three types depending upon the type of transformation zone, i.e. Excision type 1, 2, and 3 corresponding to TZ 1, TZ2, and TZ3, respectively. The length and thickness should be mentioned. The length corresponds to the distance from the distal margin to internal margin. The thickness of the specimen is the distance from the stromal margin to the surface of the excised specimen. If possible, the circumference of the specimen should be mentioned which refers to the perimeter of the excised specimen [28].

7.2.1 Loop Electrosurgical Excision Procedure/LEEP

LEEP, also called large loop excision of transformation zone(LLETZ), involves electrosurgical excision with minimal thermal injury with a thin loop of wire (Fig. 6) attached to electrosurgical unit(ESU) set at 35–55 watts. Cervix is visualized and TZ are identified. Appropriate

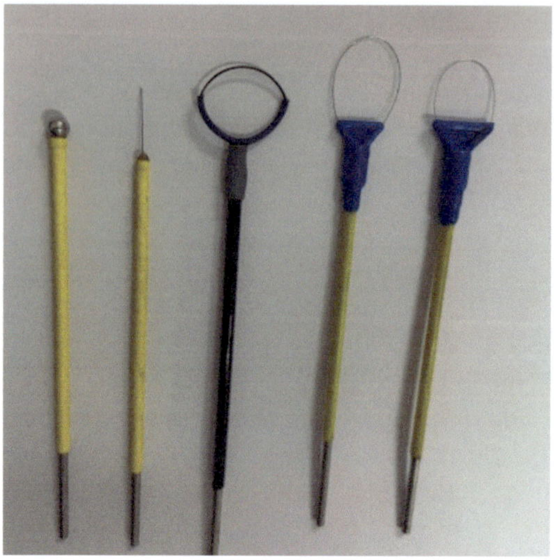

Fig. 6 Different sizes of Loops and ball electrode

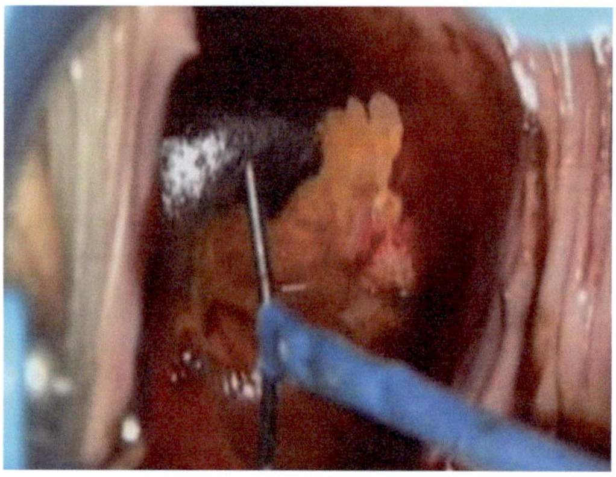

Fig. 7 Excision procedure using loop

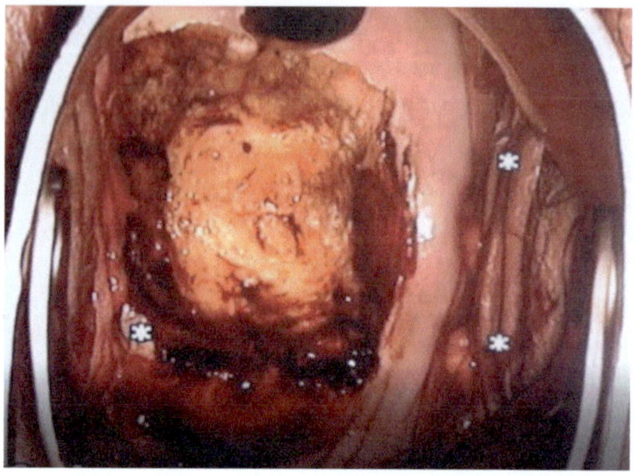

Fig. 8 Post procedure image of the cervix

loop size is selected (Fig. 4). After administering the local anaesthetics and setting the ESU with pure cutting or blended current set at 35–55 W, the specimen is excised by advancing the loop from 2 to 3 mm lateral to the TZ (Fig. 7) and cervical depth of 5 to 7 mm, to the opposite side (Fig. 7). If the lesion is large, procedure can be repeated. Haemostasis obtained by ball cautery (Fig. 8) or haemostatic agents like Monsel's paste, etc.

7.2.2 Cold Knife Conization

It involves excision of a cervix with scalpel in the shape of a cone. Under general or regional anaesthesia, colposcopy is conducted. Lateral sutures are applied at 3'O and 6'O clock position. Vasopressors may be used to supplement the control of bleeding. After sounding the endocervical canal, the specimen is excised using 11 scalpel blade in sawing motion until a whole circle is completed. The 12'O clock position of cervix is tagged. Endocervical and endometrial curettage for indicated cases may be done, perimenopausal patients, menopausal with glandular lesions and patients who have risks of endometrial pathology. Haemostasis is achieved by coagulation or suturing.

7.2.3 Laser Conization

It requires more expertise and a specialized set up. Under colposcopy, a series of dots delineating the outer limit of TZ is mapped out with CO2 laser. Black speculums and tenaculum should be used. The base diameter of the cone should be large.

Postprocedure, sexual abstinence, and avoidance of tampons for at least 4 weeks should be followed. Complications like intraoperative bleeding, even though uncommon, may require systemic devascularization or even hysterectomy. Delayed bleeding may occur 1–2 weeks and can be treated conservatively. Infection may occur. Late complications like cervical stenosis and cervical insufficiency carry adverse reproductive outcome. Cervical stenosis may affect menstrual flow and require dilatation. Treatment of CIN has been associated with second trimester pregnancy loss and preterm births are noted [66–68].

7.2.4 Hysterectomy

Hysterectomy in CIN is considered in case of coexisting gynaecologic indications like fibroids, prolapse, etc. The ASCCP considers hysterectomy for cases with recurrent or residual diseases or where repeat diagnostic excisional procedure is indicated but not feasible [41]. After hysterectomy, follow-up should continue.

7.3 Medical Therapy

Imiquimod and 5 FU are used as alternative or complement to excisional or ablative therapies in some studies. Some studies also explore the role of interferons, retinoids, antivirals, and hormonal therapy in the treatment of CIN [69, 70].

References

1. Sung H, Ferlay J, et al. Global Cancer Statistics 2020: GLOBOCAN estimates of incidence and mortality worldwide for 36 cancers in 185 countries. CA Cancer J Clin. 2021;71:209–49.
2. ICO/IARC Information Centre on HPV and Cancer. India human papillomavirus and related cancers, Fact Sheet 2018 (2019-06-17).
3. Who.int. Cervical cancer elimination initiative. [online]. 2021. https://www.who.int/initiatives/cervical-cancer-elimination-initiative>. Accessed 22 Dec 2021.
4. Hatch KD. Handbook of colposcopy. Diagnosis and treatment of lower genital tract neoplasia and infections. Boston: Little Brown; 1987. p. 7–19.
5. Coppleson M, Pixley E, Reid BL. Colposcopy: a scientific approach to the cervix uteri in health and disease. Springfield, IL: Charles C Thomas; 1986.
6. Kolstad P, Stafl A. Atlas of colposcopy. Oslo: Universitetsforlaget; 1982.
7. Coppleson M, Reid BL. Aetiology of the squamous cell carcinoma of the cervix. Obstet Gynecol. 1968;32:432–6.
8. Coppleson M, Reid B. Interpretation of changes in the uterine cervix. Lancet. 1969;2(7613):216–7.
9. Zur Hausen H. Immortalization of human cells and their malignant conversion by high risk human papillomavirus genotypes. Semin Cancer Biol. 1999;9(6):405–11.
10. Zur Hausen H. Papillomaviruses and cancer: from basic studies to clinical application. Nat Rev Cancer. 2002;2:342–50.
11. Doorbar J. Molecular biology of human papillomaviruses and cervical cancer. Clin Sci. 2006;110(5):525–41.
12. de Villiers E-M, Fauquet C, Broker TR, Bernard H-U, Hausen HZ. Classification of papillomaviruses. Virology. 2004;324(1):17–27. https://doi.org/10.1016/j.virol.2004.03.033.
13. Burchell AN, Weiner RL, de Sanjose S, et al. Chapter 6: Epedimiology and transmission dynamics of genital HPV infection. Vaccine. 2006;24(suppl 3):52–61.
14. Plummer M, Schiffman M, Castle PE, et al. A 2-year prospective study of human papillomavirus persistence among women with a cytological diagnosis of atypical squamous cells of undetermined significance or low grade squamous intraepithelial lesion. J Infect Dis. 2007;195(11):1582–9.
15. Schiffman M, Herrero R, Desalle R, et al. The carcinogenicity of human papillomavirus types reflects viral evolution. Virology. 2005;337(1):76–84.
16. Mayers ER, McCrory DC, Nanda K, Bastian L, Matchar DB. Mathematical model for the natural history of human papilloma virus infection and cervical carcinogenesis. Am J Epidemiol. 2000;1:1158–71.
17. Munger K, Phelpps WC, Bubb V, et al. The E6 and E7 genes of the human papillomavirus type 16 together are necessary and sufficient for transformation of primary human keratinocytes. J Virol. 1989;63(10):4417–21.
18. McCance DJ, Kopan R, Fuchs E, et al. Human Papillovirus type 16 alters human epithelial differentiation in vitro. Proc Natl Acad Sci U S A. 1988;85(19):7169–73.
19. Paquette RL, Lee YY, Wilczynski SP, et al. Mutations of p53 and human papillomavirus infection in cervical carcinoma. Cancer. 1993;72(4):1272–80.
20. Berezutskaya E, Yu B, Morozov A, et al. Differential regulation of the pocket domains of the retinoblastoma family proteins by the HPV 16 E7 oncoprotein. Cell Growth Differ. 1997;8(12):1277–86.
21. Bosch FX, de Sanjose S. Chapter 1: Human papillomavirus and cervical-burden and assessment of causality. J Natl Cancer Inst Monogr. 2003;31:3–13.
22. McCredie MR, Sharples KJ, Paul C, et al. Natural history of cervical neoplasia and risk of invasive cancer in women with cervical intraepithelial neoplasia 3: a retrospective cohort study. Lancet Oncol. 2008;9:425–34.
23. Koutsky LA, Holmes KK, Critchlow CW, Stevens CE, Paavonen J, Becicman AM. A cohort of study of the risk of cervical intraepithelial neoplasia grade 2 or 3 in relation to papillomavirus infection. N Engl J Med. 1992;327:1272–8.
24. Bauer HM, Ting Y, Greer CE, Chambers JC, Tashiro CJ, Chimera J, et al. Genital human papillomavirus infection in female university students as determined by a PCR-based method. JAMA. 1991;265:472–7.
25. International Collaboration of Epidemiological Studies of Cervical Cancer. Cervical cancer and

hormonal contraceptives: collaborative reanalysis of individual data for 16 573 women with cervical cancer and 35 509 women without cervical cancer from 24 epidemiological studies. The Lancet. 2007;370(9599):1609–21.
26. Nayar R, Wilbur DC. The pap test and Bethesda 2014: "the reports of my demise have been greatly exaggerated (after a quotation from Mark Twain)". J Low Genit Tract Dis. 2015;19(175):175.
27. Darragh TM, Colgan TJ, Cox JT, et al. The lower Anogenital squamous terminology standardization project for HPV-associated lesions: background and consensus recommendations from the College of American Pathologists and the American Society for Colposcopy and Cervical pathology. J Low Genit Dis. 2012;16:205–42.
28. Bornstein J, Bentley J, Bösze P, Girardi F, Haefner H, Menton M, Perrotta M, Prendiville W, Russell P, Sideri M, Strander B, Tatti S, Torne A, Walker P. 2011 colposcopic terminology of the International Federation for Cervical Pathology and Colposcopy. Obstet Gynecol. 2012;120(1):166–72. https://doi.org/10.1097/AOG.0b013e318254f90c.
29. Bowring J, Strander B, Young M, Evans H, Walker P. The swede score: evaluation of a scoring system designed to improve the predictive value of colposcopy. J Low Genit Tract Dis. 2010;14(4):301–5. https://doi.org/10.1097/LGT.0b013e3181d77756.
30. Mark Schiffman M, Wentzenson N. Human papillomavirus infection and the multistage carcinogenesis of cervical cancer. Cancer Epidemiol Biomarkers Prev. 2013;22(4):553–60.
31. International Collaboration of Epidemiological Studies of Cervical Cancer, Appleby P, Beral V, et al. Carcinoma of cervix and tobacco smoking: collaborative reanalysis of individual data on 13,541 women with carcinoma of the cervix and 23,017 women without carcinoma of the cervix from 23 epidemiological studies. Int J Cancer. 2006;118:1481.
32. Hemminki K, Chen B. Familial risks for cervical tumors in full and half siblings: etiologic apportioning. Cancer Epidemiol Biomarkers Prev. 2006;15:1413.
33. Castellsague X, Bosch FX, Munoz N, et al. Male circumcision, penile human papillomavirus infection and cervical cancer in female partners. N Engl J Med. 2002;346:1105.
34. Yu L, Sabatino SA, White MC. Rural-urban and racial/ethnic disparities in invasive cervical cancer incidence in the United States, 2010-2014. Prev Chronic Dis. 2019;16:E70.
35. Benard VB, Watson M, Castle PE, Saraiya M. Cervical carcinoma rates among young females in the United States. Obstet Gynecol. 2012;120:1117.
36. Bansal N, Wright JD, Cohen CJ, Herzog TJ. Natural history of established low grade cervical intraepithelial neoplasia (CIN1) lesions. Anticancer Res. 2008;28:1763.
37. McCredie MR, Sharples KJ, Paul C, et al. Natural history of cervical neoplasia and risk of invasive cancer in women with cervical intraepithelial neoplasia3: a retrospective cohort study. Lancet Oncol. 2008;9:425.
38. Tainio K, Athanasiou A, Tikkinen KAO, et al. Clinical course of untreated cervical intraepithelial neoplasia grade 2 under active surveillance: systemic review and meta-analysis. BMJ. 2018;360:k499.
39. Schmeink CE, Massuger LF, Lenselink CH, et al. Prospective follow up of 2,065 young unscreened women to study human papillomavirus incidence and clearance. Int J Cancer. 2013;133:172.
40. Nucci MR, Crum CP. Redefining early cervical neoplasia: recent progress. Adv Anat Pathol. 2007;14:1.
41. Perkins RB, Guido RS, Castle PE, et al. 2019 ASCCP risk-based management consensus Guidelines for abnormal cervical cancer screening tests and cancer precursors. J Low Genit Tract Dis. 2020;24:102.
42. Engemen D, Cheung LC, Chen X, et al. Risks estimates supporting the 2019 ASCCP risk-based management consensus Guidelines. J Low Genit Tract Dis. 2020;24:132.
43. Kyrgiou M, Athanasiou A, Paraskevaida M, et al. Adverse obstetric outcomes after local treatment for cervical preinvasive and early invasive disease according to cone depth: systemic review and meta-analysis. BMJ. 2016;354:i3633.
44. Tam KF, Cheung AN, Liu KL, et al. A retrospective review on atypical glandular cells of undetermined significance (AGUS) using the Bethesda 2001 classification. Gynecol Oncol. 2003;91:603.
45. McAllum B, Sykes PH, Sadler L, et al. Is the treatment of CIN 2 always necessary in women under 25 years old? Am J Obstet Gynecol. 2011;205:478.e1.
46. Douvier S, Filipuzzi L, Sagot P. Management of cervical intra-epithelial neoplasm during pregnancy. Gynecol Obstet Fertil. 2003;31:851.
47. Moscicki AB, Hills N, Shiboski S, et al. Risks for incident human papillomavirus infection and low-grade squamous intraepithelial lesion development in young females. JAMA. 2001;285:2995.
48. Ellerbrock TV, Chiasson MA, Bush TJ, et al. Incidence of cervical squamous intraepithelial lesions in HIV-infected women. JAMA. 2000;283:1031.
49. Belafsky P, Clark RA, Kissinger P, Torres J. Natural history of low-grade squamous intraepithelial lesions in women infected with human immunodeficiency virus. J Acquir Immune Defic Hum Retroviral. 1996;11:511.
50. Ahdieh-Grant L, Li R, Levine AM, et al. Highly active antiretroviral therapy and cervical squamous intraepithelial lesions in human immunodeficiency virus-positive women. J Natl Cancer Inst. 2004;96:1070.
51. Greene SA, De Vuyst H, John-Stewart GC, et al. Effect of Crotherapy vs loop electrosurgical excision procedure on cervical disease recurrence among women with HIV and high-grade cervical lesions in Kenya: a randomized control trial. JAMA. 2019;322:1570.
52. Maiman M, Watts DH, Andersen J, et al. Vaginal 5-Fuorouracil for high grade cervical dysplasia in human immunodeficiency virus infection: a randomized trial. Obstet Gynecol. 1999;94:954.

53. Marrazzo JM, Koutsky LA, Kiviat NB, et al. Papanicolaou test screening and prevalence of genital human papillomavirus among women who have sex with women. Am J Public Health. 2001;91:947.
54. Bleeker MC, Hogewoning CJ, Berkhof J, et al. Concordance of specific human papillomavirus types in sex partners is more prevalent than would be expected by chance and is associated with increases viral loads. Clin Infect Dis. 2005;41:612.
55. Hogewoning CJ, Bleeker MC, van den Brule AJ, et al. Condom use promotes regression of cervical intraepithelial neoplasia and clearance of human papillomavirus : a randomized clinical trial. Int J Cancer. 2003;107:811.
56. Lichter K, Krause D, Xu J, et al. Adjuvant human papillomavirus vaccine to reduce recurrent cervical dysplasia in unvaccinated women: a systemic review and meta-analysis. Obstet Gynecol. 2020;135(1070):1070.
57. Harrison R, Huh W. Occupational exposure to human Papilllomavirus and vaccination for health care workers. Obstet Gynecol. 2020;136:663.
58. WHO Guidelines. Use of cryotherapy for cervical intraepithelial neoplasia. Geneva: World Health Organisation; 2011.
59. D'Alessandro P, Arduino B, Borgo M, et al. Loop electrosurgical excision procedure versus cryotherapy in the treatment of cervical intraepithelial neoplasia: a systemic review and meta-analysis of randomized controlled trials. Gynecol Minim Invasive Ther. 2018;7:145.
60. Fuller TA. Laser tissue interaction: the influence of power density. In: Baggish M, editor. Basic and advanced laser surgery and gynecology. New York: Appleton-Century-Crofts; 1985. p. 51–60.
61. Duncan ID. Cold coagulation. Baillieres Clin Obstet Gynaecol. 1995;9:145.
62. Woodman CB, Jordan JA, Mylotte MJ, et al. The management of cervical intraepithelial neoplasia by coagulation electrodiathermy. Br J Obstet Gynaecol. 1985;92:751.
63. Cirisano FD. Management of pre-invasive disease of the cervix. Semin Surg Oncol. 1999;16:222.
64. Hillard PA, Biro FM, Wildey L. Complications of cervical cryotherapy in adolescents. J Reprod Med. 1991;36:711.
65. Baggish MS, Dorsey JH, Adelson M. A ten-year experience treating cervical intraepithelial neoplasia with the CO2 laser. Am J Obstet Gynecol. 1989;161:60.
66. Mathevat P, Chemali E, Roy M, Dargent D. Long-term outcome of a randomized study comparing three techniques of conisation: cold knife, laser and LEEP. Eur J Obstet Gynecol Reprod Biol. 2003;106:214.
67. Bjorge T, Skare GB, Bjorge L, et al. Adverse pregnancy outcomes after treatment for cervical intraepithelial neoplasia. Obstet Gynaecol. 2016;128:1265.
68. Zhuang H, Hong S, Zengh L, et al. Effects of cervical conisation on pregnancy outcome: a meta-analysis. J Obstet Gynaecol. 2019;39:74.
69. Desravines N, Miele K, Carlson R, et al. Topical therapies for the treatment of cervical intraepithelial neoplasia (CIN)2-3: a narrative review. Gynecol Oncol Rep. 2020;33:100608.
70. Fonseca BO, Possati-Resende JC, Saldeco MP, et al. Topical Imiquimod for the treatment of high-grade squamous intraepithelial lesions of the cervix: a randomized controlled trial. Obstet Gynaecol. 2021;137:1043.

Cancer of the Uterine Cervix

Debabrata Barmon, Amal Chandra Kataki,
Gautam Sarma, Partha Pratim Medhi,
and Umesh Mahantshetty

1 Introduction

Cervical cancer which has become a thing of the past for many developed countries but sadly enough it has become one of the commonest public health problems and greatest threat to women's life, particularly in low- and middle-income countries (LMIC). In spite of being one of the highly preventable and curable forms of cancer in its early stages, we lose one women every 2 min due to cervical cancer as almost 70–80% of the patients are presented in fairly advanced stage when the treatment becomes complicated and cure rate falls drastically.

Cervical cancer is the fourth most common cancer in females worldwide. In the LMICs it ranks second most common cancer and third most common in terms of mortality. As far as India is concerned, it is the second highest cancer in females. According to the GLOBOCON 2018 data out of the total 569,847 cases worldwide and mortality of 311,365 cases, India contributed to 96,922 new cases and 60,078 deaths [1]. Poor access to proper screening and treatment contributes to the high mortality in the low- and middle-income countries. It is estimated that almost 85% of all the new cases and 90% of all deaths due to cervical cancer occurs in the low socioeconomic sections of the population from the low-resource countries. Cervical cancer mortality contributes to 10% of all cancer related mortality in our country [2]. As per ICMR data it is more prevalent in the rural areas [3] and less common among the Muslim population [4].

2 Brief Anatomy

The cervix is also called the mouth of the uterus, it is cylindrical in shape and composed of stroma and epithelium. The cervix is divided into two parts, the ectocervix and endocervix, the exposed part of the cervix which is seen on speculum examination is called ectocervix, it is lined by squamous epithelium. The endocervical part is basically the canal which starts from the external os till the internal os, this part of the cervix is lined by columnar epithelium. Now the junction between the ectocervix and the endocervix where both the squamous and columnar epithelium

D. Barmon (✉) · A. C. Kataki
Department of Gynaecologic Oncology,
Dr. Bhubaneswar Borooah Cancer Institute
(A Unit of Tata Memorial Centre, Mumbai),
Guwahati, Assam, India
e-mail: dydiracademic@bbci.tmc.gov.in

G. Sarma · P. P. Medhi
Department of Radiation Oncology, Dr B. Borooah
Cancer Institute, Guwahati, Assam, India

U. Mahantshetty
Department of Radiation Oncology, Homi Bhabha
Cancer Hospital and Research Centre,
Vishakhapatnam, Andhra Pradesh, India
e-mail: mahantshettyum@tmc.gov.in

A. C. Kataki, D. Barmon (eds.), *Fundamentals in Gynaecologic Malignancy*,
https://doi.org/10.1007/978-981-19-5860-1_13

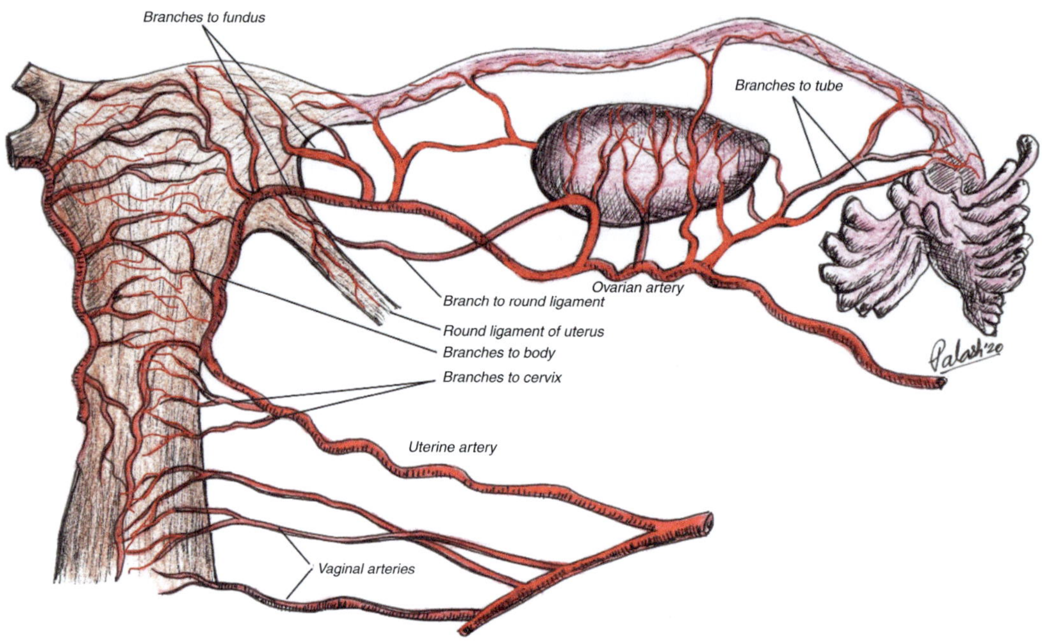

Fig. 1 Vascular supply of the uterus and cervix

meets is called squama-columnar junction. This squama-columnar junction is a dynamic entity and it moves outside in the ectocervix or inside the canal depending on the age of the individual. During the reproductive phase the SC junction shifts towards the ectocervix bringing the columnar epithelium outside the canal, once the columnar epithelium is exposed to the acidic medium of the vagina, metaplastic activity starts over the columnar epithelium, and finally the whole of exposed columnar epithelium is transformed into squamous epithelium, now the original SC junction is shifted towards the periphery away from the external os and the new SC junction is developed near the external os. The area between the original SC junction and the new SC junction is called the transformation zone. This transformation zone is of great anatomical significance as all the pre invasive lesions of the cervix starts from this zone, so a thorough understanding of this particular zone is very important.

The cervix receives its blood supply from the descending branches of the uterine arteries and venous drainage parallels the arterial system (Fig. 1). The nerve supply of the cervix comes from the pelvic autonomic system, the superior, middle, and inferior hypogastric plexuses. The lymphatic of the cervix have a dual origin from the submucosa and deep fibrous stroma [5] and both of them forms two lateral plexuses in the region of the isthmus and from here four efferent channels are formed running towards (1) the external iliac and obturator nodes (2) the hypogastric and common iliac nodes (3) the sacral nodes and (4) the nodes of the posterior wall of the urinary bladder.

2.1 Pelvic Spaces

The pelvis is divided into various avascular spaces (Fig. 2) based on their location, a thorough knowledge of these spaces is essential for performing radical surgeries because of their anatomical importance. These spaces can be classified as

1. Bilateral:
    (a) Pararectal space
    (b) Paravesical space
2. Unilateral/midline:
    (a) Prevesical space
    (b) Rectovaginal space
    (c) Retrorectal or presacral space.

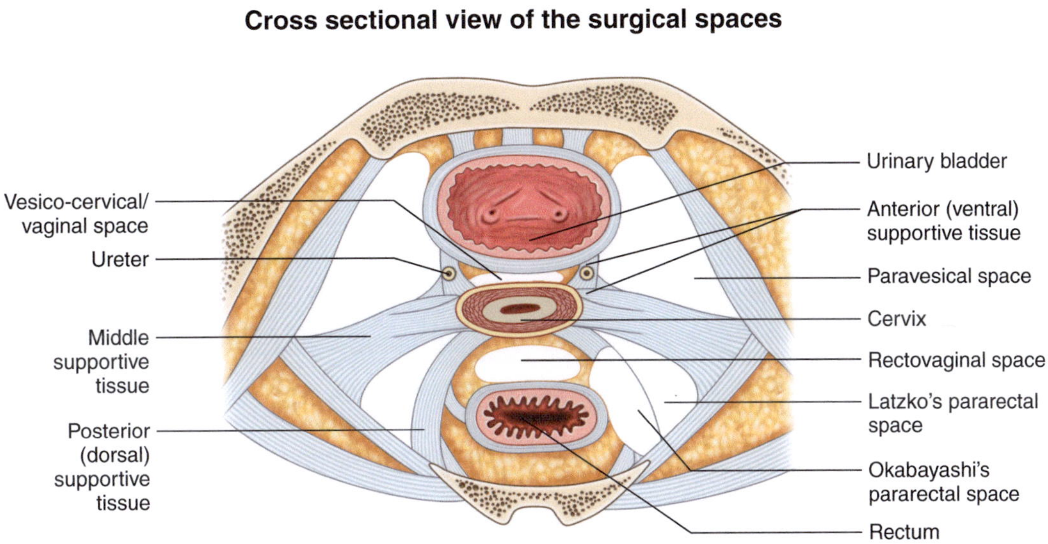

Fig. 2 Pelvic spaces and supports

The pararectal spaces lies on either side of the rectum with the ureter dividing it into the lateral (Latzko space) and medial (Okabayashi) pararectal spaces. The Okabayashi space contains the superior hypogastric nerves, which are preserved during nerve sparing radical hysterectomy.

The paravesical space lies lateral to the urinary bladder and the obliterated hypogastric artery divides this space into medial and lateral paravesical spaces. The medial paravesical space is dissected to achieve optimum oncological clearance, the lateral paravesical space contains the pelvic nodes which needs to be dissected during radical hysterectomy.

Amongst the midline spaces, the anterior most space is the prevesical space lying between the anterior abdominal wall and urinary bladder. During exenteration operation this space needs to be dissected. Another important midline space is the rectovaginal space between the rectum and uterus/vagina, bounded laterally by the uterosacral ligament. This space is bounded by the two layers of the Denonvilliers fascia, and while dissecting this space one must go between these two layers to prevent bleeding. The posterior most midline space is the retrorectal or presacral space, covered by the mesorectum anteriorly and Waldeyer fascia posteriorly. This space needs dissection during posterior exenteration operation.

3 Natural History of Cervical Cancer

The most important and necessary cause of cervical cancer is persistent infection of the cervix with certain high-risk types of HPV [6]. During the reproductive period, all women are infected with different strains of viruses, however, HPV has propensity to infect the actively dividing cells of the transformation zone of the cervix, these infections are transient and clear off within 2–5 years in 80–90% of cases, however, in the remaining women the infection persists and it progresses to the various phases of preinvasive lesions and few ultimately to invasive lesions and the whole process sometimes takes 10–30 years [7]. Older age, high-risk HPV type infection, immunosuppression, and longer duration of infection have been implicated as the main contributors of persistent infection and progression to carcinoma.

HPV infections of cervix are latent in 90% of cases and without any physical, cytological or histological manifestations. Active infection with HPV in "episomal non-integrated" state produces low-grade lesions. These lesions show characteristic cellular changes such as nuclear enlargement, multinucleation, hyperchromasia, and perinuclear cytoplasmic clearing(halo). Integration of viral genome into the host DNA is the most crucial step in cervical carcinogenesis resulting in high-grade lesions and carcinoma. This is supported by the evidence of integrated DNA in 83% of invasive cancers and only in 8% of low-grade CIN [8].

Pre-invasive lesions can regress spontaneously, persist or progress depending on the severity of CIN. ASCUS-LSIL Triage Study (ALTS) concluded that CIN1/LGSIL is a non-neoplastic lesion and not a risk factor for developing CIN3. The rate was higher in young, healthy women (>60%). On the contrary, if left untreated 30% of CIN3 will progress to invasive cancer over 30 years [9].

It is seen that HR HPV can be identified in almost all the cases of cervical cancer and it is said that association of cervical cancer and persistent ongoing infection with HPV is higher than the association of smoking with lung cancer. Although there is geographic variation in the predominant HPV types associated with cervical cancer however HPV types 16 and 18 is responsible for almost 70% of cases (http://www.iarc.fr).

4 Patho-Physiology

Among all the gynaecological cancers, the pathophysiology of cervical cancer is most well understood. The fact that almost all cervical cancers have definite pre-invasive stage, it gives us an opportunity for early identification by screening tests, treatment and vaccination.

Dr. Harald zur Hausen, isolated HPV-16 and HPV-18 in the year 1983 and 1984, respectively, and suggested it as causative agent for cervical cancer. Since then our understanding in the domain of cervical lesions (pre-invasive and invasive) has increased. Based on various epidemiological and molecular studies, HPV has been labeled as "necessary, non-sufficient cause" for cervical cancer. It has been implicated in 99.7% of cervical squamous cell cancer cases worldwide [6].

HPV (Human Papilloma Virus) is a non-enveloped, circular, double-stranded DNA virus with a proteinaceous coat. More than 200 distinct genotypes have been identified till now. HPV viruses are divided into two groups—high risk and low risk, based on their association with cervical cancer and pre-invasive lesions. High-risk HPV types include types 16, 18, 31, 33, 34, 35, 39, 45, 51, 52, 56, 58, 59, 66, 68, and 70. Low-risk HPV types include types 6, 11, 42, 43, and 44. HPV16 accounts for 50–70% of the cervical cancer cases in most countries, followed by HPV18 (10–12%) and HPV31 and 45 (4–5% each). The HPV types causing cervical adenocarcinoma are HPV16 (about 45%), HPV18 (about 40%), and HPV45 and 59 (4–5% each).

These viruses because of their epitheliotrophic nature infect the epithelial cells and mucous membrane of the ano-genital tract, specifically at the sites of micro-traumas. The most common route of HPV transmission is through sexual contact; factors such as early age at first sexual contact, multiple sexual partners, multiparity, immunocompromised state, smoking, infections with HIV, Herpes Simplex Virus, Chlamydia, combined oral contraceptive pills act as co-factors which sustain the persistence of HPV infection and allow progression of the disease.

HPV genome is composed of three regions. (1) First region, known as upstream regulatory region (URR) or long control region, is a non-coding region and contains binding sites for different activators and repressors; (2) Second region encodes for Early (E) proteins—E1, E2, E4, E5, E6, E7 which are associated with gene regulation and malignant transformation; (3) Third region codes for Late (L) proteins—Major capsid protein (L1) and minor capsid protein (L2), which help in viral attachment to the host cells (e.g., keratinocytes).

E6 and E7 are the most important viral proteins which determine the oncogenic potential of high-risk HPV. E7 protein displaces pRb (Retinoblastoma) from transcription factor E2F and leads to unregulated cell transition from G1 into S-phase. E6 inhibits apoptosis via binding to the tumour suppressor protein p53 and up-regulating the cellular telomerase activity. The HPV DNA replication is mediated by E1/E2 proteins. E1 and E2 are early events in the life cycle of HPV whereas E6 and E7 are expressed in the later stage of malignant transformation.

5 Staging

5.1 FIGO Staging

Since 2018 the new FIGO cervical cancer staging was updated (Fig. 3), where the imaging and pathologic findings were included, however, whenever these modalities were used to stage a disease, additional notation in the form of r (imaging) and p (pathology) should be used along with the stage.

Few other changes which has been recommended in the 2018 FIGO staging (Table 1) are the concept of horizontal spread in stage IA was done away and only depth of invasion was included, apart from this Stage IB is now divided into three sub-stages, stage I B1, IB2, IB3, depending on the greatest dimension of the

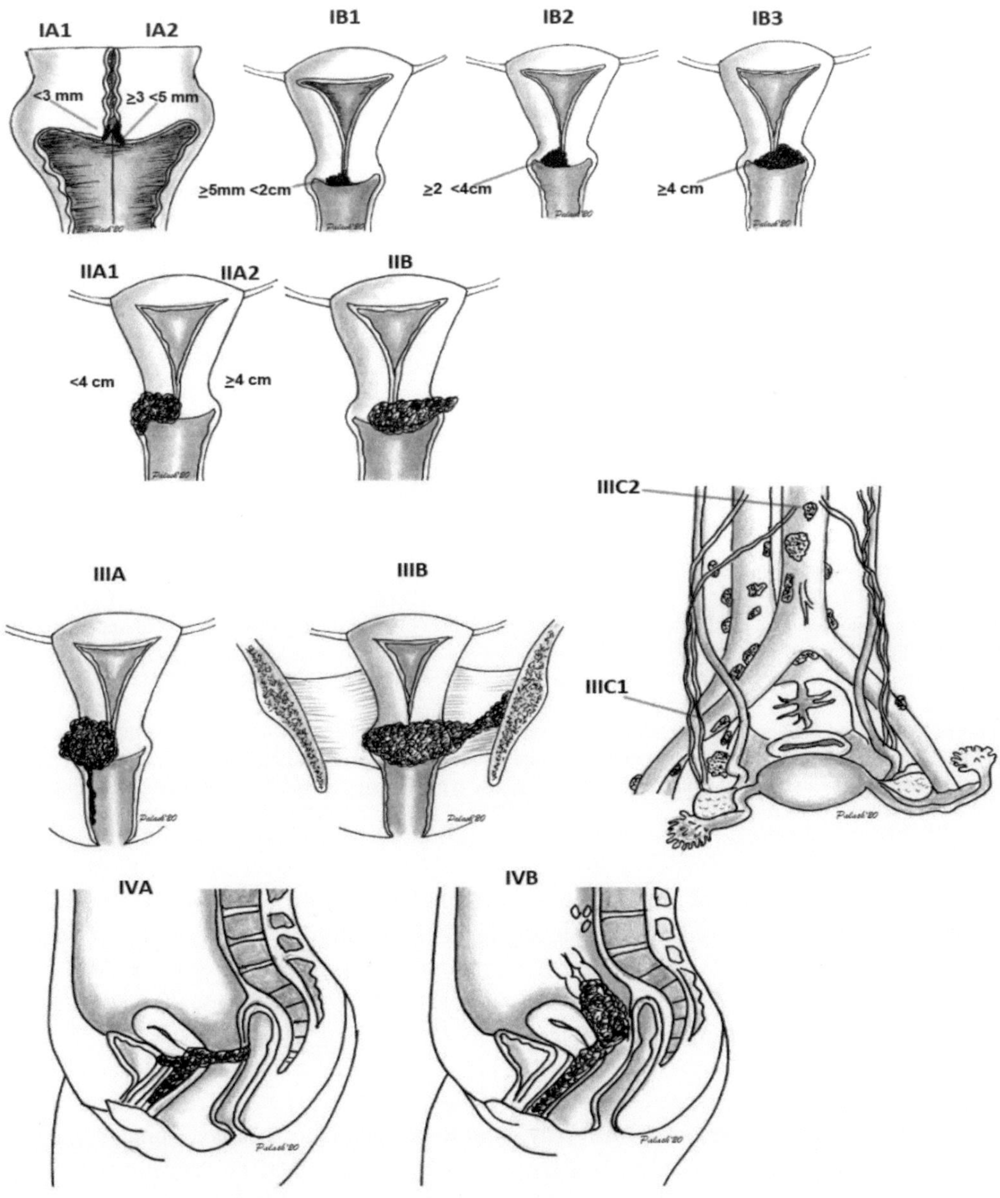

Fig. 3 Cervical cancer staging FIGO 2018

Table 1 FIGO staging of cancer of the cervix uteri (2018) [10]

Stage	Description
I	The carcinoma is strictly confined to the cervix (extension to the uterine corpus should be disregarded)
IA	Invasive carcinoma that can be diagnosed only by microscopy, with maximum depth of invasion <5 mma
IA1	Measured stromal invasion <3 mm in depth
IA2	Measured stromal invasion ≥3 mm and <5 mm in depth
IB	Invasive carcinoma with measured deepest invasion ≥5 mm (greater than Stage IA), lesion limited to the cervix uterib
IB1	Invasive carcinoma ≥5 mm depth of stromal invasion, and <2 cm in greatest dimension
IB2	Invasive carcinoma ≥2 cm and <4 cm in greatest dimension
IB3	Invasive carcinoma ≥4 cm in greatest dimension
II	The carcinoma invades beyond the uterus, but has not extended onto the lower third of the vagina or to the pelvic wall
IIA	Involvement limited to the upper two-thirds of the vagina without parametrial involvement
IIA1	Invasive carcinoma <4 cm in greatest dimension
IIA2	Invasive carcinoma ≥4 cm in greatest dimension
IIB	With parametrial involvement but not up to the pelvic wall
III	The carcinoma involves the lower third of the vagina and/or extends to the pelvic wall and/or causes hydronephrosis or nonfunctioning kidney and/or involves pelvic and/or para-aortic lymph nodesc
IIIA	The carcinoma involves the lower third of the vagina, with no extension to the pelvic wall
IIIB	Extension to the pelvic wall and/or hydronephrosis or nonfunctioning kidney (unless known to be due to another cause)
IIIC	Involvement of pelvic and/or para-aortic lymph nodes, irrespective of tumour size and extent (with r and p notations)c
IIIC1	Pelvic lymph node metastasis only
IIIC2	Para-aortic lymph node metastasis
IV	The carcinoma has extended beyond the true pelvis or has involved (biopsy proven) the mucosa of the bladder or rectum. (A bullous edema, as such, does not permit a case to be allotted to Stage IV)
IVA	Spread to adjacent pelvic organs
IVB	Spread to distant organs

When in doubt, the lower staging should be assigned

Source: Bhatla et al. [10]

[a] Imaging and pathology can be used, where available, to supplement clinical findings with respect to tumour size and extent, in all stages

[b] The involvement of vascular/lymphatic spaces does not change the staging. The lateral extent of the lesion is no longer considered

[c] Adding notation of r (imaging) and p (pathology) to indicate the findings that are used to allocate the case to Stage IIIC. Example: If imaging indicates pelvic lymph node metastasis, the stage allocation would be Stage IIIC1r, and if confirmed by pathologic findings, it would be Stage IIIC1p. The type of imaging modality or pathology technique used should always be documented

tumour size. When the size of the tumour is <2 cm in greatest dimension it is denoted as stage IBI, when the size is between ≥2 cm to <4 cm its stage IB2 and any tumour ≥4 cm will be stage IB3 [11]. The explanation behind these changes was that in stage IB1, more conservative approach as fertility sparing surgery in selected group may be tried or minimal invasive surgery (MIS) may be tried where hysterectomy is needed. In stage IB2, MIS is to be avoided and open surgery should be preferred and stage IB3 should go in favor of concurrent CTRT.

Another change which was included in the new staging system is the use of imaging/pathology for detecting enlarged pelvic and paraaortic LN. If on imaging there is any enlarged suspicious nodes and on FNAC/Tru-cut biopsy it turns out to be metastatic, then depending on the location of the node it may be staged as stage III C1 (Pelvic nodes metastasis) and stage III C2

(Paraaortic LN metastasis). Although there is no single perfect imaging technique for diagnosing metastatic LN, however, PET/CT imaging is by far the most sensitive modality in detecting metastatic LN when compared to PET alone. Final confirmation can be done by image guided FNAC/Tru-cut biopsy.

5.2 TNM System

TNM classification system which is devised by IUCC and American Joint Committee on Cancer, is a system which is parallel to FIGO system. Clinically TNM and FIGO staging system are the same. The T stages corresponds to the FIGO stages except Carcinoma In-situ (CIS). The TNM system in post-operative cases of hysterectomy also includes pathologic staging system as pTNM.

6 Risk Factors

The most important risk factor or rather the necessary causative factor for the occurrence of cervical cancer is the presence of high risk HPV infection. Studies have found out that 99% of women having squamous cell carcinoma of cervix are high risk HPV positive. Therefore, it is said that HPV is the causative agent in both squamous and adenocarcinoma of cervix, although they may follow different carcinogenic pathways [12].

Apart from HPV the other associated risk factor for cervical cancer are young age at first intercourse, especially when the age is <18 years, young age <20 years at first pregnancy, multiple pregnancy within short interval, multiple sexual partners, low socio-economic status, poor genital hygiene, race, cigarette smoking (although this hypothesis is not always supported in literature). Chronic immune suppression and infection with other co-existent sexually transmitted disease as HIV, Herpes virus, and Chlamydia trachomatis which generally acts as cofactors. HIV infection may lead to immune suppression and ultimately may cause persistence of HPV infection leading to cervical cancer.

7 Clinical Evaluation and Staging Procedure

As we know staging of cervical cancer is basically based on clinical examinations, so per speculum (PS), per vaginal (PV), per rectal (PR) examination remains the gold standard evaluation protocol.

To start with the clinical evaluation in a suspected case of carcinoma cervix, a thorough general/physical examination is done looking for enlarged supraclavicular, axillary and inguino-femoral lymph node to rule out any metastatic disease. This is followed by pelvic examination, which starts with the PS examination. On PS examination a detail inspection of the cervical anatomy is carried out looking for suspicious areas, any abnormal growth which may be proliferative/infiltrative/ulcerative, then we should look for the involvement of the fornices and vaginal walls. All the positive findings should be correlated with digital per vaginal examination to confirm the PS findings. Finally, PR examination is carried out to look for parametrial extension of the disease, which gives a feeling of nodularity or induration beyond the cervix laterally, which may extend up to the lateral pelvic wall and also involvement of rectal mucosa if any. Sometimes PR examination may also be helpful in post-menopausal ladies to look for cervical size and extension, when there is vaginal adhesions and cervix cannot be inspected properly.

Once the local physical examination is done then we should carry out a biopsy procedure, when the tumour is seen on PS examination the biopsy procedure can be done in an OPD setting, however, in very early cases when no obvious tumour is seen then colposcopic guided biopsy or endocervical curettage may be required and in some cases even conization/LEEP may be needed to establish a diagnosis. Other investigations that may be needed to aid our diagnosis and staging process are endoscopy procedures such as hysteroscopy, cystoscopy, and proctoscopy. Imaging techniques like CT Scan which can nicely detect lymph nodes involvement and MRI (Fig. 4) can be done to determine the tumour size, extent of

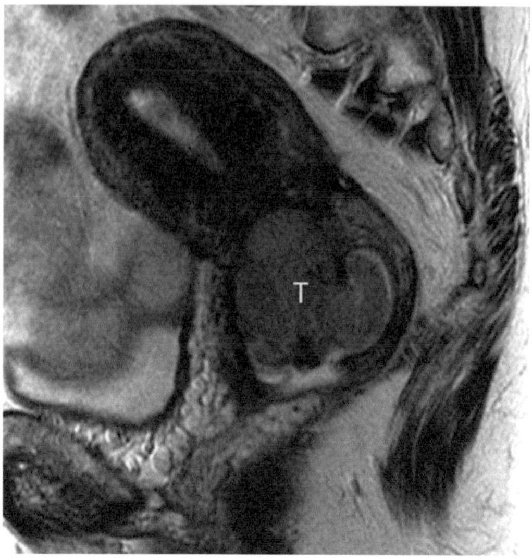

Fig. 4 MRI image showing cervical growth

parametrial invasion, vaginal involvement, and uterine involvement with accuracy [13].

A systemic review comparing CT Scan and MRI has shown excellent sensitivity on T2 weighted image of MRI in the detection of parametrial disease and MRI is significantly more sensitive with comparable specificity [14].

PET Scan on the other hand is useful in detecting distant metastasis, disease extent and particularly nodal status in normal sized nodes with high sensitivity and specificity. A meta-analysis of 72 studies found that the sensitivity and specificity of PET for detection of lymph node metastasis was 75% and 98% compared to CT which was 58% and 92%, MRI with sensitivity and specificity of 56% and 93% [15]. PET Scan is also helpful in detecting recurrence and to determine treatment outcome.

8 Histopathology

Microscopic confirmation of malignancy is the most essential diagnostic test for starting cancer treatment. The site of the primary growth determines the cancer site and in cervical cancer either the ectocervix or the endocervix must be biopsied to come to a diagnosis. Various histologic types that has been described by the World Health Organization's 2014 Tumours of the Female Reproductive Organs [16] are:

1. Squamous cell carcinoma (keratinizing, non-keratinizing; papillary, basaloid, warty, verrucous, squamotransitional, lymphoepithelioma-like)
2. Adenocarcinoma (mucinous, villoglandular, endometrioid)
3. Clear cell adenocarcinoma
4. Serous carcinoma
5. Adenosquamous carcinoma
6. Glassy cell carcinoma
7. Adenoid cystic carcinoma
8. Adenoid basal carcinoma
9. Small cell carcinoma
10. Undifferentiated carcinoma.

Grading by any of several methods is encouraged, but it is not a basis for modifying the stage groupings in cervical carcinoma. Histopathologic grades are as follows:

1. GX: Grade cannot be assessed
2. G1: Well differentiated
3. G2: Moderately differentiated
4. G3: Poorly or undifferentiated.

Squamous cell carcinoma of cervix contributes to almost 75% of all invasive carcinoma of cervix. It may be keratinizing variety (Fig. 5) where we get the typical keratin pearls and the non-keratinising variety (Fig. 6). The cell variants may be large cell and small cell variety which has a very poor prognosis. SCC has three grades as well differentiated, moderately differentiated, and poorly differentiated and the prognosis corresponds to their grades.

Adenocarcinoma of cervix (Fig. 7) contributes for 15–25% of all cervical carcinomas. It arises in the endocervix, hence sometimes it is very difficult to detect, by the time it is detected majority has already invaded the parametrium with metastatic lymph nodes. Histologic variants of this type include endometroid adenocarcinoma, villoglandular, mucinous, etc.

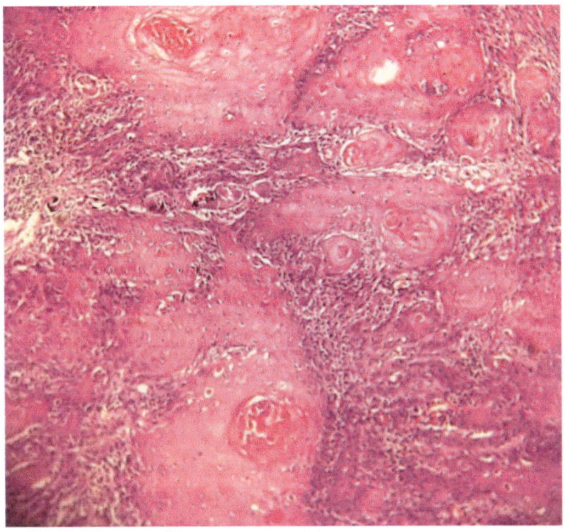

Fig. 5 Microscopic appearance of keratinizing squamous cell carcinoma of cervix

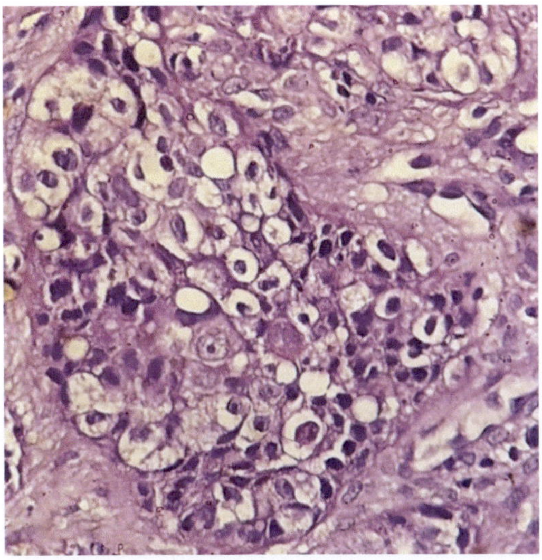

Fig. 6 Microscopic appearance of non-keratinizing large cell squamous cell carcinoma of cervix

Since 2020 WHO has come up with a new classification of histological types of Female Genital Tumours.

The histopathologic types, as described in the WHO Classification of Female Genital Tumours [17]:

1. Squamous epithelial tumours
   (a) Squamous cell carcinoma, HPV-associated

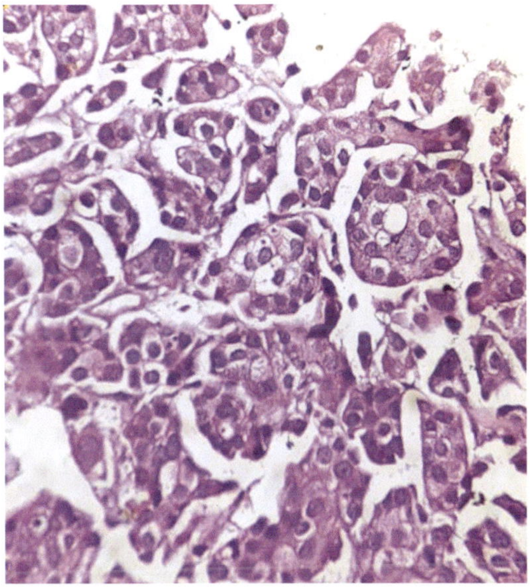

Fig. 7 Microscopic appearance of endocervical adenocarcinoma usual type

   (b) Squamous cell carcinoma, HPV-independent
   (c) Squamous cell carcinoma NOS
2. Glandular tumours
   (a) Adenocarcinoma NOS
   (b) Adenocarcinoma, HPV-associated
   (c) Adenocarcinoma, HPV-independent, gastric type
   (d) Adenocarcinoma, HPV-independent, clear cell type
   (e) Adenocarcinoma, HPV-independent, mesonephric type
   (f) Adenocarcinoma, HPV-independent, NOS
   (g) Endometrioid adenocarcinoma NOS
   (h) Carcinosarcoma NOS
   (i) Adenosquamous carcinoma
   (j) Mucoepidermoid carcinoma
   (k) Adenoid basal carcinoma
   (l) Carcinoma, undifferentiated, NOS
3. Mixed epithelial and mesenchymal tumours
   (a) Adenosarcoma
4. Germ cell tumours
   (a) Endodermal sinus tumour
   (b) Yolk sac tumour NOS
   (c) Choriocarcinoma NOS.

9 Management of Early Stage Cervical Cancer

Early stage cervical cancer comprises of all stages from IA to IIA, excluding Stage IB3 as per the new FIGO 2018 staging system. Surgery and radiation therapy are the two main treatment options, surgery comprises of fertility sparing surgery or radical surgery and radiation therapy may be with or without concurrent chemotherapy. The treatment options will depend on the stage, performance status, fertility status, age, and comorbidities.

9.1 Management of Stage IA1

Since this is a very early disease with stromal invasion less than 3 mm, the risk of lymph node metastasis is <1%. Hence fertility preservation may be offered in women desiring fertility conservation.

For patients desiring fertility preservation, conization remains the mainstay of treatment [18, 19] and following conization if the margins are negative with the absence of LVSI then observation is advised. If the margin is positive, then repeat conization is recommended and in patients where LVSI is positive radical trachelectomy along with pelvic lymph node dissection is advised [20]. Treatment remains the same for both squamous and adenocarcinoma histopathology.

Patients not desirous of fertility preservation extrafascial hysterectomy with ovarian conservation is recommended in young patients, if LVSI is present, then lymphadenectomy is advised and subsequent adjuvant concomitant CTRT will depend on lymph node status.

9.2 Management of Stage IA2

Compared to stage IA1, here due to the increased stromal invasion from 3 to ≤5 mm the incidence of lymph node metastasis is higher and there are reports which suggests lymph node involvement to be as high as 12% when LVSI is positive. The final treatment plan depends on the fertility status of the woman.

Patients desiring fertility preservation radical trachelectomy along with pelvic lymph node dissection may be done. In some patients conization may be tried along with extraperitoneal/laparoscopic pelvic lymphadenectomy but margin has to be negative, LVSI negative along with negative endocervical curettage histology [11].

Patients who do not want fertility preservation either surgery or radiation therapy may be tried however when there is no contraindications for surgery, modified radical hysterectomy along with pelvic lymph node dissection with or without para aortic lymph node sampling is preferred and depending on the lymph node status, adjuvant radiation therapy may be required. Patients who are unfit for surgery or refuses surgery, primary radiation therapy may be offered with equal survival.

9.3 Management of Stage IB1

Both radical hysterectomy and radiotherapy may be offered to this group of patients with equal survival and recurrence rates. As majority of the patients are in the reproductive age group so surgery has the advantage of ovarian preservation along with avoiding vaginal stenosis secondary to radiation therapy. Primary radiation therapy is only offered when there is some contraindications for surgery or patients unwilling for surgery.

For patients not desiring fertility and when the largest tumour diameter is less than 2 cm, cervical stromal invasion less than 50% with no suspicious nodes on imaging, it is considered as a low risk disease and modified radical hysterectomy may be performed in lieu of type C radical hysterectomy, however, pelvic lymphadenectomy is always included in the procedure [21]. Pelvic lymphadenectomy should be done first and sent for frozen section and if the nodes are negative, then radical hysterectomy is completed and if the nodes turns out to be positive, then radical hysterectomy should be abandoned and these patients should receive concomitant CTRT. Primary radiotherapy with or without concomitant chemotherapy is another option for the treatment of stage IB1 disease with equal survival. The concept of sentinel lymph node mapping is emerging in this group of patients and studies have shown that when the tumour size is less than 2 cm the detection rate is significant [22–24]. Another recommended technique is nerve sparing radical hysterectomy where we preserve the autonomic nerve supply from the hypogastric, splanchnic, and pelvic plexus leading to improved urination, defecation, and sexual functions postoperatively.

Patients desiring fertility, radical trachelectomy is recommended, where we remove the cervix along with the parametrium and finally anastomosis is performed between the uterus and the vagina. This procedure is always preceded by pelvic lymphadenectomy done either laparoscopically or extraperitoneal approach and if the nodes are negative, then radical trachelectomy is performed either vaginally or abdominally. Based on histopathology both squamous cell carcinoma and adenocarcinoma showed negligible survival difference, so the treatment remains same for both these histologies, however, fertility sparing is not recommended in small cell neuroendocrine tumour and adenocarcinoma with a deviation [25].

9.4 Management of Stage IB2 and IIA1

When the size of the tumour is from 2 cm to <4 cm either surgery or radiotherapy may be considered as primary treatment, based on patient factors and resources available with equal outcome. The surgical mode of treatment is the preferred mode and it constitutes the Type C radical hysterectomy (Figs. 8 and 9) where we remove the uterus, parametrium, upper vagina, and a part of the paracolpium, along with pelvic lymphadenectomy. All the attachments or supports of the uterus as the anterior vesico-uterine ligament (anterior and posterior leaf), lateral cardinal ligaments, and posterior sacro-uterine and recto-vaginal ligaments are ligated keeping a margin from the uterus and cervix. The pelvic lymph nodes with or without para aortic lymph node sampling is also performed along with the procedure. Pelvic lymphadenectomy consists of removal of the parametrial nodes, external iliac, internal iliac, common iliac, and obturator nodes.

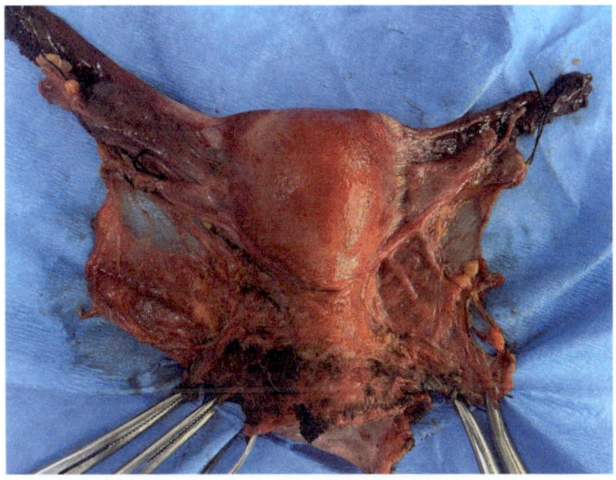

Fig. 8 Specimen of radical hysterectomy

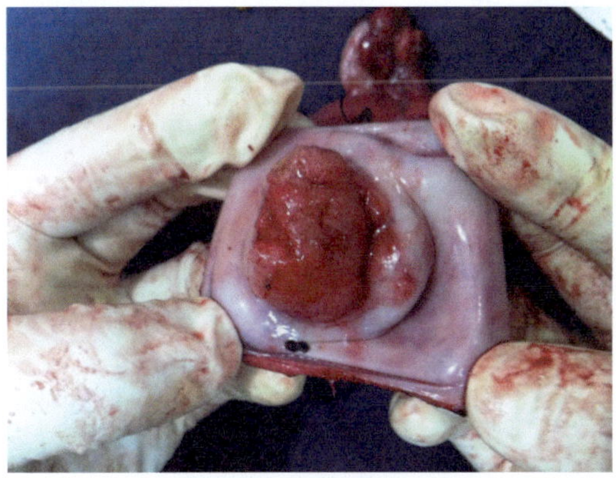

Fig. 9 Specimen showing vaginal cut margin

Since majority of the patients are in the reproductive age group so surgery is the preferred choice of treatment as it preserves the sexual functions by ovarian preservation which is done during the surgery by transpositioning the ovaries in the paracolic gutter below the ninth coastal rib and away from the radiation field in case the patient needs adjuvant radiotherapy based on histopathological findings which can precisely tell us the postoperative stage of the disease. Therefore, the advantages of surgical treatment are accurate staging of the disease and subsequent adjuvant treatment if needed, surgical removal can prevent some of the treatment failures associated with resistance to radiotherapy and finally the preservation of hormonal functions to some extent.

Sentinel lymph node (SLN) mapping in cervical cancer is still experimental and is not recommended in routine practice. Whatever evidence we have at present, tells us that it may have some role in early stage cervical cancer, i.e. FIGO Stage IA, IB1, and IB2 [26–28].

9.5 Management of Stage IB3 and IIA2

Studies have shown that when the tumour size is more than 4 cm then the chances of post-operative recurrence are high and the need for adjuvant radiotherapy also increases due to the presence of high risk factors such as positive lymph nodes, positive surgical margins, and positive parametrium along with other risk factors like LVSI, cervical stromal invasion apart from the size [29, 30]. Hence the dual mode of treatment if administered may lead to enhanced morbidity. Therefore, based on the available resources, patient factors and tumour stage primary concurrent platinum-based chemoradiation (CCRT) is preferred for all Stage IB3 to IIA2 cervical cancers. Concurrent CTRT is preferred over radiation alone as it has been demonstrated that the prognosis is more favorable with CCRT, rather than radiotherapy alone in terms of progression free survival, overall survival, and recurrences both local and distant. The role of NACT followed by surgery is reserved for research settings and low resource countries where there is scarcity of radiation facility and in patients with very large tumours or adenocarcinoma, which have lower response rates [31].

So to summarize surgical treatment is preferred from stage IA through stage IIA1 excluding stage IB3. Although there is some role of surgery in stage IVA where exenteration may be tried after fulfilling all the criteria.

10 Radical Hysterectomy

10.1 History

Ernst Wertheim in the year 1911 first described the technique of Radical Hysterectomy but during those days due to the lack of good antibiotics and anesthetics, the mortality and morbidity was very high, so the vaginal techniques gained acceptance but subsequently with the advent of improved anesthesia techniques and good antibiotics the abdominal approach regained its popularity and Meigs subsequently in 1940s improved his technique by combining bilateral pelvic lymph node dissection, and he reported an intraoperative death rate of <1%. Then in 1974 came the Piver–Rutledge–Smith classification which is divided into class I to V. Class I is the extrafacial hysterectomy to class V which is total exenteration, however, this classification became outdated over time. In the year 2008 Querleu and Morrow came out with their classification which was published in Lancet Oncology and it gained lot of publicity due to its subtypes with practical implications involving preservation of autonomic nerves and paracervical lymphadenectomy. The latest update of this classification came in 2017 (Table 2), which is widely used by everyone [32].

Radical hysterectomy is considered as the gold standard treatment for operable cervical cancer. It is indicated in all cases with stage IA2 to IIA1, except stage IB3. However, during the procedure if we come across bladder invasion (not detected during preoperative imaging) or bowel infiltration or suspicious lymph nodes which is positive on frozen section/clinical suspicion where frozen section is not available, then it is contraindicated to perform the hysterectomy. We must abandon the surgery and prefer CTRT in these patients.

10.2 Route of Surgery

- Conventional Laparotomy
- Minimal Invasive Surgery (MIS)—Laparoscopic or Robotic

In cancer cervix we prefer to do either type B/C depending on the clinical extent.

10.3 Pre-operative Preparation in OT

- Consent for surgery with proper counseling regarding loss of reproductive function/loss of reproductive organs in young patients.

Table 2 Summary of the main landmarks in each type of radical hysterectomy on each part of the parametria [32]

Dimension Type of radical hysterectomy	Paracervix or lateral parametrium	Ventral parametrium	Dorsal parametrium
A	Halfway between the cervix and ureter (medial to the ureter–ureter identified but not mobilized)	Minimal excision	Minimal excision
B1	At the ureter (at the level of the ureteral bed–ureter mobilized from the cervix and lateral parametrium)	Partial excision of the vesicouterine ligament	Partial resection of the rectouterine-rectovaginal ligament and uterosacral peritoneal fold
B2	Identical to B1 plus paracervical lymphadenectomy without resection of vascular/nerve structures	Partial excision of the vesicouterine ligament	Partial resection of the rectouterine-rectovaginal ligament and uterosacral fold
C1	At the iliac vessels transversally, caudal part is preserved	Excision of the vesicouterine ligament at the bladder. Proximal part of the vesicovaginal ligament (bladder nerves are dissected and spared)	At the rectum (hypogastric nerve is dissected and spared)
C2	At the level of the medial aspect of iliac vessels completely (including the caudal part)	At the bladder (bladder nerves are sacrificed)	At the sacrum (hypogastric nerve is sacrificed)
D	At the pelvic wall, including resection of the internal iliac vessels and/or components of the pelvic sidewall	At the bladder. Not applicable if part of exenteration	At the sacrum. Not applicable if part of exenteration

- Counseling regarding preservation of bilateral ovaries in young patients.
- Indwelling catheterization with vaginal packing.
- Patient in lithotomy position.
- DVT prevention—stocking/pneumatic compression devices.
- Patient under General anesthesia/Epidural anesthesia.

10.4 Surgical Steps

The step by step surgical approach is as follows:

- Incision—Midline vertical incision or transverse pfannenstiel suprapubic incision may need Maylard/Cherney's procedure. For Laparoscopy four entry points are created at the discretion of surgeon and patient's built.
- After opening the abdomen the entire abdominal cavity is exposed and bowel packed into the upper abdomen.
- Once no gross metastatic disease is ensured, then the broad ligaments are opened and examined for any suspicious lymph nodes, if detected, they should be taken out and sent for frozen section—if frozen section report is positive then surgery should be abandoned. If not suspicious then complete bilateral pelvic lymph nodes dissection is done.
- Next, we should open the uterovesical fold and mobilize the bladder. If there is no gross or doubtful infiltration seen, then we are good to proceed with the surgery but few surgeons may do it at a later stage of the surgery due to the improved imaging techniques available at our disposal which can precisely tell us regarding bladder and rectal invasion.
- The further steps will include dissection of the bilateral ureters, defining the ureteric tunnel

and deroofing the tunnel followed by lateralization of the ureters, and exposing the cardinal ligaments.

- Then the dissection proceeds posteriorly and the rectovaginal space is opened and after proper dissection both the uterosacral ligaments are identified to gain further access to the rectovaginal space, which is developed by sharp dissection in between the Denonvilliers fascia.
- The pelvic peritoneum over the uterosacral are divided posterolaterally thus completely exposing the rectovaginal and pararectal spaces. Then the rectum is retracted posteriorly and uterus anteriorly, so that the uterosacral ligament can be clamped.
- Following this the vaginal pack is removed then the uterus which is attached laterally by the cardinal ligaments and posteriorly by the uterosacral ligaments are clamped and cut near its origin in type III and midway in type II and the cardinal ligaments are then clamped, cut and transfixed near the pelvic side wall in type III and at the level of uterine artery crossing over the ureter in type II hysterectomy.
- The bladder is then retracted anteriorly and anterior colpotomy is performed keeping 1–1.5 cm margin from the tumour ensuring adequate vaginal cuff margin circumferentially. The vaginal vault is then closed by interrupted or continuous delayed absorbable sutures. Once the hemostasis is checked, if no bleeding then abdomen is closed in layers.

11 Radiotherapy in CA Cervix

Radiation therapy in the form of external beam radiotherapy and brachytherapy are the cornerstones in the management of carcinoma cervix. Different radiotherapy techniques have been used to deliver an optimal dose of radiation to the target volume with a minimum dose to the surrounding normal structures.

11.1 External Beam Radiation Therapy

EBRT has been used for the curative treatment of cervical cancer especially for stage IB3 to IVA. It can also be used for medically inoperable cases of IA to IB2. EBRT in palliative intent is often offered to patients with stage IVB disease with symptoms such as vaginal bleeding, pain, or urethral obstruction from extrinsic compression.

11.2 Patient Positioning

The patient can be positioned in supine or prone depending upon the different techniques used in radiation treatment. The Belly board is usually used in a prone position to shift the small bowel out of the pelvis. In the case of IMRT, the supine position is preferred with immobilization devices surrounding the pelvis so that there is minimal displacement during the treatment process. IV contrast along with oral contrast should be used to delineate pelvic vessels and small bowel, respectively, for contouring purposes.

11.3 Simulation

In this technique, plain radiographic simulation of the pelvis is done with the X-rays. Soft tissues cannot be visualized in X-ray simulation for which barium in rectum or wire marker can be placed at the scar site. Conventional planning is done either by a two-field technique (Figs. 10 and 11) or four-field technique (box technique) (Fig. 12). The superior border is placed at L4-L5 interspace so that common iliac nodes can be covered, and the inferior border should cover at least the obturator foramen or 2 cm below the lower extent of disease. The lower border can be modified according to the distal extent of growth. At the lower extent of growth, a radiopaque clip or bead should be placed during the simulation process. When the tumour involves the lower vagina, the inferior border of the portal should be extended to include inguinal lymph nodes.

The posterior border of the lateral field should be placed in such a way that the entire sacrum should be covered because there are high chances of microscopic extension to the uterosacral ligament. The anterior border of the lateral field should be placed anterior to the pubic symphysis to cover the external iliac lymph nodes. When paraaortic nodes are involved then the superior border should be placed at T12-L1 interspace, the anterior border should be at 2 cm in front of the vertebral body or the enlarged nodes and posteriorly the border bisects mid vertebral body (Fig. 13).

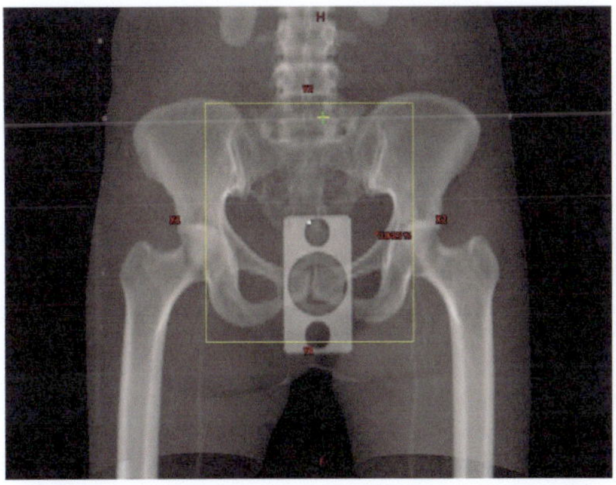

Fig. 10 Antero-posterior portal simulation film of the pelvis

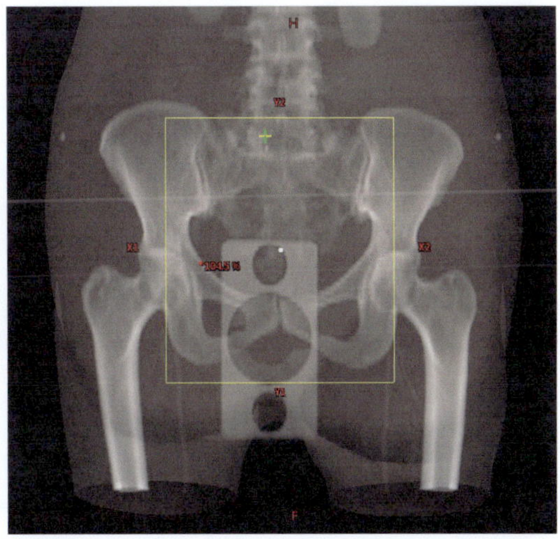

Fig. 11 Postero-anterior portal simulation film of the pelvis

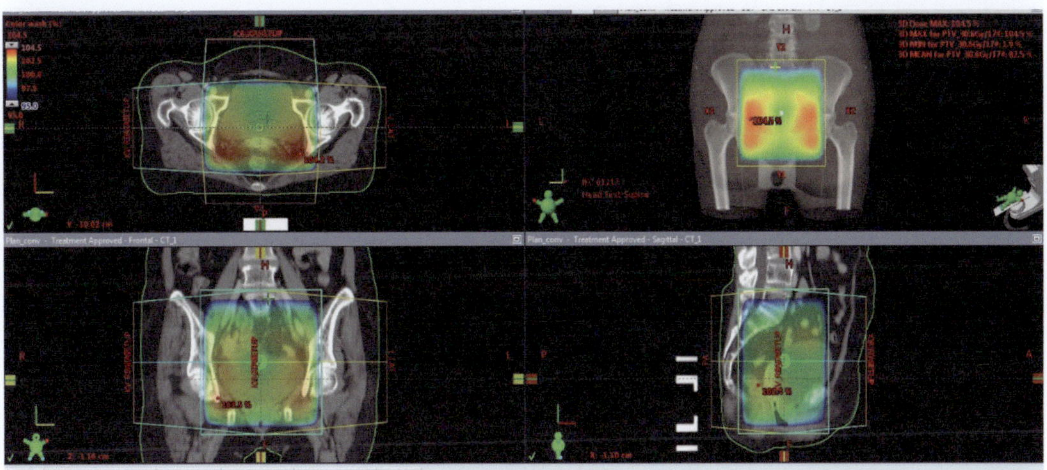

Fig. 12 Four fields (Box technique) portal simulation film of the pelvis along with dose color wash

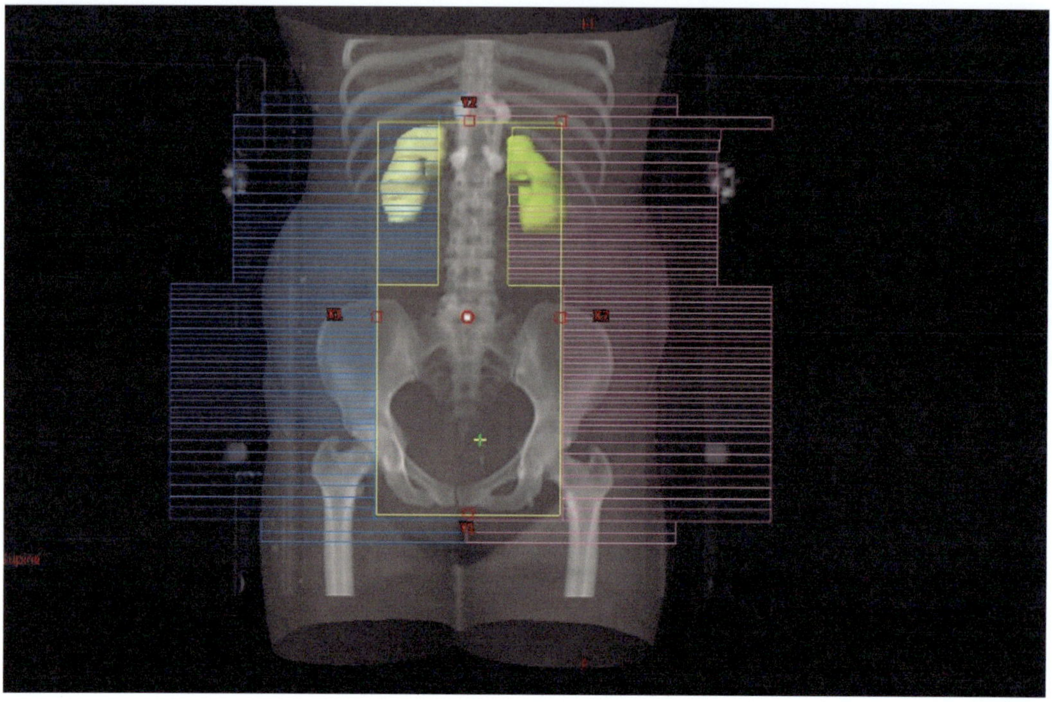

Fig. 13 Extended-field portal simulation film of the pelvis and para-aortic lymph nodes

In CT simulation there is better visualization of tumour size, pelvic vessels, pelvic nodes, and para-aortic nodal involvement. Oral contrast can be used to delineate the small bowel. Multi-leaf collimators are used to block the rectum, small bowel, soft tissue, and muscles to reduce toxicity. The superior border, inferior border, anterior border, and posterior border are usually the same, as in conventional simulation.

A review done by Bonin et al. [33], among 22 patients found that in ten patients (45%) had inadequate lymph node irradiation. The lymph nodes incompletely irradiated were the lower lateral external group. However, contouring with CT-simulation can lead to adequate coverage of these nodes.

It was found by Zunino et al. [34] that if the posterior border is placed at S2-S3 interspace, 50% of patients of FIGO stage IB, and 67% of patients with stage IIA disease, the posterior border will not adequately cover the PTV. In the patients of stage IIB and IVA disease, the PTV was not encompassed at all.

Finlay et al. [35] contoured pelvic vessels, they found that it was more accurate for field delineation as compared to bony landmarks. 96% of the total patients planned with conventional field had inadequate coverage of lymph nodes and 56% of the normal tissue, received radiation that didn't require at all. Therefore, many centers of the world use 3-D simulation for treating ca cervix.

Taylor et al. [36] used a 7 mm margin around the pelvic vessels which resulted in 99% of the nodal coverage along with very little radiation to the small bowel.

Yamazaki et al. compared 34 patients and 40 patients treated with irregular four-field technique and whole pelvis EBRT using parallel opposed fields simultaneously in post-operative patients receiving radiation to a dose 50 Gy in 25 fractions in 6 weeks. After a follow-up of 60 months, 5-year pelvic control rates were 94% and 100% with parallel opposed field and irregular four-field box technique, respectively. The incidence of small bowel toxicity significantly decreased in parallel opposed field technique.

11.4 Intensity-Modulated Radiotherapy

Most of the gynaecologic malignancies are now treated with IGRT/IMRT including VMAT in different parts of the world. It significantly reduces the dose of radiation received by the small bowel and bone marrow. It should be kept in mind to cover the full uterosacral ligament and to keep sufficient anterior margin to account for shifts.

Tyagi et al. [37] show that a uniform CTV margin of 1.5 cm would not include cervical CTV in 32% fractions with the IMRT technique. For the rapid regression of the tumour and its internal motion, IMRT re-planning at least in every other 2 weeks has to be done. PTV Margin of 1.0–1.5 cm, results in significant underdosing of CTV. That is why margins of 2–3 cm in antero-posterior direction are recommended and bladder volume at 150–300 cm^3 are recommended.

After the simulation, the images are transferred to the treatment planning station. GTV may include the cervix, uterus, and vagina.

In post-operative cases, CTV for the pelvic lymph nodes was based on RTOG atlas. In these patient's vagina is contoured after fusion of full bladder fusion with empty bladder fusion to account for vaginal mobility because of bladder filling.

The vaginal target volume is referred to as an integrated target volume. Adequate margin to CTV and PTV should be given. In trial RTOG 0921 post-operative trial, PTV of 7 mm around nodal contour is recommended and the prescribed dose should cover 97% of the vaginal PTV and nodal PTV. Dose to the normal tissue should be carefully recommended (V30% of small bowel receive <40 Gy), (V60% of rectosigmoid receive <40 Gy), (35% of bladder receive <45 Gy), and (15% of femoral head receive <35 Gy).

When a nodal boost is required, PET-scan fused based contouring should be done. To minimize small bowel toxicity, it is recommended that the absolute volume of small bowel receiving >15 Gy should be less than 120 cm^3.

Dose distribution with the IMRT technique is significantly better than those received by two-field or four-field conventional techniques. Ahmed et al. [38] found that for patients with para-aortic nodal involvement, the dose should be escalated to 60 Gy while sparing kidneys, spinal cord, small bowel, and bone marrow. Heron et al. [39] concluded that with the use of the IMRT technique reduction of dose 52% in small bowel, 66% for the rectum, and 36% for the bladder as compared with the 3D-CRT technique. The use of belly board in a prone position significantly reduces the dose received by the small bowel but it is highly unreproducible because of daily large anatomic shifts. Brixey et al. [40] and Lujan et al. [41] used the IMRT technique to spare bone marrow. Guerrero et al. [42] proposed IMRT with SIB. A dose of 50 Gy followed by a boost to 60–65 Gy to pelvic and para-aortic nodes. IMRT has a dosimetric advantage but it increases the incidence of a radiation-induced second cancer.

11.5 Image-Guided Radiation Therapy

In-room IGRT permits the visualization of bladder and rectum with the help of daily cone-beam CT. In young women with a large, mobile uterus, if an extended field is used, then there is concern uterus may be out of the field. At that time IGRT is used to confirm full coverage of CTV daily. Daily IGRT in-room demonstrates organ motion.

11.6 Sterotactic Body Radiotherapy

In SBRT highly conformal large fractions sizes are used for the nodal boost in isolated para-aortic node involvement. It should be noted that SBRT should be used after treating para-aortic node to a dose of 45 Gy by IMRT or four-field technique box. SBRT should not be the replacement of brachytherapy as it results in a significant increase in normal tissue doses with SBRT as compared to brachytherapy.

11.7 Midline Shielding in AP-PA Portals and Use of Parametrial Boost

Traditionally on the basis of institution and how much dose is delivered in brachytherapy midline shielding blocks used for the portion of the dose delivered with AP-PA portals. In the modern era of 3D Brachytherapy, midline shielding results in significant underdosing of the tumour and contributing large doses to the bladder, sigmoid, and rectum.

Many institutions previously placed midline block after completing the dose of EBRT of 45 Gy in 25 fractions to boost parametria or pelvic nodes in patients of persistent disease. For boost, the dose should be escalated to 50–60 Gy with a reduced AP/PA field. Fenkell et al. [43] compared parametrial midline shielding block in six patients with locally advanced cervical cancer treated with definitive chemoradiotherapy and MRI-based guided brachytherapy. Three planning was done, i.e. 45 Gy by four-field box technique, 9 Gy by AP/PA fields, and intracavitary MRI-guided brachytherapy boost of 28 Gy. After midline block, HR-CTV D90 remained less than 85%, and D2cc of bladder, rectum, and sigmoid increased by more than 50% of the boost dose. Therefore, the authors concluded that midline AP/PA block was not beneficial in patients receiving 3D image-planned brachytherapy.

11.8 Para-Aortic Node Irradiation

Patients are treated with 45–50 Gy to the para-aortic area followed by a sequential boost of 5–10 Gy to the enlarged lymph node preferably to be done with the IMRT technique. The 2-year local control after dose escalation to 63 Gy is 85% [44]. With the use of highly conformal techniques sparing of the stomach, liver, colon, and spinal cord were achieved. In the conventional technique, using the four-field box technique, para-aortic nodes can be irradiated. This can be done either with a long field or a separate pelvic or para-aortic field. This requires a gap calculation between the pelvic and the para-aortic portals to avoid overlap and excessive dose to the small intestine. The superior boundary of the para-aortic field is at T12-L1 interspace, lower margin at L5-S1. The width of para-aortic portals determined by different modalities like CT scan, MRI, Lymphangiography, FDG-PET Scans, or IV pyelography outlined the ureters with the goal to treat all tissue between the right and left psoas muscle. The spinal dose can be kept at <45 Gy by placing a 2 cm wide 5-half-value layer shield on the posterior portal. Rates of toxicity with IMRT are very less compared with the conventional four-field box technique but in case of dose escalation with the simultaneous integrated boost to large nodes next to duodenum must be given cautiously given the risk of duodenal perforation.

A high energy photon beam of 10 MV or higher than this should be used. As it decreases the dose of radiation peripheral normal tissue and provides more homogenous dose distribution in the central pelvis.

11.9 Hyperfractinated or Accelerated Hyperfractionated Radiation Therapy

RTOG 88-05 conducted a phase II study of hyper fractionation. In this study 1.2 Gy to the whole pelvis twice daily at 4–6 h intervals, 5 days/week with brachytherapy to 81 patients with locally advanced carcinoma of the cervix. The total dose to the whole pelvis was 24–48 Gy followed by LDR brachytherapy to deliver 85 Gy to point A and 65 Gy to the lateral pelvic nodes. Grigsby et al. updated results and noted that EBRT was completed in 71 patients (88% of cases). The 5-year cumulative rate of grade 3 and 4 late effects in patients with stage IB2 or IIB was 7% and for stage IIIA or IV A was 12%. The absolute survival was 48% at 8 years and disease-free survival was 33%.

12 General Management

12.1 Invasive Disease

The integrated approach consists of a gynaecologic oncologist and radiation oncologist should be used in treating the patient to ca cervix. The standard treatment for patients with stage IB2 to IVA cervical cancer is the use of concurrent chemoradiotherapy. It is recommended to use cisplatin-based-concurrent chemoradiation.

12.2 Stage IA

Micro invasive carcinoma stage IA includes invasive carcinoma diagnosed only by microscopically. The diagnosis can be confirmed by conization. In stage IA lesion >1 mm in depth can be treated with conization with clear margins and the patient should be in careful follow-up [45]. According to guidelines minimum, an 8–10 mm margin should be there in conization for clearance [46]. The prognostic factor for recurrence is close margins and lymph vascular invasion.

Early invasive carcinoma of cervix [Stage IA2] was treated with total abdominal hysterectomy or modified radical hysterectomy or simple conization or radical trachelectomy [47]. Inoperable patients treated with intracavitary radioactive sources 60–75 Gy to point A using LDR brachytherapy in 2 fractions or with HDR brachytherapy, approximately 10 fractions of 5 Gy per fraction. When the depth of penetration of the tumour is less than 3 mm, the incidence of lymph node metastasis is less than 1%. Therefore, lymph node dissection and pelvic radiotherapy are generally not required [48]. Tumour control with all the methods is more than 95%. Vaginal trachelectomy and laparoscopic lymphadenectomy should be used in young patients to preserve fertility.

12.3 Stage IB to IIA

The treatment of choice for patients of stage IB to IIA is either radical surgery or chemoradiation. The preference to choose one treatment over others depends on many factors like the combined opinion of the gynaecological oncologist and radiation oncologist, the general condition of the patient, and the characteristics of the lesion. An operation is done usually in young patients to reserve ovaries and to avoid premature menopause. But it has been seen that ovarian function is preserved in only 50–60% of patients treated with surgery instead of irradiation. The survival benefit found in postmenopausal women treated with chemoradiation as compared to the surgery along with no postoperative complications is same. In RTOG 90-01 for IB to IIA patients, 8-year overall survival was 55% with RT alone versus 78% with concurrent chemoradiation [49].

One of the randomized study done by Landoni et al. [50], randomized patients to surgery and radiotherapy. Post-operative irradiation was delivered to women with surgical stage pT2 or greater, <3 mm of cervical stromal invasion or cut through positive margins or positive pelvic nodes. After a median follow-up of 87 months, 5-year overall survival and DFS rates were nearly identical in surgery and radiotherapy. The recurrence rate is 25% in surgery and 26% in the RT group. The surgery group had severe morbidity compared to the irradiation group. In a meta-analysis done for patients' stage IA2, IB1 and IIA cervical cancer showed significant benefit in survival when chemotherapy was given concurrently with radiation.

A prospective randomized study done by Perez et al. [51] in patients with stage IB or IIA ca cervix treated with RT alone and irradiation and surgery (20 Gy to the whole pelvis, one ICRT followed by radical hysterectomy with pelvic lymphadenectomy 2–6 weeks later).

The 10-year cancer-specific survival (CSS) rates for patients with stage IB non-bulky tumours treated with RT alone or RT with surgery was 84% with either modality. For stage IB bulky tumours, 10-year CSS was 61% and 68%, respectively. For patients with stage IIb non-bulky tumours treated with RT or combined with surgery, 10-year CSS rates were 72% and 65%, respectively.

Patients who have undergone radical hysterectomy are considered for post-operative radiotherapy if they have high-risk features like positive pelvic lymph nodes, positive margins, or parametrial extension. Patients with deep stromal invasion, vascular/lymphatic permeation, and large tumour size are candidates for postoperative irradiation. Chemoradiation after operation significantly reduces the pelvic recurrences and distant metastasis as compared to RT only and there was no significant difference in gastrointestinal side effects. A study was done by Rotman et al. [52] in patients of stage IB cervical cancer treated by radical hysterectomy and pelvic lymphadenectomy followed by postoperative radiation in the presence of positive pelvic nodes or node-negative high-risk factors like greater than one-third stromal invasion, LVI, and large size tumour. He concluded that statistically significant reduction in recurrence in the irradiation group, with a recurrence-free rate at 2 years of 88% versus 79% for the irradiation and no further treatment groups, respectively. There is no significant difference in the survival group. A meta-analysis of trials done of stage IB1 to IIA cervical cancer found that women who received postoperative RT had a lower risk of disease progression at 5 years.

After surgery depending on the extent of resection of the vagina, there is an increased risk of recurrences at the vaginal cuff. Although vaginal brachytherapy for cervical cancer is most commonly used as a boost after EBRT. According to the American brachytherapy society guidelines vaginal cuff boost should be given to patients with less than radical hysterectomy, close or positive margins, large or deeply invasive tumours, parametrial or vaginal involvement, and extensive LVI. In the patients receiving postoperative radiation care should be taken in case of designing treatment techniques including intracavitary insertions because, after removal of the uterus, bladder and rectosigmoid may be closer to the radioactive source. Vascular supply is affected, and adhesions can prevent the mobilization of the small bowel. HDR-brachytherapy is useful in the patients after surgery because it prevents the prolonged immobilization that is required in LDR brachytherapy.

12.4 Stage I B2 to IV A

The standard treatment for the patients of stage IB2 to IV A is external radiotherapy and brachytherapy combined followed by concurrent chemotherapy. It has been found that when cisplatin is used with radiation concomitantly, the substantial effect of cell killing is observed. Coughlin and Richmond [53, 54] suggested two mechanisms of radiation enhancement with the use of cisplatin i.e. hypoxic or oxygenated cells, free radicals with the altered binding of cisplatin to DNA are formed at the time of radiation and secondly, interaction inhibits the repair of sublethal damage.

In a meta-analysis done, suggested concomitant chemotherapy and radiation improved tumour control and overall survival. The maximal benefit was found in early stage disease (stage I and II). The absolute survival benefit was 12% but patients receiving chemoradiation have a higher incidence of hematologic toxicities and gastrointestinal toxicities.

Patients with Stage IV disease can be treated either EBRT to pelvis with concurrent chemotherapy followed by intracavitary or interstitial brachytherapy and additional parametrial irradiation or with pelvic exenteration.

There are many randomized trials supporting chemoradiation in patients of ca cervix. The GOG 85, Whitney et al. [55] conducted a randomized trial in which patients of stage IIB to IV A and negative para-aortic irradiation treated with EBRT (51 Gy) combined with 30 Gy to point A with LDR brachytherapy. 127 patients received 5-FU (1 g/m^2 for 4 days) and cisplatin (50 mg/m^2 on Day 1, 29, and 30–33) and 191 patients received hydroxyurea (80 mg/kg orally twice weekly). After a median follow-up of 8.7 years, the 5-year survival rate in the cisplatin/5-FU arm was 60% compared with 47% with the hydroxyurea arm.

After that three-arm randomized trial, i.e. GOG 120 done by Rose et al. [56] comparing irradiation with cisplatin, irradiation with hydroxyurea, and irradiation with cisplatin, hydroxyurea, and 5-FU. Overall survival is more in two groups receiving cisplatin drugs.

Hematological toxicity is more in the group treated with three drugs.

The RTOG 90-01 conducted a randomized study in patients of stage IB to IIA with positive pelvic nodes and patients of stage IIB to IV A treated with pelvic and para-aortic irradiation or pelvic irradiation with three cycles of concurrent chemotherapy with cisplatin (75 mg/m^2) and 4-day infusion of 5-FU (1000 mg/m^2). Results published by Eifel et al. [49], i.e. after a median follow-up of 6.6 years overall survival rate with irradiation with chemotherapy arm was 67% compared with 41% in the irradiation only arm. DFS rates were 66% and 36%, respectively.

Southwest oncology group 8797, i.e. Peters et al. [57] did a study on patients with stage IA1, IB, or IIA carcinoma of the cervix with pelvic lymph nodes, positive parametrial involvement, and positive surgical margins at the time of primary radical hysterectomy with total pelvic lymphadenectomy. In this 127 patients are treated with EBRT with 5-FU infusion and cisplatin and 116 were treated with irradiation alone. They concluded the 3-year survival rate for women on the chemotherapy arm was 87% compared with 77% for women on the pelvic irradiation arm. An updated analysis done with a median follow-up of 5.2 years, they reported 5-year survival of 80% versus 66% favoring the chemoradiation arm.

In GOG 123, i.e. by Keys et al. [58] enrolled 369 women in their study. 183 patients of bulky disease (>4 cm) of stage IB cervix cancer with negative pelvic and para-aortic lymph nodes radiologically and surgically determined were randomized to treated with EBRT and brachytherapy followed by extra fascial hysterectomy and 186 received EBRT and brachytherapy with weekly cisplatin (40 mg/m^2) followed by extra fascial hysterectomy. After a median follow-up of 101 months, the 6-year progression-free survival rate for women treated with irradiation and cisplatin was 71% compared with 61% for patients treated with RT alone. The 6-year overall survival rates were 78% and 64%, respectively.

In 2005 Meta-analysis of concurrent chemoradiation and radiation therapy found and concluded that chemoradiation improves overall survival and PFS whether or not cisplatin was used, with absolute benefits of 10% and 13%, respectively.

Another Meta-analysis done in 2008 compared chemoradiotherapy to radiation found that there was a 6% improvement in 5-year overall survival with concurrent chemoradiation. There was a reduction in both local and distant recurrences. But the use of Chemoradiation leads to increased hematologic and gastrointestinal toxicity.

In multivariate analyses, the number of chemotherapy cycles was independently predictive of PFS and overall survival. Patients who received fewer than six cycles of chemotherapy had a worse PFS and overall stage. Advanced stage of cancer, longer time taken for RT completion, and absence of brachytherapy were also associated with decreased overall survival and Progression-free survival.

13 Side Effects of Radiation

In the case of post-operative radiation, complications of additional therapy are always expected. The main side effects of radiation are bowel, bladder, skin changes, lymphedema, and sexual function. In the presence of intestinal adhesions in the pelvis, enteric complications such as obstruction, fistula, or dysfunctions were reported in 24% of the patients [59].

Lower BMI is associated with an increase in toxicity. BMI of less than 18.5 was also associated with a decrease in overall survival. The complication rate tends to be higher when irradiation is combined with surgery because of increased incidence of injury to the ureter and bladder which can lead to urethral stricture or uretero-vaginal or vesicovaginal fistula.

14 Brachytherapy in Cervical Cancer

Brachytherapy is an integral part of treatment to deliver optimal curative doses of radiotherapy for Cervical cancer in both radical and adjuvant setting. It has been used for the treatment of cervical cancer since the first medical uses of radium after its discovery. In modern radiotherapy, brachytherapy is mainly used as a technique to boost the primary tumour to high doses (Equivalent dose up to 90 Gy) after 45–50 Gy EBRT to the pelvis. Even in this era of conformal EBRT techniques, Brachytherapy still remains quintessential to deliver best conformal radiotherapy doses to the cervix while respecting normal tissue tolerances. This is because the cervix is ideal in many ways for delivering intracavitary brachytherapy [60], viz:

1. The endocervical canal and vaginal vault have a very favorable anatomy that allows placement of radioactive sources with specifically designed applicators.
2. The mucosa of the cervix and vaginal fornices have very high tolerance to radiation doses.
3. Rapid dose fall off with distance from brachytherapy applications is particularly advantageous in limiting dose to nearby organs at risk (bladder, rectum) while delivering high dose to the tumour in the cervix.

Over the century, however, brachytherapy for cervical cancer has undergone paradigm changes in terms of better understanding of dose prescription, modernization of applicators and treatment planning, and incorporation of newer imaging modalities into its armory. When radium was first used for treatment of cervical cancer, there was a lack of knowledge about the radiation effects on the tumour and the normal tissues. In the absence of clear understanding, brachytherapy treatments were mostly empirical with definite amounts of radium (milligram) being applied to patients in specific applicators over a period of time (hours). Gradually, experts began to realize the need for standardization of brachytherapy treatments and the concept of "Dosimetric Systems" was introduced. Some of the most popular intracavitary and interstitial dosimetric systems developed around the world are enlisted below.

Intracavitary Dosimetric Systems

1. Stockholm System: Developed by Gosta Forrsell in 1913 at Radiumhemmet, Stockhlom and later modified by James Heyman and Hans Kottmeier.
2. Paris system (Claude Regard): Developed by Claude Regaud in 1922 in Institut du Radium, Paris.
3. Manchester system (Todd and Meredith) [61, 62]: Developed by M.C. Todd and W.J. Meredith in 1938 in Holt Radium Institute, Manchester and subsequently revised in 1953

Interstitial Dosimetric Systems

1. Quimby System [63]: Developed by Edith Quimby at Memorial Hospital, New York in 1930s
2. Manchester System (Patterson and Parker) [64]
3. Paris System (Pierquin and Dutreix) [65]

Most of these systems used fixed geometry sources and applicators and hence in today's era of modern image based brachytherapy are no longer relevant and shall not be discussed further. However, the Manchester System (by Todd and Meredith) of intracavitary brachytherapy which first described dose prescription based on patient's anatomy paved the way for further standardization of brachytherapy in cervical cancer [62]. They had opined that the dose limiting area when prescribing radiation to carcinoma cervix by intracavitary brachytherapy was a region in the medial edge of the broad ligament where the uterine vessels cross the ureter. This roughly pyramidal shaped area with its base resting on the lateral fornix of vagina and apex curving around the anteverted uterus was defined as the "paracervical triangle" (Fig. 14). The tolerance of this region was thought to be the main limiting factor in brachytherapy of cervix and hence they defined a point in this area for dose prescription, which could be anatomically compared from patient to patient. This "Point A" was defined to be located 2 cm lateral to the central canal of the uterus and 2 cm from the mucous membrane of the lateral fornix in the axis of the uterus (Fig. 14).

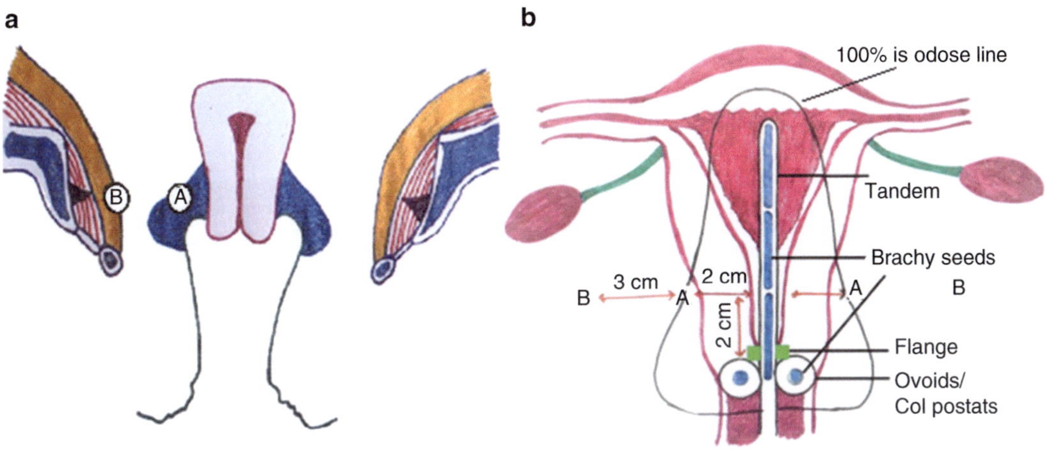

Fig. 14 Sketch representing Points and areas defined by Manchester System of Intracavitary Brachytherapy for Carcinoma Cervix. (**a**) Paracervical triangle (in blue) and Points A and B in relation to the cervix uteri and pelvis. (**b**) Points A and B in relation to the intrauterine tube and vaginal ovoids. (Artwork: Dr. Faridha Jane Momin)

Intrauterine tubes supported by a flange at the cervix and vaginal ovoid applicators of various lengths and diameters, respectively, were loaded with units of radium. The loading of applicators was based on a set of rules defining the relationship, position and activity of the radium sources to achieve consistent dose rates at Point A. They prescribed a dose of 8000 Roentgen in two sessions of 72 h each separated by 4–7 days. Along with the dose limiting Point A, another point in the pelvis was defined to estimate the lateral fall off of brachytherapy dose which was also considered clinically important. This point, "Point B," located 5 cm from the mid-line and on the same level as Point A, is representative of the dose received by obturator nodes near the pelvic sidewall (Fig. 14).

The definition of Point A was subsequently modified in 1953 by Todd and Meredith as the lateral vaginal fornix was not properly visualized on a radiograph. The modified point A (designated Ao) was defined 2 cm lateral to the central canal of the uterus and 2 cm from the external os which corresponded with the flange [61]. The concept of dose prescription to a point made Manchester system the most acceptable of all dosimetric systems of its time and thereafter. The idea was to deliver a specific dose rate to Point A (55 R per hour) by strict rules of applicator loading, no matter which combination of intrauterine tube and ovoids was used. The contribution of total dose at Point A was two-thirds from the intrauterine tube loading and one-third from radium in the vaginal ovoids. Based on these principles of Manchester Dosimetric System, with the improvement in technology and use of radioactive sources other than radium, the brachytherapy applications in cervical cancer was improvized.

The International Commission on Radiation Units and Measurements (ICRU) report no. 38 was published in 1985 with an aim to further standardize dose and volume specifications in gynaecological brachytherapy [66]. Apart from points A and B already established in intracavitary brachytherapy, this report introduced a few more critical points with regards to dose received by organs at risk (Rectal Point and Bladder Point) and draining lymph nodes (Lymphatic Trapezoid and Pelvic Wall reference Point). The location of these points were defined on orthogonal radiographs (antero-posterior and lateral views) with reference to loading of sources in the tandem and ovoid and visualized bony landmarks on X-ray. The Bladder and Rectal points served as surro-

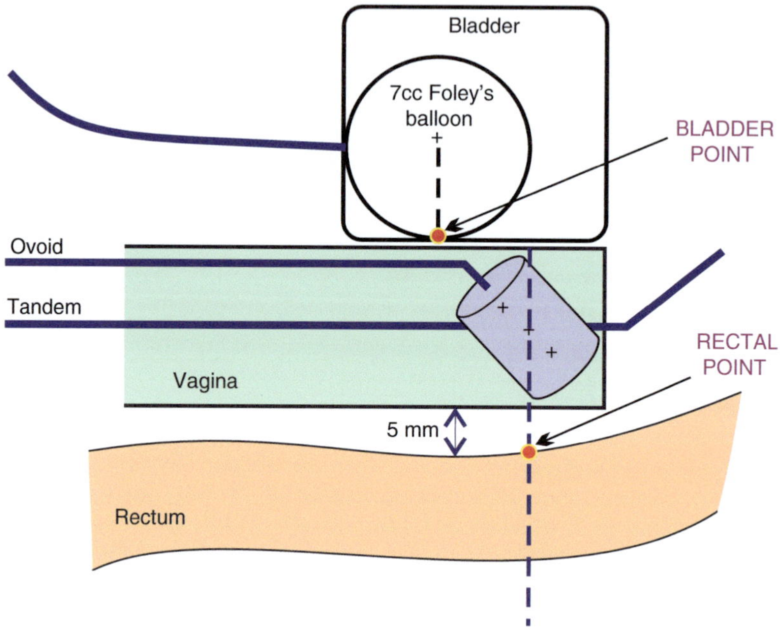

Fig. 15 Schematic representative diagram showing location of the ICRU 38 Bladder and Rectal Point on a lateral radiograph. The Bladder point is obtained on the posterior surface of the Foley's catheter balloon (filled up to 7 cm³) on a line drawn antero-posteriorly through the center of the balloon. The Rectal point is located on a line drawn from the middle of the ovoid sources, 5 mm behind the posterior vaginal wall. (Artwork: Ph. Surachandra Singha)

gates for representation and recording the dose received and subsequent toxicity correlation in these two critical organs at risk. The Lymphatic Trapezoid was representative of the lower para-aortic, common iliac and external iliac lymph nodes while the Pelvic Wall Reference Point represented absorbed dose to the lateral parametrium and obturator nodes. These points are shown schematically in Figs. 15 and 16.

14.1 Basic Principles of Intracavitary Brachytherapy (ICBT)

All ICBT applications should be performed under anesthesia/sedation. The applicator geometry consists of an intrauterine central tandem with a flange at the level of the cervix accompanied by two ovoids/colpostats in lateral vaginal fornices. Some of the basic requirements of an ideal ICBT application are:

1. The position of the tandem relative to the pelvis should be optimum: it should be midway between bladder and S1-S2 and one-third of the way between S1-S2 and pubic symphysis.
2. The tandem should bisect the ovoids. The axis of the tandem should be central to the ovoids
3. The maximum diameter of the ovoids that can fit into the fornix should be applied (Diameter may be increased by adding caps). They should be separated by 0.5–1 cm to allow for insertion of the flange on the tandem.
4. The tandem should be as long as the anatomy of the patient permits. Increase in tandem length increases the "lateral throw-off" of the dose thus increasing the dose contribution at point B relative to the uterine cavity surface dose. The concept is illustrated in Fig. 17a.
5. The ovoids with the largest possible diameter that allows insertion of the tandem flange between them without causing their downward displacement should be used. This limits dose mucosal dose to the normal vaginal fornices. The concept is illustrated in Fig. 17b.
6. The bladder and rectum should be pushed as far away from the implant as possible by packing.

The goal of the implant dosimetry is to deliver highest possible dose to the cervix and the para-cervical area, while respecting the mucosal tolerance of the lower vagina, bladder, and rectum. With the development of newer technologies and

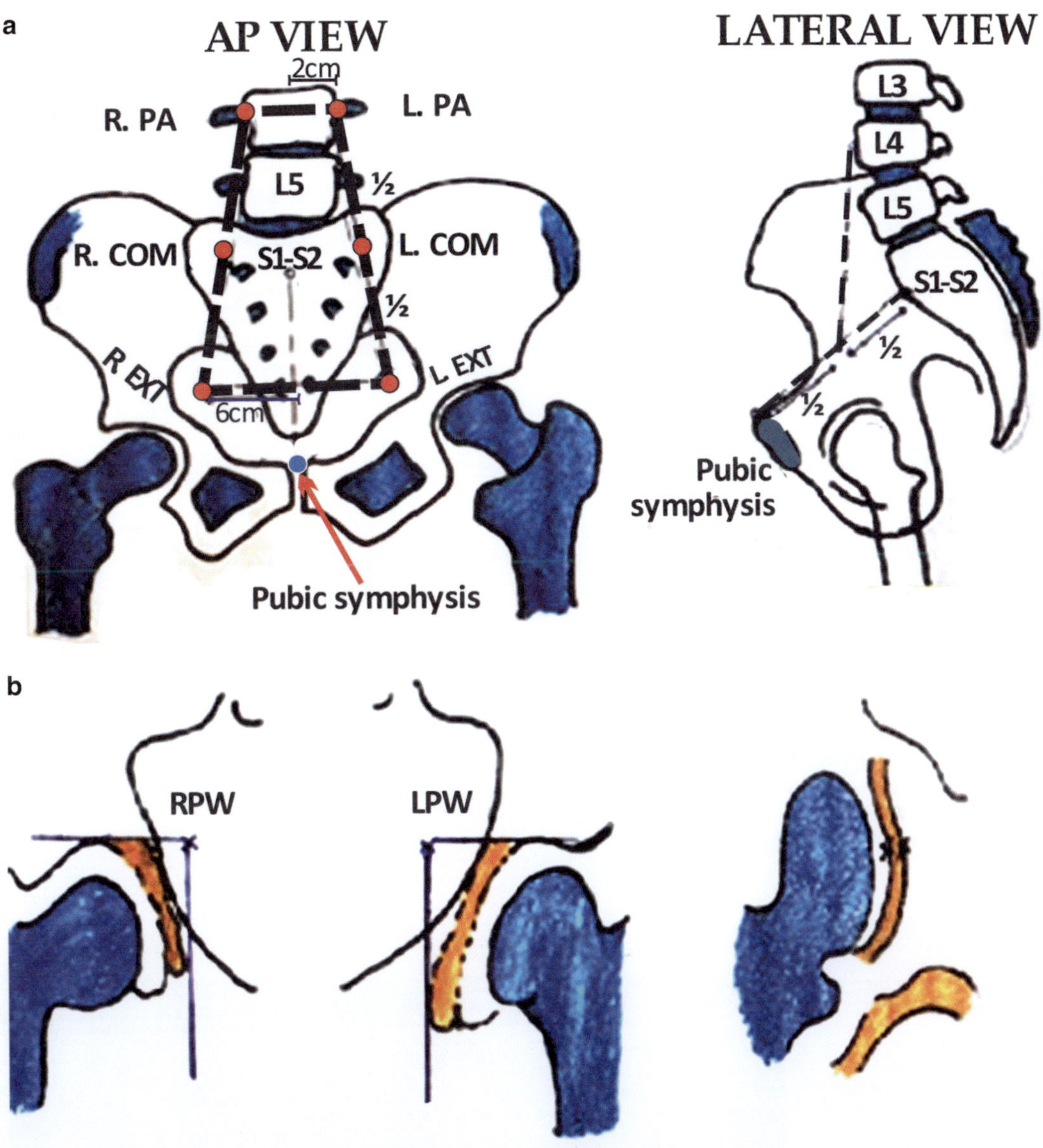

Fig. 16 The locations of the Lymphatic Trapezoid (**a**) and the Pelvic Wall Reference Point (**b**) on the antero-posterior and lateral radiographs as per ICRU [107]. (Artwork: Dr. Faridha Jane Momin and Ph. Surachandra Singha)

the herald of HDR afterloading stepping sources which were smaller in size, the ICBT applicators also were modified and developed. Yet the basic concept and design mimicked the established methods of the classical ICBT systems. The modern HDR ICBT applicators are now smaller in diameter than those used in LDR era and are compatible to imaging by Computed Tomography (CT) or Magnetic Resonance Imaging (MRI). Figure 18 shows some of the most popular modern ICBT applicators commonly used. The ideal dosimetry that should be achieved in a proper ICBT application is shown in Fig. 19a, b. Optimal placement and Point A dose prescription shows a "pear shaped" dose distribution encompassing the cervix and the paracervical area on the coronal plane and a "banana shaped" dose distribution on the sagittal plane that limits dose to large

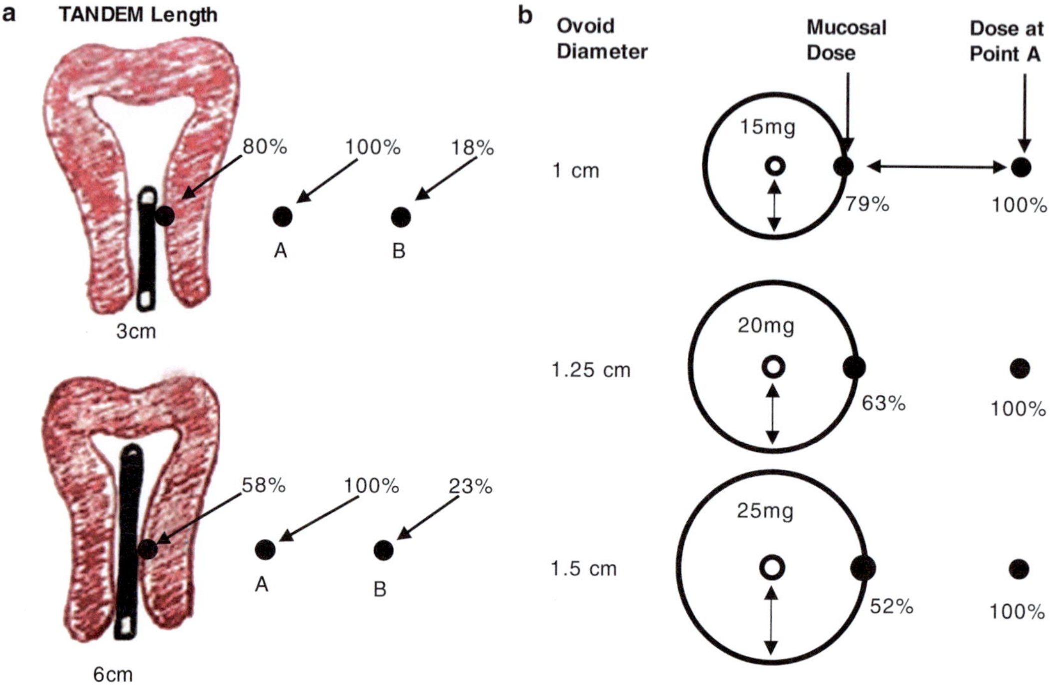

Fig. 17 Sketch representing basic principles of Intracavitary brachytherapy application. (**a**) Increase in Point B dose (18–23%) with relative decrease in uterine cavity surface dose (80–58%) as intrauterine tandem length increases from 3 to 6 cm with the same prescription at Point A. (**b**) Decrease in vaginal mucosal dose observed with increasing ovoid diameter with Point A dose remaining the same. (Artwork: Dr. Faridha Jane Momin and Ph. Surachandra Singha)

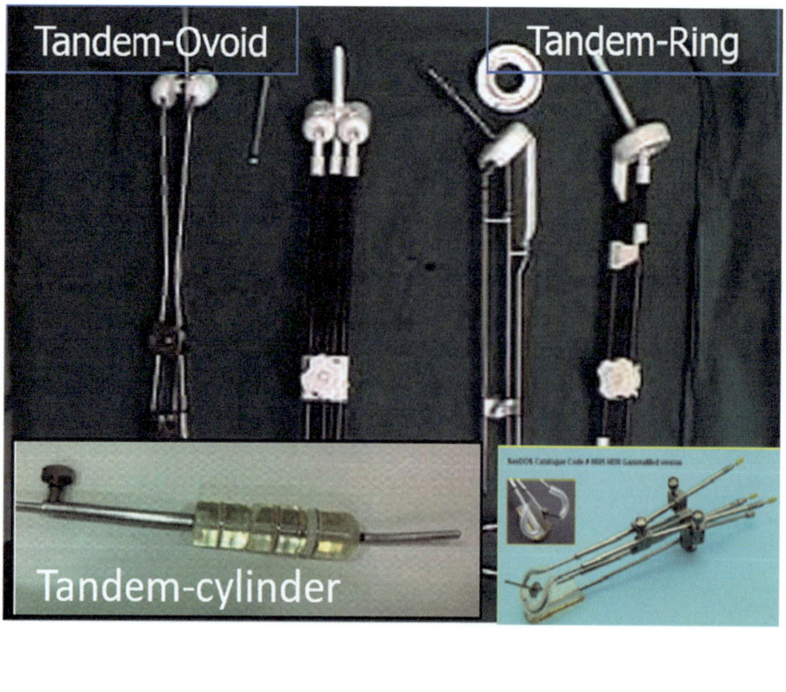

Fig. 18 Some of the widely used intracavitary brachytherapy applicators designed to obtain source geometry as per the historic dosimetry systems. (Image: Courtesy, Dr. Umesh Mahantshetty—Director, Homi Bhabha Cancer Hospital and Research Centre, Vishakhapatnam and Ex-Professor, Radiation Oncology, Tata Memorial Hospital, Mumbai)

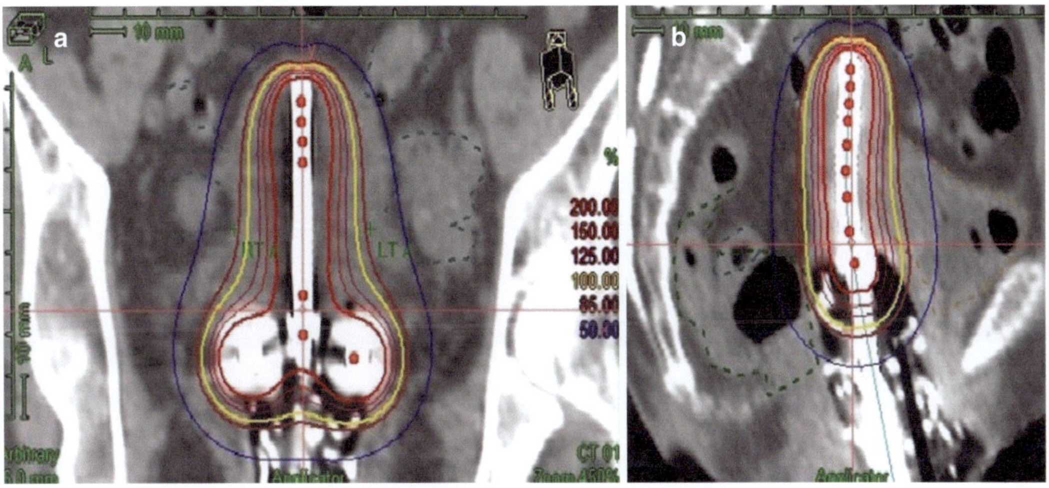

Fig. 19 Ideal intracavitary brachytherapy dosimetry in carcinoma cervix with standard applicators. (**a**) "Pear-shape" dose profile in coronal section, (**b**) "Banana-shape" dose profile in sagittal section. The different colors represent different isodose lines—Navy blue: 50%, Yellow: 100%, Red: 200% isodose lines

areas of rectum and bladder in the immediate vicinity of the applicators [60, 66].

14.2 Image Based Brachytherapy and Prescription to Volumes

With incorporation of volumetric imaging like CT scan or MRI and development of new computerized treatment planning systems for brachytherapy, it was understood that prescription to point A was not accurately representative of the dose received by the tumour in the cervix and parametrium. These reference points A and B showed significant variation in position from patient to patient and even for the same patient for different fractions of applications, leading to inconsistency in dose prescriptions. Thus the need to shift dose prescription from points to volumes was felt. In fact, ICRU 38 had introduced the concept of reference volume in treatment of cervical carcinoma in brachytherapy first in 1985. In the early twenty-first century Haie-Meder et al. [67] and Potter et al. [68], on behalf of the Groupe Europeen de Curietherapie and the European Society for Radiotherapy and Oncology (GEC-ESTRO) working group, proposed the target concept and reporting recommendations for brachytherapy in cervical cancer using 3D image based treatment planning. They emphasized the need for MRI assessment of cervical cancer to delineate the gross tumour volume (GTV) and clinical target volume (CTV) before and after EBRT and also during each fraction of brachytherapy so that dose prescription can be optimally adapted to the actual tumour volume. They also introduced concepts of dose volume parameters for dose prescription and recording of doses for the organs at risks.

The prerequisites for Image Guided Intracavitary Brachytherapy (IGBT) includes:

- Proper clinical examination and documentation of the disease at baseline, after EBRT and at each brachytherapy application.
- MRI at diagnosis, prior to brachytherapy and after each brachytherapy application.
- Advanced treatment planning system that allows 3D delineation of the tumour and OARs and compatible with planning and optimization of dose
- HDR brachytherapy applicators that are MRI compatible
- HDR brachytherapy afterloader treatment unit

The volume concepts of GEC-ESTRO for IGBT [67] is depicted diagrammatically in Fig. 20. The region depicted as high risk (HR) is

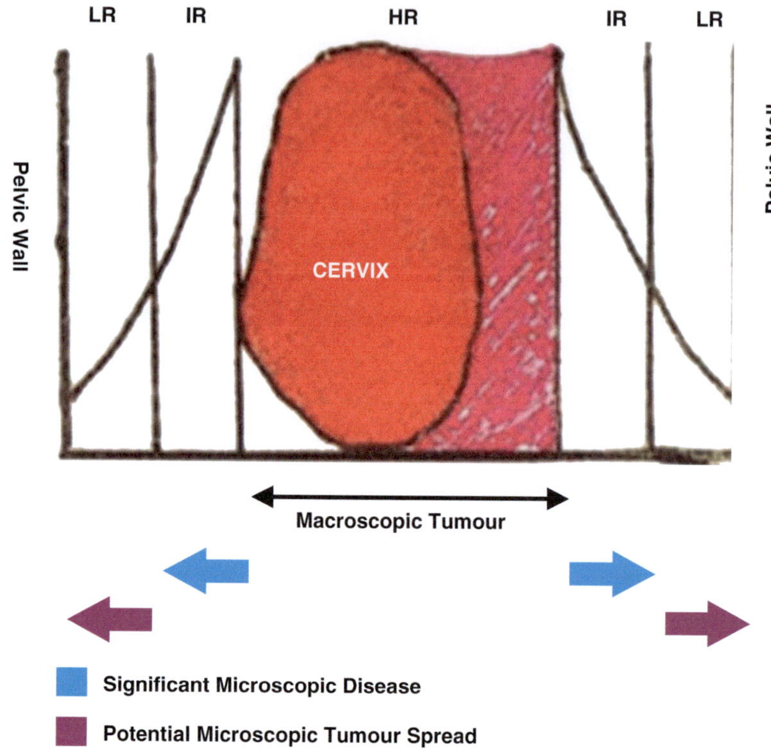

Fig. 20 Sketch representing the volume concepts of GEC-ESTRO for Image Guided Brachytherapy in cervical cancer. HR: High Risk, IR: Intermediate Risk, LR: Low Risk. (Artwork: Dr. Faridha Jane Momin and Ph. Surachandra Singha)

the area harboring the macroscopic tumour (GTV) and presumed extra cervical lesions (resolving tumour tissue) at the time of brachytherapy that needs to receive maximum permissible dose, while the intermediate risk region (IR) is the region of initial tumour prior to EBRT that is presumed to harbor significant microscopic disease. The low risk (LR) area that stretches up to the pelvic sidewall is generally not encompassed in brachytherapy. Based on these concepts of high risk CTV (HR-CTV) and intermediate risk CTV (IR-CTV) have been proposed for dose prescription by them [68]. The HR-CTV includes the GTV at brachytherapy by clinical and radiological assessment to include the whole cervix and presumed residual disease extensions (gray zones) on MRI. The planning aim is usually to deliver a total dose (combined EBRT and BT doses) of 80–90 Gy EQD2. The IR-CTV is HRCTV plus safety margins in the direction of disease extent at diagnosis and represents the GTV at diagnosis. The safety margin for IR-CTV is usually 1–1.5 cm cranially, 0.5 cm antero-posteriorly and 1 cm laterally. The dose delivered to IRCTV should be at least 60 Gy EQD2 (similar to 60 Gy volume concept of ICRU 38) [67, 68]. These concepts are depicted in Fig. 21.

14.3 Brachytherapy Planning and Dose Prescription in IGBT

Once the appropriate applicators are applied for adequate coverage of the tumour, MRI imaging is done. The dosimetrist reconstructs the applicators and planning principles include standard tandem and vaginal source loading (as per Institutional practice), interstitial needle/tube loading if applicable, optimization of doses (dwell positions and dwell times) to achieve optimum doses to the target (HR CTV) and OAR. Inverse or graphical optimization is usually discouraged for cervical cancer brachytherapy planning due to the advantages of desired high dose gradient and heterogeneity within the target.

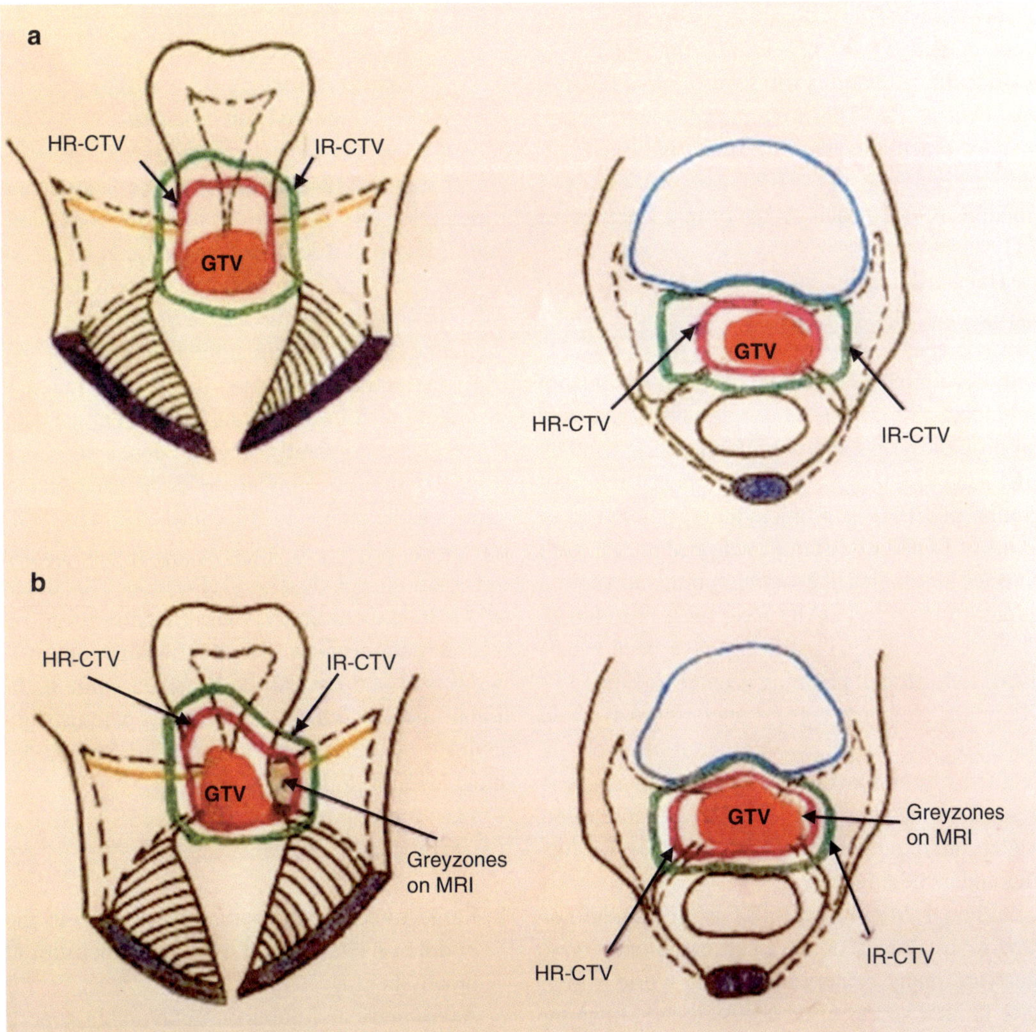

Fig. 21 Diagrammatic representation of GEC-ESTRO recommendation for Image Guided Brachytherapy planning in cervical carcinoma (Coronal: Left, Axial: Right). The GTV represents the gross tumour in the cervix in the two clinical scenarios (**a**) and (**b**). Pink outline shows the High Risk-CTV, Green outline shows the Intermediate Risk-CTV. In the clinical scenario (**a**), the GTV at brachytherapy is confined to the cervix. In scenario (**b**), there are residual gray zones in the left parametrium (seen in MRI) and hence the HR-CTV is extended to include this region. (Artwork: Dr. Faridha Jane Momin)

Various dose volume parameters related to the target and OAR are recorded and reported as per the GEC-ESTRO/ICRU 89 recommendations (references—Radiother. Oncol 2006, ICRU 89) [68, 69]. For target, the minimum dose within most exposed 90% of the volume of interest (D90) of the HR-CTV and IR-CTV are used as indices for target coverage evaluation. For organs at risk, i.e. bladder, rectum and sigmoid the minimum dose to the most irradiated tissue volume of 0.1 cm^3, 1 cm^3, and 2 cm^3 volumes (D 0.1 cm^3, D 1 cm^3, D 2 cm^3, respectively) are recommended for recording and reporting since they correlate with the spectrum of late toxicities including fistula, ulceration and telangiectasis [69].

There are no strict recommendations for the doses to target and OAR. However, with the limited literature published so far, a minimum total dose (EBRT + BT) of 80–85 Gy EQD2 to HR CTV achieves excellent local control rates and D

2 cm^3 doses of less than 65–70 Gy EQD2 for Rectum and 75–90 Gy EQD2 for bladder to restrict the probability of severe late toxicities less than 3–5%. The most popular and recommended brachytherapy dose fractionation schedules after 45–50 Gy EBRT are: 30 Gy in 5 fractions of 6 Gy each or 28 Gy in 4 fractions of 7 Gy each.

The ICRU report 89 published in 2013 has amalgamated the concepts of IGBT laid down by GEC-ESTRO [67, 68] and other groups [70, 71] with its original ICRU 38 report [66]. Apart from upholding the volume concepts and parameters for dose prescription and evaluation proposed by GEC-ESTRO, they have also proposed the integration of EBRT and brachytherapy volumes in terms of EQD2 of different volumes at risk [69]. New terminologies like vaginal point and vaginal reference length as OARs have been introduced. Three levels of dose reporting have been established for different planning scenarios: Level 1—Minimum requirements, Level 2—Advanced standard, and Level 3—Research-oriented. A detailed discussion of this exhaustive report is beyond the scope of this chapter and interested readers are requested to refer to the report for further understanding [69].

Although MRI based IGBT is the standard of care in treatment of cervical carcinoma now, there are many centers across the world which have limited access or no access to MR Imaging for brachytherapy planning. CT volumetric Imaging seems to be a practical alternative. As compared to MRI, CT imaging has its limitations in defining the targets at brachytherapy. However, in the recent past several publications suggest that with careful consideration to clinical examination and documentation, appropriate CT protocol (IV contrast, bladder/rectal contrast) with or without use of real-time trans-rectal ultrasonography during brachytherapy shows comparable results for target delineation [72]. Based on clinical scenarios, several guidelines and recommendations have been reported now for CT based contouring which may help to improve the quality of brachytherapy across the globe [73–75]. Further research and clinical evidence with CT based IGABT for cervical cancer is warranted.

14.4 Interstitial Combined with Intracavitary Brachytherapy (IS + ICBT) for Cervical Carcinoma

Using standard tandem and ovoid or tandem and ring applicators and optimization, the maximum lateral width of 100% isodose line can be safely achieved up to 2.5 cm from the tandem. In clinical situations where the HRCTV volume is contoured beyond 2–2.5 cm at the level of point “A” from the tandem, standard ICBT planning will invariably result in either sub-optimal target coverage or significantly higher doses to OAR (Fig. 10). In these clinical scenarios, use of interstitial needles/tubes in the parametria with optimization helps to achieve adequate lateral throw-off of high doses and also reduce the doses to OAR. Accordingly, with needles/tubes in medial parametrium, target coverage up to a width of 3–3.5 cm can be achieved while additional needles/tubes in lateral parametrium achieves adequate coverage of 3.5–4.5 cm width at the level of point “A.”

The most common indications of IS + ICBT in gynaecological malignancy are [69]:

1. Large tumour bulk with extension up to the middle or lateral third of the parametrium at brachytherapy
2. Asymmetrical tumours—unfavorable topography of target and OAR in relation to standard applicators
3. Tumour extending up to distal vagina or into the paracolpos
4. Large tumours in vaginal vault—post-hysterectomy recurrence.

Classical approach for advanced Intracavitary + Interstitial BT implantation includes use of perineal templates like Syed Neblett [76] or Martinez Universal Perineal Interstitial Template (MUPIT) [77]. However, these procedures are associated with limitations including loss of parallelism, many more needles to cover small targets, inaccurate geometry since needle entry is far away from the target etc. Moreover, there is a large learning curve to establish the use of these

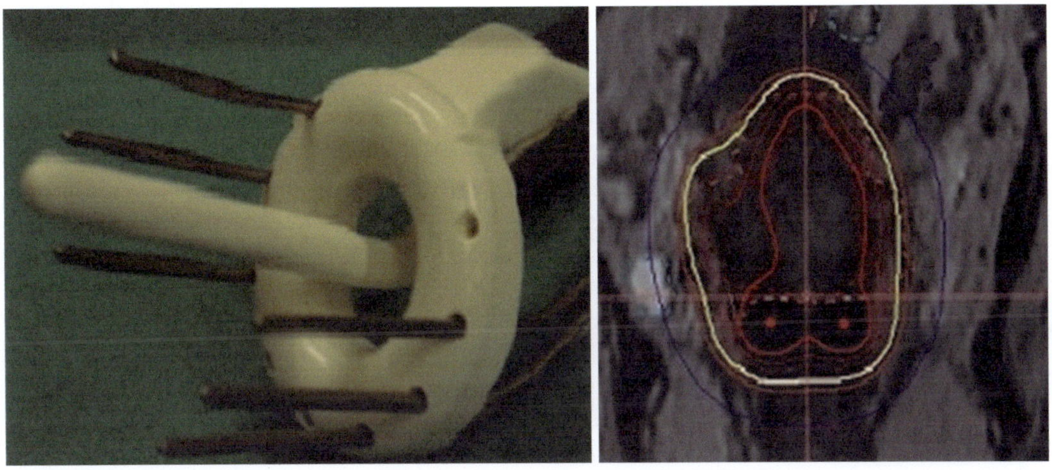

Fig. 22 The Vienna applicator (on the left): a modified intracavitary plus interstitial tandem-ring applicator with holes drilled into the ring that accommodates needles parallel to the plane of the tandem. The isodose profile of a case treated with Vienna applicator (on the right) with the 100% isodose line (yellow colored) showing a more lateral throw-off than the standard pear-shaped dose distribution due to the additional needles. (Credits: Dr. Umesh Mahantshetty Director, Homi Bhabha Cancer Hospital and Research Centre, Vishakhapatnam and Ex-Professor, Radiation Oncology, Tata Memorial Hospital, Mumbai)

classical implantation techniques which are also associated with higher severe late complications. Modern interstitial techniques generally employ specially designed applicators suited for dose delivery to such tumours. These applicators have a standard tandem and ovoid/ring assembly which is reinforced with positions for insertion of straight and oblique needles that can safely achieve dose delivery in the parametrium (Fig. 22). Examples of such applicators include Vienna [78], Utrecht [79], Venezia applicators [80], etc. Their advantages over classical templates are fewer number of required needles, close proximity of the interstitial component to the target, greater accuracy and reproducibility in subsequent fractions. Ultrasonography or fluoroscopy guided insertion further improves the accuracy and safety of these applicators.

14.5 Vaginal Cuff Brachytherapy After Hysterectomy in Carcinoma Cervix

Vaginal cuff brachytherapy after hysterectomy for cervical carcinoma is used in the following clinical situations [81]:

1. Patients with inadequate surgery—less than a radical hysterectomy.
2. Close/Positive margins.
3. Vaginal/Parametrial involvement.
4. Extensive Lymphovascular invasion.

In such situations, vaginal brachytherapy is used as a boost to the vaginal cuff along with EBRT in order to improve tumour control and limit side effects [81]. The applicators used are vaginal cylinders or ovoids which have been described in the section on Endometrial cancer brachytherapy below. Dose used is 6 Gy in 2–3 fractions of HDR brachytherapy along with 45–50.4 Gy EBRT to the pelvis.

15 Post-treatment Follow-Up

All patients treated for cervical cancer should undergo routine follow-up every 3–4 months for the first 2–3 years when the chances of recurrence is maximum, this is based on the systemic review of 17 retrospective studies of women treated for cervical cancer where the median time to recurrence ranged from 7 to 36 months following primary treatment [82]. After 3 years she is asked to come for her follow-up every 6-months until 5 years, and then annually for life. During her follow-up visit, proper symptom related history is taken and clinical examination comprising of examination of breasts, axillary and supraclavicular lymph nodes, look for lower limb swelling, palpation of liver, abdomen and groin, inspection of vulva, vagina and cervix, and finally rectovaginal pelvic examination are carried out to look for treatment related complications and early recurrences both local/distant or persistent disease. Another important component of this visit is evaluation of psychosexual morbidity and counseling done accordingly. Studies have shown that the sensitivity and specificity of clinical follow-up examination varies from 0% to 71% and the recurrences detected on routine clinical follow-up have better prognosis compared to recurrences detected with symptoms [83]. It is seen that 25% of recurrences are detected in asymptomatic women while 82% in symptomatic women.

The role of routine imaging is indicated only in special circumstances, when there is involvement of high pelvic/para-aortic lymph nodes, justifying interval imaging of the abdomen to look for potentially curable progression of disease or when she comes with specific symptoms. Clinical examination remains the gold standard for follow-up examinations specially in asymptomatic women which is evident from a systematic review, where asymptomatic recurrent disease was detected using physical exam (29–71%), chest X-ray (20–47%), CT (0–34%), and vaginal vault cytology (0–17%).

Apart from the routine follow-up, all women below 50 years of age should receive hormonal replacement therapy, if indicated. As the women continues her follow-up and as she ages her routine checkup should include age related well-woman checks including her thyroid, renal functions to ensure good quality of life.

16 Recurrent Disease

Any patient presenting with a new local or distant metastasis after 6 months of completion of treatment is termed as recurrent disease, it may be local/distant recurrence or both. Most of the recurrences occur within the first 3 years and the most common cause of mortality is uremia [82, 84]. The management of recurrent disease depends on various factors starting from patient's performance status, prior treatment received and the site and extent of the recurrent disease [85]. So depending on the ECOG score and extent of the metastatic disease a trial of palliative chemotherapy with platinum doublet may be tried with good performance status and limited metastatic disease. However, it must be emphasized that the response rate and progression free survival is not very encouraging so with the patient and family member's consent this can be tried [86].

For limited local recurrence when it is potentially curable, surgery or radiotherapy may be tried depending on the primary treatment received by the patient. As most of the local recurrence are in the pelvis and when the tumour is an isolated central pelvic recurrence less than 3 cm with a disease free interval of 24 months, its prognosis is favorable [87, 88]. Recurrence following primary surgery may be treated by radical chemoradiation or pelvic exenteration after biopsy confirmation of recurrent disease. When radiation is indicated, to prevent radiation doses over the small bowel, rectum and bladder, image guided radiotherapy or intensity modulated radiotherapy is said to be superior in comparison to conventional radiotherapy with improved 5-year overall survival and progression-free survival rates of 35.4% vs. 26.1% and 26.1% vs. 15.1%, respectively.

For isolated central recurrence free from pelvic sidewall with no evidence of intraperitoneal or extra pelvic disease, pelvic exenteration may be tried [87, 89–92] after proper counseling regarding the associated morbidity, stoma care, expenditures involved and psychological factors. One of the prerequisite before performing this exenterative surgery is getting a PET/CT scan if feasible to rule out distant metastasis [93, 94]. In carefully selected patients the 5-year survival after pelvic exenteration is about 30–60% [89, 90] with overall survival of 10% and operative mortality of less than 10% [95].

For isolated para-aortic nodal recurrence, radiation therapy or chemoradiation with a curative intent results in a long term survival of around 30% [96] and the survival improves in asymptomatic low volume disease with a disease free interval of more than 24 months.

17 Special Circumstances

17.1 Cervical Cancer with Pregnancy

Cervical cancer with pregnancy is a special condition which needs multidisciplinary team approach and the tumour board decision should be discussed with the patient and her partner. The final treatment plan must have the concurrence of the stake holders.

Basically the management of cervical cancer in pregnancy will depend on the duration of pregnancy and broadly any pregnancy less than 20 weeks, treatment of cervical cancer gets the priority while any pregnancy more than 20 weeks preservation of pregnancy is considered. Surgery or chemoradiation remains the mainstay of treatment in early pregnancy up to 20 weeks, depending on the stage of cervical cancer. Radical hysterectomy along with the fetus in situ may be an option in early second trimester pregnancy (Fig. 23) Radiation in these cases will result in spontaneous abortion. Any pregnancy beyond 20 weeks or late second trimester we can delay the treatment only in stage IA2, IB1, and IB2 with similar survival as non-pregnant women [97–99].

Delivery of these patients should ideally be carried out in a tertiary care center with well-equipped neonatal services, classical cesarean section along with radical hysterectomy is done in the same sitting latest by 34 weeks of pregnancy.

For locally advanced cervical cancer when treatment delay is planned, neoadjuvant chemotherapy can be tried [100, 101] however there is no established data to support the impact of treatment delay on survival.

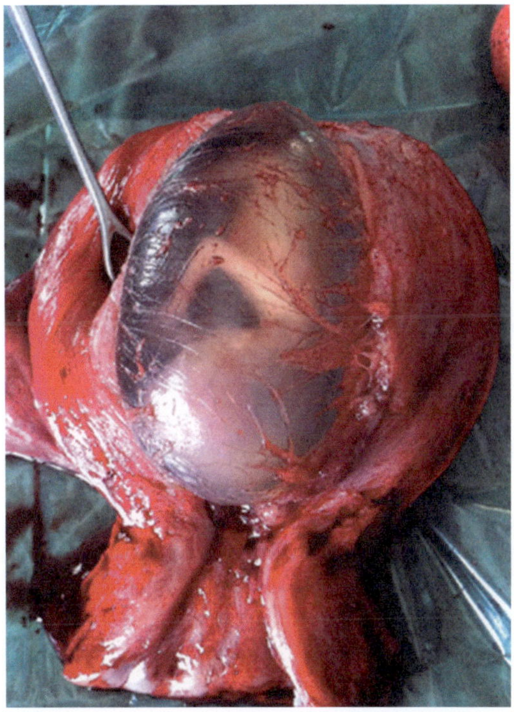

Fig. 23 Hysterectomy specimen of carcinoma uterine cervix Stage IA2 with 16 weeks pregnancy

17.2 Inadvertent Simple Hysterectomy in Carcinoma Cervix

In spite of well accepted clinical guidelines, lot of patients are subjected to inadvertent simple hysterectomies in stage IB or higher stages. The main reasons for this suboptimal treatment are [102] inadequate evaluation of abnormal PAP smears or cervical biopsies, failure to perform cone biopsy, endocervical curettage after cone biopsies, deliberate hysterectomies for gross invasive cancers, lack of preoperative PAP smears, misinterpretation of pathology results, colposcopic errors, failure to check cytology before surgery, failure to take biopsy sample of gross disease, emergency operations for bleeding or perforations and sometimes negative cytology with no clinical evidence of disease. So careful preoperative patient evaluation along with strict adherence of screening guidelines may be helpful in minimizing suboptimal surgeries in carcinoma cervix.

The treatment options for this group of patients are postoperative radiotherapy or radical parametrectomy where we remove the parametrium, upper vagina, and pelvic/paraaortic lymphadenectomy. In comparison to radiation therapy radical parametrectomy is a difficult procedure and needs highly technical skills which may not be available everywhere hence physicians tend to offer radiation therapy or concurrent chemoradiation therapy in most of these cases [103, 104]. Both of these treatment options has high rates of complications as early and late effects.

So when we compare both these options it is observed that there is no survival advantage of one treatment option over the other with similar disease stage, tumour size, tumour grade, depth of stromal invasion, LVSI, and positive resection margin. However, with the advent of latest electrosurgical machines and surgical techniques few studies has come up where they have recommended radical parametrectomy as the preferred choice.

18 Recent Important Trial Updates

18.1 Randomized Study Between Radical Surgery and Radiotherapy for the Treatment of Stage IB–IIA Cervical Cancer: 20-Year Update

Landoni et al. in 2017 published his study comparing between radical surgery and radiotherapy for the treatment of stage IB–IIA cervical cancer, a 20-year update published in 2017. Altogether 343 patients of stage IB-IIA were enrolled, 172 underwent radical surgery and 171 patients received radiation therapy. The minimum follow-up was 19 years. The primary objective was 5-year overall survival (OS) and complications rate and secondary objective was disease recurrence. It was observed that 20 year overall survival in the surgery and radiotherapy group was 72% and 77%, respectively (p = 0.008), and median time to relapse was 13.5 months and 11.5 months (p = 0.100), respectively.

The present study suggests both surgery and radiotherapy may be offered as treatment of choice for early stage cervical carcinoma in terms of survival. The treatment plan should consider factors like menopausal status, comorbidities, histological types, and tumour size.

18.2 Minimally Invasive Versus Abdominal Radical Hysterectomy for Cervical Cancer

Ramirez et al. in the year 2019 published their retrospective studies comparing the survival outcomes after laparoscopic or robot-assisted radical hysterectomy (minimally invasive surgery) with those after open abdominal radical hysterectomy (open surgery) among women with early stage cervical cancer. In this study patients were randomly assigned to undergo minimally invasive surgery or open surgery. Disease free survival at the end of 4.5 years was the primary objective and secondary objectives included comparison of recurrence rates and the overall survival rate between the two groups. Around 319 patients were assigned to minimally invasive surgery and 312 to open surgery. At the end of 4.5 years the study concluded that minimally invasive radical hysterectomy in patients with early cervical cancer was associated with a higher rate of recurrence and a lower rate of disease-free survival than the open approach, and the rate of overall survival was lower in the minimally invasive surgery group.

18.3 SUCCOR study

An international European cohort observational study comparing minimally invasive surgery versus open abdominal radical hysterectomy in patients with stage IB1 (FIGO 2009, <4 cm) cervical cancer operated in 2013–2014.

It is a cohort study involving 582 women who underwent radical hysterectomy for stage IB1 cervical cancer during the 2013–2014 period in 89 centers belonging to 23 European countries. The primary outcome was the rate of disease-free survival at 4.5 years between MIS vs. open surgery. Final analysis after a median follow-up of 58 months, showed that patients who underwent open surgery had a DFS at 4.5 years of 93% vs. 82% in the group of MIS ($p = 0.023$, HR 3.48; 95% CI: 1.17–9.48). The DFS was further worsened by the use manipulators in the MIS group (HR 2.38; 95% CI: 1.32–4.29). Overall survival at 4.5 years was significantly lower (96% vs. 88%) in the group of MIS ($p = 0.016$). The study concluded that the risk of relapse and death in the group of MIS was significantly higher and it was further worsened by the use of manipulator among MIS patients.

18.4 OUTBACK Trial

(Adjuvant chemotherapy following chemoradiation as primary treatment for locally advanced cervical cancer compared to chemoradiation alone: The randomized phase III trial) [105].

Phase III randomized trial of the Gynaecologic Cancer InterGroup (GCIG) published in 2021 included women ($n = 919$) with locally advanced cervical cancer (FIGO 2008 stage IB_1 and node positive, IB_2, II, IIIB or IVA) from April 2011 to June 2017. The control group ($n = 456$) received standard cisplatin-based chemoradiation (control) and the other group received standard cisplatin-based chemoradiation followed by adjuvant chemotherapy (ACT) ($n = 463$) with four cycles of carboplatin and paclitaxel. The primary objective was 5-year overall survival (OS) and secondary objectives were progression-free survival (PFS); adverse events (AE); and patterns of disease recurrence. The study showed no difference in Overall or Progression free survival in the two groups. The adverse events beyond 1 year of randomization and pattern of recurrence were also similar. Thus, there is no role of Adjuvant chemotherapy after standard Chemoradiation in locally advanced cervical cancer.

GOG 240 Trial adding Bevacizumab to chemotherapy in recurrent and metastatic cervical cancer:

This study is a randomized, controlled, open-label phase 3 trial comprising of 452 patients, being randomized 1:1:1:1 between April 2009 to January 2012. Study was designed to receive cisplatin plus paclitaxel or topotecan plus paclitaxel with ($n = 227$) or without ($n = 225$) bevacizumab in 21 day cycles until disease progression, unacceptable toxic effects, voluntary withdrawal, or complete response. The primary endpoint was to determine whether addition of bevacizumab to chemotherapy improves OS and secondary endpoint was to determine the impact of bevacizumab and nonplatinum doublet on PFS and overall response rate (ORR) by RECIST v1.0.

It was concluded that Bevacizumab plus chemotherapy significantly improves OS in stage IVB, recurrent or persistent cervical carcinoma by nearly 4-month which was clinically significant. There was an increase in median PFS and ORR. The Cisplatin + paclitaxel arm which is the current standard of care and did not underperform as compared to Topotican plus Paclitaxel. Although bevacizumab treatment was associated with a higher rate of adverse events, the improvement in OS with bevacizumab was not associated with decrease in health-related quality of life. Hence bevacizumab was shown to be the first targeted agent to improve OS in cervical cancer.

18.5 EMBRACE I Trial

(MRI-guided adaptive brachytherapy in locally advanced cervical cancer (EMBRACE-I): a multicenter prospective cohort study) [106].

Richard Pötter et al. studied the local tumour control and morbidity after chemoradiotherapy and MRI-based Image-guided adaptive brachytherapy (IGABT). A prospective, multicentric, observational study was done from July 30, 2008 to December 29, 2015, including Cervical cancer Stage IB-IVA or FIGO stage IVB disease restricted to paraaortic lymph nodal metastasis below the L1–L2 interspace, suitable for curative treatment. Patients received chemoradiotherapy (weekly intravenous cisplatin 40 mg/m^2, 5–6 cycles, 1 day per cycle, plus 45–50 Gy external-beam radiotherapy delivered in 1.8–2 Gy/fractions) followed by MRI-based IGABT. The primary endpoints were local control and late morbidity in all patients available for analysis.

After applying exclusion criteria, data from 1341 patients were available for analysis of disease and data from 1251 patients were available for assessment of morbidity outcome. The overall local control achieved across all stages were excellent with limited severe morbidity per organ (grade ≥3, 3.2–8.5%; grade ≥4, 0.5–3.0%), but considerable overall morbidity (grade ≥3, 18.4%; grade ≥4, 5.2%), especially for patients with stage III–IVA disease. Thus, MRI-based IGABT in combination with chemoradiotherapy leads to positive local and pelvic disease control and survival throughout all stages of locally advanced cervical cancer, with limited severe morbidity per organ.

18.6 Current Ongoing Trials

18.6.1 Surgical Treatment Related Trials

Few important trials currently being studied regarding less extensive surgery in early cervical cancer.

1. SHAPE (Simple Hysterectomy And Pelvic lymph node dissection in Early cervix cancer) study, it is a phase III randomized trial comparing type B radical hysterectomy and pelvic lymph node dissection with simple hysterectomy and pelvic lymph node dissection in stage IA2-IB1 disease with favorable pathologic characteristics. The primary objective of the study is to show that simple hysterectomy in low risk cervical cancer is safe and is associated with low morbidity with almost equal overall survival.
2. "Application of Sentinel Lymph Node Biopsy (SLNB) in Early stage Cervical Cancer: A Prospective Study": In this study early cervical cancer less than 3 cm are subjected to SLNB and based on the frozen section report impact of doing formal pelvic lymph node dissection and omitting the procedure is studied with primary endpoints of PFS and retroperitoneal lymph node recurrence and secondary endpoint of overall survival, quality of life and long term outcome of SLNB procedure.
3. "Conservative surgery for women with low risk, early stage Cervical cancer" being studied at the University of Texas MD Anderson Cancer Centre. It is a multicentric trial evaluating the safety and feasibility of performing conservative surgery in tumours less than 2 cm. It consists of two arms, patients desiring fertility will undergo cervical conization and pelvic lymph node dissection with lymphatic mapping and the other arm with patients not desiring fertility will undergo simple hysterectomy with pelvic lymph node dissection and lymphatic mapping. Evaluation of the safety and feasibility of conservative surgery in this group of patients is the primary objective.
4. GOG protocol 278: "Evaluation of physical function and quality of life before and after non-radical surgical therapy for stage IA1 (LVSI +ve) and IA2-IB1 (≤2 cm) cervical cancer". A multicentric trial with a primary objective to determine the impact of non-radical surgery on bladder, bowel, sexual functions and severity of lymphedema.

18.6.2 Trials Associated with Chemotherapy/Immunotherapy in Cervical Cancer

Various trials are currently undertaken to look for the role of chemotherapeutic/immunotherapeutic agents in cervical cancer and most of the studies are being tried in recurrent and metastatic settings. Mention must be made of the following ongoing trials.

INTERLACE Induction Chemotherapy Plus Chemoradiation as First Line Treatment for Locally Advanced Cervical Cancer (https://clinicaltrials.gov/ct2/show/NCT01566240).

A Phase III multicentric trial of 6 cycles of weekly Paclitaxel and Carboplatin (Induction chemotherapy) followed by standard Chemoradiation versus standard Chemoradiation alone in patients with Locally Advanced Cervical Cancer (FIGO stage IB2-IVA, stage IB1 and positive lymph nodes). The primary outcome is 5-year overall survival and secondary outcomes are progression free survival, adverse events, Quality of Life (QOL), patterns of first relapse (local and/or systemic). The final results of the study are expected in May 2026.

The EMBRACE II study The outcome and prospect of two decades of evolution within the GEC-ESTRO GYN working group and the EMBRACE studies [106].

EMBRACE II study is an interventional and observational multicentric study. The study is designed to benchmark the clinical outcome of the overall approach of advanced radio-chemotherapy and brachytherapy. Interventions address local, nodal and systemic treatment as well as exposure of Organ at risk (OARs). Endpoints include local and nodal (pelvic) control within the specific EBRT and brachytherapy targets, physician-assessed morbidity and patient-reported outcome (PRO) related to OAR in the pelvis and the para-aortic region, quality of life (QoL) indicators, as well as systemic control, overall survival, disease free survival, and cancer-specific survival. The study aims to recruit 1000 patients from at least 30 institutions in 4 years and to monitor them for at least 5 years.

EMBRACE III The study is designed to identify patient-related, disease-related, and treatment-related risk factors and biomarkers for outcome to define risk groups, which can be used for intensification of multimodality treatment in high-risk patients and de-escalation of treatment in low-risk patients [106].

References

1. Bray F, Ferlay J, Soerjomataram I, Siegel RL, Torre LA, Jemal A, et al. Global cancer statistics 2018: GLOBOCAN estimates of incidence and mortality worldwide for 36 cancers in 185 countries. CA Cancer J Clin. 2018;68:394–424.
2. World Health Organisation. The global burden of disease: 2004 update. Geneva: WHO; 2009.
3. Karthigeyan K, et al. Cervical cancer in India and HPV vaccination. Indian J Med Paediatr Oncol. 2012;33(1):7–12.
4. Dikshit R, Gupta PC, Ramasundarahettige C, et al. Cancer mortality in India: a nationally representative survey. Lancet. 2012;379(9828):1807–16.
5. Reiffenstuhl G. The lymphatics of the female genital organs. 1st ed. Philadelphia, PA: J. B. Lippincott; 1964.
6. Walboomers JM, Jacobs MV, Manos MM, Bosch FX, Kummer JA, et al. Human papillomavirus is a necessary cause of invasive cervical cancer worldwide. J Pathol. 1999;189:12–9.
7. Wright TC, Kurman RJ. A critical review of the morphologic classification systems of preinvasive lesions of the cervix: the scientific basis for shifting the paradigm. Papillomavirus Rep. 1994;5:175–82.
8. Hopman AH, Smedts F, Dignef W, Ummelen M, Sonke G, Mravunac M, et al. Transition of high-grade cervical intraepithelial neoplasia to micro-invasive carcinoma is characterized by integration of HPV 16/18 and numerical chromosome abnormalities. J Pathol. 2004;202(1):23–33.
9. McCredie MR, Sharples KJ, Paul C, Baranyai J, Medley G, Jones RW, Skegg DC. Natural history of cervical neoplasia and risk of invasive cancer in women with cervical intraepithelial neoplasia 3: a retrospective cohort study. Lancet Oncol. 2008;9(5):425–34.
10. Bhatla N, Berek J, Cuello M, et al. New revised FIGO staging of cervical cancer (2018). Abstract S020.2. Presented at the FIGO XXII World Congress of Gynecology and Obstetrics. Rio de Janeiro, Brazil, October 14-19, 2018. Int J Gynecol Obstet. 2018;143(Suppl 3):22.
11. Milliken DA, Shepherd JH. Fertility preserving surgery for carcinoma of the cervix. Curr Opin Oncol. 2008;20:575–80.
12. Reimers LL, Anderson WF, Rosenberg PS, et al. Etiologic heterogeneity for cervical cancer by histopathologic type, using comparative age-period-cohort models. Cancer Epidemiol Biomark Prev. 2009;18:792–800.
13. Wagenaar HC, Trimbos JB, Postema S, et al. Tumor diameter & volume assessed by magnetic resonance imaging in the prediction of outcome of invasive cervical cancer. Gynecol Oncol. 2001;82:474–82.
14. Bipat S, Glas AS, Velden J, et al. Computed tomography and magnetic resonance imaging in staging of uterine cervical carcinoma: a systemic review. Gynecol Oncol. 2003;91:59–66.
15. Selman TJ, Mann C, Zamora J, et al. Diagnostic accuracy of tests for lymph node status in primary cervical cancer: a systemic review & metaanalysis. CMAJ. 2008;178:855–62.
16. Kurman RJ, Carcangiu ML, Herrington CS, Young RH. WHO classification of tumours of female reproductive organs. 4th ed. Lyon: IARC; 2014.
17. Bhatla N, Aoki D, Sharma DN, Sankaranarayanan R. Cancer of the cervix uteri: 2021 update. Int J Gynecol Obstet. 2021;155:28–44.
18. Andikyan V, Khoury-Collado F, Denesopolis J, et al. Cervical conization and sentinel lymph node

mapping in the treatment of early stage I cervical canceris less enough? Int J Gynecol Cancer. 2014;24:113–7.
19. Wright JD, Nathavith AR, Lewin SN, et al. Fertility conserving surgery for young women with stage IA cervical cancer; safety and access. Obstet Gynecol. 2010;115:585–90.
20. Tinelli R, Malzoni M, Cosentino F, et al. Robotics versus laparoscopic radical hysterectomy with lymphadenectomy in patients with early cervical cancer: a multicenter study. Ann Surg Oncol. 2011;18:2622–8.
21. Kato T, Takashima A, Kasamatsu T, et al. Gynecologic Oncology Study Group of the Japan Clinical Oncology Group. Clinical tumor diameter and prognosis of patients with FIGO stage IB1 cervical cancer (JCOG0806-A). Gynecol Oncol. 2015;137:34–9.
22. Tax C, Rovers MM, de Graaf C, et al. The sentinel node procedure in early stage cervical cancer, taking the next step; a diagnostic review. Gynecol Oncol. 2015;139:559–67.
23. Wu Y, Li Z, Wu H, et al. Sentinel lymph node biopsy in cervical cancer: a meta-analysis. Mol Clin Oncol. 2013;1:1025–30.
24. Kadkhodayan S, Hasanzadeh M, Treglia G, et al. Sentinel node biopsy for lymph nodal staging of uterine cervix cancer: a systemic review and meta-analysis of the pertinent literature. Eur J Surg Oncol. 2015;41:1–20.
25. Fujiwara H, Yokota H, Monk B, et al. Gynecologic Cancer InterGroup (GCIG) consensus review for cervical adenocarcinoma. Int J Gynecol Cancer. 2014;24:S96–101.
26. Martínez-Palones JM, Gil-Moreno A, Pérez-Benavente MA, Roca I, Xercavins J. Intraoperative sentinel node identification in early stage cervical cancer using a combination of radiolabeled albumin injection and isosulfan blue dye injection. Gynecol Oncol. 2004;92:845–50.
27. van de Lande J, Torrenga B, Raijmakers PG, et al. Sentinel lymph node detection in early stage uterine cervix carcinoma: a systematic review. Gynecol Oncol. 2007;106:604–13.
28. Gortzak-Uzan L, Jimenez W, Nofech-Mozes S, et al. Sentinel lymph node biopsy vs. pelvic lymphadenectomy in early stage cervical cancer: is it time to change the gold standard? Gynecol Oncol. 2010;116:28–32.
29. Rotman M, Sedlis A, Piedmonte MR, et al. A phase III randomized trial of postoperative pelvic irradiation in Stage IB cervical carcinoma with poor prognostic features: follow-up of a gynecologic oncology group study. Int J Radiat Oncol Biol Phys. 2006;65:169–76.
30. Sedlis A, Bundy BN, Rotman MZ, Lentz SS, Muderspach LI, Zaino RJ. A randomized trial of pelvic radiation therapy versus no further therapy in selected patients with stage IB carcinoma of the cervix after radical hysterectomy and pelvic lymphadenectomy: a Gynecologic Oncology Group Study. Gynecol Oncol. 1999;73:177–83.
31. Dastidar GA, Gupta P, Basu B, Shah JK, Seal SL. Is neo-adjuvant chemotherapy a better option for management of cervical cancer patients of rural India? Indian J Cancer. 2016;53–1:56–9.
32. Querleu D, Cibula D, et al. Update on the Querleu–Morrow classification of radical hysterectomy. Ann Surg Oncol. 2017;24:3406–12.
33. Bonin S, Lanciano R, Corn B, Hogan W, Hartz W, Hanks G. Bony landmarks are not an adequate substitute for lymphangiography in defining pelvic lymph node location for the treatment of cervical cancer with radiotherapy. Int J Radiat Oncol Biol Phys. 1996;34(1):167–72.
34. Zunino S, Rosato O, Lucino S, Jauregui E, Rossi L, Venencia D. Anatomic study of the pelvis in carcinoma of the uterine cervix as related to the box technique. Int J Radiat Oncol Biol Phys. 1999;44(1):53–9.
35. Finlay M, Ackerman I, Tirona R, Hamilton P, Barbera L, Thomas G. Use of CT simulation for treatment of cervical cancer to assess the adequacy of lymph node coverage of conventional pelvic fields based on bony landmarks. Int J Radiat Oncol Biol Phys. 2006;64(1):205–9.
36. Taylor A, Rockall A, Reznek R, Powell M. Mapping pelvic lymph nodes: guidelines for delineation in intensity-modulated radiotherapy. Int J Radiat Oncol Biol Phys. 2005;63(5):1604–12.
37. Tyagi N, Lewis J, Yashar C, Vo D, Jiang S, Mundt A, et al. Daily online cone beam computed tomography to assess interfractional motion in patients with intact cervical cancer. Int J Radiat Oncol Biol Phys. 2011;80(1):273–80.
38. Ahmed R, Kim R, Duan J, Meleth S, De Los Santos J, Fiveash J. IMRT dose escalation for positive para-aortic lymph nodes in patients with locally advanced cervical cancer while reducing dose to bone marrow and other organs at risk. Int J Radiat Oncol Biol Phys. 2004;60(2):505–12.
39. Heron D, Gerszten K, Selvaraj R, King G, Sonnik D, Gallion H, et al. Conventional 3D conformal versus intensity-modulated radiotherapy for the adjuvant treatment of gynecologic malignancies: a comparative dosimetric study of dose–volume histograms☆. Gynecol Oncol. 2003;91(1):39–45.
40. Brixey C, Roeske J, Lujan A, Yamada S, Rotmensch J, Mundt A. Impact of intensity-modulated radiotherapy on acute hematologic toxicity in women with gynecologic malignancies. Int J Radiat Oncol Biol Phys. 2002;54(5):1388–96.
41. Lujan A, Mundt A, Yamada S, Rotmensch J, Roeske J. Intensity-modulated radiotherapy as a means of reducing dose to bone marrow in gynecologic patients receiving whole pelvic radiotherapy. Int J Radiat Oncol Biol Phys. 2003;57(2):516–21.
42. Guerrero M, Li X, Ma L, Linder J, Deyoung C, Erickson B. Simultaneous integrated intensity-modulated radiotherapy boost for locally advanced

gynecological cancer: radiobiological and dosimetric considerations. Int J Radiat Oncol Biol Phys. 2005;62(3):933–9.
43. Fenkell L, Assenholt M, Nielsen S, Haie-Meder C, Pötter R, Lindegaard J, et al. Parametrial boost using midline shielding results in an unpredictable dose to tumor and organs at risk in combined external beam radiotherapy and brachytherapy for locally advanced cervical cancer. Int J Radiat Oncol Biol Phys. 2011;79(5):1572–9.
44. Townamchai K, Lee L, Poorvu P, Viswanathan A. Clinical outcomes with dose escalation using intensity modulated radiation therapy for node-positive endometrial and cervical cancer. Int J Radiat Oncol Biol Phys. 2012;84(3):S454.
45. Kolstad P. Follow-up study of 232 patients with stage Ia1 and 411 patients with stage Ia2 squamous cell carcinoma of the cervix (microinvasive carcinoma). Gynecol Oncol. 1989;33(3):265–72.
46. Raspagliesi F, Ditto A, Quattrone P, Solima E, Fontanelli R, Dousias V, et al. Prognostic factors in microinvasive cervical squamous cell cancer: long-term results. Int J Gynecol Cancer. 2005;15(1):88–93.
47. Abu-Rustum N, Sonoda Y. Fertility-sparing surgery in early-stage cervical cancer: indications and applications. J Natl Compr Cancer Netw. 2010;8(12):1435–8.
48. Brunschwig A. The surgical treatment of cancer of the cervix: stage I and II. Am J Roentgenol. 1968;102(1):147–51.
49. Eifel PJ, Winter K, Morris M, Levenback C, Grigsby PW, Cooper J, et al. Pelvic irradiation with concurrent chemotherapy versus pelvic and para-aortic irradiation for high-risk cervical cancer: an update of Radiation Therapy Oncology Group Trial (RTOG) 90-01. J Clin Oncol. 2004;22(5):872–80.
50. Landoni F, Maneo A, Colombo A, Placa F, Milani R, Perego P, et al. Randomised study of radical surgery versus radiotherapy for stage Ib-IIa cervical cancer. Lancet. 1997;350(9077):535–40.
51. Perez CA, Camel HM, Kao MS, Hederman MA. Randomized study of preoperative radiation and surgery or irradiation alone in the treatment of Stage IB and IIA carcinoma of the uterine cervix: final report. Gynecol Oncol. 1987;27(2):129–40.
52. Rotman M, Sedlis A, Piedmonte MR, Bundy B, Lentz SS, Muderspach LI, et al. A phase III randomized trial of postoperative pelvic irradiation in stage IB cervical carcinoma with poor prognostic features: follow-up of a gynecologic oncology group study. Int J Radiat Oncol Biol Phys. 2006;65(1):169–76.
53. Coughlin CT, Richmond RC. Biologic and clinical developments of cisplatin combined with radiation: concepts, utility, projections for new trials, and the emergence of carboplatin. Semin Oncol. 1989;16(4 Suppl 6):31–43.
54. Douple EB. Platinum-radiation interactions. NCI Monogr. 1988;(6):315.
55. Whitney C, Sause W, Bundy B, Malfetano J, Hannigan E, Fowler W Jr, et al. Randomized comparison of fluorouracil plus cisplatin versus hydroxyurea as an adjunct to radiation therapy in stage IIB-IVA carcinoma of the cervix with negative para-aortic lymph nodes: a Gynecologic Oncology Group and Southwest Oncology Group Study. J Clin Oncol. 1999;17(5):1339.
56. Rose P, Bundy B, Watkins E, Thigpen J, Deppe G, Maiman M, et al. Concurrent cisplatin-based radiotherapy and chemotherapy for locally advanced cervical cancer. N Engl J Med. 1999;340(15):1144–53.
57. Peters W, Liu P, Barrett R, Stock R, Monk B, Berek J, et al. Concurrent chemotherapy and pelvic radiation therapy compared with pelvic radiation therapy alone as adjuvant therapy after radical surgery in high-risk early-stage cancer of the cervix. J Clin Oncol. 2000;18(8):1606–13.
58. Keys H, Bundy B, Stehman F, Muderspach L, Chafe W, Suggs C, et al. Cisplatin, radiation, and adjuvant hysterectomy compared with radiation and adjuvant hysterectomy for bulky stage IB cervical carcinoma. N Engl J Med. 1999;340(15):1154–61.
59. Magrina J, Goodrich M, Weaver A, Podratz K. Modified radical hysterectomy: morbidity and mortality. Gynecol Oncol. 1995;59(2):277–82.
60. Gerbaulet A, Potter R, Haie-Meder C. Cervix cancer. In: Gerbaulet A, Potter R, Mazeron JJ, Meertens H, Limbergen EV, editors. The GEC ESTRO handbook of brachytherapy. Leuven: ACCO, ESTRO; 2002. p. 301–64.
61. Tod M, Meredith WJ. Treatment of cancer of the cervix uteri, a revised Manchester method. Br J Radiol. 1953;26(305):252–7. https://doi.org/10.1259/0007-1285-26-305-252.
62. Tod MC, Meredith WJ. A dosage system for use in the treatment of cancer of the uterine cervix. Br J Radiol. 1938;11(132):809–24. https://doi.org/10.1259/0007-1285-11-132-809.
63. Quimby EH, Castro V. The calculation of dosage in interstitial radium therapy. Am J Roentgenol Radium Therapy, Nucl Med. 1953;70:739–40.
64. Paterson R, Parker HM. A dosage system for interstitial radium therapy. Br J Radiol. 1938;11:313–39.
65. Pierquin B, Dutreix A, Paine CH, Chassagne D, Marinello G, Ash D. The Paris system in interstitial radiation therapy. Acta Radiol Oncol Radiat Phys Biol. 1978;17(1):33–48. https://doi.org/10.3109/02841867809127689.
66. International Commission on Radiation Units and Measurements. Dose and volume specification for reporting intracavitary therapy in gynecology. ICRU report 38. Bethesda, MD: ICRU; 1985.
67. Haie-Meder C, Potter R, Van Limbergen E, Briot E, De Babandere M, Dimopoulos J, et al. GEC-ESTRO Working Group Recommendations (I): concepts and terms in 3D image-based 3D treatment planning in cervix cancer brachytherapy with emphasis on MRI assessment of GTV and CTV. Radiother Oncol. 2004;74:235–45.

68. Potter R, Haie-Meder C, Van Limbergen E, Barillot I, De Brabandere M, Dimopoulos J, et al. GEC ESTRO Working Group. Recommendations from gynaecological (GYN) GEC ESTRO working group (II): concepts and terms in 3D image-based treatment planning in cervix cancer brachytherapy-3D dose volume parameters and aspects of 3D image based anatomy, radiation physics, radiobiology. Radiother Oncol. 2006;78:67–77.
69. International Commission on Radiation Units and Measurements. Prescribing, recording and reporting brachytherapy for cancer of the cervix. ICRU report no. 89. J ICRU. 2013;13(1–2):1.
70. Viswanthan A, Thomasden B. American Brachytherapy Society consensus guidelines for locally advanced carcinoma of the cervix. Part I: general principles. Brachytherapy. 2012;11:47–52.
71. Viswanthan AN, Beriwal S, De Los Santos JF, Demanes DJ, Gaffney D, Hansen J, et al. American Brachytherapy Society consensus guidelines for locally advanced carcinoma of the cervix. Part II: high dose rate brachytherapy. Brachytherapy. 2012;11:33–46.
72. Mahantshetty U, Naga CP, Khadanga CR, et al. A prospective comparison of computed tomography with transrectal ultrasonography assistance and magnetic resonance imaging-based target-volume definition during image guided adaptive brachytherapy for cervical cancers. Int J Radiat Oncol Biol Phys. 2018;102(5):1448–56. https://doi.org/10.1016/j.ijrobp.2018.05.080.
73. Viswanathan AN, Dimopoulos J, Kirisits C, Berger D, Pötter R. Computed tomography versus magnetic resonance imaging-based contouring in cervical cancer brachytherapy: results of a prospective trial and preliminary guidelines for standardized contours. Int J Radiat Oncol Biol Phys. 2007;68(2):491–8. https://doi.org/10.1016/j.ijrobp.2006.12.021.
74. Mahantshetty U, Poetter R, Beriwal S, et al. IBS-GEC ESTRO-ABS recommendations for CT based contouring in image guided adaptive brachytherapy for cervical cancer. Radiother Oncol. 2021;160:273–84. https://doi.org/10.1016/j.radonc.2021.05.010.
75. Ohno T, Wakatsuki M, Toita T, et al. Recommendations for high-risk clinical target volume definition with computed tomography for three-dimensional image-guided brachytherapy in cervical cancer patients. J Radiat Res. 2017;58(3):341–50. https://doi.org/10.1093/jrr/rrw109.
76. Syed AMN, Puthawala AA, Neblett D, et al. Transperineal interstitial-intracavitary "Syed-Neblett" applicator in the treatment if carcinoma of the uterine cervix. Endoc Hypertherm Oncol. 1986;2:1–13.
77. Martinez A, Cox RS, Edmundson GK. A multiple-site perineal applicator (MUPIT) for treatment of prostatic, anorectal, and gynecologic malignancies. Int J Radiat Oncol Biol Phys. 1984;10(2):297–305. https://doi.org/10.1016/0360-3016(84)90016-6.
78. Kirisits C, Lang S, Dimopoulos J, Berger D, Georg D, Pötter R. The Vienna applicator for combined intracavitary and interstitial brachytherapy of cervical cancer: design, application, treatment planning, and dosimetric results. Int J Radiat Oncol Biol Phys. 2006;65(2):624–30. https://doi.org/10.1016/j.ijrobp.2006.01.036.
79. Nomden CN, de Leeuw AA, Moerland MA, Roesink JM, Tersteeg RJ, Jürgenliemk-Schulz IM. Clinical use of the Utrecht applicator for combined intracavitary/interstitial brachytherapy treatment in locally advanced cervical cancer. Int J Radiat Oncol Biol Phys. 2012;82(4):1424–30. https://doi.org/10.1016/j.ijrobp.2011.04.044. Epub 12 Jun 2011. PMID: 21669505.
80. Walter F, Maihöfer C, Schüttrumpf L, et al. Combined intracavitary and interstitial brachytherapy of cervical cancer using the novel hybrid applicator Venezia: clinical feasibility and initial results. Brachytherapy. 2018;17(5):775–81. https://doi.org/10.1016/j.brachy.2018.05.009.
81. Small W Jr, Beriwal S, Demanes DJ, et al. American Brachytherapy Society consensus guidelines for adjuvant vaginal cuff brachytherapy after hysterectomy. Brachytherapy. 2012;11(1):58–67. https://doi.org/10.1016/j.brachy.2011.08.005.
82. Elit L, Fyles AW, Devries MC, Oliver TK, Fung-Kee-Fung M. Follow-up for women after treatment for cervical cancer: a systematic review. Gynecol Oncol. 2009;114:528–35.
83. Sartori E, Pasinetti B, Carrara L, et al. Pattern of failure and value of follow-up procedures in endometrial and cervical cancer patients. Gynecol Oncol. 2007;107:241–7.
84. Eifel PJ, Jhingran A, Brown J, Levenback C, Thames H. Time course and outcome of central recurrence after radiation therapy for carcinoma of the cervix. Int J Gynecol Cancer. 2006;16:1106–11.
85. Eralp Y, Saip P, Sakar B, et al. Prognostic factors and survival in patients with metastatic or recurrent carcinoma of the uterine cervix. Int J Gynecol Cancer. 2003;13:497–504.
86. Moore DH, Blessing JA, McQuellon RP, et al. Phase III study of cisplatin with or without paclitaxel in stage IVB, recurrent, or persistent squamous cell carcinoma of the cervix: a gynecologic oncology group study. J Clin Oncol. 2004;22:3113–9.
87. Estape R, Angioli R. Surgical management of advanced and recurrent cervical cancer. Semin Surg Oncol. 1999;16:236–41.
88. Friedlander M, Grogan M, U.S. Preventative Services Task Force. Guidelines for the treatment of recurrent and metastatic cervical cancer. Oncologist. 2002;7:342–7.
89. Shingleton HM, Soong SJ, Gelder MS, Hatch KD, Baker VV, Austin JM Jr. Clinical and histopathologic factors predicting recurrence and survival after pelvic exenteration for cancer of the cervix. Obstet Gynecol. 1989;73:1027–34.

90. Rutledge FN, Smith JP, Wharton JT, O'Quinn AG. Pelvic exenteration: analysis of 296 patients. Am J Obstet Gynecol. 1977;129:881–92.
91. Morley GW, Hopkins MP, Lindenauer SM, Roberts JA. Pelvic exenteration, University of Michigan: 100 patients at 5 years. Obstet Gynecol. 1989;74:934–43.
92. Benn T, Brooks RA, Zhang Q, et al. Pelvic exenteration in gynecologic oncology: a single institution study over 20 years. Gynecol Oncol. 2011;122:14–8.
93. Sun SS, Chen TC, Yen RF, Shen YY, Changlai SP, Kao A. Value of whole body 18F-fluoro-2-deoxyglucose positron emission tomography in the evaluation of recurrent cervical cancer. Anticancer Res. 2001;21(4B):2957–61.
94. Husain A, Akhurst T, Larson S, Alektiar K, Barakat RR, Chi DS. A prospective study of the accuracy of 18Fluorodeoxyglucose positron emission tomography (18FDG PET) in identifying sites of metastasis prior to pelvic exenteration. Gynecol Oncol. 2007;106:177–80.
95. Höckel M, Dornhöfer N. Pelvic exenteration for gynaecological tumours: achievements and unanswered questions. Lancet Oncol. 2006;7:837–47.
96. Niibe Y, Kenjo M, Kazumoto T, et al. Multi-institutional study of radiation therapy for isolated para-aortic lymph node recurrence in uterine cervical carcinoma: 84 subjects of a population of more than 5,000. Int J Radiat Oncol Biol Phys. 2006;66:1366–9.
97. Duggan B, Muderspach LI, Roman LD, Curtin JP, d'Ablaing G III, Morrow CP. Cervical cancer in pregnancy: reporting on planned delay in therapy. Obstet Gynecol. 1993;82(4 Pt 1):598–602.
98. Nevin J, Soeters R, Dehaeck K, Bloch B, Van Wyk L. Advanced cervical carcinoma associated with pregnancy. Int J Gynecol Cancer. 1993;3:57–63.
99. Hunter MI, Tewari K, Monk BJ. Cervical neoplasia in pregnancy. Part 2: Current treatment of invasive disease. Am J Obstet Gynecol. 2008;199:10–8.
100. Tewari K, Cappuccini F, Gambino A, Kohler MF, Pecorelli S, DiSaia PJ. Neoadjuvant chemotherapy in the treatment of locally advanced cervical carcinoma in pregnancy: a report of two cases and review of issues specific to the management of cervical carcinoma in pregnancy including planned delay of therapy. Cancer. 1998;82:1529–34.
101. Boyd A, Cowie V, Gourley C. The use of cisplatin to treat advanced-stage cervical cancer during pregnancy allows fetal development and prevents cancer progression: report of a case and review of the literature. Int J Gynecol Cancer. 2009;19:273–6.
102. Munstedt K, Johnson P, von Georgi R. Consequencies of inadvertent, suboptimal primary surgery in carcinoma of the uterine cervix. Gynecol Oncol. 2004;94:515–20.
103. Park JY, Kim DY, Kim JH, Kim YM, Kim YT, Nam JH. Management of occult invasive cervical cancer found after simple hysterectomy. Ann Oncol. 2010;21:994–1000.
104. Leath CA III, Straughn JM, Bhoola SM, et al. The role of radical parametrectomy in the treatment of occult cervical carcinoma after extrafascial hysterectomy. Gynecol Oncol. 2004;92:215–9.
105. Mileshkin LR, Moore KN, Barnes E, Gebski V, Narayan K, Bradshaw N, Lee YC, Diamante K, Fyles AW, Small W, Gaffney DK. Adjuvant chemotherapy following chemoradiation as primary treatment for locally advanced cervical cancer compared to chemoradiation alone: the randomized phase III OUTBACK Trial (ANZGOG 0902, RTOG 1174, NRG 0274). J Clin Oncol. 2021;39(18_suppl):LBA3.
106. Pötter R, Tanderup K, Kirisits C, et al. The EMBRACE-II study: the outcome and prospect of two decades of evolution within the GEC-ESTRO GYN working group and the EMBRACE studies. Clin Transl Radiat Oncol. 2018;9:48–60.
107. Koh WJ, Abu-Rustum NR, Bean S, et al. Uterine neoplasms, version 1.2018, NCCN clinical practice guidelines in oncology. J Natl Compr Cancer Netw. 2018;16(2):170–99. https://doi.org/10.6004/jnccn.2018.0006.

Endometrial Cancer

Amal Chandra Kataki, Upasana Baruah, Amita Maheshwari, Partha Medhi, and Kaushik Jaganath Kataki

1 Epidemiology and Risk Factors

Endometrial cancer has been traditionally associated amongst women with obesity and is regarded having a good prognosis as majority of women are symptomatic at an early stage. Statistically it ranks sixth among all the cancer occurring in females. According to facts derived from Globocan for the year 2020, the overall incidence was 417,367 and 97,370 died due to it [1]. Geographical distribution is skewed towards western countries with high incidence noted in North American, Eastern and Northern European countries. In comparison incidence is lowest in several African and Asian countries including India which may be related to the higher prevalence of obesity in the west. However, the risk seems to have increased over the years, even in the Asian and African countries which is contemplated to be the result of the rapid socio-economic growth occurring in these regions [2]. In India, the incidence is low, with 16,413 new cases as per Globocan 2020 data [3]. Chennai has the highest incidence with an AAR of 6 per 100,000 population, followed by Delhi (AAR 5.5) and Thiruvananthapuram (AAR5.1) [4]. In comparison, North America has an AAR of 26 per 100,000 population, making it the second most common malignancy occurring in females after breast cancer [5]. The risk of endometrial cancer increases as age advances and the median age of onset has been shown to be at 63 years as per the SEER data with a range of 55–64 years [5]. In India, the median age of onset is 54 years which is similar to median age reported from studies of other Asian countries [6–8]. Increased prevalence of obesity and higher life expectancy are the two major contributing factors in the increasing prevalence of endometrial cancers in high-income countries [9]. It is, therefore, a disease occurring mainly in the postmenopausal women and is rare before 30 years of age. Majority of the patients are symptomatic and present as postmenopausal bleeding. The overall 5-year survival rate is estimated to be 81.2%, and in patients where the disease is confined to the uterus, it is more than 90% [5]. This fact, however, cannot be generalized as prognosis may be poor in patients having unfavourable characteristics such as high grade, aggressive histology, and advanced age.

A. C. Kataki (✉) · U. Baruah · P. Medhi
Department of Gynaecologic Oncology, Dr. Bhubaneswar Borooah Cancer Institute (A Unit of Tata Memorial Centre, Mumbai), Guwahati, Assam, India

A. Maheshwari
Department of Gynaecological Oncology, Tata Memorial Hospital, Mumbai, India

K. J. Kataki
Department of Radiation Oncology, Princess Margaret Cancer Centre, Toronto, ON, USA
e-mail: kaushik.kataki@rmp.uhn.ca

A. C. Kataki, D. Barmon (eds.), *Fundamentals in Gynaecologic Malignancy*,
https://doi.org/10.1007/978-981-19-5860-1_14

Apart from age and obesity, prolonged oestrogen exposure to the uterus is the most significant risk factor. It is the reason patients with chronic anovulation, early menarche, and late menopause have an increased association of endometrial hyperplasia and endometrial cancer [10]. Likewise, hormone replacement therapy and tamoxifen use are associated with an increased risk [11, 12]. Risk of endometrial cancer increases with the increasing duration of use of tamoxifen in breast cancer patients. The relative risk is 2.0 for 2–5 years of use as compared to non-users and some have been documented to have an unfavourable outcome due to less favourable histology and higher stage [12]. Factors that reduce circulating oestrogen levels like weight reduction, physical exercise, cigarette smoking appear to be protective against endometrial cancer. Likewise, progestins antagonize the effects of oestrogen on the endometrium and prevent the development of hyperplasia and cancer.

1.1 Hereditary Risk

Genetic predisposition of developing endometrial cancer is less as compared to ovarian cancer, and the majority of the cases are sporadic. Only 2–5% of endometrial cancers are due to Lynch syndrome, also known as hereditary nonpolyposis colorectal cancer/HNPCC. The inheritance is autosomal dominant and is due to a mutation in one of the several DNA mismatch repair genes called the MMR genes, which are MLH1, MSH2, MSH6, and PMS 2. Dysfunction of any of these leads to repair complex failure and results in the accumulation of numerous DNA replication errors, microsatellite instability (MSI), and cancer formation [13]. In patients less than 50 years of age it accounts for nearly 10% of cases of endometrial cancer [14, 15]. The name Lynch Syndrome is derived after Hendry T. Lynch, who reported data based on study of more than 650 family members susceptible for genetic inheritance of colon cancers. Initially a predominance of colon, uterine, and stomach cancers was found, however, subsequently cancers of the small intestine, liver, gall bladder, ovaries, urinary tract, brain, and skin were found to be associated with it. Women with this syndrome have a higher overall risk of developing cancer than men because of the added risk of cancers of the female genital system [16]. Ovarian cancers in Lynch syndrome are mostly of clear cell variety with a lifetime risk of 9–12% [17]. Recently it was found that patients have a 40–60% probability of developing endometrial cancer as their first clinical manifestation with Lynch syndrome and can serve as the sentinel cancer for the patients and of their family members [15]. The risk of developing a second malignancy is estimated at 25% in 10 years and 50% at 15 years following an initial endometrial cancer diagnosis [17].

Lynch syndrome (LS) can be suspected on the basis of the Amsterdam II or Bethesda criteria [18].

Women with Lynch syndrome should be counselled about the need to undergo periodic screening and seek medical attention in case of abnormal uterine bleeding. Surveillance of the endometrium with annual pelvic examination, transvaginal ultrasound, and endometrial biopsy should be done 1–2 years interval beginning at the age of 30–35 years or 10 before the age of first diagnosis of Lynch associated cancer in the family [19, 20]. Likewise, colonoscopy should be performed every 1–2 years. Surveillance should be continued till risk-reducing hysterectomy is performed after childbearing is completed at 35–45 years of age. Hysterectomy should also include removal of bilateral tubes and ovaries as they may be involved later. This is also supported by the fact that there are no dependable screening tests to detect ovarian cancer which generally present at an advanced stage, unlike endometrial cancer. In young patients, counselling should be done about the limited data available about the future risk of ovarian cancer against the risk of developing premature menopause and risks associated with hormone replacement therapy. Women not planning a pregnancy may reduce their risk of developing endometrial and ovarian cancer by using hormonal contraception in addition to ongoing surveillance [21].

2 Etiopathogenesis

Dualistic model: Based on the clinical and pathologic factors, endometrial cancer is traditionally classified into two groups (Bokhman 1984) [22]. Type I cancers make up 85% of all endometrial cancers and are related to endogenous or exogenous oestrogen exposure. This group has cancers with endometrioid histology, are low-grade and carry a good prognosis due to their early diagnosis. Atypical endometrial hyperplasia's (AEH) or endometrial intraepithelial neoplasia's (EIN) are considered to be the precursor lesion [23, 24]. In contrast, Type II tumours are high grade and primarily include papillary serous (10%) and clear cell carcinomas. Undifferentiated cancers also fall into this category though they are less common. These tumours are aggressive, mostly present at an advanced age and are seen in the background of an atrophic endometrium. Molecular pathogenesis is also different in these two types of cancers with Type I cancers showing MSI, mutations in PTEN, PIK3CA, K-RAS, and beta-catenin. Type II tumours display alterations of p53, loss of heterozygosity (LOH) on several chromosomes and are associated with alterations in STK15, p16, E-cadherin, and c-erb-B2 [25]. Although most patients with Lynch syndrome exhibit MSI, both types of endometrial cancers are associated with it. However, the mean age of diagnosis of these non-endometrioid tumours in patients with Lynch syndrome is 46.4 years, which is lesser than the average age of Type II tumours in the general population [17].

In recent years genomic studies have divided endometrial cancers into four molecular subgroups based on underlying genomic aberrations. The classification aims to provide prognostic as well as predictive information and is a significant leap in information in the last few years. Combining clinicopathological parameters and molecular features may become an essential part of endometrial cancer management in near future.

The TCGA (The cancer genome atlas) network defined four distinct classes of endometrial cancers with unique genomic changes, breaking the traditional dualistic view [26]. It is based on classification at molecular levels. **The first group** has copy number-stable, but ultramutations in the DNA polymerase enzyme. Histologically these cancers are typically high-grade endometrioid cancers with a classical superficial broad front pattern of invasion, and presence of tumour giant cells and tumour-infiltrating lymphocytes (TIL). **The second group** reported by the TCGA was cancers with microsatellite instability (MSI) due to dysfunctional MMR proteins. Histologically they are mostly endometrioid cancers, but non-endometrioid subtypes have also been described. Like *POLE*-mutant endometrial cancers, these tumours typically display TILs and peri-tumoural lymphocytes and have a so-called 'microcystic elongated and fragmented (MELF) pattern of invasion. **The third group** is genomically relatively stable (copy number-low), MMR-proficient, with moderate number of mutations in the PI3K/Akt and Wnt signalling pathways. This variety is almost exclusively composed of endometrioid cancers with oestrogen and progesterone receptor positivity. **The fourth group has high somatic copy number alterations (SCNA)** and has frequent *TP53* mutations (92%). Morphologically, these consist of high-grade (grade 3) endometrial cancers, including most serous cancers, but 26% of endometrioid variety were also classified in this group [27].

For use in routine clinical practice immunohistochemical surrogates of molecular prognostic markers have been proposed, as immunohistochemistry is faster, less expensive and more widely available than sequencing analyses. A molecular classifier known as the Proactive Molecular Risk Classifier for Endometrial Cancer (ProMisE) has recently been validated. It is based on immunohistochemistry for MMR proteins, p53, and POLE sequencing [28].

3 Histopathological Features of Endometrial Cancers

Malignant change may occur in any part of the endometrium. It may involve the entire endometrium or may be localized as a polyp. Grossly it appears as irregular and shaggy with polypoidal areas and necrosis.

3.1 Endometrioid Carcinomas (Type I) (Figs. 1 and 2)

Endometrioid histology is the most common variety of endometrial adenocarcinomas and has a good prognosis as the disease is mostly confined to the endometrium or is minimally invasive at presentation. Atypical hyperplasia (AH) or endometrial intraepithelial lesion (EIN) is the direct precursor and is associated with occult endometrioid carcinoma in 29% to 40% of the cases [29–31].

Overgrowth of oval or round endometrial glands with smooth inner contour is characteristics of this variety. Solid areas varying in distribution can be seen along with glandular areas. Depending on the number of solid areas three grades are described. Up to 5% of solid or non-squamous constitute grade I, 6–50% of solid / non-squamous component is grade II and 50% of solid, non-squamous, component falls under grade III. The presence of severe nuclear atypia in majority of cells raises the grade of the tumour by one [32].

Apart from the usual variant of endometroid adenocarcinomas, other variants such as villoglandular pattern, intermediate grade papillary endometrioid cancer, micro-glandular like pattern, and secretory carcinomas are also seen [32].

Villoglandular pattern has tumour architecture resembling finger-like papillae with fibrovascular core. The cells lining it are of columnar variety with mild atypia only. Although there is higher incidence of lymph nodal metastasis in this variety, the behaviour is similar to that of nonvilloglandular endometrioid carcinomas and should be considered to carry a similar prognosis [33].

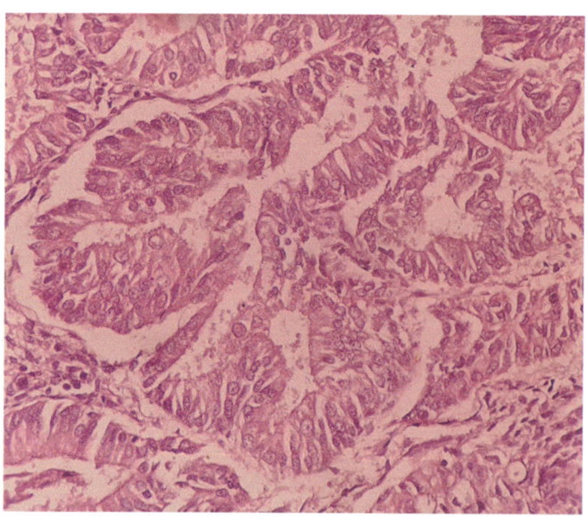

Fig. 1 (Grade 1 Endometrioid adenocarcinoma)

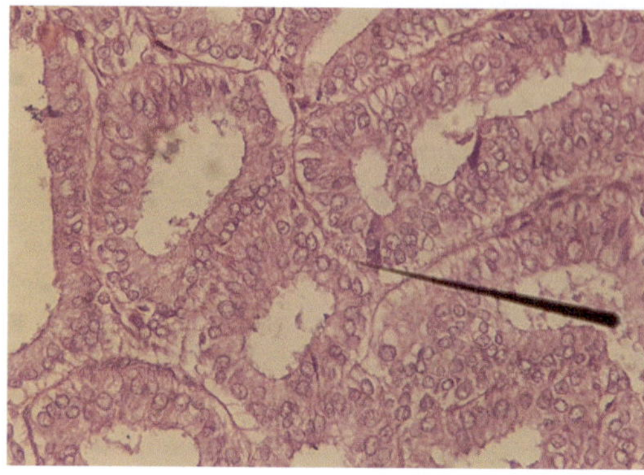

Fig. 2 Grade 1 Endometroid adenocarcinoma

Papillary endometrioid adenocarcinomas of intermediate grade are characterized by papillary structures, which can be mistaken for papillary serous adenocarcinoma. It is also associated with significant vascular/lymphatic invasion and lymph node metastasis [32, 34].

Microglandular-like pattern typically occurs after menopause and is associated hormonal therapy [32].

3.1.1 Endometrioid Adenocarcinomas with Clear Cells

Presence of clear cells may sometime be found with endometrioid variety and may cause confusion with clear cell carcinoma. However, these clear changes most commonly are due to presence of glycogen or secretory vacuoles. It may also be related to nonspecific clear cell changes or by an artifact [32].

3.1.2 Ciliated Cell Carcinoma

This variety is extremely uncommon but has a good prognosis. It is reported to have a strong correlation with oestrogen exposure as normally formation of cilia by endometrial cells occur after oestrogen use [35].

3.1.3 Endometrioid Adenocarcinoma with Squamous Differentiation

This is noted in about 25% of cases. Endometrial adenocarcinomas with benign-appearing squamous elements are usually associated with well-differentiated glandular components and have a prognosis identical to that of typical well-differentiated adenocarcinoma [36].

3.2 Non-endometrioid Carcinomas (Type II)

Non-endometrioid endometrial cancers comprise of mucinous, squamous, serous, clear cell, neuroendocrine, and undifferentiated carcinomas.

Serous carcinoma (Fig. 3) accounts for less than 10% of endometrial malignancies and closely resemble serous carcinoma of the ovary. Endometrial intraepithelial carcinoma (EIC) is considered to be the precursor lesion which is characterized by epithelial cells with marked nuclear abnormalities. They have a poor prognosis and may have distant metastasis even when serous carcinoma is confined to the endometrium [37]. They have marked and diffuse cytologic atypia with a papillary, glandular or solid architecture pattern. They generally develop in the background of atrophic endometrium or in a polyp. Psammoma bodies are found in one-third of cases. Numerous mitotic figures are usually found. Sometimes diagnosis may be confused with high grade endometrioid carcinomas where in that case immunohistochemistry (IHC) may aid in the diagnosis. Serous carcinoma is favoured by the expression of P16 with weak or absent staining for oestrogen and progesterone receptors [38].

3.2.1 Clear Cell Carcinomas (Fig. 4)

They are uncommon, occur in older age group, and are aggressive like serous carcinomas. The term clear cell carcinoma was first defined by Scully and Barlow, who described these tumours to be originated from the Mullerian epithelium. Under microscopy, the tumours show tubulocystic, papillary, or solid patterns. They have a clear appearance because of their high glycogen content and not due to intracellular mucin. They sometimes include eosinophilic cells and hobnail cells [39]. As it may sometimes be confused with Grade III endometrioid carcinomas and with those having clear cell changes IHC is required. They are ER, PR negative unlike endometrioid carcinomas, HNF1B-positive, Napsin A-positive [40, 41]. In contrast to serous carcinoma, strong p53 expression occurred less frequently in clear cell carcinoma and predominantly in clear cell carcinoma with serous features suggesting a molecular pathway different from those of endometrioid and serous carcinoma [42].

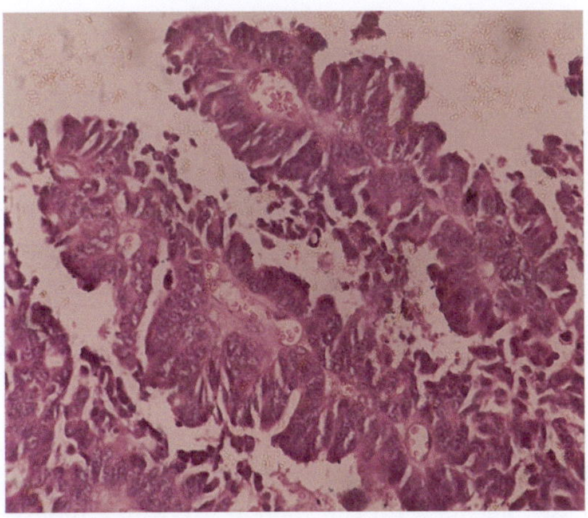

Fig. 3 High grade serous papillary carcinoma of endometrium

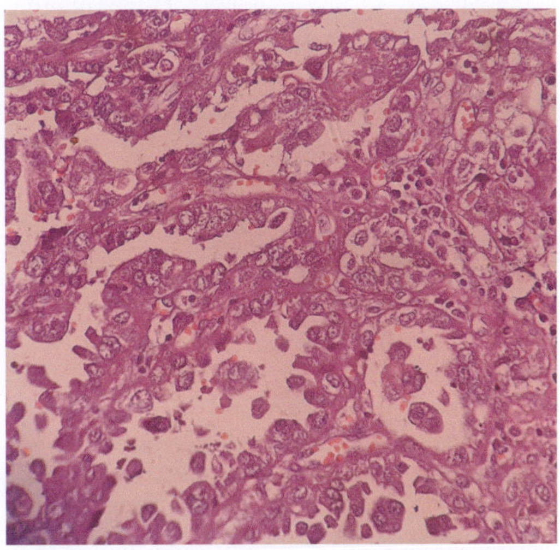

Fig. 4 Clear cell carcinoma with hobnail appearance

3.2.2 Squamous Cell Carcinomas of Endometrium

Primary squamous carcinoma of the endometrium is very rare and may be confused with cervical carcinoma. Three pathological criteria have been described for its diagnosis which are absence of **coexistent adenocarcinoma of the endometrium, absence of connection between the tumour in the endometrium and cervical squamous epithelium, and absence of primary squamous cell carcinoma of the cervix** [43]. The role of immunohistochemistry is limited, with most studies demonstrating a mutation of the p53 tumour suppressor gene, high Ki-67, positive immunoreactivity for the cytokeratin 7, p63 and p16INK4a proteins, but not for cytokeratin 20 or the oestrogen and progesterone receptors. Lack of oestrogen cannot be completely ruled out as an aetiological factor since most patients diagnosed are postmenopausal [44, 45].

Mucinous carcinoma is diagnosed when there is more than 50% of tumour cells containing intracytoplasmic mucin [46]. They are rare and the outcomes are similar to endometrioid adenocarcinomas of endometrium [46].

3.2.3 Undifferentiated Carcinoma

Undifferentiated carcinoma of the endometrium is defined as a malignant neoplasm with no differentiation. It displays solid patternless growth and has worse clinical outcome than high grade endometrioid adenocarcinoma. Differentiating between them is important because of the fulminant clinical outcomes and poorer prognosis than high grade endometrioid carcinoma. IHC reveals absence of epithelial markers (CK 18 &EMA), ER, PR, Vimentin or PAX 8. They may be associated with DNA mismatch repair deficiencies but cannot be used to make diagnosis as it may found in other endometrial cancers [38, 47].

4 Diagnosis and Screening, Imaging, Tumour Markers

The initial workup includes a thorough history, general, systemic examination, and pelvic examination with imaging and endometrial biopsy. It should be remembered that imaging does not compensate for lack of physical examination.

More than 90% of patients with endometrial cancers present with postmenopausal bleeding or abnormal uterine bleeding [48]. However, the risk of endometrial cancer in a woman presenting with postmenopausal bleeding is 8–11% [49]. Although not absolute, presentation may vary in high grade non-endometrioid varieties where patients may present with signs and symptoms of advanced disease.

Routine screening for endometrial cancer does not improve the survival and is not indicated. Asymptomatic women with high risk of developing endometrial cancer like unopposed oestrogen therapy, late menopause, tamoxifen therapy, nulliparity, infertility, obesity, diabetes or hypertension should be explained of the risks and associated symptoms. They should be advised to report any unexpected bleeding or spotting to their physicians [50]. Screening is recommended for patients with Lynch Syndrome.

Cervical cytology has limited role in diagnosis of endometrial cancer but the detection of abnormal glandular cells on cervical smear implies a high grade or advanced stage disease [51].

All women with abnormal uterine bleeding and postmenopausal bleeding should **undergo office endometrial biopsy or endometrial curettage** as a part of evaluation. Office endometrial biopsy with a Pipelle is an acceptable diagnostic procedure and has been shown to have sensitivity more than 90% in many studies. It can be performed without cervical dilatation and use of anaesthesia. Studies have shown that adequate tissue sampling is obtained in around 97% of cases and endometrial polyps and atrophic endometrium were the most common cause of inadequate sampling [52–54]. It, however, cannot be performed in patients with stenotic cervical os in whom dilatation and curettage under anaesthesia needs to be done. It has been seen that in Pipelle biopsy sensitivity of diagnosing atypical hyperplasia and malignancy is higher than benign diseases and hence even though a positive biopsy can be taken as conclusive for endometrial cancer a negative biopsy cannot rule it out completely and further evaluation with dilatation and curettage with hysteroscopic assistance should be done in cases with high suspicion [55–57]. Hysteroscopy is associated with intraperitoneal dissemination of tumour cells but prognosis has not been shown to be worsened in patients who have undergone the procedure [58, 59].

Transvaginal ultrasound (TVS) is the imaging procedure of choice for initial evaluation of patients with postmenopausal bleeding [60, 61]. According to American College of Obstetricians and Gynecologist (ACOG) guidelines endometrial thickness (ET) of 4 mm or less has more than 99% negative predictive value for endometrial cancer and has been mentioned as a reasonable alternative to endometrial sampling as a first approach in evaluating a postmenopausal woman with an initial episode of bleeding [62]. Cut-off values of 3 mm and 5 mm have also been shown in literature and there seems to be lack of consensus about the exact value [63, 64]. In an asymptomatic women measurement greater than 4 mm that is incidentally discovered should not always trigger evaluation, but an individualized assessment based on patient characteristics and risk factors is required [62]. It must, however, be remembered that type 2 endometrial cancers can occur in the background of atrophic endometrium and in patients with persistent bleeding endometrial biopsy is mandatory [62]. It has been seen that higher tumour grade was associated with larger tumour, higher prevalence of non-uniform endometrial morphology and heterogeneous endometrium without cystic areas, and lower prevalence of regular endometrial–myometrial junction and no detectable vascularization [65].

On confirmation of malignancy on endometrial biopsy further imaging is required to evaluate the extent of spread of disease. Imaging is not the substitute for surgical staging but helps in tailoring the treatment. **X-ray chest** is recommended for ruling out lung metastasis.

CT/MRI scan is advised depending on the clinical or laboratory findings. CT is used to rule out nodal metastases and distant spread in endometrial cancer. However, it been considered inferior to MRI for characterization of uterine abnormalities due to lower soft-tissue contrast resolution [66]. Additionally, CT scan is useful for excluding unexpected anatomy that may result in modification of planned surgery [67]. If MRI is available, it is preferred to detect the extent of myometrial invasion, cervical stromal involvement, and parametrial extension. In fact, it is the only imaging which is recommended to rule out the involvement of myometrium in grade 1 endometrioid carcinomas in women who desire fertility [68] (Figs. 5 and 6). **PET-CT** demonstrated a high diagnostic performance in identifying lymph node metastasis preoperatively. However, most patients of endometrial cancers present with early stage disease and are at low risk for lymph node metastases. Therefore, it cannot be routinely recommended in all patients for preoperative staging. Presently it is mainly limited in detecting recurrence after endometrial carcinoma surgery with curative intent [69].

Serum Ca 125 is frequently elevated in patients of endometrial cancer, but its role is not well defined as in cases of ovarian malignancies. Elevated CA-125 levels are shown to

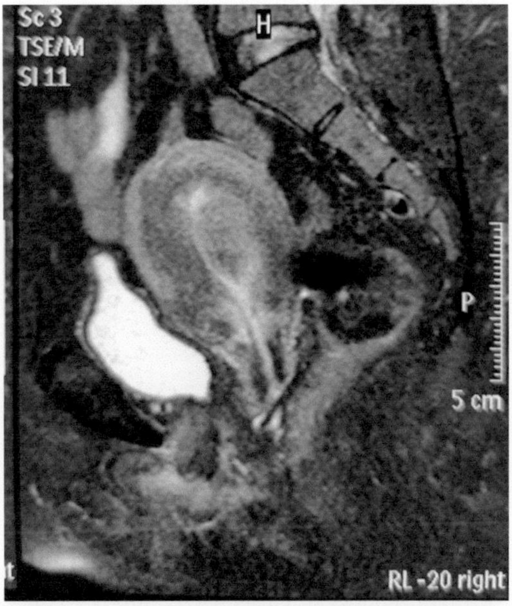

Fig. 5 MRI image showing heterogenous endometrium without myometrial infiltration

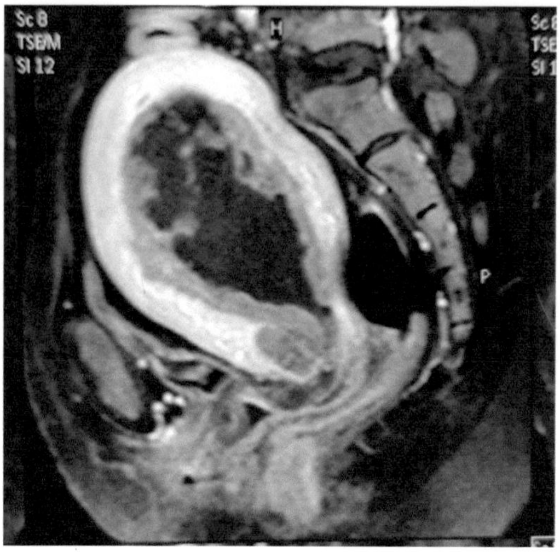

Fig. 6 MRI showing cervical stromal involvement

have significant correlation with lymph node metastasis, depth of invasion, cervical invasion, and advanced stage and few studies have suggested that in these patients a complete surgical staging should be undertaken [70–72]. CA125 level can help in monitoring clinical response in patients with metastatic disease. HE4 is also elevated in endometrial cancers and combination of preoperative HE4 and CA125 has been shown to be a better predictor of metastatic disease than either one alone in endometrial carcinoma [73]. Other molecular-based predictors are still far from having a practical application and only preoperative radiological scans are recommended for detection of metastatic disease.

5 Staging

Surgical staging replaced clinical staging of endometrial cancer in the year 1988 and was again revised in 2009. Histologic verification of grading is included with the extent of the tumour. Clinical staging may still be considered for small number of cases where surgery is not possible.

FIGO Stage 2009 (Reproduced from International Federation of Gynaecology and Obstetrics. Annual report on the results of treatment in gynaecologic cancer.) [74]

I[a]	Tumour confined to the corpus uteri
IA[a]	No or less than half myometrial invasion
IB[a]	Invasion equal to or more than half of the myometrium
II[a]	Tumour invades cervical stroma, but does not extend beyond the uterus[b]
III[a]	Local and/or regional spread of the tumour
IIIA[a]	Tumour invades the serosa of the corpus uteri and/or adnexae[c]
IIIB[a]	Vaginal involvement and/or parametrial involvement[c]
IIIC[a]	Metastases to pelvic and/or para-aortic lymph nodes[c]
IIIC1[a]	Positive pelvic nodes
IIIC2[a]	Positive para-aortic nodes with or without positive pelvic lymph nodes
IV[a]	Tumour invades the bladder and/or bowel mucosa, with or without distant metastasis.
IVA[a]	Tumour invasion of the bladder and/or bowel mucosa
IVB[a]	Distant metastasis, including intra-abdominal metastases and/or inguinal nodes

[a] Either G1, G2, or G3
[b] Endocervical glandular involvement only should be considered as Stage I and no longer as Stage II
[c] Positive cytology has to be reported separately without changing the stage

5.1 Histopathologic grades (G)

1. GX: Grade cannot be assessed.
2. G1: Well-differentiated.
3. G2: Moderately differentiated.
4. G3: Poorly or undifferentiated.

Degree of differentiation of the adenocarcinoma is also used for classification carcinoma of the corpus, which are grouped as follows:

1. G1: less than 5% of a Non-squamous or Nonmorular solid growth pattern.
2. G2: 6%–50% of a Non-squamous or non-morular solid growth pattern.
3. G3: greater than 50% of a Non-squamous or Non-morular solid growth pattern.

5.2 Pathologic Grading Notes

Notable nuclear atypia (pleomorphism and prominent nucleoli), which is not appropriate for the architectural grade, raises the grade of a grade 1 or grade 2 tumour by 1. Most authors consider serous and clear cell carcinomas high grade by definition. Grading of adenocarcinomas with squamous differentiation is allocated according to the nuclear grade of the glandular component.

6 Route of Spread

Endometrial cancer spreads mainly by local invasion, lymphatic spread, and hematogenous spread.

Endometrial cancer initially invades the myometrium and majority of patients have disease limited to uterus at the time of diagnosis. Exfoliated cells can be disseminated into the abdominal cavity via retrograde flow into the fallopian tubes [75, 76]. Lymphatic dissemination occurs via the infundibulopelvic and parametrium. Sometimes tumour may disseminate to paraaortic areas via the infundibulopelvic ligament [77, 78]. Invasion of the para-aortic lymph nodes without pelvic lymph nodes involvement is not a common clinical finding, with reports suggesting it occurs in only 1% to 6% of cases. Direct embolization to the para-aortic lymph nodes from the corpus, without coursing through commonly shared pelvic routes, is probably a late and relatively uncommon event [79–81].

Although vagina is an adjacent organ direct spread without the involve of cervix does not occur. When it does occur, it is considered to be the result of lymphatic spread as the cervix is spared [82, 83].

Hematogenous spread is a late and uncommon occurrence with endometrioid variety.

7 Prognostic Factors

Patients of endometrial cancer mostly present in early stage are type 1 variety and associated with good prognosis. Apart from stage and grade of tumour certain other clinicopathological factors also influence the overall prognosis and outcome. Patients with endometrial cancer can be categorized into prognostic risk groups based on clinicopathologic findings and prognostication helps to ensure that patients receive optimal treatment.

7.1 Age

Advanced age is considered to be a poor prognostic factor. Older patients generally present with advanced clinical stage, higher grade, and increased depth of myometrial infiltration [84, 85]. After deducing data from a GOG study Zaino et al. had found that the 5-year survival is more than 95% in age group less than 50 years but drops down by almost 10% for every 10 years rise in age group and is only approximately 50% over 80 years of age [86]. Similar finding was reported from the PORTEC-1 study where it was reported that locoregional relapse rate was threefold higher for patients aged 60 years and GOG-99 study which identified that increasing age of 70 years and above was a poor prognostic factor in addition to other high-risk pathologic features [87, 88].

7.2 Histologic Type, Grade, and Myometrial Invasion

Type II non-endometroid tumours like serous and clear cell carcinomas are associated with poor prognosis. In 2017 clinical pathological relationships associated with extra uterine disease spread of endometrial cancer was published by GOG10. More than thousand patients with poor histological type were available for analysis and it was found that in these tumours greater number of patients had more than 50% myometrial invasion (33–44%). Pelvic nodal metastasis was associated in 21–25% of patients and paraaortic nodal metastasis in 15–17% [89]. The chances of nodal metastasis increased considerably with increasing depth of myometrial invasion. With only endometrial involvement, 2.6% of pelvic lymph node and 1.2% of para-aortic node metastasis was detected but increased to 31% and 20% respectively when outer one-half of the myometrium or serosa was involved [89]. Same study showed Grade 1 tumours which were limited to the endometrium had only 0.8% pelvic nodal metastasis whereas with involvement of the outer half of myometrium, 15.4% had pelvic nodal metastasis. For grade 3 tumours limited to endometrium, 1.7% had pelvic nodal metastasis which increases to 29.1% with the outer half of myometrial involvement. These finding are similar to previous GOG findings of surgical pathologic spread patterns of endometrial cancer [90]. Compared to histological grade nuclear grading is more accurate and presence of nuclear atypia inappropriate for histological grade raises the grade by one [91]. Atrophic endometrium is regarded as an independent prognostic factor with grade 1 endometroid cancers by one study [92].

7.3 Lymphovascular Space Invasion

This appears to be an independent risk factor of endometrial carcinoma for all histologic types [86, 93]. In node negative patients with disease limited to uterus, the 5-year overall survival was 97.3% in patients without lymphovascular space invasion and 90.9% in those with lymphovascular space invasion [94].

7.4 Positive Peritoneal Cytology

The prognostic significance of positive peritoneal cytology is controversial as it depends on the presence of other risk factors like higher grade and stage, but studies have also reported that positive peritoneal cytology is an independent factor for survival in patients with surgically staged endometrial cancer [95–98]. However, investigators also found that malignant peritoneal cytology has poor prognostic value and adjuvant therapy based on positive peritoneal cytology was not beneficial for long-term survival [99, 100]. Also, it was found that endometrial cancer cells found in the peritoneal cavity usually disappeared within a short time and seemed to have a low malignant potential and only malignant cells from special cases, such as adnexal metastasis are capable of independent growth, and are possibly associated with intraperitoneal recurrence [101]. Although peritoneal cytology has no effect on staging, it is a mandatory component of the 2009 International Federation of Gynaecology and Obstetrics (FIGO) staging system [74].

7.5 Hormonal Receptor Status

Hormonal receptor status may have a role in predicting survival in endometrial cancer patients. Results of a metanalysis have shown that higher levels of ER and PR were significantly associated with a favourable survival whereas increased level of HER2 receptors predicted a poorer survival [102].

7.6 Tumour size

In a study by Schink et al. tumour size was considered independently associated with risk of lymph node metastasis. Only 4% of patients with tumour size less than or equal to 2 cm had lymph node metastasis whereas it was 15% for tumours more than 2 cm and increased further to 35% when the entire uterine cavity was involved [103]. Vargas et al. evaluated the risk of nodal metastasis in patients with endometrial cancer, using the Mayo criteria. Study group consisted of 19,329 women with surgically staged endometrial cancer from the data collected from National Cancer Institute's SEER registry. The low-risk group, as per the Mayo criteria, was defined by: grade 1 or 2 tumour histology; less than 50% myometrial invasion; and tumour size less than or equal to 2 cm. The high-risk group was comprised of tumours with myometrial invasion more than 50%, grade 3 histology, or tumour size more than 2 cm. In this large series of 381 patients having Grade 1/2 endometrioid cancers and less than 50% myometrial invasion, no patients with tumour size less than 2 cm had lymph node involvement. When patients with grade 1 tumours were analysed separately, lymph node involvement remained below 2% until tumour size exceeded 4 cm. Even in tumours greater than 5 cm in size, the rate of lymph node involvement remained below 3%. They concluded it was reasonable to defer lymph node dissection in all grade 1 tumours with less than 50% invasion, irrespective of tumour size [104].

7.7 Molecular Subgroups

A study by Raffone et al. provided a pooled data about prognosis of TCGA groups, in order to support future clinical trials and to better understand the usefulness of molecular risk stratification in patients with endometrial cancer. Data from this metanalyses has shown that p53 mutated group had the worst prognosis which was further worsened by unfavourable clinicopathological factors. Prognosis of MSI group overlapped with low copy number group but was worsened by unfavourable clinicopathological factors. Prognosis of POLE mutated group was the best one and did not seem to be significantly affected by clinicopathological factors [105].

8 Surgical Management

Majority of endometrial cancer patients undergo surgery as a part of their treatment. Patients with significant medical comorbidities who are not acceptable candidates for surgery (markedly advanced age, diminished performance status, severe cardiac/pulmonary disease, massive obesity) may still be managed by primary radiation therapy without surgery.

For patients presenting with disseminated or nonresectable disease, nonsurgical options including radiation, chemotherapy, or hormonal therapy are used. Surgery with palliative intent may be required to control vaginal bleeding in some of these cases.

The initial approach for patients who are medically fit should be extra fascial hysterectomy with bilateral salphingo-oophorectomy. Removal of the tubes and ovaries is recommended even if they appear normal, as they may contain micrometastases. However, in very selected cases in premenopausal women with low grade early stage disease, ovarian preservation may be considered based on few studies [106, 107]. Traditionally with cervical stromal involvement a Type 2 hysterectomy is performed. But recently after evidence by Phelippeau et al. and Takano et al. was published where no survival benefit from radical hysterectomy was found a simple extrafascial hysterectomy with free margins is also recommended [108, 109]. This recommendation was also included in the ESMO-ESGO-ESTRO report [50].

A lower midline abdominal incision is preferred which allows easy access and inspection of the upper abdomen. For patients with grade 1 or 2 tumours and less than 50% myometrial infiltration evident on MRI a lower transverse abdominal incision may be used.

After opening the abdomen, peritoneal washings are taken and sent for cytological analysis. Exploration of the abdomen and pelvis is done in a systematic manner and any suspicious lesions are biopsied. After completion of hysterectomy the uterus is then cut open on the operating table to determine whether surgical staging is required in patients with grade 1 or 2 tumours as surgical staging will be needed in cases with more than 50% myometrial infiltration. Intraoperative frozen section is not recommended nowadays. For patients with serous or clear cell carcinomas a comprehensive surgical staging like ovarian cancer is mandatory (Figs. 7 and 8).

8.1 Pelvic Lymphadenectomy

The paradigm of routine complete retroperitoneal lymphadenectomy was challenged with the publication of two randomized trials. These trials demonstrated that systemic lymphadenectomy did not offer a survival advantage in women with endometrial cancer.

ASTEC trial which is the acronym for 'A Study in the Treatment of Endometrial Cancer' successfully randomized participants to postoperative external beam radiotherapy to pelvis independent

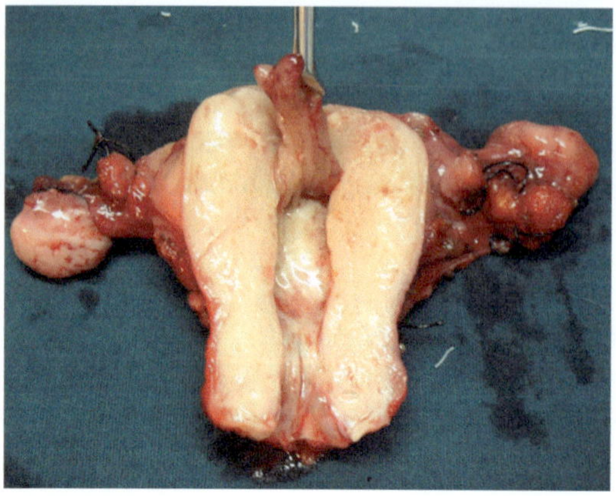

Fig. 7 Intraoperative cut section of uterus showing polypoid growth limiting to the endometrium

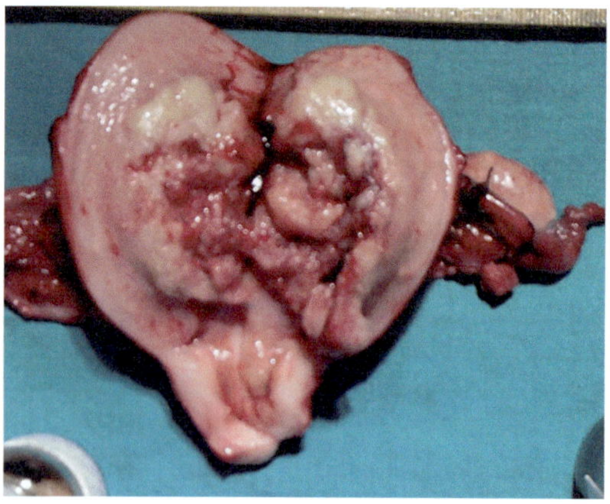

Fig. 8 Endometrial growth showing myometrial infiltration (Frozen section confirmed more than 50% infiltration)

of lymph-node status. This randomized trial showed no evidence of a benefit for systematic lymphadenectomy for endometrial cancer in terms of overall, disease-specific, and recurrence-free survival [110]. The second trial was the Italian CONSORT trial where patients were assigned to hysterectomy with or without pelvic lymphadenectomy. Systematic pelvic lymph node dissection was considered to have been performed appropriately and according to protocol when at least 20 pelvic lymph nodes were removed and analysed by the pathologist. The 5-year disease-free and overall survival rates analysis were similar between arms and was concluded that although systematic pelvic lymphadenectomy statistically significantly improved surgical staging, it did not improve disease-free or overall survival [111].

However, both these trials have been criticized due to many factors. Patients identified with positive nodes were not given adjuvant therapy, poor quality of the lymph node dissection in ASTEC trial, absence of para-aortic nodal dissection, lack of quality-of-life assessment evaluating effect of both surgery and downstream use of adjuvant therapy, and the over representation of low-risk patients [112, 113].

The Mayo criteria is widely used for selecting patients requiring pelvic lymphadenectomy during surgical staging. In 2000, Mariani et al. from the Mayo clinic demonstrated in their study patients with favourable characteristics which included three low-risk features: tumour size ≤2 cm, grade 1 or 2 tumours, and depth of invasion ≤50%. They concluded that patients who have FIGO grade 1 or 2 endometrioid cancer with greatest surface dimension ≤2 cm, myometrial invasion ≤50%, and no intraoperative evidence of macroscopic disease can be treated optimally with hysterectomy only [114].

The Mayo criteria has been validated by many studies and shown that in the absence of these factors, the risk of retroperitoneal lymph node metastasis is approximately 1% [104–116].

Sampling of lymph nodes results inaccurate information as micro-metastasis cannot be determined. Therefore, if staging has to be performed a comprehensive lymphadenectomy should be done. Anatomic boundaries for pelvic lymphadenectomy include common iliac bifurcation superiorly, deep circumflex vein inferiorly, genitofemoral nerve on the iliopsoas muscle laterally, and obliterated umbilical artery medially.

8.2 Paraaortic Nodal Dissection (Fig. 9)

Factors associated with para-aortic lymph node dissemination include advanced stage, adnexal involvement, high grade, deep myometrial invasion, cervical involvement, lymph vascular space involvement, and the presence of pelvic lymph node metastases. In a GOG study the highest cor-

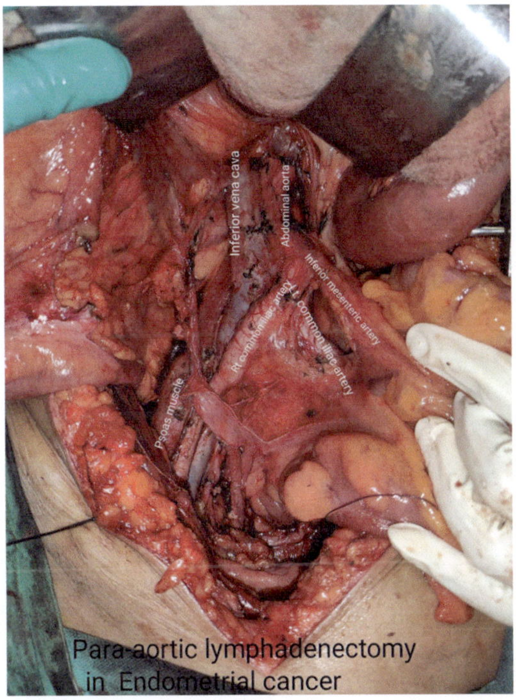

Fig. 9 Paraaortic nodal dissection

relation was seen with pelvic node metastasis with 32.3% of pelvic nodes metastasis also having paraaortic node metastases [117].

In the survival effect of paraaortic lymphadenectomy in endometrial cancer study 2010(SEPAL) it was seen that patients with intermediate or high risk of recurrence, pelvic, and para-aortic lymphadenectomy reduced the risk of death compared with pelvic lymphadenectomy alone [118]. The SEPAL study suggests that high-risk patients may benefit from aggressive surgery.

8.3 Sentinel Node Biopsy

Sentinel lymph node dissection can be considered as an alternative to complete lymphadenectomy. If sentinel is negative, it is unlikely for the remaining nodes to be involved. Complete lymphadenectomy can thus be avoided resulting a significant reduction in surgery-related morbidity. Studies have shown that sentinel node biopsy is a feasible technique and can triage patients even for high-risk endometrial cancer patients [119–123].

Lymphatic mapping with technetium-99m (99mTc) is the most common radiolabelled colloid injected for sentinel node detection. Blue-coloured dyes like 1% isosulfan blue and 1% methylene blue are also used for direct visualization of lymphatic channels and sentinel lymph nodes. FIRES trial published in 2017 provided a strong evidence in favour of sentinel node biopsy. This trial was designed with the primary objective to estimate the sensitivity and negative predictive value of sentinel-lymph-node mapping using robotic assisted fluorescence imaging of the tracer indocyanine green. Among 385 patients who were enrolled, 29% had high grade endometrial pathology. They concluded that sentinel lymph nodes identified with indocyanine green have a high degree of diagnostic accuracy in and can safely replace lymphadenectomy in the staging of endometrial cancer [124]. Three injection sites mainly used are the uterine fundus, the endometrium using hysteroscopy, and the cervix. Cervical injection technique is the most convenient because of easy access to the cervix [124–128].

8.4 Omentectomy

Omentectomy as part of surgical staging plays a significant role in patients with adnexal involvement, macroscopic peritoneal metastasis, high grade and deeply invasive lesions [129, 130]. In cases with gross omental or intraperitoneal disease spread, cytoreductive surgery with total omentectomy, radical peritoneal stripping, and occasionally bowel resection is required.

8.5 Minimal Invasive Surgery

Minimal invasive surgery for endometrial cancer is now an established procedure with many studies establishing the feasibility and outcome comparable with open surgeries. However, it has been suggested that obese patients are poor laparoscopic candidates because of difficulties in establishing pneumoperitoneum, poorer visualization, inability to tolerate the steep Trendelenburg positioning, and difficulties with ventilation [131–134].

There are three main trials addressing the MIS approach for endometrial cancer surgery. First was a feasibility trial also known as the LAP1 trial. It has fewer number of cases and had only 84 patients. LAP-1 showed that laparoscopic staging in patients with presumed stage 1 endometrial cancer can be done safely and this led to the phase III GOG LAP-2 trial [135]. LAP-2 study had a larger patient cohort where 2616 women were randomly assigned to laparoscopic or open surgery. Among patients who underwent laparoscopy almost 25% were converted to laparotomy. Most commonly the conversion rate was attributed to poor exposure, tumour spread, excessive bleeding, and equipment failure. Increasing BMI and age were found to be statistically correlated with the need to perform a laparotomy. Complication rates for those who had an open procedure were 7.6%, compared to 9.5% of patients randomized to laparoscopy. Comparing patients who underwent open surgery versus successful completion of laparoscopy, operative time was longer (median 70 min), but hospital time was shorter (2 days vs. 4 days) with laparoscopy. The authors concluded that laparoscopic surgical staging is an acceptable and possibly a better option, particularly when the surgery can be successfully completed laparoscopically [136].

The LACE (Laparoscopic Approach to Carcinoma of the Endometrium trial) trial addressed quality-of-life outcomes and disease-free survival in patients with early endometrial cancer. Conversions were lower when compared to LAP trials as they excluded cases with uterine size more than 10 weeks and included only those surgeons with expertise in laparoscopy. Moreover, for grade 1/2 tumours with less than 50% myometrial invasion nodal dissection was not carried out. The trial results favoured laparoscopic approach similar to LAP trials [137].

Robotic Surgery for endometrial cancer surgery is a safe and effective surgical practice but its large-scale application still faces a series of challenges, such as a high cost, testing, maintenance costs, and surgical costs. The advantages include improved visualization with 3-D optics, wrist-like motion of instruments allowing greater dexterity, reduction in tremor, easier learning curve for adoption compared to straight-stick laparoscopy, and more comfortable ergonomics. Published data suggest comparable outcomes with laparoscopy with regard to blood loss, nodal counts, and operative time. Robotic surgery may offer unique opportunities for obese patients as the flexibility and stability of robotic surgery makes lymphadenectomy more thorough [138–143].

8.6 Role of Cytoreductive Surgery

The percentage of patients presenting with advanced endometrial cancer is low and as a result any study on the role of extensive surgery has limited number of patients. Most of the data either in favour for upfront surgical approach or following neoadjuvant chemotherapy is derived from management of ovarian cancer. Greer and Hamberger had published outcomes of debulking surgery in a group of 31 patients and they found that when debulking was done to less than 2 cm followed by radiation therapy a survival of more than 70% was obtained [144]. Similar to this study Martinez et al. which had 25 patients presented similar conclusion [145]. Bristow et al. had slightly a greater number of patients ($n = 65$) and optimal cytoreduction was achieved 55%. They showed a definite benefit following optimal cytoreduction where a median survival of approximately 34 months was achieved. In contrast patients with suboptimal surgery only 11 months of median survival could be achieved [146]. Cytoreduction to no visible disease is associated with improved overall survival in advanced stage and is the cornerstone of management [147].

9 Adjuvant Treatment

Surgically staged patients with disease confined to the uterine corpus have a small risk of recurrence and various trials have been conducted to study the benefit of teletherapy and brachytherapy in postoperative setting for disease confined to the uterus. For the purpose of allocating adjuvant treatment postoperatively endometrial cancer has been subclassified into various risk groups. What constitutes low, intermediate or high risk has been defined differently by different trials over the years. Risk classification became more confusing after revision of FIGO staging in 2009. Recently risk stratification and required adjuvant therapy is suggested based on molecular markers. The ESMO/ESTRO guidelines recommend that when the molecular classification is unknown, Stage IA endometroid, low grade (comprising Grade I & II), LVSI negative or focal tumours may be stratified as low risk. When the molecular classification is known, Stage I–II POLE mutated Endometrial carcinoma with no residual disease as well as Stage IA low grade tumours with no or focal LVSI which are mismatch repair deficient (MMRd) or have nonspecific molecular profile (NSMP) are also considered low risk. These patients are to be kept on follow-up and no adjuvant therapy is recommended [148].

For the ease of understanding various landmark trials addressing requirement of adjuvant radiation and chemotherapy are briefly described in this chapter. One of the first attempts to evaluate the benefit of pelvic radiotherapy for surgically staged patients with intermediate risk endometrial adenocarcinoma was made by GOG 99. Intermediate risk endometrial adenocarcinoma in this trial was defined based on data from a surgical staging protocol of GOG 33 [117]. All women found to have any degree of myometrial invasion with adenocarcinoma of any grade and no evidence of lymph node involvement (initial FIGO stage IB, IC, IIA occult, and IIB occult) were considered to be in the intermediate risk group. In this study as clear cell and serous adenocarcinomas of the endometrium were associated with a relatively high risk of recurrence they were excluded. A high intermediate risk group was defined as (1) Grade II/III tumour with presence of LVSI, or myometrial infiltration of outer one third. (2) Age 50 or more required two risk factors, (3) Age 70 years or more with any one risk factor mentioned above. This trial had more than 400 women who were divided in two arms based on whether adjuvant radiation was received or not. After a median follow-up of 69 months the radiation arm showed less incidence of pelvic recurrence (12% in observation arm and 3% in the radiotherapy arm). The treatment difference was significant among the high intermediate risk group with recurrence in observation versus radiotherapy group being 26% versus 6%. The impact of decreased pelvic recurrence after radiation therapy did not translate to improved overall survival when compared to observation arm. The 4-year survival was 86% in the no adjuvant radiation arm and 92% for the radiotherapy arm which was not significantly different. They concluded that adjunctive radiotherapy should be recommended for high intermediate risk patients [88].

PORTEC 1 (Post-Operative Radiation Therapy in Endometrial Carcinoma) had drawn similar conclusion like GOG 99 where parameters like locoregional control, overall survival, and treatment-related morbidity of patients with stage-1 endometrial carcinoma, treated with postoperative pelvic radiotherapy or surgery alone was studied. The 5-year locoregional recurrence rates were 4% in the radiotherapy group and 14% in the control group. The rates of distant metastases (6% and 5%) and of endometrial-cancer-related death (11% and 8%) were similar with and without radiotherapy. The 5-year overall survival rates were similar in the two groups: 81% (radiotherapy) and 85% (controls). The study concluded that postoperative radiotherapy in stage-1 endometrial carcinoma reduces locoregional recurrence but has no effect on overall survival and is not indicated in stage-1 endometrial carcinoma below 60 years and patients with grade-2 tumours with superficial invasion [87].

After the question of requirement of pelvic radiation was addressed, it became important to find out whether the same benefit could be delivered by vaginal brachytherapy alone and thereby reduce the toxicity associated with whole pelvic RT. The answer to this question was PORTEC II trial where patients with stage I or IIA endometrial carcinoma with features of high-intermediate risk were randomly assigned to pelvic EBRT or VBT (vaginal brachytherapy). The primary endpoint was vaginal recurrence. **This trial concluded that VBT is effective for vaginal control, resulting in lesser gastrointestinal side effects than with EBRT and recommended that VBT should be the adjuvant treatment of choice for patients with endometrial carcinoma of high-intermediate risk** [149].

The GOG 249 trial was conducted for determining if vaginal brachytherapy with chemotherapy could improve survival in patients with high-intermediate risk early endometrial carcinoma. Chemotherapy was initiated up to 3 weeks from start of brachytherapy. No benefit could be demonstrated with the addition of chemotherapy and it was found that it added to more frequent and severe acute toxicity [150].

Adjuvant therapy for advanced endometrial cancer requires a combination of both radiation and chemotherapy. This is to achieve both local and systemic control as well as prevent recurrence in both sites. GOG 122 showed superiority with systemic chemotherapy in these patients. It was shown that chemotherapy (doxorubicin 60 mg/m [2] and cisplatin 50 mg/m [2] given every 3 weeks for seven cycles, followed by one cycle of cisplatin) had better survival than whole abdomen radiation therapy when an optimal surgery was done [151].The phase II RTOG-9708 trial assessed the response along with safety and feasibility when chemotherapy was combined with adjuvant radiation for patients with high-risk endometrial cancer. Radiation included 45 Gy in 25 fractions to the pelvis along with cisplatin (50 mg/m^2) on days 1 and 28. Vaginal brachytherapy was performed after the external beam radiation. Four courses of cisplatin (50 mg/m [2]) and paclitaxel (175 mg/m [2]) were given at 4-week intervals following completion of radiotherapy. This trial demonstrated 4-year disease-free survival of 85%and overall survival of 81% favouring good locoregional control with combined approach [152].

Based on the success of these trials similar regimen was used by GOG 258 and PORTEC 3. GOG 258 examined the role of combined chemotherapy and radiation in patients with stage III/IVA uterine cancer. The primary endpoint of this randomized trial was to determine whether treatment with cisplatin and radiation followed by carboplatin and paclitaxel for 4 cycles (C-RT, experimental arm) resulted in reduced risk of recurrence or death when compared to carboplatin and paclitaxel for six cycles (CT, control arm) in patients with stages III-IVA (<2 cm residual disease) or FIGO 2009 stage I/II serous or clear cell UC and positive cytology. Secondary objectives were assessment of overall survival (OS), acute and late toxicities, and quality of life. At 60 months of follow-up patients who were alive and recurrence-free was 59% in the CTRT arm and 58% in the CT-only arm. The trial concluded that chemotherapy combined with radiation did not result in a longer progression-free survival than chemotherapy alone in patients with stage III or IVA endometrial carcinoma [153].

In PORTEC 3 trial women were randomly assigned to receive radiotherapy or radiotherapy and chemotherapy (consisting of two cycles of cisplatin 50 mg/m^2 given during radiotherapy, followed by four cycles of carboplatin AUC5 and paclitaxel 175 mg/m^2). The cohort of patients ranged from high grade early stage to stage III and IV. After a median follow-up was 60 months overall survival was 81.8% with chemoradiotherapy versus 76.7% with radiotherapy alone which was not statistically significant. In contrast 5-year failure-free survival difference was significant which was 75.5% in chemoradiotherapy arm versus 68.6%in radiotherapy arm respectively. Adverse events were more common when both radiation and chemotherapy was given and occurred in 60% of patients who received chemoradiotherapy versus 12% who received radiotherapy only. Although there was no significant benefit demonstrated between the two groups on overall survival subset analysis showed that stage III patients fared better with both radiotherapy and chemotherapy [154].

The NCCN recommends that systemic therapy with or without vaginal brachytherapy or EBRT with or without vaginal brachytherapy for adjuvant therapy of advanced stage endometrial cancer [155].

To summarize after surgery, we need to decide whether.

- No adjuvant treatment is required.
- Only Vaginal Brachytherapy.
- EBRT and vaginal brachytherapy with or without chemotherapy.
- Sequential chemotherapy and radiotherapy.
- Systemic Chemotherapy alone.

Both NCCN and ESGO /ESTO guideline address the questions but later has the advantage that it takes in account molecular parameters based on TGCA classification.

10 Radiotherapy in Endometrial Cancer

Radiotherapy delivery in Endometrial Cancer patients involves Teletherapy in combination with Brachytherapy techniques depending upon the clinical scenario. Besides being an effective adjuvant therapy for achieving superior local control, radiotherapy has also been used with radical intent in primary inoperable endometrial cancers, as a neoadjuvant therapy prior to surgery and for recurrent disease.

10.1 External Beam Radiotherapy (EBRT) in Endometrial Cancer

EBRT target volume consists of the vaginal cuff, proximal two-thirds of the vagina and the pelvic lymph nodes- encompassing the sites of known or suspected tumour involvement as specified by histopathology and imaging findings. The obturator, external, internal, and lower common iliac group of lymph nodes are routinely included in the EBRT fields while presacral nodes are also included in cases with involvement of the cervix. Historically, conventional planning with X-ray based simulation has been used for pelvic radiotherapy treatment with considerable success. In conventional radiotherapy, a four-field box technique is used to deliver pelvic radiotherapy for endometrial cancer. Two radiation fields—one in the anterio-posterior (AP) direction and other in the postero-anterior (PA) direction, are combined with two beams in bilateral direction to achieve target coverage. The superior borders of the AP/PA fields are placed at L5-S1 junction while the inferior border is placed at the bottom of the obturator foramen with the lateral borders placed 2 cm beyond the maximum diameter of the inlet of the true bony pelvis. For the bilateral fields, the anterior border lies anterior to the pubis symphysis and the posterior border is placed at S2–S3 junction while their superior and inferior borders coincide with that of the AP/PA fields. All the fields are treated daily. In cases with para-aortic lymph node involvement, an Extended Field technique of EBRT needs to be used. In such a scenario, along with the pelvic RT volume, the paracaval, para-aortic, and inter-aortocaval nodes also need to be encompassed within the RT portals with the upper border of the fields at least 1–2 cm above the level of renal vessels (T12-L1 level). The greatest drawback in conventional planning in adjuvant radiotherapy of endometrial cancers is the increased rates of small bowel toxicity [87, 148]. This risk increases further when extended fields are used as the volume of small bowel included in the RT portals becomes higher. Hence, Intensity Modulated Radiotherapy (IMRT) technique is preferred nowadays for pelvic EBRT that reduces the small bowel irradiation by 50–60% as compared to conventional planning [156, 157] resulting in significant reduction of radiation induced acute gastrointestinal toxicities [158].

In IMRT, the radiation delivery to the target is in the form of multiple small beamlets of varying intensities achieved in specialized linear accelerators equipped with multi-leaf collimators, thereby providing superior target coverage while sparing surrounding normal tissue considerably. With IMRT, proper delineation of the target volume is imperative for successful treatment- which requires proper imaging and knowledge of surgical pathology findings. Small et al. [159] published a consensus guideline on delineation of clinical target volume (CTV) for IMRT use in pelvic radiotherapy for postoperative endometrial cancer. CT based simulation of the pelvic region in the treatment position is obtained with intravenous contrast. Generally two scans are obtained—once with full bladder and another with bladder empty. The CTV of the vaginal cuff, upper vagina, and parametrium may undergo daily variations due to differential bladder filling. Hence contouring them in both the bladder full and empty scans helps generate an internal target volume (ITV) which is then used to generate the CTV to ensure that the target always remains inside the treated volume irrespective of daily bladder variations. The nodal CTV is drawn by using the contrast enhanced pelvic vessels as a surrogate and adding an isotropic margin of 7 mm around them while excluding the bowel and muscles-as advocated by Taylor et al. [160] and Small et al. [161] Planning target volume (PTV) is generated by addition of setup margins as per institutional protocols. An example of an IMRT treatment using Volumetric Modulated Arc Therapy (VMAT) in a case of endometrial carcinoma is shown in Fig. 10.

External beam radiotherapy dose to the target volume defined above is usually 45–50.4 Gy at 180 to 200 cGy per fraction that accounts for microscopic residual in the pelvis. However, in cases with grossly involved/enlarged residual pelvic or para-aortic nodes, a boost to these regions with IMRT to a dose of 14.4 Gy in 8 fractions as per RTOG 0921 can be considered [161].

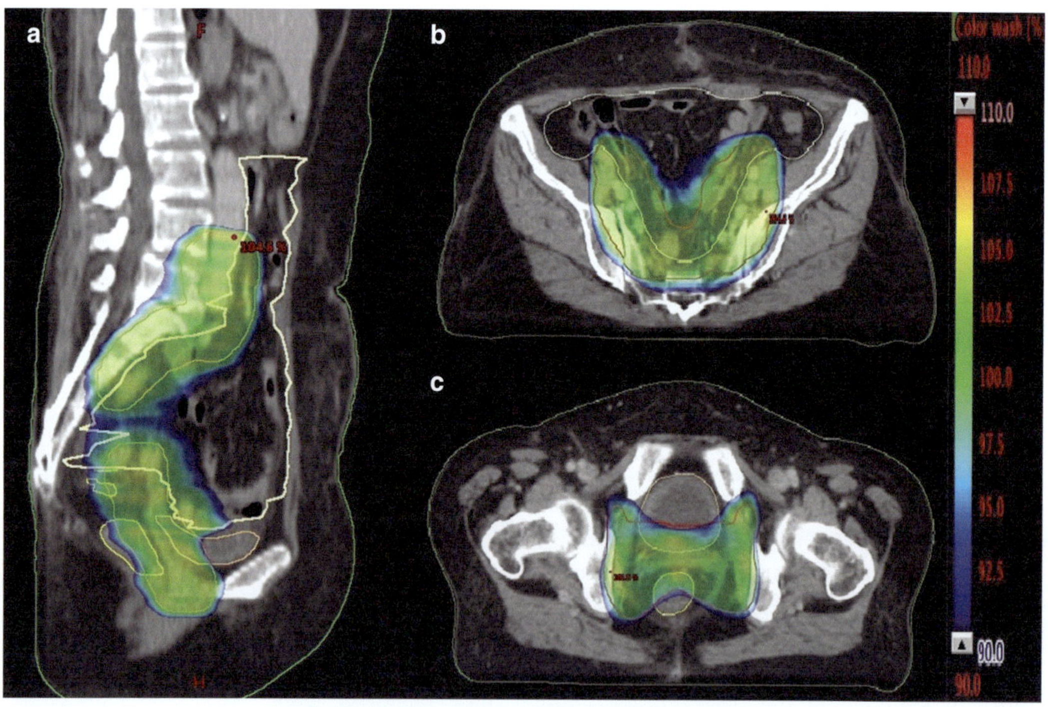

Fig. 10 Shows the isodoses of radiotherapy planning by Volumetric Modulated Arc Therapy (VMAT) technique in a post operative case of Endometrial Carcinoma. Note the homogeneous coverage of the Planning Target Volume (contoured in red) with significant sparing of the small bowel (contoured in yellow) from irradiation to high doses (**a**: Sagittal View & **b**: Axial view-upper pelvis). Adequate coverage of the vaginal cuff and obturator nodes with significant sparing of urinary bladder and posterior wall of rectum is also depicted (**c**: Axial view- lower pelvis) [Credits: Mr. Shashi B. Sharma]

10.2 Brachytherapy in Endometrial Cancer

Brachytherapy is an integral component of treatment of endometrial cancer. Modern radiotherapy uses high dose rate (HDR) sources like Cobalt-60 and Iridium-192. These sources can deliver radiotherapy doses at more than 12 Gy per hour which has substantially reduced the treatment time of brachytherapy as compared to the low dose rate (LDR) era. Also advancements in imaging, computerized treatment planning, and after loading techniques have further improved the efficacy and safety of brachytherapy. The indications of brachytherapy in endometrial cancer are as follows [155, 162]:

1. As adjuvant therapy for the treatment of the vaginal cuff after radical hysterectomy- as the sole modality or in combination with EBRT.
2. Treatment of recurrences in the vaginal cuff after previous treatment.
3. Treatment of primary inoperable endometrial cancer.

10.2.1 Adjuvant Brachytherapy Post-hysterectomy

The American Brachytherapy Society has laid down guidelines for endometrial cancer brachytherapy in the HDR era [162]. The choice of the optimum HDR brachytherapy applicator for treatment of the vaginal vault is imperative and must take into account the variations in disease presentation and patient anatomy. Some of the widely used applicators in brachytherapy treatment of vaginal vault post hysterectomy are vaginal cylinders, vaginal ovoids, and Houdek applicator. The utility of these applicators depend on the clinical scenario- whether to treat only the vaginal cuff or the whole length of vagina up to introitus, shape of the vagina (wide or narrow) and the shape of the vaginal cuff (symmetric or "dog-eared" configuration). Thus, a detailed visual and manual examination of the vaginal vault is a must before deciding upon the type of applicator to be used. Placement of radio-opaque seeds/clips at the vaginal apex is suggested by some authors to verify the correct position of the applicator to the vaginal mucosa.

Vaginal cylinders are preferred when the treatment of the entire vaginal canal is indicated and in cases with narrow vagina. They are available in various diameters ranging from 1.5 to 4 cm and the cylinders are usually segmented such that they can be assembled for required length of treatment. The largest diameter cylinder that can comfortably be accommodated in the vaginal canal of the patient should be used. The mucosa of the apex and canal of the vagina should be in firm contact with the surface of the cylinder. The cylinder must lie in the midline and be secured in a neutral position for adequate dose distribution. Most widely used cylinders have a single, central channel for entry and dwell positions of the source. Multi-channel vaginal cylinders containing up to six peripheral channels along the applicator surface together with a central channel have also been designed. Such applicators allow shaping of the dose distribution according to disease extent by differential loading of the channels while also accounting for the anisotropy of dose at the vaginal apex with single channel applicators.

Fletcher-type and Henschke-type shielded or unshielded vaginal ovoids of varying diameters (2–3 cm) are available for treatment of vaginal cuff with HDR brachytherapy. Unlike cylinders, ovoids can be used along with rectal separators and anterior packing to displace the rectum and bladder from the high dose region. They are particularly useful in treating assymetric vaginal cuffs with "dog-ear" configuration but the disadvantage is that treatment of the entire vaginal canal with ovoids is not possible. Care must be taken such that the medial aspects of the ovoids are touching each other after placement so as to avoid a cold spot in the vaginal mucosa between them.

After insertion of the applicators, imaging is done to ensure their proper localization and proper planning of brachytherapy dose. The methods of vaginal applicator localization include fluoroscopy/ plain-film radiography, CT scan or MRI with dummy sources placed inside

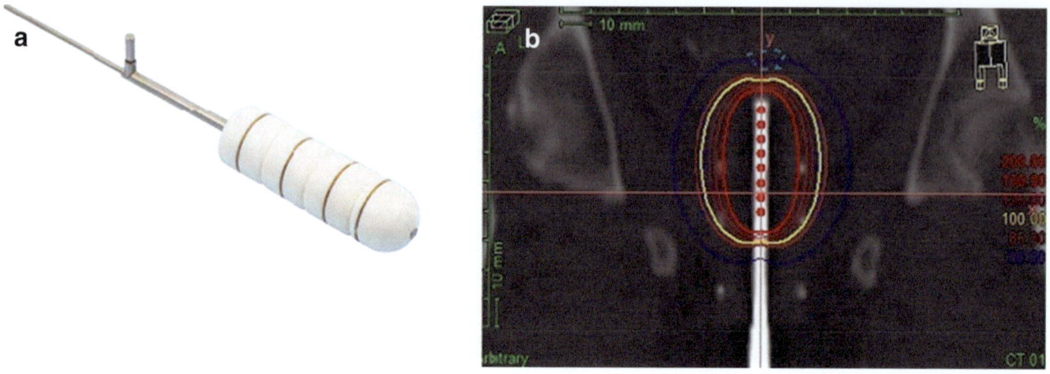

Fig. 11 (**a**) A segmented single-channel vaginal cylinder applicator used for adjuvant vaginal vault brachytherapy. (**b**) The dosimetry of a brachytherapy treatment using the same applicator on a localization planning CT scan. Red dots represent the dwell positions of the HDR stepping source. Yellow line depicts the 100% isodose prescription which lies at a depth of 5 mm from the applicator surface

the applicator. Localization imaging should be obtained in the treatment position with radio-opaque contrast material inside bladder foley catheter balloon and standard rectal markers to allow the bladder and rectal doses to be estimated as per ICRU 38 recommendations [163]. Although X-ray based simulation and planning is most widely used, the incorporation of CT based localization and planning provides better delineation of the vaginal mucosa and normal organs. The information may allow better treatment dosimetry by optimization of dose based on proximity to the rectum and bladder and thickness of the vaginal wall. The proximal 3–5 cm of the vagina is usually treated except in serous and clear cell histologies where treatment of the entire vaginal canal is recommended. Dose is prescribed and optimized either at the surface of the cylinder/ovoid or at a depth of 0.5 cm from the vaginal mucosa. ABS recommends recording of dose at both these points regardless of prescription [162]. As fixed geometry applicators are used for vaginal brachytherapy, a customized treatment plan is generally calculated for the patient on the first fraction and the same plan used for all subsequent treatment fractions. Optimization in vaginal cuff brachytherapy in generally done to shape the dose distribution to the curve of the cylinder. The ABS recommends placing optimization points both at the apex and along the curved portion of the cylinder dome in addition to the lateral vaginal mucosa and the use of proper anisotropic dose calculation model. The most commonly prescribed dose fraction for HDR brachytherapy in post-op endometrial cancer after 45 Gy EBRT dose is 7Gy x 3 fractions at 0.5 cm depth of prescription. Figure 11 depicts the adjuvant brachytherapy treatment of a case of post-operative endometrial carcinoma with vaginal cylinder applicator.

10.2.2 Brachytherapy for Vaginal Vault Recurrence

Brachytherapy to the vaginal vault is used as a boost after 45–50 Gy EBRT to the pelvis in vaginal recurrences post-hysterectomy in endometrial cancer patients who have not received radiotherapy previously. A careful examination of the local extent of the recurrent disease by clinical examination and imaging needs to be done prior to choosing brachytherapy as treatment in such cases. The choice of applicator and dose will depend on thickness and location of the recurrence as well as previous radiotherapy received. Apart from the general principles of adjuvant vault brachytherapy stated above, the following principles outlined by ABS guides brachytherapy treatment in this clinical scenario [162, 164]:

(A) For non-bulky recurrences (thickness less than 5 mm) brachytherapy with appropriate vaginal applicator should be used.
(B) For bulky recurrences (thickness more than 5 mm) and previously irradiated cases, interstitial brachytherapy in a centre with considerable experience is advisable.
(C) For recurrences in only one wall of the vagina, due measures should be taken to limit dose to the opposite wall.
(D) Radio-opaque markers/clips should be placed at the margins of the gross disease before EBRT treatment to guide proper applicator placement at the time of brachytherapy.

The dose specification and optimization is similar to the post-operative adjuvant treatment of endometrial cancer. Brachytherapy dose prescribed with 45 Gy EBRT is 6 Gy × 4 fractions or 7 Gy × 3 fractions when prescribed at 0.5 cm depth.

10.2.3 Brachytherapy for Primary Inoperable Endometrial Cancer

Primary endometrial cancer patients who are poor candidates for surgery or EBRT due to advanced age and/or presence of co-morbidities may be offered definitive HDR brachytherapy with fairly high local control rates. Unlike in adjuvant brachytherapy, HDR applicators for treatment of the intact uterus resembles those of cervical carcinoma (tandem and ovoids/ring etc.). Dedicated endometrial applicators can be used that offer more homogeneous dose distribution over the uterine walls. The placement of applicators is carried out under sedation or spinal anaesthesia. A thorough examination to determine the size and position of the uterus relative to the cervix and vagina is done. Ultrasound guidance during uterine sounding and placement of intrauterine tandem is helpful. Placement of two 15 degree tandems rotated by 30–45 degrees such that each fits into the two cornua of the uterine fundus helps to deliver better dose distribution at the fundus [162]. Proper dose distribution at the vagina is usually not achieved by ovoids, hence vaginal cylinders are used with the tandem(s).

The target volume here is the entire uterus, cervix, and the upper 3–5 cm of the vagina. The irregular shape of the target volume presents a challenge towards achieving satisfactory dose distribution from brachytherapy. The ABS guidelines recommend that treatment planning should be image and target based and should ensure the coverage of entire uterine serosa and the vaginal wall (to a depth of 0.5 cm) within the prescription isodose [162]. The dose is to be prescribed at a point 2 cm from the central axis at the midpoint along the uterine applicator and the isodose should be widened at the uterine fundus to account for the increased width at that level. At vaginal level, the dose distribution should be optimized to deliver prescribed dose at 0.5-cm depth of the vaginal mucosal surface. ICRU reported bladder and rectum point doses should be recorded and sigmoid colon localization and dose reporting should preferably be done [163]. Scwarz et al. [165] have published a recommendation for brachytherapy in inoperable endometrial carcinoma and suggested that MRI or CT scan should be used for target volume and OAR delineation for planning purposes. The GTV defined as the visible abnormality on T2 weighted MRI should be contoured. The CTV which includes the entire uterus, cervix, and 1–2 cm of proximal vagina along with nearby organs at risk like bladder, rectum, sigmoid, normal vagina, and bowel should also be delineated. The panel recommended the EQD2 dose in Stage I endometrial cancer should be at least 48 Gy for brachytherapy alone and at least 65 Gy for the combination of external beam plus brachytherapy to 90% of the (D90) CTV volume with the GTV receiving more than 80 Gy [165].

11 Neoadjuvant Therapy in Endometrial Cancer

Neoadjuvant radiotherapy with or without chemotherapy followed by a less extensive extrafascial hysterectomy is an approach sometimes adopted for locally advanced endometrial cancer clinically extending to the cervix and parametrium. The dose of neoadjuvant radiation used is 45–50 Gy EBRT followed by image based HDR brachytherapy 5–6 Gy per fraction for 3–4 fractions [166]. Platinum based concurrent chemotherapy is generally used along with EBRT. Iheagwara et al. [167] reported 94% rate of downstaging with negative surgical margins in extrafascial hysterectomy in 34 patients of locally advanced type II endometrial cancer using this approach. Vargo et al. [166] also reported in their series of 36 patients that neoadjuvant chemoradiotherapy was associated with 24% pathologic complete response rate with 3-year local control, overall survival and grade 3+ toxicity rates of 96%, 100%, and 11%, respectively. However, in the absence of any randomized clinical trial evaluating this approach, there is dearth of data to recommend neoadjuvant therapy in locally advanced endometrial cancer patients.

12 Treatment of Metastatic Endometrial Cancer

In patients with metastatic endometrial cancer surgical cytoreduction is preferred if optimal cytoreduction can be achieved. Patients who are not fit for surgery should be offered medical therapy. Such patients have a poor prognosis and whatever treatment modality is chosen should have the aim of balancing disease control and maintaining quality of life. Patients with metastatic endometrial cancer are treated with systemic therapy either following surgical cytoreduction or as primary therapy. Treatment of stage IV disease must be individualized but usually involves a combination of surgery, radiation therapy and either hormonal therapy or chemotherapy. A major goal of therapy should be to try to achieve local disease control in the pelvis, in order to palliate bleeding, vaginal discharge, pain, and fistula formation. Carboplatin and paclitaxel are preferred chemotherapeutic regimen although triple regimen comprising doxorubicin, cisplatin and paclitaxel can be used. Both are similar in efficacy but the latter is associated with more serious toxicity [168–170].

13 Role of Hormonal Therapy

Type I endometrial cancers express oestrogen and progesterone and therefore they are sensitive to hormonal agents. Apart from its use in fertility preservation for Grade 1 endometrioid variety limited to endometrium, it is used in disseminated disease and when systemic chemotherapy cannot be used [171]. Progesterone alone or in combination with tamoxifen is commonly preferred in the metastatic setting.

Medroxyprogesterone acetate 200 mg daily is recommended by a GOG study if the tumour shows positivity for hormonal receptors and are of low grade [172]. Medroxyprogesterone acetate 160 mg in single or in divided dose is used more commonly and it is continued till disease progression. However, side effects from high dose progestins like oedema, thrombophlebitis, tremor, hypertension, and thromboembolism can occur and should be explained to the patients [173].

14 Recurrent Endometrial Cancer

Though endometrial cancer has a good overall prognosis there can be recurrence specially if the disease is high grade or if was advanced at presentation. Patient should be kept on follow-up and clinical examination should focus on detecting both locoregional and distant metastasis. Patients should be made aware of the possible symptoms they may have during recurrence and clinical history should be obtained at each visit. We recommend periodic visit at 3 monthly intervals during the first 2 years following treatment followed by 6 monthly visit for the next 3 years followed by annual visit. Relapse is commonly seen within lymph nodes, the vagina, the peritoneum, and the lung. Unusual sites of disease include spleen, pancreas, rectum, muscle, and brain [172]. Data suggest vaginal smears are ineffective in the detection of recurrences compared with physical examination alone [174–177]. In patients with elevated CA-125 at presentation it may be used to monitor recurrence. Imaging studies such as chest radiography, CT, magnetic resonance imaging should be performed for patients who are symptomatic or have abnormal findings on physical examination.

Treatment approach in recurrent setting depends on the site of recurrence and previous treatment undertaken. It also depends of the general condition of the patient as patient with poor performance status cannot withstand any form of extensive surgery or chemotherapy. Locoregional recurrence mostly involves the vagina and if radiation was not given previously it is used to treat it. This approach is preferred and evidence comes from a follow-up analysis of the PORTEC-1 study where it was found that survival after vaginal relapse was better for patients that had not received adjuvant radiation (65% vs. 43%) [176].

Surgery should only be advised if complete resection is feasible in a previously irradiated patient. Extent of resection depends on the volume of disease. For instance, vaginectomy may be sufficient to remove small focus of disease whereas in some patients more radical procedure such as exenteration will be required. The complication rate post-surgery may be as high as 60–80% as evident from case series studies and may achieve an overall 5-year survival of 20–45% [178, 179].

The management for disseminated disease is difficult and there is no definite guideline for curative treatment. Chemotherapy is commonly preferred although there is also benefit seen after optimal cytoreduction [180–182]. Most commonly a combination of carboplatin and paclitaxel is used and recently Bevacizumab is also used [183, 184]. These group of patients have poor prognosis which worsens if the disease worsens during treatment or there is a recurrence. Similar to ovarian cancer treatment response to previous platinum therapy is taken as a reference for further treatment in such situations and a response of 60% is obtained if there was a disease free interval of more than a year [185, 186].

Trastuzumab and lapatinib are also considered an option due to the moderate expression of HER 2 neu and EGRF receptors by these tumours [187–191]. PTEN mutations are common with type I endometrioid cancers and they act as a regulatory protein of mTOR which is studied as a therapeutic target [192–194].

Temsirolimus and deforolimus which are mTOR inhibitors have also shown appreciable activity in recurrent and metastatic settings [195, 196].

15 Management of Endometrial Carcinoma in Young Women

Although endometrial cancer is a disease of older women it sometimes does occur. Though options for management are similar to older patients the morbidity associated with surgical menopause is troublesome and difficult to manage. Most of these women are nulliparous and consideration for fertility preservations has to be made. Conservative management involves intake of high dose progesterone and can be done in very selected cases. It is only considered in case of Grade 1 endometrioid cancers which is limited to the endometrium. MRI is the imaging recommended to rule out myometrial invasion.

Initially a 3-month trial of megestrol acetate orally is given in the dosage of 160,320 mg daily. Alternatively, medroxyprogesterone acetate 200–500 mg daily is also [197, 198]. Close monitoring with endometrial sampling every 3–6 months is recommended. Hysterectomy and salpingo-oophorectomy with staging is recommended after childbearing is complete or if patients have documented progression with biopsies and if endometrial cancer is still present after 6–12 months of progestin-based therapy. Bilateral ovaries can be preserved in low grade tumours with less than 50% infiltration. Levonorgestrel-releasing intrauterine device (LNG-IUD) as an option for conservative management of endometrial hyperplasia and early endometrial cancer. However, results of small studies which have used LNG-IUD for endometrial cancer have inconclusive results [172, 199].

16 Synchronous Primary Cancers of the Endometrium and Ovary

Synchronous primary cancers of the endometrium and ovary occur in approximately 10% of all women with ovarian cancer and 5% of all women with endometrial cancer [200]. Whenever both the organs are involved, it is important to rule out metastasis from either organ as the management will differ. In 1985, Ulbright and Roth delineated a set of pathologic criteria to help distinguish metastatic disease from synchronous primary tumours [201]. Different histological types, grade or DNA ploidy, absence of invasion or only superficial myometrial invasion of endometrial cancer, absence of LVSI in endometrial or ovarian tumour and unilateral ovarian involvement are suggestive of synchronous tumours [202]. Metastatic disease to the ovary, rather than a synchronous primary, should be suspected when ovarian disease is small, bilateral, or multinodular with surface implants and angiolymphatic invasion at the ovarian cortex [202]. The incidence is higher in premenopausal women and 5–29% have a synchronous ovarian malignancy [203]. In cases with synchronous primary tumours of both ovary and endometrium, treatment is based on the combined treatment recommendations for each cancer according to stage.

17 Summary and Conclusion

Management of endometrial cancer has come a long way over the years. Minimal invasive surgery is preferred over laparotomy for surgical staging in selected patients to prevent postoperative morbidity. Risk stratification for adjuvant therapy for stage I endometrial cancers based on molecular markers is a new advent. Diagnostic algorithm using three immunohistochemical markers (p53, MSH6, and PMS2) and mutation analysis of the exonuclease domain of POLE to identify prognostic groups analogous to the TCGA molecular-based classification is commonly utilized. Molecular classification is now encouraged in all endometrial carcinomas, especially high grade tumours. PORTEC IVa is an ongoing randomized controlled trial that attempts to tailor adjuvant radiation therapy in high-intermediate risk endometrial cancer with molecular-integrated risk profile-based recommendations. It aims to identify favourable molecular subgroups which can be managed by observation or vaginal brachytherapy to prevent overtreatment. Treatment of patients based on histopathology and molecular profiling will lead to a better biological understanding of the disease and lead to an individualized therapy in near future.

References

1. Sung H, Ferlay J, Siegel RL, Laversanne M, Soerjomataram I, Jemal A, Bray F. Global cancer statistics 2020: GLOBOCAN estimates of incidence and mortality worldwide for 36 cancers in 185 countries. CA Cancer J Clin. 2021;71(3):209–49.
2. Lortet-Tieulent J, Ferlay J, Bray F, Jemal A. International patterns and trends in endometrial cancer incidence, 1978–2013. J Natl Cancer Inst. 2018;110(4):354–61.
3. Globocan 2020. Globocan 2020: India factsheet - India Against Cancer [Internet]. [cited 2021 Mar 20]. Available from: http://cancerindia.org.in/globocan-2020-india-factsheet/
4. National Cancer Registry Programme (NCRP I. consolidated report of population based cancer registries 2012–2014. Bangalore: NCRP; 2016.
5. Uterine Cancer — Cancer Stat Facts [Internet]. [cited 2020 Jun 9]. Available from: https://seer.cancer.gov/statfacts/html/corp.html
6. Maheshwari A, Kumar N, Mahantshetty U. Gynecological cancers: a summary of published Indian data. South Asian J Cancer. 2016;5(3):112.
7. Hong XW, Bing Xiang Y, Zheng W, Zhang X, Xian Ruan Z, Rong Cheng J, et al. Weight history and risk of endometrial cancer among Chinese women. Int J Epidemiol. 2006;35:159–66.
8. Inoue M, Okayama A, Fujita M, Enomoto T, Tanizawa O, Ueshima H. A case-control study on risk factors for uterine endometrial cancer in Japan. Japanese J Cancer Res. 1994;85(4):346–50.
9. Amant F, Mirza MR, Koskas M, Creutzberg CL. Cancer of the corpus uteri. Int J Gynecol Obstet. 2015;1(131):S96–104.
10. Ali AT. Reproductive factors and the risk of endometrial cancer. Int J Gynecol Cancer. 2014;24(3):384–93.
11. Wartko P, Sherman ME, Yang HP, Felix AS, Brinton LA, Trabert B. Recent changes in endometrial can-

cer trends among menopausal-age US women. Cancer Epidemiol. 2013;37(4):374–7.
12. Bergman L, Beelen ML, Gallee MP, Hollema H, Benraadt J, van Leeuwen FE. Risk and prognosis of endometrial cancer after tamoxifen for breast cancer. Comprehensive cancer Centres' ALERT Group. Assessment of Liver and Endometrial cancer Risk following Tamoxifen. Lancet (London, England). 2000;356(9233):881–7.
13. Walsh S. The pathology of lynch syndrome. Diagnostic Histopathol. 2015;21(4):161–4.
14. Meyer LA, Broaddus RR, Lu KH. Endometrial cancer and Lynch syndrome: clinical and pathologic considerations. Cancer Control. 2009;16(1):14–22.
15. Rodabaugh KJ, Lu KH, Schorge JO, Daniels MS, Sun CC, Soliman PT, et al. Prospective determination of prevalence of Lynch Syndrome in young women with endometrial cancer gynecologic cancers: mechanisms and treatments view project genomic characterization of agressive endometrial tumors view project prospective determination of. Artic J Clin Oncol. 2007;25:5158–64.
16. Boland CR, Lynch HT. The history of Lynch syndrome. Familial Cancer. 2013;12(2):145–57.
17. Wang Y, Wang Y, Li J, Cragun J, Hatch K, Chambers SK, et al. Lynch syndrome related endometrial cancer: clinical significance beyond the endometrium equal contributors. J Hematol Oncol. 2013;6:22.
18. Lynch HT, Snyder CL, Shaw TG, Heinen CD, Hitchins MP. Milestones of Lynch syndrome: 1895-2015. Nat Rev Cancer. 2015;15(3):181–94.
19. Provenzale D, Gupta S, Ahnen DJ, Bray T, Cannon JA, Cooper G, David DS, Early DS, Erwin D, Ford JM, Giardiello FM. Genetic/familial high-risk assessment: colorectal version 1.2016, NCCN clinical practice guidelines in oncology. J Natl Compr Canc Netw. 2016;14(8):1010–30.
20. Syndrome L. Practive bulletin 147. Obstet Gynecol. 2014;124(5):1042–54.
21. Lu KH, Loose DS, Yates MS, Nogueras-Gonzalez GM, Munsell MF, Chen LM, et al. Prospective multicenter randomized intermediate biomarker study of oral contraceptive versus depo-Provera for prevention of endometrial cancer in women with Lynch syndrome. Cancer Prev Res. 2013;6(8):774–81.
22. Bokhman JV. Two pathogenetic types of endometrial carcinoma. Gynecol Oncol. 1983;15(1):10–7.
23. Passarello K, Kurian S, Villanueva V. Endometrial cancer: an overview of pathophysiology, management, and care. Semin Oncol Nurs. 2019;35(2):157–65.
24. Cohen IR, Lambris JD. Advances in experimental medicine and biology editorial board. Berlin: Springer; 2017. p. 47–74.
25. Santaballa A, Matías-Guiu X, Redondo A, Carballo N, Gil M, Gómez C, et al. SEOM clinical guidelines for endometrial cancer (2017). Clin Transl Oncol. 2018;20(1):29–37.
26. Getz G, Gabriel SB, Cibulskis K, Lander E, Sivachenko A, Sougnez C, et al. Integrated genomic characterization of endometrial carcinoma. Nature. 2013;497(7447):67–73.
27. McAlpine J, Leon-Castillo A, Bosse T. The rise of a novel classification system for endometrial carcinoma; integration of molecular subclasses. J Pathol. 2018;244(5):538–49.
28. Kommoss S, McConechy MK, Kommoss F, Leung S, Bunz A, Magrill J, et al. Final validation of the ProMisE molecular classifier for endometrial carcinoma in a large population-based case series. Ann Oncol. 2018;29(5):1180–8.
29. Kurman RJ, Kaminski PF, Norris HJ. The behavior of endometrial hyperplasia. Cancer. 1985;56(2):403–12.
30. Trimble CL, Kauderer J, Zaino R, Silverberg S, Lim PC, Burke JJ, et al. Concurrent endometrial carcinoma in women with a biopsy diagnosis of atypical endometrial hyperplasia: a gynecologic oncology group study. Cancer. 2006;106(4):812–9.
31. Lacey JV, Ioffe OB, Ronnett BM, Rush BB, Richesson DA, Chatterjee N, et al. Endometrial carcinoma risk among women diagnosed with endometrial hyperplasia: the 34-year experience in a large health plan. Br J Cancer. 2008;98(1):45–53.
32. Malpica A. How to approach the many faces of endometrioid carcinoma. Mod Pathol. 2016;29(S1):S29–44.
33. Zaino RJ, Kurman RJ, Brunetto VL, Morrow CP, Bentley RC, Cappellari JO, et al. Villoglandular adenocarcinoma of the endometrium: a clinicopathologic study of 61 cases: a gynecologic oncology group study. Am J Surg Pathol. 1998;22(11):1379–85.
34. Pavlakis K, Messini I, Vrekoussis T, Panoskaltsis T, Chrysanthakis D, Yiannou P, et al. MELF invasion in endometrial cancer as a risk factor for lymph node metastasis. Histopathology. 2011;58(6):966–73.
35. Hendrickson MR, Kempson RL. Ciliated carcinoma—a variant of endometrial adenocarcinoma. Int J Gynecol Pathol. 1983;2(1):1–12.
36. Zaino RJ, Kurman RJ. Squamous differentiation in carcinoma of the endometrium: a critical appraisal of adenoacanthoma and adenosquamous carcinoma. Semin Diagn Pathol. 1988;5:154–71.
37. Hamilton CA, Cheung MK, Osann K, Chen L, Teng NN, Longacre TA, et al. Uterine papillary serous and clear cell carcinomas predict for poorer survival compared to grade 3 endometrioid corpus cancers. Br J Cancer. 2006;94(5):642–6.
38. Hanley KZ, Birdsong GG, Mosunjac MB. Recent developments in surgical pathology of the uterine corpus. Arch Pathol Lab Med. 2017;141(4):528–41.
39. Scully RE, Barlow JF. "Mesonephroma" of ovary. Tumor of müllerian nature related to the endometrioid carcinoma. Cancer. 1967;20(9):1405–17.
40. Yamamoto S, Tsuda H, Aida S, Shimazaki H, Tamai S, Matsubara O. Immunohistochemical detection of

hepatocyte nuclear factor 1β in ovarian and endometrial clear-cell adenocarcinomas and nonneoplastic endometrium. Hum Pathol. 2007;38(7):1074–80.
41. Hoang LN, Han G, McConechy M, Lau S, Chow C, Gilks CB, et al. Immunohistochemical characterization of prototypical endometrial clear cell carcinoma-diagnostic utility of HNF-1β and oestrogen receptor. Histopathology. 2014;64(4):585–96.
42. Lax SF, Pizer ES, Ronnett BM, Kurman RJ. Clear cell carcinoma of the endometrium is characterized by a distinctive profile of p53, Ki-67, estrogen, and progesterone receptor expression. Hum Pathol. 1998;29(6):551–8.
43. Zhang C, Zhang H, Yang L, Wang Y, Li X, Guo J, et al. Primary squamous cell carcinoma of the endometrium in a woman of perimenopausal age: a case report. Medicine. 2018;97:48.
44. Giordano G, D'Adda T, Merisio C, Gnetti L. Primary squamous cell carcinoma of the endometrium: a case report with immunohistochemical and molecular study. Gynecol Oncol. 2005;96(3):876–9.
45. Lee SJ, Choi HJ. Primary endometrial squamous cell carcinoma: a case report and review of relevant literature on Korean women. Korean J Pathol. 2012;46(4):395–8.
46. Galic V, Schiavone MB, Herzog TJ, Holcomb K, Lewin SN, Lu YS, et al. Prognostic significance of mucinous differentiation of endometrioid adenocarcinoma of the endometrium. Cancer Investig. 2013;31(7):500–4.
47. Han J, Ki EY, Rha SE, Hur SY, Lee A. Dedifferentiated endometrioid carcinoma of the uterus: report of four cases and review of literature. World J Surg Oncol. 2017;15(1):1–9.
48. Kimura T, Kamiura S, Yamamoto T, Seino-Noda H, Ohira H, Saji F. Abnormal uterine bleeding and prognosis of endometrial cancer. Int J Gynecol Obstet. 2004;85(2):145–50.
49. Clarke MA, Long BJ, Del Mar MA, Arbyn M, Bakkum-Gamez JN, Wentzensen N. Association of endometrial cancer risk with postmenopausal bleeding in women a systematic review and meta-analysis. JAMA Intern Med. 2018;178(9):1201–8.
50. Colombo N, Creutzberg C, Amant F, Bosse T, González-Martín A, Ledermann J, et al. ESMO-ESGO-ESTRO consensus conference on endometrial cancer: diagnosis, treatment and follow-up. Int J Gynecol Cancer. 2016;26(1):2–30.
51. Gu M, Shi W, Barakat RR, Thaler HT, Saigo PE. Pap smears in women with endometrial carcinoma. Acta Cytol. 2001;45(4):555–60.
52. Guido RS, Kanbour-Shakir A, Rulin MC, Christopherson WA. Pipelle endometrial sampling: sensitivity in the detection of endometrial cancer. J Reprod Med Obstet Gynecol. 1995;40(8):553–5.
53. Fakhar S, Saeed G, Khan AH, Alam AY. Validity of pipelle endometrial sampling in patients with abnormal uterine bleeding. Ann Saudi Med. 2008;28(3):188–91.
54. Abdelazim IA, Aboelezz A, Abdulkareem AF. Pipelle endometrial sampling versus conventional dilatation & curettage in patients with abnormal uterine bleeding. J Turkish Ger Gynecol Assoc. 2013;14(1):1–5.
55. Kremer C, Duffy S. A randomised controlled trial comparing transvaginal ultrasound, outpatient hysteroscopy and endometrial biopsy with inpatient hysteroscopy and curettage. BJOG An Int J Obstet Gynaecol. 2000;107(8):1058.
56. Alfhaily F, Ewies AAA. The first-line investigation of postmenopausal bleeding: transvaginal ultrasound scanning and endometrial biopsy may be enough. Int J Gynecol Cancer. 2009;19(5):892–5.
57. Clark TJ. Hysteroscopy or curettage? In: Hysteroscopy. Cham: Springer International Publishing; 2018. p. 141–8.
58. Chen J, Clark LH, Kong WM, Yan Z, Han C, Zhao H, et al. Does hysteroscopy worsen prognosis in women with type II endometrial carcinoma? PLoS One. 2017;12(3):1–12.
59. Polyzos NP, Mauri D, Tsioras S, Messini CI, Valachis A, Messinis IE. Intraperitoneal dissemination of endometrial cancer cells after hysteroscopy: a systematic review and meta-analysis. Int J Gynecol Cancer. 2010;20(2):261–7.
60. Ewies AAA, Musonda P. Managing postmenopausal bleeding revisited: what is the best first line investigation and who should be seen within 2 weeks? A cross-sectional study of 326 women. Eur J Obstet Gynecol Reprod Biol. 2010;153(1):67–71.
61. Wong ASW, Lao TTH, Cheung CW, Yeung SW, Fan HL, Ng PS, et al. Reappraisal of endometrial thickness for the detection of endometrial cancer in postmenopausal bleeding: a retrospective cohort study. BJOG An Int J Obstet Gynaecol. 2016;123(3):439–46.
62. ACOG Committee Opinion No. 734: the role of transvaginal ultrasonography in evaluating the endometrium of women with postmenopausal bleeding. Obstet Gynecol. 2018;131(5):e124–9.
63. Jokubkiene L, Sladkevicius P, Valentin L. Transvaginal ultrasound examination of the endometrium in postmenopausal women without vaginal bleeding. Ultrasound Obstet Gynecol. 2016;48(3):390–6.
64. Timmermans A, Opmeer BC, Khan KS, Bachmann LM, Epstein E, Clark TJ, et al. Endometrial thickness measurement for detecting endometrial cancer in women with postmenopausal bleeding: a systematic review and meta-analysis. Obstet Gynecol. 2010;116:160–7.
65. Epstein E, Fischerova D, Valentin L, Testa AC, Franchi D, Sladkevicius P, et al. Ultrasound characteristics of endometrial cancer as defined by international endometrial tumor analysis (IETA) consensus nomenclature: prospective multicenter study. Ultrasound Obstet Gynecol. 2018;51(6):818–28.

66. Haldorsen IS, Salvesen HB. What is the best preoperative imaging for endometrial cancer? Curr Oncol Rep. 2016;18(4):1–11.
67. Lin MY, Dobrotwir A, McNally O, Abu-Rustum NR, Narayan K. Role of imaging in the routine management of endometrial cancer. Int J Gynecol Obstet. 2018;143:109–17.
68. Nougaret S, Horta M, Sala E, Lakhman Y, Thomassin-naggara I, Kido A, et al. Endometrial Cancer MRI staging: Updated Guidelines of the European Society of Urogenital Radiology. Eur Radiol. 2019;29:792–805.
69. Bollineni VR, Ytre-Hauge S, Bollineni-Balabay O, Salvesen HB, Haldorsen IS. High diagnostic value of 18F-FDG PET/CT in endometrial cancer: systematic review and meta-analysis of the literature. J Nucl Med. 2016;57(6):879–85.
70. Wang Y, Han C, Teng F, Bai Z, Tian W, Xue F. Predictive value of serum HE4 and CA125 concentrations for lymphatic metastasis of endometrial cancer. Int J Gynecol Obstet. 2016;136(1):58–63.
71. Hapsari K, Makin J, Dreyer G. The accuracy of preoperative serum CA-125 levels to predict lymph node metastasis in a population of south African women with endometrial carcinoma. South African J Gynaecol Oncol. 2019;11(1):7–10.
72. Modarres-Gilani M, Vaezi M, Shariat M, Zamani N, Nourizadeh R. The prognostic role of preoperative serum CA125 levels in patients with advanced endometrial carcinoma. Cancer Biomark. 2017;20(2):135–41.
73. Saarelainen SK, Peltonen N, Lehtimäki T, Perheentupa A, Vuento MH, Mäenpää JU. Predictive value of serum human epididymis protein 4 and cancer antigen 125 concentrations in endometrial carcinoma. Am J Obstet Gynecol. 2013;209(2):142.e1–6.
74. Amant F, Mirza MR, Koskas M, Creutzberg CL. Cancer of the corpus uteri. Int J Gynecol Obstet. 2018;143:37–50.
75. Berry E, Lindheim SR, Connor JP, Hartenbach EM, Schink JC, Harter J, et al. Sonohysterography and endometrial cancer: incidence and functional viability of disseminated malignant cells. Am J Obstet Gynecol. 2008;199(3):240.e1–8.
76. Guralp O, Kushner DM. Iatrogenic transtubal spill of endometrial cancer: risk or myth. Arch Gynecol Obstet. 2011;284(5):1209–21.
77. Burke TW, Levenback C, Tornos C, Morris M, Wharton JT, Gershenson DM. Intraabdominal lymphatic mapping to direct selective pelvic and paraaortic lymphadenectomy in women with high-risk endometrial cancer: results of a pilot study. Gynecol Oncol. 1996;62(2):169–73.
78. Mariani A, Webb MJ, Keeney GL, Podratz KC. Routes of lymphatic spread: a study of 112 consecutive patients with endometrial cancer. Gynecol Oncol. 2001;81(1):100–4.
79. Hirahatake K, Hareyama H, Sakuragi N, Nishiya M, Makinoda S, Fujimoto S. A clinical and pathologic study on Para-aortic lymph node metastasis in endometrial carcinoma. J Surg Oncol. 1997;65(2):82–7.
80. Yokoyama Y, Maruyama H, Sato S, Saito Y. Indispensability of pelvic and paraaortic lymphadenectomy in endometrial cancers. Gynecol Oncol. 1997;64(3):411–7.
81. Abu-Rustum NR, Gomez JD, Alektiar KM, Soslow RA, Hensley ML, Leitao MM, et al. The incidence of isolated paraaortic nodal metastasis in surgically staged endometrial cancer patients with negative pelvic lymph nodes. Gynecol Oncol. 2009;115(2):236–8.
82. Rutledge FN, Tan SK, Fletcher GH. Vaginal metastases from adenocarcinoma of the corpus uteri. Am J Obstet Gynecol. 1958;75(1):167–74.
83. Phillips GL, Prem KA, Adcock LL, Twiggs LB. Vaginal recurrence of adenocarcinoma of the endometrium. Gynecol Oncol. 1982;13(3):323–8.
84. Aziz H, Hussain F, Edelman S, Cirrone J, Aral I, Fruchter R, Homel P, Rotman M. Age and race as prognostic factors in endometrial carcinoma. Am J Clin Oncol. 1996;19(6):595–600.
85. Vance S, Yechieli R, Cogan C, Hanna R, Munkarah A, Elshaikh MA. The prognostic significance of age in surgically staged patients with type II endometrial carcinoma. Gynecol Oncol. 2012;126(1):16–9.
86. Zaino RJ, Kurman RJ, Diana KL, Morrow CP. Pathologic models to predict outcome for women with endometrial adenocarcinoma: the importance of the distinction between surgical stage and clinical stage—a gynecologic oncology group study. Cancer. 1996;77(6):1115–21.
87. Creutzberg CL, van Putten WL, Koper PC, Lybeert ML, Jobsen JJ, Wárlám-Rodenhuis CC, De Winter KA, Lutgens LC, van den Bergh AC, van de Steen-Banasik E, Beerman H, van Lent M. Surgery and postoperative radiotherapy versus surgery alone for patients with stage-1 endometrial carcinoma: multicentre randomised trial. PORTEC Study Group. Post Operative Radiation Therapy in Endometrial Carcinoma. Lancet. 2000;355:1404–11.
88. Keys HM, Roberts JA, Brunetto VL, Zaino RJ, Spirtos NM, Bloss JD, et al. A phase III trial of surgery with or without adjunctive external pelvic radiation therapy in intermediate risk endometrial adenocarcinoma: a gynecologic oncology group study. Gynecol Oncol. 2004;92(3):744–51.
89. Creasman WT, Ali S, Mutch DG, Zaino RJ, Powell MA, Mannel RS, et al. Surgical-pathological findings in type 1 and 2 endometrial cancer: an NRG oncology/gynecologic oncology group study on GOG-210 protocol. Gynecol Oncol. 2017;145(3):519–25.
90. Creasman WT, Morrow CP, Bundy BN, Homesley HD, Graham JE, Heller PB. Surgical pathologic spread patterns of endometrial cancer: a gynecologic oncology group study. Cancer. 1987;60(8 S):2035–41.

91. Nielsen AL, Thomsen HK, Christian H, Nyholm J. Evaluation of the reproducibility of the revised 1988 international federation of gynecology and obstetrics grading system of endometrial cancers with special emphasis on nuclear grading. Cancer. 1991;68:2303–9.
92. Geels YP, Pijnenborg JMA, Van Den Berg-Van Erp SH, Bulten J, Visscher DW, Dowdy SC, et al. Endometrioid endometrial carcinoma with atrophic endometrium and poor prognosis. Obstet Gynecol. 2012;120(5):1124–31.
93. Weinberg LE, Kunos CA, Zanotti KM. Lymphovascular space invasion (LVSI) is an isolated poor prognostic factor for recurrence and survival among women with intermediate-to high-risk early-stage endometrioid endometrial cancer. Int J Gynecol Cancer. 2013;23(8):1438–45.
94. Cusano E, Myers V, Samant R, Sudai T, Keller A, Le T, et al. Prognostic significance of Lymphovascular space invasion in the absence of lymph node metastases in Early-stage endometrial cancer. Int J Gynecol Cancer. 2018;28(5):890–4.
95. Takeshima N, Nishida H, Tabata T, Hirai Y, Hasumi K. Positive peritoneal cytology in endometrial cancer: enhancement of other prognostic indicators. Gynecol Oncol. 2001;82(3):470–3.
96. Mariani A, Webb MJ, Keeney GL, Aletti G, Podratz KC. Assessment of prognostic factors in stage IIIA endometrial cancer. Gynecol Oncol. 2002;86(1):38–44.
97. Tanaka K, Kobayashi Y, Sugiyama J, Yamazaki T, Dozono K, Watanabe M, et al. Histologic grade and peritoneal cytology as prognostic factors in type 1 endometrial cancer. Int J Clin Oncol. 2017;22(3):533–40.
98. Yildirim N, Bilgi A, Gokulu SG, Akman L, Zekioglu O, Serin G, et al. Lymphovascular space invasion and positive peritoneal cytology are independent prognostic factors for lymph node metastasis and recurrence in endometrial cancer. Eur J Gynaecol Oncol. 2018;39(6):977–83.
99. Yazigi R, Piver MSBL. Malignant peritoneal cytology as prognostic indicator in stage I endometrial cancer. Obstet Gynaecol. 1983;62:359–62.
100. Konski A, Poulter C, Keys H, Rubin P, Beecham J, Doane K. Absence of prognostic significance, peritoneal dissemination and treatment advantage in endometrial cancer patients with positive peritoneal cytology. Int J Radiat Oncol Biol Phys. 1988;15:135–40.
101. Hirai Y. Malignant potential of positive peritoneal cytology in endometrial cancer. Obstet Gynecol. 2001;97(5):725–8.
102. Zhang Y, Zhao D, Gong C, Zhang F, He J, Zhang W, et al. Prognostic role of hormone receptors in endometrial cancer: a systematic review and meta-analysis. World J Surg Oncol. 2015;13(1):1–12.
103. Schink JC, Miller DS, Lurain JR, Rademaker AW. Tumor size in endometrial cancer. Cancer. 1991;67(11):2791–4.
104. Vargas R, Rauh-Hain JA, Clemmer J, Clark RM, Goodman A, Growdon WB, et al. Tumor size, depth of invasion, and histologic grade as prognostic factors of lymph node involvement in endometrial cancer: a SEER analysis. Gynecol Oncol. 2014;133(2):216–20.
105. Raffone A, Travaglino A, Mascolo M, Carbone L, Guida M, Insabato L, et al. TCGA molecular groups of endometrial cancer: pooled data about prognosis. Gynecol Oncol. 2019;155(2):374–83.
106. Gonthier C, Trefoux-Bourdet A, Koskas M. Impact of conservative managements in young women with grade 2 or 3 endometrial adenocarcinoma confined to the endometrium. Int J Gynecol Cancer. 2017;27(3):493–9.
107. Koskas M, Bendifallah S, Luton D, Daraï E, Rouzier R. Safety of uterine and/or ovarian preservation in young women with grade 1 intramucous endometrial adenocarcinoma: a comparison of survival according to the extent of surgery. Fertil Steril. 2012;98(5):1229–35.
108. Phelippeau J, Koskas M. Impact of radical hysterectomy on survival in patients with stage 2 Type1 endometrial carcinoma: a matched cohort study. Ann Surg Oncol. 2016;23(13):4361–7.
109. Takano M, Ochi H, Takei Y, Miyamoto M, Hasumi Y, Kaneta Y, et al. Surgery for endometrial cancers with suspected cervical involvement: is radical hysterectomy needed (a GOTIC study)? Br J Cancer [Internet]. 2013;109(7):1760–5. https://doi.org/10.1038/bjc.2013.521.
110. Kitchener H, Swart AM, Qian Q, Amos CPM. Efficacy of systematic pelvic lymphadenectomy in endometrial cancer (MRC ASTEC trial): a randomised study. Lancet. 2009;373(9658):125–36.
111. Panici PB, Basile S, Maneschi F, Lissoni AA, Signorelli M, Scambia G, et al. Systematic pelvic lymphadenectomy vs no lymphadenectomy in early-stage endometrial carcinoma: randomized clinical trial. J Natl Cancer Inst. 2008;100(23):1707–16.
112. Creasman WT, Mutch DE, Herzog TJ. ASTEC lymphadenectomy and radiation therapy studies: are conclusions valid? Gynecol Oncol. 2010;116(3):293–4.
113. Seamon LG, Fowler JM, Cohn DE. Lymphadenectomy for endometrial cancer: the controversy. Gynecol Oncol. 2010;117(1):6–8.
114. Mariani A, Webb MJ, Keeney GL, Haddock MG, Calori G, Podratz KC. Low-risk corpus cancer: is lymphadenectomy or radiotherapy necessary? Am J Obstet Gynecol. 2000;182(6):1506–19.
115. Ben-Shachar I, Pavelka J, Cohn DE, Copeland LJ, Ramirez N, Manolitsas T, et al. Surgical staging for patients presenting with grade 1 endometrial carcinoma. Obstet Gynecol. 2005;105(3):487–93.
116. Milam MR, Java J, Walker JL, Metzinger DS, Parker LP, Coleman RL. Nodal metastasis risk in endometrioid endometrial cancer. Obstet Gynecol. 2012;119(2):286–92.

117. Morrow CP, Bundy BN, Kurman RJ, Creasman WT, Heller P, Homesley HD, et al. Relationship between surgical-pathological risk factors and outcome in clinical stage I and II carcinoma of the endometrium: a gynecologic oncology group study. Gynecol Oncol. 1991;40(1):55–65.
118. Todo Y, Kato H, Kaneuchi M, Watari H, Takeda M, Sakuragi N. Survival effect of Para-aortic lymphadenectomy in endometrial cancer (SEPAL study): a retrospective cohort analysis. Lancet. 2010;375(9721):1165–72.
119. Schlappe BA, Weaver AL, Ducie JA, Eriksson AGZ, Dowdy SC, Cliby WA, et al. Multicenter study comparing oncologic outcomes between two nodal assessment methods in patients with deeply invasive endometrioid endometrial carcinoma: a sentinel lymph node algorithm versus a comprehensive pelvic and paraaortic lymphadenectomy. Gynecol Oncol. 2018;151(2):235–42.
120. Buda A, Gasparri ML, Puppo A, Mereu L, De Ponti E, Di Martino G, et al. Lymph node evaluation in high-risk early stage endometrial cancer: a multi-institutional retrospective analysis comparing the sentinel lymph node (SLN) algorithm and SLN with selective lymphadenectomy. Gynecol Oncol. 2018;150(2):261–6.
121. Brugger S, Hamann M, Mosner M, Beer M, Braun M, Pölcher M. Endometrial cancer-how many patients could benefit from sentinel lymph node dissection? World J Surg Oncol. 2018;16(1):1–7.
122. Tschernichovsky R, Diver EJ, Schorge JO, Goodman A. The role of lymphadenectomy versus sentinel lymph node biopsy in Early-stage endometrial cancer. Am J Clin Oncol Cancer Clin Trials. 2016;39(5):516–21.
123. Ballester M, Dubernard G, Lécuru F, Heitz D, Mathevet P, Marret H, et al. Detection rate and diagnostic accuracy of sentinel-node biopsy in early stage endometrial cancer: a prospective multicentre study (SENTI-ENDO). Lancet Oncol. 2011;12(5):469–76.
124. Rossi EC, Kowalski LD, Scalici J, Cantrell L, Schuler K, Hanna RK, et al. A comparison of sentinel lymph node biopsy to lymphadenectomy for endometrial cancer staging (FIRES trial): a multicentre, prospective, cohort study. Lancet Oncol. 2017;18(3):384–92.
125. Cormier B, Rozenholc AT, Gotlieb W, Plante M, Giede C. Sentinel lymph node procedure in endometrial cancer: a systematic review and proposal for standardization of future research. Gynecol Oncol. 2015;138(2):478–85.
126. Martinelli F, Ditto A, Bogani G, Signorelli M, Chiappa V, Lorusso D, et al. Laparoscopic sentinel node mapping in endometrial cancer after hysteroscopic injection of indocyanine green. J Minim Invasive Gynecol. 2017;24(1):89–93.
127. Martinelli F, Ditto A, Signorelli M, Bogani G, Chiappa V, Lorusso D, et al. Sentinel node mapping in endometrial cancer following hysteroscopic injection of tracers: a single center evaluation over 200 cases. Gynecol Oncol. 2017;146(3):525–30.
128. Gezer S, Duman Öztürk S, Hekimsoy T, Vural Ç, Işgören S, Yücesoy I, et al. Cervical versus endometrial injection for sentinel lymph node detection in endometrial cancer: a randomized clinical trial. Int J Gynecol Cancer. 2020;30(3):325–31.
129. Sakai K, Yamagami W, Susumu N, Nomura H, Kataoka F, Banno K, et al. Pathological factors associated with omental metastases in endometrial cancer. Eur J Gynaecol Oncol. 2015;36(4):397–401.
130. Metindir J, Dilek GB. The role of omentectomy during the surgical staging in patients with clinical stage I endometrioid adenocarcinoma. J Cancer Res Clin Oncol. 2008;134(10):1067–70.
131. Spirtos NM, Schlaerth JB, Gross GM, Spirtos TW, Schlaerth AC, Ballon SC. Cost and quality-of-life analyses of surgery for early endometrial cancer: laparotomy versus laparoscopy. Am J Obstet Gynecol. 1996;174(6):1795–800.
132. Malur S, Possover M, Michels W, Schneider A. Laparoscopic-assisted vaginal versus abdominal surgery in patients with endometrial cancer - a prospective randomized trial. Gynecol Oncol. 2001;80(2):239–44.
133. Tozzi R, Malur S, Koehler C, Schneider A. Laparoscopy versus laparotomy in endometrial cancer: first analysis of survival of a randomized prospective study. J Minim Invasive Gynecol. 2005;12(2):130–6.
134. Zullo F, Palomba S, Falbo A, Russo T, Mocciaro R, Tartaglia E, et al. Laparoscopic surgery vs laparotomy for early stage endometrial cancer: long-term data of a randomized controlled trial. Am J Obstet Gynecol. 2009;200(3):296.e1–9.
135. Homesley HD, Boike G, Spiegel GW, Mackey D. Feasibility of laparoscopic management of presumed stage I endometrial carcinoma and assessment of accuracy of myoinvasion estimates by frozen section: a gynecologic oncology group study. Int J Gynecol Cancer. 2004;14(2):341–7.
136. Walker JL, Piedmonte MR, Spirtos NM, Eisenkop SM, Schlaerth JB, Mannel RS, et al. Laparoscopy compared with laparotomy for comprehensive surgical staging of uterine cancer: gynecologic oncology group study LAP2. J Clin Oncol. 2009;27(32):5331–6.
137. Obermair A, Janda M, Baker J, Kondalsamy-Chennakesavan S, Brand A, Hogg R, et al. Improved surgical safety after laparoscopic compared to open surgery for apparent early stage endometrial cancer: results from a randomised controlled trial. Eur J Cancer. 2012;48(8):1147–53.
138. Bell MC, Torgerson J, Seshadri-Kreaden U, Suttle AW, Hunt S. Comparison of outcomes and cost for endometrial cancer staging via traditional laparotomy, standard laparoscopy and robotic techniques. Gynecol Oncol. 2008;111(3):407–11.

139. Lim PC, Kang E, Park DH. A comparative detail analysis of the learning curve and surgical outcome for robotic hysterectomy with lymphadenectomy versus laparoscopic hysterectomy with lymphadenectomy in treatment of endometrial cancer: a case-matched controlled study of the first o. Gynecol Oncol. 2011;120(3):413–8.
140. Cardenas-Goicoechea J, Adams S, Bhat SB, Randall TC. Surgical outcomes of robotic-assisted surgical staging for endometrial cancer are equivalent to traditional laparoscopic staging at a minimally invasive surgical center. Gynecol Oncol. 2010;117(2):224–8.
141. Boggess JF, Gehrig PA, Cantrell L, Shafer A, Ridgway M, Skinner EN, et al. A comparative study of 3 surgical methods for hysterectomy with staging for endometrial cancer: robotic assistance, laparoscopy, laparotomy. Am J Obstet Gynecol. 2008;199(4):360.e1–9.
142. Corrado G, Cutillo G, Pomati G, Mancini E, Sperduti I, Patrizi L, et al. Surgical and oncological outcome of robotic surgery compared to laparoscopic and abdominal surgery in the management of endometrial cancer. Eur J Surg Oncol. 2015;41(8):1074–81.
143. Johnson L, Bunn WD, Nguyen L, Rice J, Raj M, Cunningham MJ. Clinical comparison of robotic, laparoscopic, and open hysterectomy procedures for endometrial cancer patients. J Robot Surg. 2017;11(3):291–7.
144. Greer BE, Hamberger AD. Treatment of intraperitoneal metastatic adenocarcinoma of the endometrium by the whole-abdomen moving-strip technique and pelvic boost irradiation. Gynecol Oncol. 1983;16(3):365–73.
145. Martinez A, Podratz K, et al. Results of whole Abdomsnopelvic irradiation with nodal boost for patients with endometrial cancer at high risk of failure in the peritoneal cavity: a prospective clinical trial at the Mayo Clinic. Hematol Oncol Clin North Am. 1998;2(3):431–46.
146. Bristow RE, Zerbe MJ, Rosenshein NB, Grumbine FC, Montz FJ. Stage IVB endometrial carcinoma: the role of cytoreductive surgery and determinants of survival. Gynecol Oncol. 2000;78(2):85–91.
147. Vitale SG, Valenti G, Gulino FA, Cignini P, Biondi A. Surgical treatment of high stage endometrial cancer: current perspectives. Updat Surg. 2016;68(2):149–54.
148. Colombo N, Creutzberg C, Amant F, Bosse T, González-Martín A, Ledermann J, Marth C, Nout R, Querleu D, Mirza MR, Sessa C. ESMO-ESGO-ESTRO consensus conference on endometrial cancer: diagnosis, treatment and follow-up. International journal of gynecologic. Cancer. 2016;26(1)
149. Nout RA, Smit VTHBM, Putter H, Jürgenliemk-Schulz IM, Jobsen JJ, Lutgens LCHW, et al. Vaginal brachytherapy versus pelvic external beam radiotherapy for patients with endometrial cancer of high-intermediate risk (PORTEC-2): an open-label, non-inferiority, randomised trial. Lancet. 2010;375(9717):816–23.
150. Randall ME, Filiaci V, McMeekin DS, Von Gruenigen V, Huang H, Yashar CM, et al. Phase III trial: adjuvant pelvic radiation therapy versus vaginal brachytherapy plus paclitaxel/ carboplatin in high-intermediate and high-risk early stage endometrial cancer. J Clin Oncol. 2019;37(21):1810–8.
151. Randall ME, Filiaci VL, Muss H, Spirtos NM, Mannel RS, Fowler J, et al. Randomized phase III trial of whole-abdominal irradiation versus doxorubicin and cisplatin chemotherapy in advanced endometrial carcinoma: a gynecologic oncology group study. J Clin Oncol. 2006;24(1):36–44.
152. Greven K, Winter K, Underhill K, Fontenesci J, Cooper J, Burke T. Final analysis of RTOG 9708: adjuvant postoperative irradiation combined with cisplatin/paclitaxel chemotherapy following surgery for patients with high-risk endometrial cancer. Gynecol Oncol. 2006;103(1):155–9.
153. Matei D, Filiaci V, Randall ME, Mutch D, Steinhoff MM, DiSilvestro PA, Moxley KM, Kim YM, Powell MA, O'Malley DM, Spirtos NM. Adjuvant chemotherapy plus radiation for locally advanced endometrial cancer. N Engl J Med. 2019;380(24):2317–26.
154. de Boer SM, Powell ME, Mileshkin L, Katsaros D, Bessette P, Haie-Meder C, et al. Adjuvant chemoradiotherapy versus radiotherapy alone for women with high-risk endometrial cancer (PORTEC-3): final results of an international, open-label, multicentre, randomised, phase 3 trial. Lancet Oncol. 2018;19(3):295–309.
155. Koh WJ, Abu-Rustum NR, Bean S, Bradley K, Campos SM, Cho KR, Chon HS, Chu C, Cohn D, Crispens MA, et al. Uterine neoplasms, version 1.2018, NCCN clinical practice guidelines in oncology. J Natl Compr Cancer Netw. 2018;16(2):170–99.
156. Portelance L, Chao KS, Grigsby PW, Bennet H, Low D. Intensity-modulated radiation therapy (IMRT) reduces small bowel, rectum, and bladder doses in patients with cervical cancer receiving pelvic and Para-aortic irradiation. Int J Radiat Oncol Biol Phys. 2001;51:261–6.
157. Roeske JC, Lujan A, Rotmensch J, Waggoner SE, Yamada D, Mundt AJ. Intensity-modulated whole pelvic radiation therapy in patients with gynecologic malignancies. Int J Radiat Oncol Biol Phys. 2000;48:1613–21.
158. Mundt AJ, Mell LK, Roeske JC. Preliminary analysis of chronic gastrointestinal toxicity in gynecology patients treated with intensity-modulated whole pelvic radiation therapy. Int J Radiat Oncol Biol Phys. 2003;56(5):1354–60. https://doi.org/10.1016/s0360-3016(03)00325-0.
159. Small W Jr, Mell LK, Anderson P, et al. Consensus guidelines for delineation of clinical target volume for intensity-modulated pelvic radiotherapy in postoperative treatment of endometrial and cervical can-

cer. Int J Radiat Oncol Biol Phys. 2008;71(2):428–34. https://doi.org/10.1016/j.ijrobp.2007.09.042.
160. Taylor A, Rockall AG, Reznek RH, Powell ME. Mapping pelvic lymph nodes: guidelines for delineation in intensity-modulated radiotherapy. Int J Radiat Oncol Biol Phys. 2005;63(5):1604–12. https://doi.org/10.1016/j.ijrobp.2005.05.062.
161. Viswanathan AN, Moughan J, Miller BE, et al. NRG oncology/RTOG 0921: a phase 2 study of post-operative intensity-modulated radiotherapy with concurrent cisplatin and bevacizumab followed by carboplatin and paclitaxel for patients with endometrial cancer. Cancer. 2015;121(13):2156–63.
162. Nag S, Erickson B, Parikh S, Gupta N, Varia M, Glasgow G. The American brachytherapy society recommendations for high-dose-rate brachytherapy for carcinoma of the endometrium. Int J Radiat Oncol Biol Phys. 2000;48(3):779–90. https://doi.org/10.1016/s0360-3016(00)00689-1.
163. International Commission on Radiation Units and Measurements. Dose and volume specification for reporting intracavitary therapy in gynecology. ICRU report 38. Bethesda, MD: ICRU; 1985.
164. Small W Jr, Beriwal S, Demanes DJ, et al. American brachytherapy society consensus guidelines for adjuvant vaginal cuff brachytherapy after hysterectomy. Brachytherapy. 2012;11(1):58–67. https://doi.org/10.1016/j.brachy.2011.08.005.
165. Schwarz JK, Beriwal S, Esthappan J, et al. Consensus statement for brachytherapy for the treatment of medically inoperable endometrial cancer. Brachytherapy. 2015;14(5):587–99. https://doi.org/10.1016/j.brachy.2015.06.002.
166. Vargo JA, Boisen MM, Comerci JT, et al. Neoadjuvant radiotherapy with or without chemotherapy followed by extrafascial hysterectomy for locally advanced endometrial cancer clinically extending to the cervix or parametria. Gynecol Oncol. 2014;135(2):190–5. https://doi.org/10.1016/j.ygyno.2014.09.001.
167. Iheagwara UK, Vargo JA, Chen KS, et al. Neoadjuvant chemoradiation therapy followed by Extrafascial hysterectomy in locally advanced type II endometrial cancer clinically extending to cervix. Pract Radiat Oncol. 2019;9(4):248–56. https://doi.org/10.1016/j.prro.2019.02.007.
168. Miller D, Filiaci V, Fleming G, Mannel R, Cohn D, Matsumoto T, et al. Late-breaking abstract 1: randomized phase III noninferiority trial of first line chemotherapy for metastatic or recurrent endometrial carcinoma: a gynecologic oncology group study. Gynecol Oncol. 2012;125(3):771.
169. Fleming GF. Systemic chemotherapy for uterine carcinoma: metastatic and adjuvant. J Clin Oncol. 2007;25(20):2983–90.
170. Hoskins PJ, Swenerton KD, Pike JA, Wong F, Lim P, Acquino-Parsons C, et al. Paclitaxel and carboplatin, alone or with irradiation, in advanced or recurrent endometrial cancer: a phase II study. J Clin Oncol. 2001;19(20):4048–53.
171. Markman M. Hormonal therapy of endometrial cancer. Eur J Cancer. 2005;41(5):673–5.
172. Thigpen JT, Brady MF, Alvarez RD, Adelson MD, Homesley HD, Manetta A, Soper JT, Given FT. Oral medroxyprogesterone acetate in the treatment of advanced or recurrent endometrial carcinoma: a dose-response study by the gynecologic oncology group. J Clin Oncol. 1999;17(6):1736.
173. Sohaib SA, Houghton SL, Meroni R, Rockall AG, Blake P, Reznek RH. Recurrent endometrial cancer: patterns of recurrent disease and assessment of prognosis. Clin Radiol. 2007;62(1):28–34.
174. Salani R, Backes FJ, Fung Kee Fung M, Holschneider CH, Parker LP, Bristow RE, et al. Posttreatment surveillance and diagnosis of recurrence in women with gynecologic malignancies: Society of Gynecologic Oncologists recommendations. Am J Obstet Gynecol. 2011;204(6):466–78.
175. Novetsky AP, Kuroki LM, Massad LS, Hagemann AR, Thaker PH, Powell MA, et al. The utility and management of vaginal cytology after treatment for endometrial cancer. Obstet Gynecol. 2013;121(1):129–35.
176. Bristow RE, Purinton SC, Santillan A, Diaz-Montes TP, Gardner GJ, Giuntoli RL. Cost-effectiveness of routine vaginal cytology for endometrial cancer surveillance. Gynecol Oncol. 2006;103(2):709–13.
177. Creutzberg CL, Van Putten WLJ, Koper PC, Lybeert MLM, Jobsen JJ, Wárlám-Rodenhuis CC, et al. Survival after relapse in patients with endometrial cancer: results from a randomized trial. Gynecol Oncol. 2003;89(2):201–9.
178. Barakat RR, Goldman NA, Patel DA. Pelvic exenteration for recurrent pelvic cancer. Gynecol Oncol. 1999;75:99–102.
179. Morris M, Alvarez RD, Kinney WK, Wilson TO. Treatment of recurrent adenocarcinoma of the endometrium with pelvic exenteration. Gynecol Oncol. 1996;60(2):288–91.
180. Barlin JN, Puri I, Bristow RE. Cytoreductive surgery for advanced or recurrent endometrial cancer: a meta-analysis. Gynecol Oncol. 2010;118(1):14–8.
181. Turan T, Tasci T, Karalok A, Ureyen I, Kocak O, Turkmen O, et al. Salvage cytoreductive surgery for recurrent endometrial cancer. Int J Gynecol Cancer. 2015;25(9):1623–32.
182. Papadia A, Bellati F, Ditto A, Bogani G, Gasparri ML, Di Donato V, et al. Surgical treatment of recurrent endometrial cancer: time for a paradigm shift. Ann Surg Oncol. 2015;22(13):4204–10.
183. Aghajanian C, Sill MW, Darcy KM, Greer B, McMeekin DS, Rose PG, et al. Phase II trial of bevacizumab in recurrent or persistent endometrial cancer: a gynecologic oncology group study. J Clin Oncol. 2011;29(16):2259–65.
184. Simpkins F, Drake R, Escobar PF, Nutter B, Rasool N, Rose PG. A phase II trial of paclitaxel, carboplatin, and bevacizumab in advanced and recurrent

endometrial carcinoma (EMCA). Gynecol Oncol. 2015;136(2):240–5.
185. Fleming GF. Second-line therapy for endometrial cancer. Obstet Gynecol Surv. 2016;71(7):406–8.
186. Nagao S, Nishio S, Michimae H, Tanabe H, Okada S, Otsuki T, et al. Applicability of the concept of "platinum sensitivity" to recurrent endometrial cancer: the SGSG-012/GOTIC-004/intergroup study. Gynecol Oncol. 2013;131(3):567–73.
187. Santin AD, Bellone S, Gokden M, Palmieri M, Dunn D, Agha J, et al. Overexpression of HER-2/neu in uterine serous papillary cancer. Clin Cancer Res. 2002;8(5):1271–9.
188. Grushko TA, Filiaci VL, Mundt AJ, Ridderstråle K, Olopade OI, Fleming GF. An exploratory analysis of HER-2 amplification and overexpression in advanced endometrial carcinoma: a gynecologic oncology group study. Gynecol Oncol. 2008;108(1):3–9.
189. Villella JA, Cohen S, Smith DH, Hibshoosh H, Hershman D. HER-2/neu overexpression in uterine papillary serous cancers and its possible therapeutic implications. Int J Gynecol Cancer. 2006;16(5):1897–902.
190. Odicino FE, Bignotti E, Rossi E, Pasinetti B, Tassi RA, Donzelli C, et al. HER-2/neu overexpression and amplification in uterine serous papillary carcinoma: comparative analysis of immunohistochemistry, real-time reverse transcription-polymerase chain reaction, and fluorescence in situ hybridization. Int J Gynecol Cancer. 2008;18(1):14–21.
191. Fleming GF, Sill MW, Darcy KM, McMeekin DS, Thigpen JT, Adler LM, et al. Phase II trial of trastuzumab in women with advanced or recurrent, HER2-positive endometrial carcinoma: a gynecologic oncology group study. Gynecol Oncol. 2010;116(1):15–20.
192. Mutter GL, Lin M, Fitzgerald JT, Jennifer B, Baak JP, Jacqueline A, et al. Altered PTEN expression as a diagnostic marker for the earliest endometrial precancers. J Natl Cancer Inst. 2000;92(11):924–30.
193. Lax SF, Kendall B, Tashiro H, Slebos RJC, Ellenson LH. The frequency of p53, K-ras mutations, and microsatellite instability differs in uterine endometrioid and serous carcinoma: evidence of distinct molecular genetic pathways. Cancer. 2000;88(4):814–24.
194. Cantley LC. The phosphoinositide 3-kinase pathway. Science. 2002;296(5573):1655–7.
195. Oza AM, Elit L, Biagi J, Chapman W, Tsao M, Hedley D, et al. Molecular correlates associated with a phase II study of temsirolimus (CCI-779) in patients with metastatic or recurrent endometrial cancer—NCIC IND 160. J Clin Oncol. 2006;24(18_suppl):3003.
196. Colombo N, McMeekin S, Schwartz P, Kostka J, Sessa C, Gehrig P, et al. A phase II trial of the mTOR inhibitor AP23573 as a single agent in advanced endometrial cancer. J Clin Oncol. 2007;25(18_suppl):5516.
197. Gunderson CC, Fader AN, Carson KA, Bristow RE. Oncologic and reproductive outcomes with progestin therapy in women with endometrial hyperplasia and grade 1 adenocarcinoma: a systematic review. Gynecol Oncol. 2012;125(2):477–82.
198. Hubbs JL, Saig RM, Abaid LN, Bae-Jump VL, Gehrig PA. Systemic and local hormone therapy for endometrial hyperplasia and early adenocarcinoma. Obstet Gynecol. 2013;121(6):1172–80.
199. Fan Z, Li H, Hu R, Liu Y, Liu X, Gu L. Fertility-preserving treatment in young women with grade 1 presumed stage IA endometrial adenocarcinoma: a meta-analysis. Int J Gynecol Cancer. 2018;28(2):385–93.
200. Zaino R, Whitney C, Brady MF, Ph D, Degeest K, Burger RA, et al. Simultaneously Detected Endometrial and Ovarian Carcinomas—A Prospective Clinicopathologic Study of 74 Cases: A Gynecologic Oncology Group Study 1. Gynecol Oncol. 2001;83:355–62.
201. Ulbright TM, Roth LM. Metastatic and independent cancers of the endometrium and ovary: a clinicopathologic study of 34 cases. Hum Pathol. 1985;16(1):28–34.
202. Scully RE, PBC RHY. In: Scully RE, Young RH, Philip B, editors. Tumors of the Ovary, Maldeveloped Gonads, Fallopian Tube, and Broad Ligament. Clement, Armed Forces Institute of Pathology (U.S.), Universities Associated for Research and Education in Pathology—Googl; 1998.
203. Walsh C, Holschneider C, Hoang Y, Tieu K, Karlan B, Cass I. Coexisting ovarian malignancy in young women with endometrial cancer. Obstet Gynecol. 2005;106(4):693–9.

Uterine Sarcoma

Aparajita, Pallavi Ramchandra,
Debabrata Barmon, and Amal Chandra Kataki

1 Introduction

Uterine sarcomas are rare gynaecological cancer with an aggressive clinical course and poor prognosis. It is a heterogeneous group of tumours of mesenchymal origin constituting 1% of female genital tract malignancies and 3–7% of uterine malignancies [1].

2 Clinical Presentation

Although it can occur in women of any age, the peak incidence is between the fifth and seventh decade of life. They usually present with vague symptoms mimicking benign conditions. Nevertheless, abnormal uterine bleeding (86%), pain abdomen (24%), and/or pelvic mass (15%) are the chief complaints [2].

Aparajita (✉) · D. Barmon · A. C. Kataki
Department of Gynaecologic Oncology,
Dr. Bhubaneswar Borooah Cancer Institute
(A Unit of Tata Memorial Centre, Mumbai),
Guwahati, Assam, India
e-mail: dydiracademic@bbci.tmc.gov.in

P. Ramchandra
Department of Gynaecological Oncology,
Kidwai Memorial Institute of Oncology,
Bengaluru, Karnataka, India

3 Risk Factors

Risk factors were explained in previous research [3–5]. They are indicated in the following points:

1. Pelvic radiation: 5–25 years after radiation therapy for another pelvic cancer
2. Race: Twice as common in African-American women as they are in white or Asian women
3. Combined hormonal replacement therapy in postmenopausal women for 5 years or longer
4. Prolonged use of tamoxifen
5. Inherited genetic syndromes—hereditary retinoblastoma, Li-Fraumeni syndrome

4 Classification

Uterine sarcomas are classified into three major groups—leiomyosarcomas (LMS—63%), endometrial stromal sarcomas (ESS—21%), and undifferentiated uterine sarcoma (UUS) [6]. In 2009, carcinosarcoma (malignant mixed Müllerian tumour) was excluded from the diagnostic category and is now considered in tumours of the endometrial epithelium [7]. The World Health Organization classifies tumours of the uterine corpus into different types as given in Table 1 [8].

A. C. Kataki, D. Barmon (eds.), *Fundamentals in Gynaecologic Malignancy*,
https://doi.org/10.1007/978-981-19-5860-1_15

Table 1 WHO classification of uterine mesenchymal tumours (2014)

Mesenchymal tumours specific to the uterus	Mixed epithelial and mesenchymal tumours
Leiomyoma NOS Intravenous leiomyomatosis Smooth muscle tumour of uncertain malignant potential (STUMP) Metastasizing leiomyoma Leiomyosarcoma Spindle leiomyosarcoma Epithelioid leiomyosarcoma Myxoid leiomyosarcoma Endometrial stromal nodule Endometrial stromal al sarcoma, low grade Endometrial stromal sarcoma, high grade Undifferentiated uterine sarcoma Uterine tumour resembling ovarian sex cord tumour Perivascular epithelioid cell tumour, benign Perivascular epithelioid cell tumour, malignant Inflammatory myofibroblastic tumour	Adenomyoma Atypical polypoid adenomyoma Adenosarcoma

Table 2 Various molecular markers of uterine sarcomas

LMS [9]	Gain or loss of tumour suppressor genes/ hyperactivation of cell proliferation pathway	TP53 (51%), RB1 (15.3%), and ATRX (13.3%) (www.cbioportal.org), TP53 (24%), MED12 (7%), and KRAS (7%)
HG-ESS [10, 11]	Fusion genes	YWHAE-NUTM2A/B (also known as YWHAE-FAM22A/B) gene fusion; t(10;17) (q22;p13) and ZC3H7B-BCOR
LG-ESS [12]	Fusion genes	JAZF1 rearrangements- [t(7;17) (p15;q21)] JAZF1-SUZ12 (formerly JAZF1-JJAZ1) fusion and PHF1 rearrangements- [t(6;7) t(6;10)] JAZF1- PHF1, and the much less common EPC1- PHF1, MEAF6-PHF1ZC3H7-BCOR, and MBTD1-CXorf67
UUS	Complex genetic alterations [12]	No specific translocation pattern

5 Biological and Molecular Behaviour

The distinct biological and molecular profiles of these tumours as given in Table 2 may determine their behaviour under treatment.

The genetic fusion between YWHAE and FAM22A/B, harbouring t(10;17)(q22;p13) in a sub-set of HG-ESS, has an intermediate prognosis between LG-ESS and UUS. Unlike the conventional low-grade areas, the high-grade areas of the tumour show the presence of cyclin D1. The CD10, ER, and PR expressions are not observed in these cases. This strongly indicates the onset of a high-grade sarcoma and appears not to respond to the usual treatment for low-grade ESS [13].

6 Leiomyosarcoma

It constitutes up to 80% of uterine sarcomas when carcinosarcomas are excluded [9]. It presents most commonly in 45–55 years and arises de-novo from uterine smooth muscle. This contradicts the previous notion of their origin from uterine myomas, which may occur rarely. With a pre-operative diagnosis of fibroids, there is a 0.7% chance of revelation of LMS in the final histopathological report. A rapid increase in the size of the fibroid or pain should raise the suspicion of the development of LMS. Uterine curetting diagnostic rate is 10–20% only.

Grossly, they are mostly solitary with a fleshy appearance. More than 75% have sizes exceeding 5.0 cm. Areas of necrosis, haemorrhage, or cyst

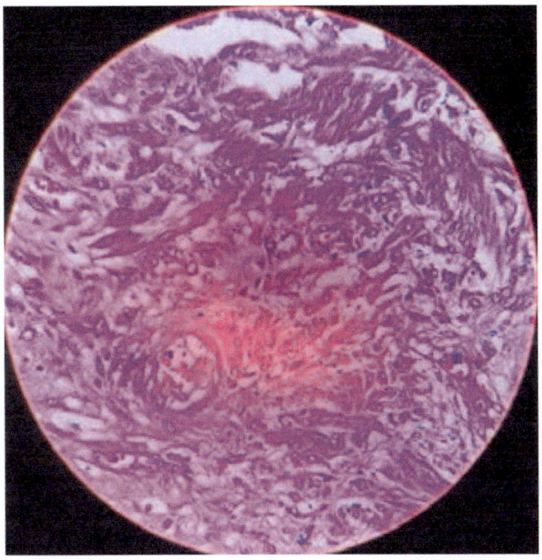

Fig. 1 Histopathological image of uterine leiomyosarcoma

Table 3 Immunohistochemical markers to differentiate LMS from leiomyoma

	LMS	Uterine myoma
SMA	+	–
Desmin	+	–
Caldesmon	+	–
ER expression	40%	78%
PR expression	38%	88%
P16	Overexpressed	
P53	Overexpressed	
Ki67 proliferation index	High	
Keratin	+ in epithelioid variant	

growth can sometimes be observed. Pathological characteristics include diffuse mild to acute cytologic atypia. They can be characterized by elevated levels of mitotic index (with values over 10 per 10 high power fields). Signs of coagulative tumour cell necrosis can also be observed in the patients (Stanford's criteria) [9]. There is no grading system for LMS as it does not correlate with survival outcomes. The microscopic appearance of LMS is as shown in Fig. 1.

Immunohistochemistry can help to differentiate LMS from leiomyoma [14]. Relevant markers are given in Table 3. Imaging features of LMS as obtained from research by Sun et al. are given in Table 4 [15].

Table 4 Imaging features of leiomyosarcomas

USG	Large heterogeneous masses with areas of central vascularity or necrosis
Colour Doppler	Irregular vessel distribution, low impedance to flow, high peak systolic velocity
MRI	T2-weighted images—heterogeneous hyperintense lesions with irregular borders and areas
	T1-weighted images—haemorrhage or necrosis
	Absence of calcifications
CE-CT	Does not reliably distinguish between leiomyoma and sarcoma

Contrast-enhanced MRI usually exhibits better diagnostic accuracy (0.94) than diffusion-weighted imaging (0.52). Specificity values are also higher (0.96 vs. 0.36) in differentiating LMS/STUMP and fibroids [16]. Contrast-enhanced CT scan of the chest and abdomen can be used to assess extra-uterine spread.

6.1 Staging

FIGO staging for LMS (Leiomyosarcomas and endometrial stromal sarcomas) as described by Pratt is shown in the following [17].

1. Stage I: Tumour limited to the uterus
   (a) Less than 5 cm
   (b) More than 5 cm
2. Stage II: Tumour extending beyond the uterus, within the pelvis
   (a) IIA: Adnexal involvement
   (b) IIB: Involvement of other pelvic tissues
3. Stage III: Tumour invading abdominal tissues (not just protruding into the abdomen)
   (a) IIIA: One site
   (b) IIIB: More than one site
   (c) IIIC: Metastasis to the pelvic and/or para-aortic lymph nodes
4. Stage IV
   (a) IVA: Tumour invading bladder and/or rectum
   (b) IVB: Distant metastasis

Table 5 Prognostic groups of LMS

	Good	Poor
Tumour diameter	<10 cm	>10 cm
Mitotic index	<20 MF/10 HPF	>20 MF/10HPF
Ki67	Negative	Positive
Bcl-2 immunostaining	Positive or negative	Negative

6.2 Prognostic Factors

Tumour progression, necrosis, mitotic count, age, co-morbidity, tumour size, lymph node involvement, positive surgical margin, and metastasis are the important prognostic factors [18]. Using histological criteria, the French Federation of Anticancer Centers (FNCLCC) have developed a scoring system. However, it has not been validated as a prognostic tool for uterine sarcomas. LMS has two different prognostic groups as given in Table 5.

6.3 Treatment

Standard treatment of early-stage LMS is en bloc total hysterectomy and complete surgical resection of all gross tumours [19]. Laparoscopic/assisted or robotic surgery can be carried out if the tumour can be resected without morcellation. Ovarian metastases of primary uterine LMS occur in less than 5% of cases. Hence, ER/PR testing is recommended to guide ovarian resection, particularly in young patients. Bilateral salpingo-oophorectomy is favoured if ER/PR is positive [6]. The recurrence rate remains high even in operable stages (stage I–III). The role of adjuvant therapy is controversial with a low level of evidence and limited by small studies. Treatment options for advanced or metastatic disease are mainly palliative with systemic chemotherapy and/or EBRT +/− brachytherapy and/or targeted agents. Surgical resection of isolated metastases can be considered. NCCN recommends additional therapy with observation for stage I and systemic therapy and/or radiation for stage II–IV disease. Observation can be the option for stage II–IVA in completely resected cases with no evidence of disease on postoperative imaging [6].

6.4 Role of Lymphadenectomy

Uterine sarcoma spreads haematogenously predominantly, and the lymphatic mode of dissemination is less common. The incidence of lymph node metastasis in uterine LMS and ESS is documented to be 6.6%–11% and ~10%, respectively [6, 20]. About 44.4% of cases showed the pelvic and/or para-aortic lymph node involvement at primary surgery. This was also observed among the UES with macroscopically completed resection [21]. Previous literature quoted no survival advantage for patients with positive lymph node dissection, though it was of prognostic significance and improved the staging [22–24]. However, a recent meta-analysis shows that it is of no therapeutic or prognostic value in early-stage LMS or ESS. Hence, routine lymphadenectomy is not advocated for uterine sarcomas.

6.5 Role of Radiotherapy

In leiomyosarcomas, smaller and retrospective studies showed better local control of the disease with adjuvant radiation without any improvement in relapse-free and overall survival. Given the aggressive nature of the disease, the extra-pelvic site has the propensity to be the eventual site of recurrence in such a setting. The European Organization for Research and Treatment of Cancer (EORTC) conducted the only randomized phase III trial regarding postoperative radiation. There was no substantial difference between the progression-free survival rate of radiotherapy and the control group (53% and 50%, respectively) in 219 assessable patients. An overall survival rate was 58% and 56%, respectively [25]. To conclude, postoperative pelvic radiation is not generally recommended in optimally resected LMS. However, its use as adjuvant RT can be considered in selected cases with risk factors, including local relapse, cervical involvement, parametrial involvement, serosal involvement, and UES histology [19].

6.6 Role of Chemotherapy

Adjuvant chemotherapy in early LMS has been used due to the high risk of systemic relapse. The first line adjuvant chemotherapy in early-stage LMS has traditionally been doxorubicin. However, after the conflicting results of the benefit of doxorubicin-based adjuvant chemotherapy, the phase II trial (SARC 005) studied four cycles of adjuvant gemcitabine and docetaxel followed by an additional four cycles of doxorubicin and reported a disease-free interval rate of 78% at 2 years and 50% at 3 years [26]. The tolerability of the regimen is proved by the completion of therapy by 89% of patients. A phase III trial (NCT01533207) which randomized women with stage I LMS to observation or the complete regimen studied in SARC 005, was closed due to slower recruitment. However, with the given number of patients, the trial did not show the superiority of adjuvant chemotherapy [27]. Systemic therapy for advanced uterine LMS, UUS, and heterologous sarcomas generally follows adult soft tissue sarcomas recommendations. Apart from doxorubicin-based therapy with ifosfamide or dacarbazine, other recommended regimens for uterine sarcoma are docetaxel/gemcitabine, gemcitabine/dacarbazine, gemcitabine/vinorelbine, and single agents like dacarbazine, epirubicin, ifosfamide, liposomal doxorubicin, pazopanib, temozolomide, trabectedin, and eribulin [6]. Chemotherapy for advanced and recurrent disease with doxorubicin or docetaxel/gemcitabine have showed response rates being 27–36%.

6.7 Role of Targeted Therapy and Immunotherapy

Olaratumab is a human anti-platelet-derived growth factor receptor-α monoclonal antibody [6]. After the positive result of a phase II study on survival, the FDA approved its combination with doxorubicin for advanced unresectable soft tissue sarcomas [28]. The NCCN also offers the regimen as a preferred one.

Trabectedin [6, 29]. It is recommended for unresectable or metastatic LMS patients after exhaustion from an anthracycline-based regimen. Pazopanib is a second-generation small-molecule selective tyrosine kinase inhibitor that shows activity against LMS with effects similar to other soft tissue sarcomas [30]. Nivolumab—LMS expresses the T-cell checkpoint protein, PD-1 [31]. Nivolumab is an anti-PD1 antibody with activity against refractory LMS and other soft tissue sarcomas. Pembrolizumab was advocated by FDA for its use for tumours with mismatch repair deficiency or high microsatellite instability [32]. It got its approval for solid tumours and advanced cervical cancer with progression on chemotherapy in 2017 and 2018, respectively. A phase 2 trial in 86 metastatic or surgically unresectable soft tissue or bone sarcoma patients (out of which ten patients had LMS) after up to three prior lines of chemotherapy reported no clinically significant objective response.

Anti-CD47 monoclonal antibodies, CD47, a cell surface marker protein is overexpressed in 87% of cancer cells. It forms a signalling complex with signal-regulatory protein α (SIRPα), enabling these cancer cells to escape from macrophage-mediated phagocytosis. LMS shows high levels of macrophage infiltration. Inhibition of the anti-phagocytic functions of CD47 is hypothesized to result in the restoration of the anti-tumour function of responsible macrophages. In vitro studies have confirmed the efficacy of anti-CD47 antibodies, while in vivo studies have also shown a significant reduction in tumour volume. The response to metastatic disease was as high as 70-fold. Several anti-CD47 monoclonal antibodies are currently under investigation in phase I trials [33].

Recent advancements in cancer therapy have shifted to developments of agents targeting molecular pathways depending on the tumour biomarker characterization. The Cancer Genome Atlas (TCGA) Research Network (2017) reported LMS to carry a majority of mutations in tumour suppressor genes RB1, TP53, and PTEN. Whole-exome sequencing demonstrated alterations in ATRX and MED12 [34]. The PI3K/AKT and mTOR pathway is activated by dele-

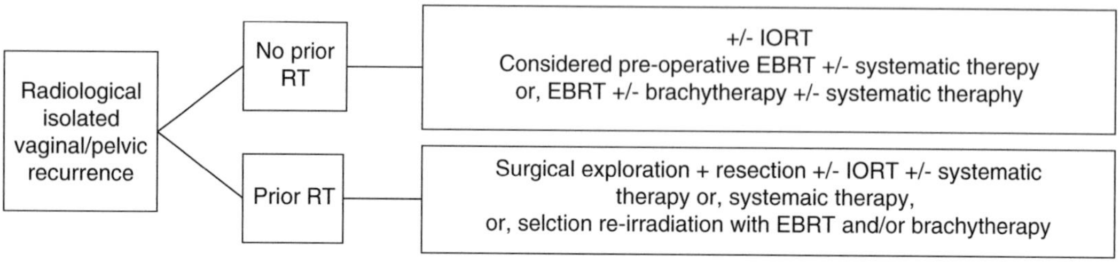

Fig. 2 Scheme of recurrence management

tions in the long arm of chromosome 10 leading to PTEN disruption. The mTOR inhibitors, such as everolimus and temsirolimus, have shown modest clinical efficacy in such settings. Rb1inactivation caused by a deletion in the long arm of chromosome 13 affects G1-S checkpoint resulting in uncontrolled cell division.

Stathmin 1, another biomarker is noted to be expressed in 100% of uterine LMS cases. This protein destabilizes microtubules during the cell cycle and activates the PI3K-AKT-mTOR pathway. STMN1 expression has been associated with a poorer prognosis in all analysed endometrial cancer cases in GOG 177 [35, 36]. Paclitaxel being a microtubule-stabilizing agent may prove to be useful in stathmin overexpression. Insulin-like growth factor mRNA binding protein 3 (IMP3). More than half of uterine LMS cases show strong expression of insulin-like growth factor mRNA binding protein 3 (IMP3). Overexpression of this RNA binding carcino-embryonic protein is associated with a poor prognosis [37]. The lack of c-KIT hotspot mutations has restricted the use of imatinib (inhibitor of the tyrosine kinase activity of c-KIT) despite the expression of c-KIT in many cases of LMS [38, 39].

6.8 Recurrent Disease

Recurrence rates vary between 45% and 75%, with median intervals to recurrence of 12–24 months in LMS [6]. Local recurrence in the vagina and/or pelvis can be treated depending on the history of prior radiation exposure; Fig. 2 shows the management of recurrent disease.

6.9 Uterine Fibroids and Their Morcellation

Uterine morcellation is a surgical method of cutting the uterus to facilitate its removal through a limited incision. It may be performed abdominally, vaginally, or laparoscopically using a scalpel, scissors, or power morcellator. However, morcellation carries the risk of dissemination and upstaging of the malignant disease during procedures carried out for presumed benign diseases. There is no definite consensus on the estimated prevalence of LMS in patients undergoing hysterectomy/myomectomy for presumed leiomyoma. It ranges from 1/498 to 1/570 to 1/750 [40, 41]. AHRQ estimated this data to be 0.05–0.09% and 0.05–0.13% in prospective and retrospective studies, respectively (1 in 10,000 to 1 in 770 surgeries) [41]. After morcellation, greater than half of the patients (50–64%) are upstaged due to peritoneal dissemination, and there is a 2.5-fold worsening of overall survival compared to tumours that were removed intact [42, 43]. The expected 5-year survival for women undergoing power morcellation, scalpel morcellation, and no morcellation at all was 30% (95% BCI, 13–61%) 59% (95% BCI, 33–84%), and 60% (95% BCI, 24–98%), respectively.

Application of laparoscopic power morcellators was discouraged by the FDA in 2014 for fibroids treatment. The patients were primarily the women who underwent myomectomy or hysterectomy. This resulted in an increase in the incidence of major and minor surgical complications related to hysterectomy [44]. Usually, higher mortality is observed due to LMS morcellation than with laparoscopic hysterectomy when compared to elevated mortality of abdominal hysterectomy. This is mostly related to the procesure itself. Research indicated insignificant difference between laparoscopic and abdominal approaches in an age-specific updated analysis of prevalence and mortality. It was also concluded that the risk of death associated with laparoscopic morcellation was greater in women >50 years of age. Subsequently, FDA 2020 recommends laparoscopic power morcellation for myomectomy or hysterectomy be performed only with a tissue containment system legally marketed in the US and works with only specifically designed laparoscopic morcellator. Moreover, morcellation is not to be utilized in postmenopausal and >50 years of age and candidates for removal of tissue en bloc through the vagina or mini-laparotomy incisions for the removal of uterine tissue containing suspected leiomyomas.

Before considering morcellation of the uterus, pre-operative evaluation includes risk stratification and the appropriate use of imaging, cervical cancer screening, and endometrial tissue sampling to identify malignancy. Moreover, patients with LMS following morcellation (including the residual cervix) procedure must undergo subsequent additional resection due to increased upstaging risk. This must be done if the cervix was left in situ, peritoneal biopsies (including surrounding previous port sites), and either omental biopsy or omentectomy as part of a reexploration surgery [6]. Imaging techniques including PET/CT could also be utilized to investigate for the occurrence of the disseminated condition ahead of additional surgery.

7 Endometrial Stromal Sarcomas

ESS presents in comparatively younger women with the mean age of 42–58 years with an annual incidence of ESS being 1–2 per million women [45]. ESS was originally divided into low-grade and high-grade based on the mitotic count. Mitotic index, an indicator of proliferation and tumour grade, was not used to classify ESS according to WHO 2003 criteria as it was found to be prognostically irrelevant [46]. It removed the "high-grade" category and reclassified these tumours into ESS and undifferentiated endometrial sarcoma (UES). However, it was later evident that the UES category was too broad with various heterogeneous tumours with different clinical behaviours and outcomes.

WHO 2014 classifies Endometrial Stromal Tumours into four categories—benign endometrial stromal nodules (ESN), low-grade ESS, high-grade ESS, and undifferentiated uterine sarcoma (UUS) based on distinct translocations as well as tumour morphology and prognosis. ESN is defined as tumours with absent to at most minimal myometrial invasion (≤3 mm and <3 protrusions) and no vascular invasion. LG-ESS is a slow-growing and hormone-responsive tumour with recurrences occurring even 20 years after initial diagnosis. The exact pathogenesis is unknown, but exposure to tamoxifen and unopposed oestrogens (e.g., polycystic disease of the ovary) is implicated. It often occurs in association with endometriosis. ESN and LG-ESS are low-grade tumours that appear like the proliferative phase of endometrial stromal cells. Uterine curettage is usually diagnostic. As LG-ESS closely resembles normal endometrium, the definitive diagnosis sometimes can be made only after hysterectomy. Additionally, 30–50% are present in extra-uterine locations such as the ovary, pelvis, abdominal cavity, vulva, and vagina. MRI is a useful pre-operative diagnostic modality with the findings of low-signal intensity bands within the myometrium due to tumour permeation. LG-ESS is positive for CD 10 and inhibin. They are 75% ER and 95% PR positive showing their hormone responsiveness. Conventional ESS and USS usually do not need molecular testing for diagnosis. This, however, could verify the presence of HG-ESS in tumours with a round cell-epithelioid shape. The fibroblastic variant of conventional LG-ESS could also exhibit similar conditions.

Treatment for LG-ESS includes total hysterectomy with bilateral salpingo-oophorectomy. Bilateral salpingo-oophorectomy has a beneficial effect in most endometrial stromal tumours, owing to their hormonal responsiveness. However, it can be omitted for premenopausal women with stage-I due to the adverse effects of early surgical menopause. Hormone replacement therapy is contraindicated postoperatively. The rate of nodal metastasis was found to be 10%, and lymphadenectomy carries a prognostic value. Its therapeutic role is still unclear. Postoperative observation or oestrogen blockade is recommended for stage-I ESS. Adjuvant hormone therapy in the form of megestrol/medroxyprogesterone, gonadotropin-releasing hormone (GnRH) analogues, and aromatase inhibitors are available. Adjuvant megestrol therapy in stage-I disease cured 75% of patients, while 29% of patients who did not receive adjuvant megestrol had recurrence. NCCN recommends oestrogen blockade for stage II to IV disease. Although the role of radiation is questionable in ESS, tumour-directed radiotherapy in the form of brachytherapy +/− EBRT can be considered for stage II to IV disease or unresectable tumours. Recurrent ESS has also been treated with hormone therapy, radiation, surgical re-excision, or a combination of these. Tamoxifen is contraindicated [6]. The preferred agent for HG-ESS is gemcitabine combined with docetaxel, doxorubicin with ifosfamide/dacarbazine, etc. Additional treatment for IV B is a combination of chemotherapy and radiotherapy.

Differential diagnoses of endometrial stromal tumours are shown below [47]:

1. *ESN*: Cellular leiomyoma, LG-ESS.
2. *LG-ESS*: Gland-poor adenomyosis, Cellular leiomyoma, intravascular leiomyomatosis, LMS with an extensive intravascular component, HG-ESS, UTROSCT, PEComa, GIST.
3. *HG-ESS*: LG-ESS, LMS, UUS, GIST.
4. *UES*: LMS, HG-ESS, Undifferentiated carcinoma, Carcinosarcoma, Adenosarcoma with stromal overgrowth, Lymphoma, Melanoma, GIST, PEComa, perivascular epithelioid cell tumour; UTROSCT, uterine tumour resembling ovarian sex cord tumour.

8 Undifferentiated Uterine Sarcoma

UUS should be a diagnosis of exclusion and constitutes a heterogeneous group of high-grade tumours morphologically and immunohistochemically different from translocation positive endometrial sarcomas. There are reports of a few rare occurrences of a simultaneous LG-ESS component. They indicated a dedifferentiation path in a low-grade sarcoma leading to their onset.

Histopathologically, these tumours demonstrate an abundant mitotic activity with atypical forms and marked cellular pleomorphism. They have unusual growth pattern and vascularity of LG-ESS. Unlike the infiltrative pattern of LG-ESS, they displace the myometrium. They, frequently, are like the sarcomatous component of a carcinosarcoma. Their S-phase fraction could exceed 10%. They are mostly aneuploid and do not show the presence of ER or PR (CAP).

According to their mitotic index, Hardell et al. recently concluded that UUS should be subdivided into mitogenic and not otherwise specified [48]. Mitotic index is shown to be of prognostic importance even after neoadjuvant chemotherapy for primary, localized, high-grade soft tissue sarcomas [49]. Differences in the mitotic index are associated with different molecular subtypes of the disease that may explain the recognized prognostic significance of the mitotic index in these patients. Treatment of UUS is followed in the same line like that for LMS [6].

9 Other Tumour Types

Other mesenchymal lesions primary to the uterus include perivascular epithelioid cell tumour (PEComa) and rhabdomyosarcoma. PEComa is characterized by components of both melanocytic and smooth muscle differentiation. Though rare, rhabdomyosarcomas is the commonest uterine heterologous sarcoma which stains positive for desmin, muscle-specific actin, myogenin, Myo D1, and myoglobin and negative for smooth muscle actin. Pleomorphic and alveolar subtypes have a worse prognosis than the embryonal subtype.

10 Follow-up [6]

Patients should be educated regarding the symptoms and signs of recurrence like vaginal/rectal/urinary tract bleeding, weight loss, abdominal/pelvic/back/hip pain, decreased appetite with weight loss, and abdominal or limb swelling. NCCN recommends history and physical examination every 3–4 months for the first 2–3 years and then every 6–12 months thereafter. Chest/abdominal/pelvic CT is recommended every 3–6 months for the first 3 years and then 6–12 months for the next 2 years. 1 to 2 yearly imaging can be considered for the next 2 years. Other imaging modalities like abdominal/pelvic MRI or PET/CT can be considered as the need arises to confirm the findings.

11 Clinical Outcomes

While the FIGO stage Ia still has a 5-year survival rate of 84.3%, this dramatically decreases for stage II (43.6%), III (38.8%), and IV (19.8%) [50]. 45–75% have recurrence, with the commonest site of first recurrence being the lungs (40%) [51].

12 Conclusion

Uterine sarcomas are rare mesenchymal tumours with an aggressive course. Uterine curetting has a low diagnostic rate, with imaging serving as another limited adjunct to reach the diagnosis. Complete surgical resection of the gross tumour is the primary modality of treatment in early disease. The role of adjuvant therapy is limited by the lack of larger studies due to a limited number of cases. Palliation with systemic therapy and/or radiation and/or targeted therapy is advocated for an advanced stage. The rate of recurrence is high even after the treatment, and close follow-up is recommended. Treatment and prognosis based on molecular characterization are opening the window for a new approach to these tumours.

References

1. Mbatani N, Olawaiye AB, Prat J. Uterine sarcomas. Int J Gynaecol Obstet. 2018;143(Suppl 2):51–8.
2. Husseiny GE, Bareedy NA, Mourad WA, Mohamed G, Shoukri M, Subhi J, Ezzat A. Prognostic factors and treatment modalities in uterine sarcoma. Am J Clin Oncol. 2002;25(3):256–60.
3. Skubitz KM, D'Adamo DR. Sarcoma. Mayo Clin Proc. 2007;82(11):409–32.
4. Felix AS, Cook LS, Gaudet MM, Rohan TE, Schoten LJ, Setiawan VW, Wise LA, Anderson KE, Bernstein L, Vivo ID, Friedenreich CM, Gapstur SM, Goldbohm RA, Henderson RA, Horn-Ross PL, Kolonel L, Lacey JV, Liang X, Lissowska J, Magliocco A, McCullough ML, Miller AB, Olson SH, Palmer JR, Park Y, Patel AV, Prescott J, Rastogi R, Robien K, Robien K, Rosenberg L, Schairer C, Ou X, Brandt PA, Virkus RA, Wentzensen N, Xiang YB, Xu WH, Yang HP, Brinton LA. The etiology of uterine sarcomas: a pooled analysis of the epidemiology of endometrial cancer consortium. Br J Cancer. 2013;108(3):727–34.
5. Lavie O, Barnett-Griness O, Narod A, Rennert G. The risk of developing uterine sarcoma after tamoxifen use. Int J Gynecol Cancer. 2008;18(2):352–6.

6. NCCN. Uterine cancer: endometrical carcinoma uterine sarcoma. National Comprehensive Cancer Network; 2021.
7. Prat J. FIGO staging for uterine sarcomas. Int J Gynaecol Obstet. 2009;104(3):177–8.
8. World Health Organization, International Agency for Research on Cancer (IARC), WHO Classification of Tumours Editorial Board. WHO classification of tumours: female genital tumours, vol. 4. 5th ed. Lyon: IARC; 2020.
9. Cui RR, Wright JD, Hou JY. Uterine leiomyosarcoma: a review of recent advances in molecular biology, clinical management and outcome. BJOG. 2017;124(7):1028–37.
10. Lee C-H, Ou W-B, Mariño-Enriquez A, Zhu M, Mayeda M, Wang Y, Guo X, Brunner AL, Amant F, French CA, West RB, McAlpine JN, Gilks CB, Yaffe MB, Prentice LM, McPherson A, Jones SJM, Marra MA, Shah SP, van de Rijn M, Huntsman DG, Cin PD, Debiec-Rychter M, Nucci MR, Fletcher JA. 14-3-3 Fusion oncogenes in high-grade endometrial stromal sarcoma. Proc Natl Acad Sci U S A. 2012;109(3):929–34.
11. Lewis N, Soslow RA, Delair DF, Park KJ, Murali R, Hollmann TJ, Davidson B, Micci F, Panagopoulos I, Hoang LN, Arias-Stella JA 3rd, Oliva E, Young RH, Hensley ML, Leitao MM Jr, Hameed M, Benayed R, Ladanyi M, Frosina D, Jungbluth AA, Antonescu CR, Chiang S. ZC3H7B-BCOR high-grade endometrial stromal sarcomas: a report of 17 cases of a newly defined entity. Mod Pathol. 2018;31(4):674–84.
12. Micci F, Gorunova L, Agostini A, Johannessen E, Brunetti M, Davidson B, Heim S, Panagopoulos I. Cytogenetic and molecular profile of endometrial stromal sarcoma. Genes Chromosomes Cancer. 2016;55(11):834–46.
13. Lee C-H, Mariño-Enriquez A, Ou W, Zhu M, Ali RH, Chiang S, Amant F, Gilks CB, van de Rijn M, Oliva E, Debiec-Rychter M, Cin PD, Fletcher JA, Nucci MR. The clinicopathologic features of YWHAE-FAM22 endometrial stromal sarcomas: a histologically high-grade and clinically aggressive tumor. Am J Surg Pathol. 2012;36(5):641–53.
14. Lee C-H, Turbin DA, Sung Y-CV, Espinosa I, Montgomery K, van de Rijn M, Gilks CB. A panel of antibodies to determine site of origin and malignancy in smooth muscle tumors. Mod Pathol. 2009;22(12):1519–31.
15. Sun S, Bonaffini PA, Nougaret S, Fournier L, Dohan A, Chong J, Smith J, Addley H, Reinhold C. How to differentiate uterine leiomyosarcoma from leiomyoma with imaging. Diagn Interv Imaging. 2019;100(10):619–34.
16. Lin G, Yang LY, Huang YT, Ng K, Ng S, Ueng S, Chao A, Yen T, Chang T, Lai C. Comparison of the diagnostic accuracy of contrast-enhanced MRI and diffusion-weighted MRI in the differentiation between uterine leiomyosarcoma/smooth muscle tumor with uncertain malignant potential and benign leiomyoma. J Magn Reson Imaging. 2016;43(2):333–42.
17. Mbatani N, Olawaiye AB, Prat J. Uterine sarcomas. Int J Gynecol Obstet. 2018;143(52):51–8.
18. Seagle BL, Sobecki-Rausch J, Strohl AE, Shilpi A, Grace A, Shahabi S. Prognosis and treatment of uterine leiomyosarcoma: a National Cancer Database study. Gynecol Oncol. 2017;145(1):61–70.
19. Gronchi A, Miah AB, Tos APD, Abecassis N, Bajpai J, Bauer S, Biagini R, Bielack S, Blay JY, Bolle S, Bonvalot S, Boukovinas I, Bovee JVMG, Boye K, Brennan B, Brodowicz T, Buonadonna A, Álava ED, Muro XG, Dufrense A, Eriksson M, Fagioli F, Fedenko A, Ferraresi V, Ferrari A, Frezza AM, Gasperoni S, Gelderblom H, Gouin F, Grignani G, Haas R, Hassan AB, Hecker-Nolting S, Hindi N, Hohenberger P, Joensuu H, Jones RL, Jungles C, Jutte P, Kager L, Kasper B, Kawai A, Kopeckova K, Krakorova DA, Cesne AL, Grange FL, Legius E, Leithner A, Lopez-Pousa A, Martin-Broto J, Merimsky O, Messiou C, Mir O, Montemurro M, Morland B, Morosi C, Palmerini E, Pantaleo MA, Piana R, Piperno-Neumann S, Reichardt P, Rutkowski P, Safwat AA, Sangalli C, Sbaraglia M, Scheipl S, Schoffski P, Sleijfer S, Strauss D, Strauss S, Hall KS, Trama A, Unk M, van de Sande MAJ, van der Graaf WTA, van Houdt WJ, Frebourg T, Casali PG, Stacchiotti S, ESMO Guidelines Committee, EURACAN and GENTURIS. Soft tissue and visceral sarcomas: ESMO-EURACAN-GENTURIS clinical practice guidelines for diagnosis, treatment and follow-up. Ann Oncol. 2021;32(11):1348–65.
20. Ayhan A, Aksan G, Gultekin M, Esin S, Himmetoglu C, Dursun P, Usubutun A, Yuce K. Prognosticators and the role of lymphadenectomy in uterine leiomyosarcomas. Arch Gynecol Obstet. 2009;280(1):79–85.
21. Malouf GG, Lhommé C, Duvillard P, Morice P, Haie-Meder C, Pautier P. Prognostic factors and outcome of undifferentiated endometrial sarcoma treated by multimodal therapy. Int J Gynaecol Obstet. 2013;122(1):57–61.
22. Shah JP, Bryant CS, Kumar S, Ali-Fehmi R, Malone JM Jr, Morris RT. Lymphadenectomy and ovarian preservation in low-grade endometrial stromal sarcoma. Obstet Gynecol. 2008;112(5):1102–8.
23. Koh W, Greer BE, Abu-Rustum NR, Apte SM, Campos SM, Cho KR, Chu C, Cohn D, Crispens MA, Dizon DS, Dorigo O, Eifel PJ, Fisher CM, Frederick P, Gaffney DK, George S, Han E, Higgins S, Huh WK, Lurain JR 3rd, Mariani A, Mutch D, Fader AN, Remmenga SW, Reynolds RK, Tillmanns T, Valea FA, Yashar CM, McMillian NR, Scavone JL. Uterine sarcoma, Version 1.2016: featured updates to the NCCN Guidelines. J Natl Compr Cancer Netw. 2015;13(11):1321–31.
24. Dafopoulos A, Tsikouras P, Dimitraki M, Galazios G, Liberis V, Maroulis G, Teichmann AT. The role of lymphadenectomy in uterine leiomyosarcoma:

review of the literature and recommendations for the standard surgical procedure. Arch Gynecol Obstet. 2010;282(3):293–300.
25. Reed NS, Mangioni C, Malmstrom H, Scarfone G, Poveda A, Pecorelli S, Tateo S, Franchi M, Jobsen JJ, Coens C, Teodorovic I, Vergote I, Vermorken JB. Phase III randomised study to evaluate the role of adjuvant pelvic radiotherapy in the treatment of uterine sarcomas stages I and II: an European Organisation for Research and Treatment of Cancer Gynaecological Cancer Group Study (protocol 55874). Eur J Cancer. 2008;44(6):808–18.
26. Hensley ML, Wathen JK, Maki RG, Araujo DM, Sutton G, Priebat DA, George S, Soslow RA, Baker LH. Adjuvant therapy for high-grade, uterus-limited leiomyosarcoma: results of a phase 2 trial (SARC 005). Cancer. 2013;119(8):1555–61.
27. Hensley ML, Enserro D, Hatcher H, Ottevanger PB, Krarup-Hansen A, Blay J, Fisher C, Moxley KM, Lele SB, Lea JS, Tewari KS, Thaker PH, Zivanovic O, O'Malley DM, Robinson K, Miller DS. Adjuvant Gemcitabine Plus Docetaxel followed by Doxorubicin versus observation for high-grade uterine leiomyosarcoma: a Phase III NRG Oncology/Gynecologic Oncology Group Study. J Clin Oncol. 2018;36(33):JCO1800454.
28. Roberts ME, Aynardi JT, Chu CS. Uterine leiomyosarcoma: a review of the literature and update on management options. Gynecol Oncol. 2018;151(3):562–72.
29. Angarita FA, Cannell AJ, Razak ARA, Dickson BC, Blackstein ME. Trabectedin for inoperable or recurrent soft tissue sarcoma in adult patients: a retrospective cohort study. BMC Cancer. 2016;16:16–30.
30. Benson C, Ray-Coquard I, Sleijfer S, Litière S, Blay JY, Cesne AL, Papai Z, Judson I, Schöffski P, Chawla S, Gil T, Piperno-Neumann S, Marréaud S, Dewji MR, van der Graaf WTA. Outcome of uterine sarcoma patients treated with pazopanib: a retrospective analysis based on two European Organisation for Research and Treatment of Cancer (EORTC) Soft Tissue and Bone Sarcoma Group (STBSG) clinical trials 62043 and 62072. Gynecol Oncol. 2016;142(1):89–94.
31. Ben-Ami E, Barysauskas CM, Solomon S, Tahil K, Malley R, Hohos M, Polson K, Loucks M, Severgnini M, Patel T, Cunningham A, Rodig SJ, Hodi FS, Morgan JA, Merriam P, Wagner AJ, Shapiro GI, George S. Immunotherapy with single agent nivolumab for advanced leiomyosarcoma of the uterus: results of a phase 2 study. Cancer. 2017;127(17):3285–90.
32. Tawbi HA, Burgess M, Bolejack V, van Tine BA, Schuetze SM, Hu J, D'Angelo S, Attia S, Riedel RF, Preibat DA, Movva S, Davis LE, Okuno SH, Reed DR, Crowley J, Butterfield LH, Salazar R, Rodriguez-Canales J, Lazar AJ, Wistuba II, Baker LH, Maki RG, Reinke D, Patel S. Pembrolizumab in advanced soft-tissue sarcoma and bone sarcoma (SARC028): a multicentre, two-cohort, single-arm, open-label, phase 2 trial. Lancet Oncol. 2017;18(11):1493–501.
33. Edris B, Weiskopf K, Volkmer AK, Volkmer J, Willingham SB, Contreras-Trujillo H, Liu J, Majeti R, West RB, Fletcher JA, Beck AH, Weissman IL, van de Rijn M. Antibody therapy targeting the CD47 protein is effective in a model of aggressive metastatic leiomyosarcoma. Proc Natl Acad Sci U S A. 2012;109(17):6656–61.
34. Mäkinen N, Aavikko M, Heikkinen T, Taipale M, Taipale J, Koivisto-Korander R, Bützow R, Vahteristo P. Exome sequencing of uterine leiomyosarcomas identifies frequent mutations in TP53, ATRX, and MED12. PLOS Genet. 2016;12(2):e1005850.
35. Allen ML, Douds JJ, Liang SX, Desouki MM, Parkash V, Fadare O. An immunohistochemical analysis of stathmin 1 expression in uterine smooth muscle tumors: differential expression in leiomyosarcomas and leiomyomas. Int J Clin Exp Pathol. 2015;8(3):2795–801.
36. Reyes HD, Miecznikowski J, Gonzalez-Bosquet J, Devor EJ, Zhang Y, Theil KW, Samuelson MI, McDonald M, Stephan J, Harjani P, Guntupalli S, Tewari KS, Backes F, Ramirez N, Fleming GF, Filiaci V, Birrer MJ, Leslie KK. High stathmin expression is a marker for poor clinical outcome in endometrial cancer: an NRG oncology group/gynecologic oncology group study. Gynecol Oncol. 2017;146(2):247–53.
37. Yasutake N, Ohishi Y, Taguchi K, Hiraki Y, Oya M, Oshiro Y, Mine M, Iwasaki T, Yamamoto H, Kohashi K, Sonoda K, Kato K, Oda Y. Insulin-like growth factor II messenger RNA-binding protein-3 is an independent prognostic factor in uterine leiomyosarcoma. Histopathology. 2017;72(5):739–48.
38. Raspollini MR, Amunni G, Villanucci A, Pinzani P, Simi L, Paglierani M, Taddei GL. c-Kit expression in patients with uterine leiomyosarcomas: a potential alternative therapeutic treatment. Clin Cancer Res. 2004;10(10):3500–3.
39. Serrano C, Mackintosh C, Herrero D, Martins AS, de Alava E, Hernández T, Pérez-Fontán J, Abad M, Pérez A, Serrano E, Bullón A, Orfao A. Imatinib is not a potential alternative treatment for uterine leiomyosarcoma. Clin Cancer Res. 2005;11(13):4977–9.
40. Food and Drug Administration. Quantitative assessment of the prevalence of unsuspected uterine sarcoma in women undergoing treatment of uterine fibroids. FDA; 2014.
41. Hartmann KE, Fonnesbeck C, Surawicz T, Krishnaswami S, Andrews JC, Wilson JE, Velez-Edwards D, Kugley S, Sathe NA. Management of uterine fibroids: comparative effectiveness review, number 195. Rockville: Agency for Healthcare Research and Quality; 2017.
42. Bogani G, Cliby WA, Aletti GD. Impact of morcellation on survival outcomes of patients with unexpected uterine leiomyosarcoma: a systematic review and meta-analysis. Gynecol Oncol. 2015;137(1):167–72.
43. Seidman MA, Oduyebo T, Muto MG, Crum CP, Nucci MR, Quade BJ. Peritoneal dissemination complicat-

ing morcellation of uterine mesenchymal neoplasms. PLoS One. 2012;7(11):e50058.
44. Multinu F, Casarin J, Hanson KT, Angioni S, Mariani A, Habermann EB, Laughlin-Tommaso SK. Practice patterns and complications of benign hysterectomy following the FDA statement warning against the use of power morcellation. JAMA Surg. 2018;153(6):e180141.
45. Hanby AM, Walker C. The WHO, and what of the breast and female genital organs: part IV in the WHO classification of tumours series. Breast Cancer Res. 2004;6(3):133–4.
46. Ravid Y, Formanski M, Smith Y, Reich R, Davidson B. Uterine leiomyosarcoma and endometrial stromal sarcoma have unique miRNA signatures. Gynecol Oncol. 2016;140(3):512–7.
47. Nucci MR. Practical issues related to uterine pathology: endometrial stromal tumors. Mod Pathol. 2015;29:92–103.
48. Hardell E, Josefson S, Ghaderi M, Skeie-Jensen T, Westbom-Fremer S, Cheek EH, Bell D, Selling J, Schoolmeester JK, Måsbäck A, Davidson B, Carlson JW. Validation of a mitotic index cutoff as a prognostic marker in undifferentiated uterine sarcomas. Am K Surg Pathol. 2017;41(9):1231–7.
49. Andreou D, Werner M, Pink D, Traub F, Schuler M, Gosheger G, Jobke B, Reichardt P, Tunn PU. Prognostic relevance of the mitotic count and the amount of viable tumour after neoadjuvant chemotherapy for primary, localised, high-grade soft tissue sarcoma. Br J Cancer. 2015;112(3):455–60.
50. Kosary CL. Chapter 15: Cancer of the corpus uteri. In: LAG R, Young JL, Keel GE, Eisner MP, Lin YD, Horner M-J, editors. SEER survival monograph: cancer survival among adults: U.S. SEER Program, 1988–2001, Patient and tumor characteristics. Bethesda: SEER Program, National Cancer Institute; 2007. p. 123–32. NIH Pub. No. 07-6215.
51. D'Angelo E, Prat J. Uterine sarcomas: a review. Gynecol Oncol. 2010;116(1):131–9.

Epithelial Ovarian Cancer

Upasana Baruah, Lalit Kumar,
and Amal Chandra Kataki

1 Epidemiology and Risk Factors

Regarded as a dreaded disease amongst gynaecological cancer, epithelial ovarian cancer is second common gynaecological malignancy (after uterine in developed and after cervix in developing world) [1, 2]. It remains the major cause mortality amongst females in developed countries due to advanced stage at presentation. Worldwide 313,959 women were diagnosed with this disease in the year 2020 with an age standardized rate (ASR) of 6.6 per 100,000 [2]. Its incidence is higher in Central and Eastern Europe, with ASR of 11.4 per 100,000 women. However, an increasing trend is observed for most countries in Asia, Central and Eastern Europe, and Central and South America [3]. This has been attributed to smaller family sizes, high-fat diet, higher socioeconomic status, older age, and a predominantly Caucasian population in European countries. In India, as per the population-based cancer registry (PBCR) data in 2014 the ASR of ovarian cancer in India was 6.5 per 100,000 with highest incidence in Papumpare District (15.2) followed by Delhi PBCR (10.0) [4].

Various factors are implicated in the pathogenesis of the disease. Among these a strong family history and genetic cause is found to have a direct correlation with the probability of a woman developing the disease [5]. Other risk factors include hormonal and reproductive factors such as parity, breast-feeding, early menarche, late menopause, obesity, menopausal hormonal treatment, oral contraceptive (OCP) use, and endometriosis. Smoking is considered to be a risk factor for mucinous ovarian cancer [6]. The median age at onset is 63 years worldwide; in India median age is around 53 years [4]. However, in women with hereditary ovarian cancer it occurs approximately a decade earlier [1, 5].

2 Hereditary Ovarian Cancer

Among the different causes of epithelial ovarian cancer, genetic factor is the strongest predisposing element. Patients with family history of ovarian cancer are divided into three categories: (A) breast and ovarian cancer syndrome, (B) site-specific ovarian cancer, and (C) hereditary non-polyposis colorectal cancer (HNPCC or Lynch II syndrome). Mutations in the tumour suppressor

U. Baruah (✉) · A. C. Kataki
Department of Gynaecologic Oncology,
Dr. Bhubaneswar Borooah Cancer Institute
(A Unit of Tata Memorial Centre, Mumbai),
Guwahati, Assam, India

L. Kumar
Department of Medical Oncology, AIIMS,
New Delhi, Delhi, India

NCI-India, Delhi, India

A. C. Kataki, D. Barmon (eds.), *Fundamentals in Gynaecologic Malignancy*,
https://doi.org/10.1007/978-981-19-5860-1_16

BRCA genes are associated with the initial two categories whereas Lynch syndrome is associated with mutations in the DNA mismatch repair (MMR) genes. Approximately 10% of all epithelial ovarian malignancies are genetic, with BRCA gene mutations accounting for the majority, i.e. 90% of the cases and Lynch syndrome accounting for the other 10% [7].

Recent data have shown that BRCA mutations can be as high as 20% in high grade serous carcinomas of ovary [8, 9]. Women who are BRCA1 carriers have a lifetime risk of ovarian cancer of 40–50% and BRCA2 carriers have a risk of 20–30% [7]. Knowledge about hereditary cancer syndromes can be traced back to 1866, when a French surgeon, Pierre Paul Broca described the history of breast cancer in his wife's family. His work referred ten women with breast cancer over three generations [10]. After the observation and work of many scientists in 1994, the BRCA1 gene on chromosome 17 and BRCA2 gene in chromosome 13 was localized [10]. Normally the prevalence of BRCA1 or BRCA2 mutations in the general population is low (1:300 to 1:800) but it increases in specific ethnic populations with founder mutations such as French Canadians, Icelanders, Mexicans, and Ashkenazi Jews (approximately 2%) [11].

As the BRCA genes are inherited as autosomal dominant, every first-degree relative has a 50% probability of harbouring a mutation. Due to the extensive work published over the last two decades we now have a better understanding of the pathway involved and interventions beneficial in BRCA-related ovarian cancers. Our cells have five primary pathways of DNA repair that are responsible in probing and identifying defects protecting the genome. The major pathways involved are direct repair, mismatch repair (MMR), base excision repair (BER), nucleotide excision repair (NER), and double-strand break (DSB) recombinational repair, which includes both non-homologous end-joining (NHEJ) and homologous recombinational repair. BRCA genes are tumour suppressor genes and form a complex with Rad51, a protein that has an established role in homologous recombination. BRCA1 is also involved in complexing with and activation of p53 [12]. The function of p53 is to signal about DNA damage and temporarily arrest the cell cycle to either allow repair or trigger cell death. Normally we have two copies of BRCA genes which is inherited from each parent. Individuals inheriting BRCA mutations carry a deleterious germ-line mutation in one of the BRCA gene. When the second copy is affected due to sporadic event (second hit) cells lose the ability to repair double-strand breaks, develop increased genomic instability and a predisposition for malignant transformation [13]. Several other genes (BRIP1, PALB2, RAD51C) which are part of this pathway are also found to be mutated in epithelial ovarian cancer [14].

Majority of the patients have high-grade serous histology, but studies have also reported borderline, mucinous tumours, endometrioid and clear cell histologies [15, 16]. Although serous high-grade histology is more common among these patients it is seen that they have better overall outcomes and greater response-rates to platinum compounds as well as to other drugs commonly used for ovarian cancer. The lack of functional BRCA genes seems to provide an advantage when treated with DNA-damaging chemotherapeutic agents because the presence of defects in homologous recombination causes synthetic lethality in the cancerous cells [17, 18]. Although BRCA mutations are associated with better short-term survival, this advantage decreases over time and is, eventually reversed [19]. In these patient's breast cancer is more common, appear at an early age and usually precedes the ovarian cancer [20]. The average cumulative risks for breast and ovarian cancers were 65% and 39%, respectively, at 70 years for carriers of BRCA 1 mutation. The corresponding estimates for BRCA2 were 45 and 11% [21].

Patients with Lynch syndrome have an autosomal dominant mode of inheritance and is caused by a mutation in one of the DNA mismatch repair genes called the MMR genes which are MLH1, MSH2, MSH6, and PMS 2. Dysfunction of any of these leads to repair complex failure resulting in accumulation of numerous DNA replication errors and microsatellite instability (MSI) and cancer formation [22]. Ovarian cancers in Lynch syndrome are mostly of clear cell variety with a lifetime risk of 9–12% [23].

2.1 Management of Women with Hereditary Ovarian Cancer

The identification of a BRCA mutation may impact their treatment, because it might indicate an increased sensitivity to poly (ADP-ribose) polymerase (PARP) enzyme inhibitors as well as to platinum compounds both in the first- and second-line setting [24]. *The Society of Gynaecologic Oncology (SGO) recommends that individuals with inherited predisposition to cancer should be offered genetic counseling* [25].

Lynch syndrome (LS) can be suspected on the basis of the Amsterdam II or Bethesda criteria [26]. It requires significant time and expertise to counsel a woman at risk for hereditary cancer and a genetic counsellor with proficient experience should evaluate the risks and provide appropriate medical advice.

The current ovarian cancer screening options of transvaginal ultrasound and CA-125 have not proven to be effective in improving detection or survival in either the normal or high-risk population, as evidenced by the United Kingdom Trial of Ovarian Cancer Screening (UK-TOCS) and the United Kingdom Familial Ovarian Cancers Screening (UK-FOCS) trials [27, 28]. However, periodic screening using transvaginal ultrasound and CA-125 may be performed at the physicians discretion starting at the age of 30–35 years. Therefore, current recommendations focus on prevention with oral contraceptives and risk-reducing bilateral salpingo-oophorectomy (RRSO).

Before establishing a family, females should be advised to use oral contraceptives. Prophylactic bilateral salpingo-oophorectomy should be advocated for women who choose not to maintain her fertility or have had their children. As some ovarian malignancies develop in the fallopian tubes, risk-reducing surgery involves removing both fallopian tubes and the ovaries [29].

Prophylactic bilateral oophorectomy reduces the risk of cancer of the coelomic epithelium in BRCA carriers by about 96% and the risk of breast cancer by 53%. It implies that there is still 4% chance of peritoneal carcinomatosis after RRSO [30]. Because BRCA2 mutation carriers will develop ovarian cancer later than women with BRCA1 mutations, delaying RRSO in BRCA2 mutation carriers until age 50 can be considered. However, women with BRCA2 mutations have a 26–34% risk of developing breast cancer by the age of 50, and the evidence suggests that the breast cancer risk reduction conferred by RRSO is greater when the ovaries are removed earlier [31].

Clinical breast examination should be done every 6–12 months beginning at the age of 25 with annual breast MRI with contrast or mammogram if MRI is unavailable. At age 30–75 years annual breast MRI with contrast and mammogram should be advised [32].

Women with Lynch syndrome should be counselled about need to undergo periodic screening and seek medical attention in case of abnormal uterine bleeding. Surveillance of the endometrium with annual pelvic examination, transvaginal ultrasound, and endometrial biopsy should be done at 1–2 years interval beginning at the age of 30–35 years or 10 years before the earliest age of first diagnosis of Lynch associated cancer in the family. Likewise, colonoscopy should be performed every 1–2 years. Surveillance should be continued till risk reducing hysterectomy is performed after child bearing is completed at 35–45 years of age [33, 34].

3 Pathogenesis

The overwhelming majority of ovarian cancer incidences are epithelial in nature. According to the World Health Organization (WHO), fallopian tube, ovarian, and peritoneal cancers are classified histologically as under [35].

Serous adenocarcinoma.
Mucinous adenocarcinoma.
Endometrioid adenocarcinoma.
Clear cell carcinoma.
Brenner's tumour.
Undifferentiated carcinomas (this group are too poorly differentiated to be classified in any other group).
Mixed epithelial tumours (composed of two or more of the five major cell types).

Nearly 70–80% epithelial malignancies have a serous histologic type, with 80% of them being high-grade tumours [36].

Primary ovarian mucinous carcinomas are very rare and account for only 3% of all mucinous ovarian tumours. Frequency of mucinous subtype is higher (10–15%) in early-stage disease. Therefore, among patients with advanced stage disease, whenever mucinous histology is encountered it is essential to rule out possibility of metastatic disease from GIT/hepatobiliary system. Seidman et al. proposed an algorithm to identify primary and metastatic mucinous carcinoma based on tumour size and laterality. Tumours that were more than 10 cm in diameter and unilateral were found to be primary in 82% of cases. Unilateral tumours less than 10 cm were metastatic 87% of the time. Bilateral tumours less than 10 cm were metastatic in 92% of cases, while bilateral tumours less than 10 cm were metastatic in 95% of cases. Hence, even in the case of a unilateral tumour, the probability of metastatic mucinous carcinoma should always be considered [37].

Often patients with mucinous tumours have an elevated level of one of two tumour markers, CEA or CA19-9. Because of the large size of the primary tumour, both mucinous and endometrioid ovarian cancers have a likelihood to be discovered at an early stage.

Endometroid variety account for 10% of cases of ovarian cancer and most of them are confined to the pelvis at diagnosis (FIGO stage I or II). Clear cell, Brenner, and undifferentiated ovarian carcinomas are rare [38].

Epithelial ovarian malignancies can be split into two types based on their grade and pathogenesis: Type I and Type II tumours. The model does not substitute standard histopathologic ovarian tumour classification, but it does give a foundation for ovarian carcinogenesis research. Low-grade micropapillary serous carcinoma, endometrioid, mucinous, and clear cell carcinomas are all examples of type I tumours. They typically present as large masses that are confined to one ovary, are indolent, and have a good prognosis. Low-grade serous carcinoma develops from a well-known sequence of events, such as borderline serous tumours or endometriosis. They have mutations in a variety of genes, including PTEN, BRAF, KRAS, and beta-catenin, and are genetically stable.

Type II tumours are fast-growing, extremely aggressive tumours and no well-defined precursor lesions have been established. High-grade serous carcinoma, malignant mixed mesodermal tumours (carcinosarcomas), and undifferentiated carcinomas all are examples of type II tumours. The mutation of TP53 characterizes this category of tumours, which has a high degree of genetic instability [39, 40].

Initially ovary was originally considered to be the primary site of cancer initiation and the ovarian surface epithelium represented the cell of origin. The "incessant ovulation" hypothesis proposed that tumour developed due to repetitive injury of the ovarian surface epithelium with each ovulatory cycle [41]. Although this model could account for a number of important features associated with ovarian cancer, particularly Type I tumours, it failed to present a roadmap for understanding Type II tumours.

The Serous Tubal Intraepithelial Carcinoma (STIC): Recently the fallopian tube has emerged as likely site of origin for high-grade serous carcinoma. This theory was mainly derived from the study of the fallopian tubes, prophylactically removed during surgery, in high-risk women including BRCA carriers [42]. Subsequent studies led to the discovery of a potential premalignant lesion in the epithelium of fimbrial end of fallopian tube which was termed "serous tubal intraepithelial carcinoma (STIC)" [43, 44]. STIC is a non-invasive premalignant lesion with malignant cellular features, including enlarged nuclei, dark staining of the nucleus (hyperchromasia), coarse chromatin aggregates, and prominent nucleoli. STIC are found in 10–15% of prophylactically removed fallopian tubes from asymptomatic BRCA mutation carriers [[45–49]]. Most STICs exhibit robust immunostaining of p53 and harbour p53 mutations which are collectively termed the "p53 signature".

4 Immunohistochemistry (IHC)

IHC has a significant role in establishing or ruling out a diagnosis of ovarian primary especially in the setting of advanced disease with mucinous histology where GI primary needs to be ruled out. Serous carcinomas are usually positive for CK7, CA 125, PAX8 WT1 and negative for CK20 (Figs. 1 and 2). CK 20 and CDX2 are usually positive in adenocarcinomas originating from colorectum. HNF-1β is overexpressed in clear cell carcinoma and its overexpression is useful to differentiate from high grade serous cancer where it is negative. Clear cell carcinomas are negative for ER, PR, WT1, and p 53 in contrast to high grade serous carcinomas [50–52].

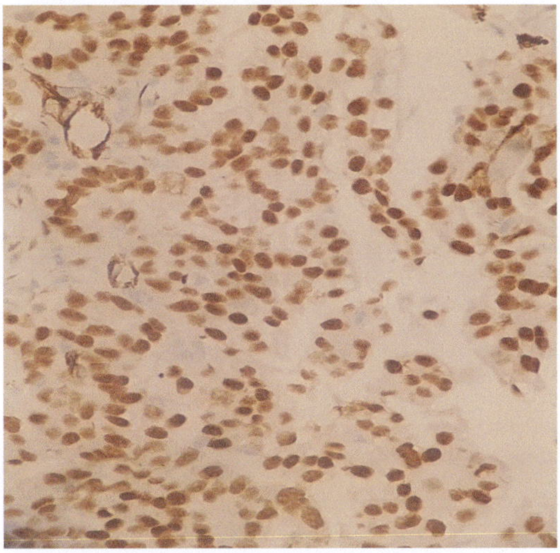

Fig. 1 Cytoplasmic positivity of CK7 in ovarian cancer

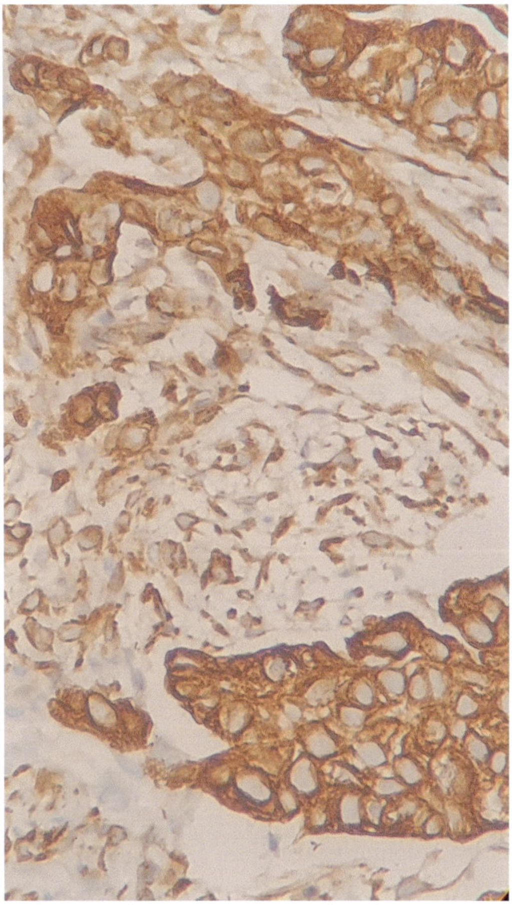

Fig. 2 WT1 nuclear positivity in ovarian cancer

5 Patterns of Spread

5.1 Trans-coelomic (Fig. 3)

It is the most common mode of dissemination for ovarian cancer. Trans coelomic spread is the result of exfoliation of cells from the tumour as spheroids that circulate in the peritoneal fluid. Due to the stresses of respiration, they migrate along a defined course from pelvis, through the paracolic gutters, notably on the right, down the intestinal mesenteries to right hemidiaphragm [53–55]. The Pouch of Douglas, right hemidiaphragm, paracolic gutters, liver surface, peritoneal surfaces of intestines and their mesenteries and omentum are all common sites for metastases [56, 57].

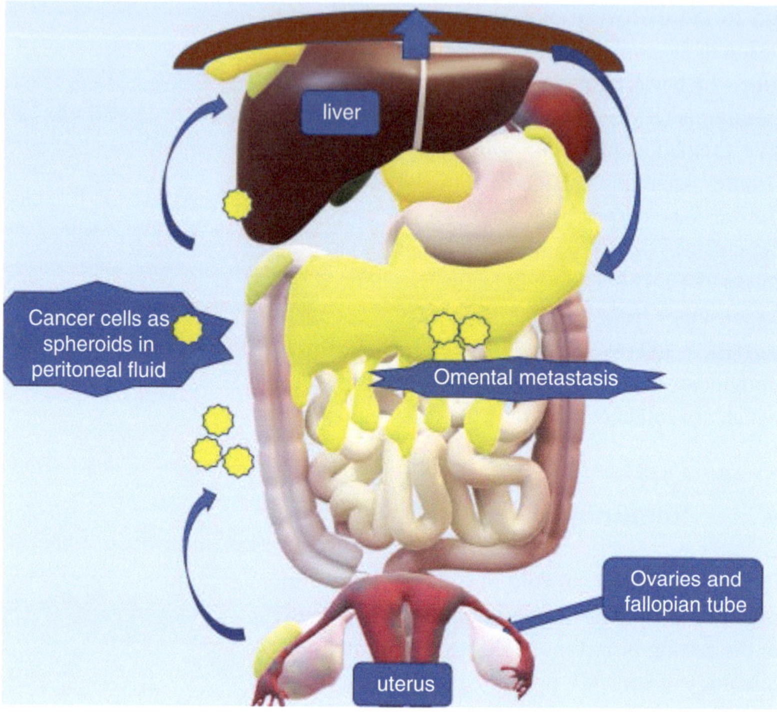

Fig. 3 Transcoelomic spread of ovarian cancer

Other than metastases to the contralateral ovary, an omental metastasis is often the largest tumour in the abdominal cavity [58, 59]. Infiltration into the intestinal lumen is an infrequent occurrence but as it is associated with disseminated surface deposits there is progressive agglutination of loops of bowel, resulting in functional intestinal obstruction known as carcinomatous ileus [60]. Women with advanced serous ovarian cancer, who have disseminated miliary disease often have large-volume ascites. Lymphatic communication through the diaphragm allows trans-diaphragmatic spread of tumour cells into the pleural space, causing a malignant pleural effusion particularly on the right side [61]. The peritoneum is the organ most commonly affected [62]. In patients with extensive pelvic disease with infiltration, it may be difficult to identify the individual organs and their anatomic boundaries.

5.2 Lymphatic

Retroperitoneal lymphatics that drain the ovary follow the infundibulopelvic ligament and terminate in nodes lying along the aorta and vena cava up to the level of the renal vessels. The next lymph node stations are at the celiac trunk from where tumour cells may continue up to the mediastinal and supraclavicular nodes. Lymphatic channels also pass laterally through the broad ligament and parametrial channels to terminate in the pelvic sidewall lymph nodal stations, namely the external iliac, obturator, and hypogastric chains [63].

Lymphatic dissemination to the pelvic and para-aortic nodes is more prevalent in advanced-stage cancer [64]. Based on a study positive para-aortic nodes were found to be 18.2% in Stage I disease, 20.0% in Stage II, 41.9% in Stage III, and 66.7% in Stage IV. Stage I disease had a 9.1% incidence of pelvic node metastases, Stage II had a 10% incidence, Stage III had 12.9% incidence, and Stage IV had a 33.3% incidence.

Grade 3 tumours had the highest incidence of nodal involvement in the study, with positive para-aortic nodal metastasis of 52.5% and pelvic nodal involvement of 15.5% [65]. Cancer cells can also disseminate via the lymphatics that drain along the round ligament to inguinal lymph nodes. It explains why inguinal lymph node metastasis is sometimes detected in patients with ovarian cancer. Retrograde lymph drainage does not occur and intrauterine or cervical metastases is rare in serous ovarian cancer.

5.3 Hematogenous

Hematogenous spread at the time of diagnosis is generally uncommon and result in intraparenchymal spread to vital organ, such as the liver, spleen, lungs, and brain [66].

6 Prognostic Factors of Epithelial Ovarian Carcinoma

Stage and residual volume of tumour after surgical cytoreduction are the most consistently reported prognostic factor [67–71]. According to a FIGO report, survival for stage IA disease is about 90%, 70–80% for stage IC, 70% for stage II disease, 30% for stage IIIC, and 18% for stage IV [72]. For stage I cancers, multivariate analyses identified grade as the most powerful prognostic indicator of disease-free survival [73]

The extent of residual disease post-cytoreductive surgery has been shown to be one of the most important parameters influencing both progression-free (PFS) and overall survival (OS). Females who had no markedly evident residual disease after first debulking surgery had considerably longer overall survival and progression-free survival. Survival estimates favoured the lower volume residual disease group when comparing greater than 1 cm against less than 1 cm of residual malignancy [74].

The prognosis of low-grade serous carcinoma is much better than that of high-grade serous carcinoma [75].

Mucinous ovarian cancer of stage III and IV have a poor prognosis when compared to similar stage of high grade serous ovarian cancers. There is also evidence that the response rate of mucinous ovarian cancer to standard platinum-based therapy is much lower than for high grade serous ovarian cancer [76, 77].

Another histological subtype which has a poor prognosis is clear cell carcinoma. Clear cell carcinoma of the ovary are generally diagnosed at a young age, are high grade, mostly unilateral, have early stage at presentation and most of the patients are negative for CA125. Advanced clear cell carcinoma is associated with a very poor prognosis as it is resistant to standard chemotherapy [78].

Furthermore, the volume of ascites, the age of the patient, and the patient's performance condition are all considered as independent prognostic variables [79]. Patients with a higher performance status have a higher tolerance for various therapeutic modalities and are more likely to complete intensive surgical and chemotherapeutic modalities [80–82].

7 Diagnosis and Staging

Ovarian cancer is surgically staged as per the FIGO staging system 2014. It combines classification of ovarian, fallopian, and peritoneal carcinomatosis [83].

Stage I cancer comprises of tumour which is confined to ovaries or fallopian tubes. It is further subdivided into three subgroups based on extracapsular spread either during (1CI) or before surgery (1C2) and presence of cancer cells in ascitic fluid or peritoneal wash taken during surgery (1C3). Preoperative FNAC or Biopsy is therefore not recommended as it upstages the disease.

Stage II refers to extension to uterus and/or fallopian tubes *and/or ovaries* (In cases of fallopian tube and peritoneal cancer) (IIA) or to other pelvic intraperitoneal organs (IIB).

Stage III implies metastasis outside the pelvis with or without retroperitoneal lymph nodal involvement. Only positive retroperitoneal nodal involvement is classified under IIIA1 which is subclassified into two groups (i and ii) based on the size of nodes up to than or more than 10 mm.

Microscopic extra pelvic peritoneal involvement with or without positive retroperitoneal lymph nodes is classified under stage IIIA2. Macroscopic peritoneal disease beyond the pelvis up to 2 cm refers to IIIB and disease more than 2 cm, with or without metastasis to the retroperitoneal lymph nodes are considered IIIC. If there is only involvement of capsule of liver and spleen without intraparenchymal spread, it falls under IIIC.

Stage IV includes distant metastasis outside the abdominal cavity. Malignant pleural effusion falls under IVA whereas metastases to extra-abdominal organs including inguinal nodes and lymph nodes outside of the abdominal cavity falls under IVB.

7.1 Clinical Presentation

Symptoms in patients with ovarian cancer are generally nonspecific and therefore diagnosis is often delayed. Most patient have dyspepsia, anorexia, fatigue, early satiety, and loss of appetite as their presenting symptom. Women with symptoms and findings suspicious of malignant ovarian mass should be evaluated with pelvic examination and pelvic imaging. The evaluation to exclude malignancy includes a comprehensive medical history, physical examination, imaging, and laboratory evaluation for tumour markers.

As majority of patients with small ovarian tumours are asymptomatic, the mass is usually discovered during a workup for other conditions. Large adnexal masses cause pain and pressure in the pelvis by compressing the surrounding structures resulting in urinary urgency, frequency, and dyspareunia. Posteriorly, a fixed pelvic tumour can compress the sigmoid colon, causing severe constipation and pain. These symptoms can occur in both benign disease and early ovarian cancer. Therefore, it is impossible to identify by clinical examination alone. Borderline ovarian tumours and low-grade cancers generally present as large masses resulting in an early diagnosis. Sometimes there may be sudden onset of abdominal pain due to rupture, torsion, infarction, and haemorrhage of the ovarian mass.

Infiltration into the peritoneum, bowel mesentery, and ascites occur as the disease advances and may result in dull aching pain and discomfort due to abdominal distention. If the tumour has metastasized to the omentum, there may be upper abdominal discomfort with nausea, belching, early satiety, and fullness. Dyspnoea occurs due to upward displacement of the diaphragm or pleural effusion. With extensive involvement of the bowel patient may present with subacute intestinal obstruction.

The probability that an adnexal mass is malignant depends mainly upon imaging findings that are consistent with malignancy and risk increases with advanced age or postmenopausal status, and raised tumour markers. Minimally invasive biopsy technique or image-guided ovarian biopsy to confirm malignancy prior to staging laparotomy results in the spillage of malignant cells and is not recommended.

Age is an important factor not only in identifying the risk of malignancy but also speculating the predominant histology prevalent in the particular age group. In premenarchal girls, an adnexal mass is often germ cell in origin. In postmenopausal patients, a complex adnexal mass is particularly concerning as a normal postmenopausal ovary is atrophic and small (1.5 × 1 × 0.5 cm). However, it should be remembered that although ovarian cancer is much more prevalent in postmenopausal women, the most common ovarian cyst in a postmenopausal patient is still a benign cyst [84]. Every postmenopausal woman with a solid adnexal mass should have a surgical exploration to determine histology as early-stage ovarian cancer has a much better prognosis than advanced-stage disease.

7.2 Tumour Markers

CA-125 is most frequently elevated in epithelial ovarian cancer. Initially described by Dr. Robert Bast it is expressed both on Mullerian (tubal, endometrial, endocervical) and coelomic (pericardium, pleura, peritoneum, ovarian surface) epithelium. Only 50% of stage I disease is associated with an elevated serum CA-125, which is one reason that CA-125 is not a good screening method for early-stage ovarian cancer and even in advanced-stage cancers the marker has a 20–25% false-negative rate [85]. CA-125 is highest in serous and lowest in mucinous ovarian cancers. Clear cell and endometrioid ovarian cancer often have lower CA-125 values [86]. Sensitivity is further decreased by the fact that several nonmalignant conditions can falsely elevate its levels like acute or chronic inflammation, peritoneal tuberculosis, endometriosis, fibroids, pregnancy, cirrhosis of the liver, systemic lupus erythematosus, and inflammatory bowel disease. Moreover, it is not specific to ovarian cancer, as it is increased in gastrointestinal, breast, and endometrial cancer [87].

Mucinous ovarian cancer is associated with elevated CEA values, but it is not diagnostic as it is also increased in patients with gastrointestinal malignancies, especially colon and gastric cancer. A ratio of CA-125/CEA > 25 is more helpful and is used clinically to exclude a gastrointestinal malignancy [88]. CA-125 is most useful in distinguishing between a benign and malignant mass when used in conjunction with clinical history (age, menopausal status, imaging) and helps triage women with an adnexal mass for surgery or observation. CA-125 is also helpful in the evaluation of response to therapy in patients with an established diagnosis of ovarian cancer and can assist in the diagnosis of recurrence.

HE4 is also elevated in ovarian cancer but is not commonly utilised. Unlike CA125 it is elevated less frequently in benign disease, particularly in premenopausal patients [89].

7.3 Transvaginal Sonography (TVS)

TVS allows better visualization of the ovaries, has shorter examination time than transabdominal ultrasound and size and morphologic characteristics of the ovary are better assessed with it [90]. When a lesion is large or extends beyond the field of view of TVS, transabdominal ultrasound is required along with it. The main objective is to ascertain if the mass is benign or malignant so that approach to surgical intervention can be made. Several ultrasound-based predictive models have been developed to differentiate between benign and malignant tumours. RMI 1 and 2 are commonly used. The RMI 1 (malignancy risk index) described by Jacobs et al. is calculated based on the serum CA 125 value, menopausal status (M), and evaluation of ultrasound (U). The ultrasound result is scored 1 point for multilocularity, solid areas, ascites, metastases, and bilaterality. If there are no such features, a score of 0 is given and score of 1 is given for single feature. For more than 1 feature a score of 3 is given. The menopausal status is scored as 1 in pre-menopausal and 3 for post-menopausal women. All women with an RMI I score of 250 or greater should be referred to a centre with specialist multidisciplinary team [91, 92]. In RMI 2, for ultrasound score of 1 is given for either 1 or none of the five features whereas with 2 or more features a score of 4 is given. For premenopausal women M is scored as 1 and for postmenopausal M is scored as 4 [93].

ROMA (risk of ovarian malignancy algorithm) incorporates cancer antigen 125 (CA125), HE4, and menopausal status. ROMA cutoff values for high-risk patients were ≥13.1% and ≥27.7% for pre-menopausal and post-menopausal women, respectively, as suggested by Moore et al. [94]. Because ultrasonography characteristics of ovarian tumours were more predictive than tumour markers, the IOTA (International Ovarian Tumour Analysis) group developed a standardized technique for preoperative categorization of adnexal masses [95]. The study's highlight was a set of ten simple ultrasonography rules with exceptional sensitivity and specificity that could be applied to a wide range of tumours. A benign feature is a unilocular cyst with solid components less than 7 mm in diameter, a smooth multilocular tumour less than 10 cm in diameter, acoustic shadows, and no detectable doppler signal (B). Malignant features (M) include an irregular multilocular-solid mass more than 10 cm in diameter, an irregular solid tumour, more than four papillary structures, ascites, and a high Doppler signal (Figs. 4 and 5). The mass is defined as malignant or benign based on the application of one or more

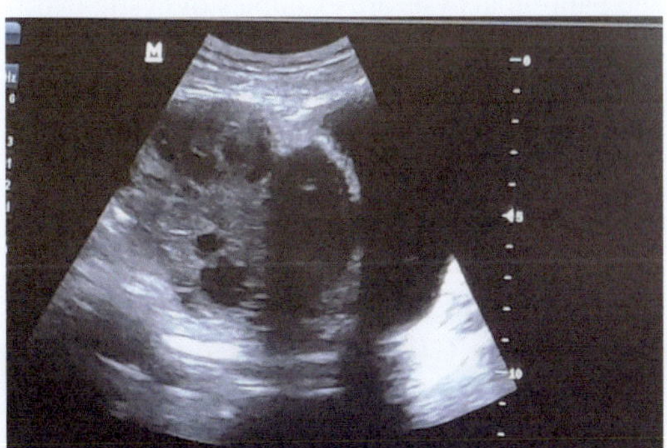

Fig. 4 Irregular multilocular-solid ovarian mass

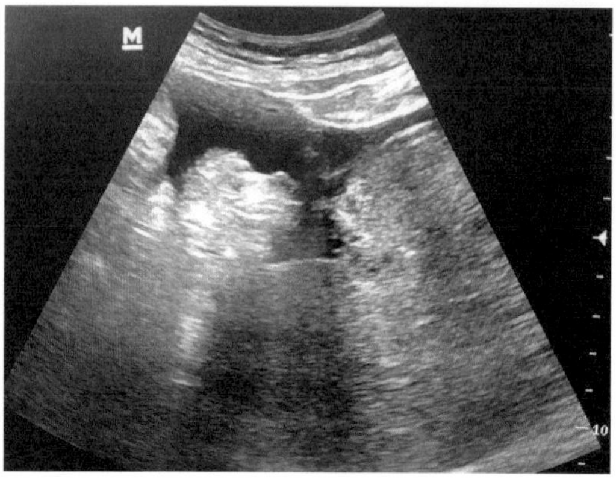

Fig. 5 Irregular solid tumour with presence of ascites

M-rules in the absence of a B-rule, or one or more B-rules in the absence of an M-rule. The mass could not be classified if both M-rules and B-rules apply, or if neither rule applies. For the detection of malignancy in cases where IOTA basic rules were applicable, the sensitivity was 91.66 %, and the specificity was 84.84 % [95].

7.4 Role of MRI, CT, PET-CT

Contrast-enhanced MRI had a sensitivity and specificity of 100% and 94%, respectively, for diagnosing malignancy when utilized to evaluate an ambiguous tumour observed on ultrasound [96]. Although MRI is excellent at predicting whether a mass is benign or malignant, it cannot distinguish between borderline and aggressive cancers. When an ambiguous adnexal lesion is discovered on ultrasonography, an MRI is recommended. Peritoneal inclusion cysts, hydrosalpinx, and para-tubal cysts are examples of cystic extra-ovarian lesions. Dermoid, exophytic uterine and broad ligament fibroids, and ovarian fibrothecomas are solid-appearing adnexal tumours [97].

Although characterization of ovarian/adnexal lesion is best with MRI it fails to detect abdominal metastasis due to prolonged image acquisition times. Therefore, for metastatic workup of ovarian cancer CT scan is utilized to determine the extent of disease specially in the upper abdomen, omental and mesenteric involvement, and intrahepatic liver involvement and retroperitoneal adenopathy. It is the most useful technique for preoperative staging of ovarian carcinoma, with reported accuracy of 70–90% [98]. Many investigators used CT scan for predicting optimal debulking before primary debulking surgery in patients with advanced ovarian cancer. Bristow et al. had reported that peritoneal thickening or implants more than 2 cm, involvement of the spleen, stomach, lesser sac, bowel mesenteric extension more than 2 cm, suprarenal paraaortic lymph nodes enlargement (≥1 cm), and pelvic sidewall involvement with or without hydroureter were the most important predictive factors for suboptimal debulking. They proposed a unique predictive index score (PIS). PIS 4 and above had the highest overall accuracy at 92.7% and identified patients undergoing suboptimal debulking with a sensitivity of 100% [98]. Various other models have been proposed but disagreements remain in literatures on the predictive value of CT findings for suboptimal cytoreduction [99].

PET CT imaging, which have a report of 83–86% sensitivity as well as a specificity of 54–86%, is not routinely indicated for ovarian cancer primary detection. There have been erroneous negative reports with borderline tumours or low-grade and early adenocarcinomas. Hydrosalpinx, endometriosis, and pedunculated fibroids have all been associated to false-positive results [100, 101]. Newer findings show that PETCT can detect lymph node and distant metastasis in ovarian cancer with high accuracy and may, therefore, alter the management to obtain better clinical outcomes. It particularly has a value to detect recurrent disease, mainly in patients with elevated serum CA-125 levels and negative or inconclusive conventional imaging test results. PET-MRI is a newer approach and may be beneficial for tumour staging because MRI has higher soft tissue contrast and no ionizing radiation exposure compared to CT [102].

8 Surgery for Early-Stage Ovarian Cancer

Thorough surgical staging is important in early ovarian cancer in order to establish the correct stage. This also provides a roadmap for subsequent treatment and may obviate the need for cytotoxic chemotherapy in many patients. Also, approximately 30% of the patients who undergo completion surgery are upstaged, with 54% of these finally diagnosed as stage III disease [103, 104].

In patients with a probable ovarian malignancy, a midline abdominal incision is preferred. Minimally invasive approaches are not preferred as there are multiple concerns like limited visibility as compared to open technique, inability to palpate tissue, tumour spillage, and longer operating time. Another concern with minimal invasive method is the possibility of port site metastasis and although this risk is small (1%), it is often a sign of disseminated intra-abdominal disease [105].

During surgery the ovarian tumours should be extracted in its entirety and examined by frozen section. If ovarian cancer is confirmed and the tumour appears to be restricted to the ovaries or pelvis, a detailed surgical staging procedure is performed. Any evident fluid should be sent for cytology, particularly within pelvis. When free fluid is not present, a peritoneal wash with 50–100 mL of saline from the Douglas pouch, paracolic gutter, and beneath the hemidiaphragm should be performed. After that, all of the peritoneal surfaces and viscera are fully investigated. It should be done clockwise from the caecum, right paracolic gutter, ascending colon, liver and gallbladder, right hemidiaphragm, the entrance to the lesser sac, over the transverse colon to the left hemidiaphragm, descending colon to the rectosigmoid colon. The small intestine and its mesentery from the Treitz tendon to the cecum must be examined. If there is no sign of disease, repeated intraperitoneal biopsies from the peritoneum of the Pouch of Douglas, both paracolic gutters, over the bladder, and the intestinal mesenteries must be taken. Either a biopsy or a scraping of the diaphragm should be performed.

Infracolic omentectomy, and a systematic pelvic and para-aortic lymph node dissection is carried out. The contralateral ovary and the uterus in young patients desiring fertility can be preserved in appropriately selected cases of early-stage epithelial invasive and borderline ovarian cancer.

Pelvic and para-aortic lymph nodal dissection is an integral part of the staging system of ovarian cancer. Both the pelvic and at least infrarenal para-aortic lymph nodes should be removed when a systematic lymphadenectomy is performed in patients with early ovarian cancer. Removal of high infrarenal para-aortic lymph nodes is also important considering the lymphatic drainage of the ovaries. The anatomic borders of a pelvic lymph node dissection are laterally, the external iliac artery and the genitofemoral nerve, superiorly, the distal half of common iliac artery, medially, the anterior division of the hypogastric artery and the ureter and deep circumflex iliac vein distally [106, 107].

Fertility Sparing Surgery's Role: As per the 2014 FIGO staging system for stage IA and IC grade 1 and 2 cancer, as well as stage IC1, conservative treatment can be carried out reliably. The safety of fertility sparing surgery in patients with less favourable prognostic factors (grade 3 or stage IC3 disease) has not been established; however, patients should be informed that radical surgery may not always optimize the oncological results, since the poorest survival observed is related to the natural course of the disease, not particularly to the use of a conservative treatment. It could be explored for stage IA clear cell tumours, but it is inappropriate for all histological subtypes in stage II/III disease [108].

Borderline Tumours: Surgical methods used to treat epithelial ovarian cancer are often employed to treat borderline ovarian tumours as well. But some patients may be over-treated as a result of this. The need for systematic lymph node dissection has been a point of contention in recent years. Despite the fact that lymph nodes are involved in 21–29% of cases, recurrence and survival rates for patients with impacted or unaffected lymph nodes are comparable [109, 110]. To rule out the risk of ovarian metastasis from mucinous appendix tumours, appendectomy is no longer generally indicated for mucinous borderline tumours [111]. Fertility-preserving surgery is critical since they occur a decade earlier than epithelial ovarian cancer. As a result, patients should be counselled about the retention of the uterus and at least one ovary, which should be considered an appropriate level of care. According to available statistics, the rate of recurrence after conservative care is around 10–20% against 5% in case of radical approach which is higher in general [112, 113]. In the German AGO ROBOT

(Residual tumour, and fertility preservation in the large cohort research on BOT of the Arbeitsgemeinschaft Gynaekologische Onkologie) study, this greater recurrence rate did not result in a higher mortality rate [114].

9 Advanced Epithelial Ovarian Cancer

The existing standard is primary debulking surgery (PDS) with the goal of optimum cytoreduction followed by paclitaxel and carboplatin-based chemotherapy. An inverse link has been established between residual tumour diameter and patient survival in a number of retrospective and prospective investigations. Patients with no visible residual tumour have a better prognosis than those with the greatest residual mass of less than 0.5 cm, who in turn have a better outcome than those with a residual mass of 0.5–1.5 cm. As a result, an aggressive surgical strategy has been advocated in order to achieve optimal cytoreduction [115].

Total abdominal hysterectomy and bilateral salpingo-oophorectomy, as well as a full omentectomy and resection of any metastatic lesions from the peritoneal surfaces or the intestines, are all part of the cytoreductive operation. Due to pelvic adhesions, a retroperitoneal approach with retrograde hysterectomy is sometimes recommended. The sigmoid colon may be involved in some situations, necessitating resection. Patients with serous malignancies, on the other hand, rarely require a colostomy because serous tumours grow above the peritoneal reflection. If the patient is left with optimum disease at the end of the cytoreduction, this is justified. The disease may spread to the splenic hilum and splenic flexure of the colon on the left, as well as the capsule of liver and hepatic flexure of the colon on the right. In cases when the tumour has spread to the splenic hilum or parenchyma, a splenectomy will be recommended. The disease typically does not spread to the liver or spleen parenchyma, and a plane can be seen between the tumour and these organs. In some circumstances, diaphragmatic stripping and resection have been employed to optimally resect upper abdominal disease (Figs. 6 and 7).

The significance of pelvic and para-aortic lymphadenectomy during debulking surgery for advanced-stage ovarian cancer remains unclear as this procedure does not influence the surgical stage and its therapeutic benefit is uncertain. The current practice in advanced ovarian cancer is to remove enlarged/suspicious lymph nodes as part of tumour debulking (Fig. 8).

It is ambiguous whether the better response is attributable to the surgeon's skill or the tumour's location and nature (Table 1). In practise, bilateral salpingo-oophorectomy and omentectomy alone can achieve optimum cytoreduction in some individuals undergoing hysterectomy. For optimal debulking, bowel resection, peritoneal/diaphragmatic stripping, or enblock resection of

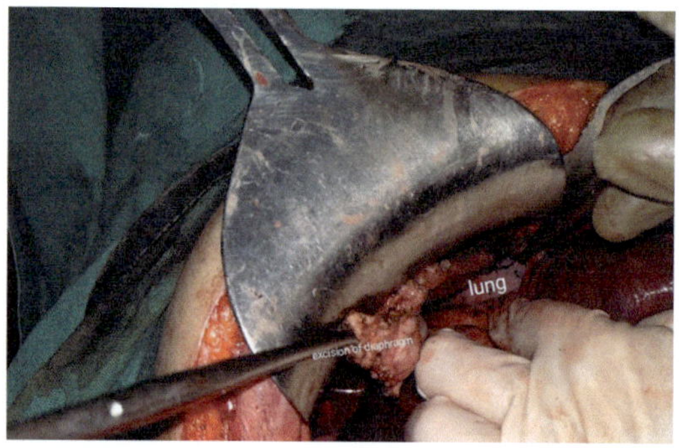

Fig. 6 Resection of diaphragm

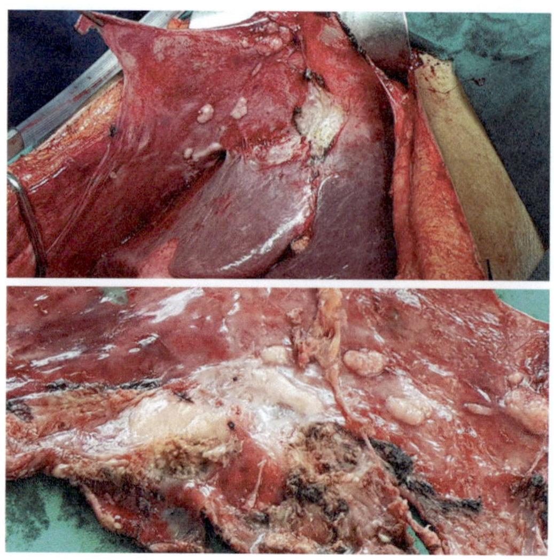

Fig. 7 Diaphragmatic stripping along with stripping of Glisson's capsule of liver

the ovaries, uterus, and sigmoid colon may be required, which may be associated with significant morbidity. Furthermore, some surgeons can undertake aggressive surgery with negligible morbidity in certain patients; however, for many surgeons and patients, morbidity can be significant, with substantial operative complications [116, 117]. This may also cause post-operative chemotherapy to be delayed.

Over the past three decades, the parameters with what constitutes an optimal debulking have evolved, from Griffith et al.'s 2 cm residual disease in 1978 to Gynaecologic Oncology Group's 1 cm residual disease in the last decade to "no visible residual tumour" in latest studies [116, 118]. The vast bulk of the literature by North America and Europe has demonstrated that 15–30% of patients can be debulked (no visible tumour) to microscopic residual disease [117]. As a result, numerous researchers have employed upfront NACT as a substitute for primary surgery in order to improve surgical efficacy.

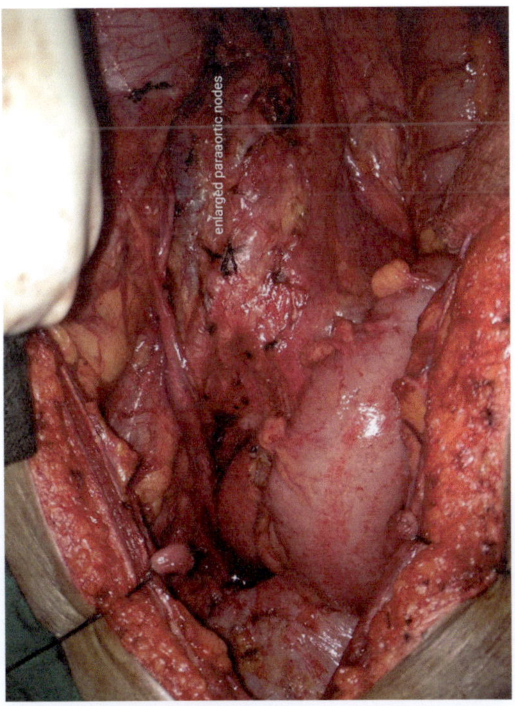

Fig. 8 Enlarged paraaortic nodes

The significance of pelvic and para-aortic lymphadenectomy during debulking surgery for advanced-stage ovarian cancer remains unclear as this procedure does not influence the surgical stage and its therapeutic benefit is uncertain. The German AGO retrospectively reviewed data from three large phase III trials (AGO-OVAR 3, 5, 7) of chemotherapy in advanced epithelial ovarian cancer. They found that in the subgroup of patients with no residual disease and no enlarged lymph nodes, a systematic lymph node dissection was associated with a small statistically significant survival benefit (median OS, 108 months vs. 83 months) [119]. In Lymphadenectomy in Ovarian Neoplasms (LION) trial, 647 patients with advanced ovarian cancer (FIGO IIB-IV) who underwent macroscopically complete debulking and clinically negative pelvic and para-aortic lymph nodes were randomized to systematic pelvic and para-aortic lymphadenectomy versus no lymphadenectomy. The primary endpoint was overall survival. The lymphadenectomy arm showed higher rates of infection, and postoperative mortality, and this did not result in prolonged progression-free or overall survival.

Table 1 Factors affecting optimum debulking rate

Surgical skills	*Experience*	*Training*	*Infrastructure*
Biology	Disease burden (stage IIIC, IV)	Location upper abdomen vs. lower abdomen	Size >5 cm
Poor performance status	Poor nutritional and immunological status	Low serum albumin, anaemia	Delayed presentation
Histopathology	*Subtype*	*Grade*	
Age	Elderly, >70 years (co-morbid conditions, morbid)	Obesity (BMI ≥40)	
Genes			
Other factors	Access to a specialized centre/high volume hospital	Low socio-economic status	

The evaluation showed that in patients with advanced ovarian cancer, systematic lymphadenectomy of clinically negative lymph nodes should be avoided to reduce post-operative morbidity and mortality [120]. In advanced ovarian cancer, enlarged/suspicious lymph nodes are removed as part of the tumour debulking procedure (Fig. 8).

9.1 Upfront Neoadjuvant Chemotherapy (NACT)

This procedure involves three to four cycles of chemotherapy and interval debulking surgery. An optimal cytoreduction (≤1 cm) is reported in 60–94% of patients [117, 119, 120]. Operative morbidity is lowered with this procedure because blood loss is minimized, ICU and post-operative hospitalization are reduced, and post-operative infections have been reduced. Patients treated with the usual strategy, i.e., primary debulking surgery followed by chemotherapy, have a similar overall and progression-free survival rate. Core biopsy of the main tumour or one of the metastatic locations is required prior to NACT treatment and is regarded the gold standard. The use of fine needle aspiration cytology (FNAC) in conjunction with a CA-125/CEA ratio of >25 is also acceptable [88].

Patient's Selection: Poor performance status (ECOG 3-4), old age patients of age above 70 years, significant co-morbid conditions, impacting them with high risk for anaesthesia, massive pleural effusion or large volume ascites, features of sub-acute intestinal obstruction, and those with evidence of liver or splenic, pleural deposits, or distant spread are all criteria used in most studies to select patients for NACT [117, 118]. The strategy of neoadjuvant chemotherapy followed by interval debulking surgery is used when the patient with advanced ovarian cancer is medically unfit for primary cytoreductive surgery or if adequate cytoreduction is not possible. Neoadjuvant chemotherapy has been demonstrated in studies to be non-inferior to initial debulking surgery and to have similar survival outcomes (Table 2).

Randomized trials have shown neoadjuvant chemotherapy is noninferior to primary debulking surgery and have similar survival outcomes (Table 2).

EORTC-GCG (The European Organization for Research and Treatment of Cancer) trial [121]: In this study the largest residual tumour after surgery was less than 1 cm in 80% of patients treated with the neo-adjuvant approach, whereas this was only accomplished in 42% of all patients who underwent up-front debulking. There were fewer complications in the NACT group, as well as a shorter operative time. There was no significant difference in PFS (12 months in both groups) and OS (29/30 months) between the two groups. The study was criticized for its low PFS and OS results and the low rate of optimal debulking. In the primary debulking group 19.4% of all patients were reduced to microscopic disease, whereas the rate was 51.2% for the neo-adjuvant group.

CHORUS trial which also randomized between two groups found no significant difference in OS between the two groups (PFS 10.7 months vs. 12 months, OS 22.6 months vs. 24.1 months) [122]. There were fewer complications in the neo-adjuvant group, and more patients in the neo-adjuvant group had an improvement in global quality of life. Fourteen patients (6%) died in the primary surgery group. Debulking to microscopic disease was accomplished in only 17% of the women who had primary surgery compared with 39% of those who had primary chemotherapy ($p = 0.0001$). In the primary surgery group 27% did not have a bilateral salpingo-oophorectomy, 24% did not have a hysterectomy, and only 20% had upper abdominal surgery. Even though these two trials showed noninferiority of NACT the increased rate of optimal cytoreduction in the NACT arm did not translate into improved over all survival.

Scorpion Trial has been published recently with analysis of peri-operative outcome and survival. They testedPDS versus NACT in patients with Fagotti scores from 8 to 12. Perioperative moderate to severe morbidity were shown to be more favourable in NACT/IDS arm than PDS arm. There was no significant difference in PFS between patients who underwent PDS versus NACT (15 months vs. 14 months). Median OS was 41 months in the PDS arm and not reached in the

Table 2 Upfront surgery vs. neoadjuvant chemotherapy: randomized trials

Country	Europe (Vergote et al.) [121]	UK, NZ (CHORUS trial) [122]	SCORPION (Italy) [123]	Japan (JCOG0602) [124]	India (Kumar L. et al) [125]
Stage	IIIC/IV	IIIC/IV	IIIC/IV	IIIC/IV	IIIC/IVa
Sites	Ovary Fallopian tube Peritoneum	Ovary Fallopian tube Peritoneum	Ovary Fallopian tube Peritoneum	Ovary Fallopian tube Peritoneum	Ovary
Primary end point	Overall survival	Overall survival	Post operative morbidity PFS	Overall survival	Optimum debulking rate Overall survival PFS QOL
Regimen	cDDP/ carbo + Paclitaxel/ docetaxel	Paclitaxel + carboplatin or Carboplatin monotherapy	Paclitaxel + carboplatin ± bevacizumab	Paclitaxel + carboplatin	Paclitaxel + Carboplatin
No. of cycles	6 (NACT-3)	6 (NACT-3)	6 (NACT3-4)	8 (NACT-4)	6 (NACT-3)
No. of patients (PDS/IDS)	336/334	276/274	47/52	149/152	65/63

NACT arm. Seven (8.3%) deaths for post-operative complications were registered in the PDS versus none in the NACT arm. They concluded that NACT was not superior to PDS in terms of PFS for patients endowed with high tumour load receiving maximal surgical effort [123].

The initial findings of the JCOG trial were discussed in the American Society of Clinical Oncology meeting in 2014 and later published in 2016. The NACT arm had a decreased rate of bowel or organ resection, as well as operational morbidity such as blood/ascitic fluid loss and albumin transfusion. When non-inferior survival was verified in the anticipated primary analysis in 2017, the authors stated that neoadjuvant treatment may become the new standard treatment for advanced ovarian cancer [124].

Interim results of a randomized trial in India by L. Kumar et al. had similar findings [125]. Patients in neoadjuvant chemotherapy arm had a higher optimal debulking rate, decreased blood loss during surgery, and reduced postoperative infections (14.8% vs. 2.5%). Median operative time and hospital stay (12 days vs. 9.4 days) were similar in both arms. At a median follow-up of 41 months, the median overall survival and disease-free survival were not different.

9.2 Number of NACT Cycles Before and After IDS

The PRIMOVAR-1 phase II RCT found that whether patients received three or two cycles of NACT had no effect on response rate, interval debulking cytoreduction, PFS, or OS [126]. According to the NCCN Guidelines, three cycles of NACT are recommended before interval debulking, while surgery after 4–6 cycles may be performed based on clinical judgement. Those with stable disease after three cycles of NACT should contemplate surgery, but additional cycles of NACT (up to a total of six cycles) before IDS should be explored. According to the NCCN guidelines, interval debulking should be followed with adjuvant chemotherapy regardless of the number of cycles of NACT received. A minimum of six cycles of treatment, including at least three cycles of adjuvant therapy after IDS, is indicated for all patients who receive NACT with Interval debulking surgery [127].

10 Chemotherapy

10.1 Recommendation for Adjuvant Treatment of Early-Stage Ovarian Cancer

The International Collaborative Ovarian Neoplasm 1 (ICON1)/Adjuvant Chemotherapy in Ovarian Neoplasm trials (ACTION trial) showed an effect on survival of adjuvant chemotherapy in early-stage ovarian cancer, but in patients who underwent adequate surgical staging, there was no additional effect [128, 129]. Based on the findings of the trials the following recommendations are made

Low-risk Early-Stage Disease: For patients with well-differentiated encapsulated unilateral illness (stage IA, grade 1) or those with fully staged IB, well or moderately differentiated (grade 1–2) disease, no adjuvant treatment is advised.

High-risk Early-Stage Disease: Stage IC (Tumour confined to the ovary with positive peritoneal washings) or stage II (tumour involving the pelvis) disease, Clear cell histology (any stage), High tumour grade (grade 3), adjuvant chemotherapy is recommended.

Whenever restaging is not a feasible, chemotherapy should be provided to patients with unstaged early cancer. Most patients receive 3–6 cycles of carboplatin and paclitaxel chemotherapy, while single-agent carboplatin might well be preferable for women with major medical co-morbidities. In selected individuals with clear cell and endometrioid tumours who are at risk for local recurrence, pelvic radiation should be considered.

No. of cycles: In Gynaecologic Oncology Group Trial 157 (GOG 157), 457 women were treated with either three or six courses of paclitaxel (175 mg/m^2) plus carboplatin (area under the curve (AUC) 7.5) given every 3 weeks to 457 women with high-risk early-stage disease [130]. Compared with three cycles, the administration of six cycles was associated with more toxicity (neurotoxicity, granulocytopenia, and anaemia). In a subsequent ad hoc analysis of the same trial, a significantly lower risk of recurrence was seen for six rather than three cycles of chemotherapy in patients with serous tumours but not for other histologic types. Because of the relatively poor prognosis for patients with a clear cell ovarian cancer, clinical trials exploring alternative or novel agents are ongoing. Such agents include temsirolimus with carboplatin and paclitaxel in GOG 268 (as a first-line therapy) and sunitinib in GOG 254 (for the treatment of recurrent disease). It is our practice to give six cycles of paclitaxel and carboplatin (AUC 6) in patients who are fit and with adequate organ functions. For elderly patients (≥70 years) and those with co-morbidities we prefer single agent chemotherapy with carboplatin (AUC 5).

10.2 Advanced-Stage Ovarian Cancer

For patients with advanced disease systemic chemotherapy remains the most important component of management. Phase III data and a meta-analysis established the superiority of intravenous cisplatin (75 mg/m^2) plus paclitaxel (135 mg/m^2) over cisplatin plus cyclophosphamide [131–133]. Subsequently it was also shown in Phase III trials that carboplatin plus paclitaxel was at least as effective as cisplatin plus paclitaxel [134, 135].

GOG 182/ICON5, the world's biggest prospective trial of first-line ovarian cancer chemotherapy, compared four treatment arms of three cytotoxic medicines to three-weekly carboplatin and paclitaxel in 2009. It was found that adding a third medication to three-weekly carboplatin and paclitaxel did not improve PFS and that this combination was the gold standard for intravenous chemotherapy [136]. The AUC (area under the curve) is the best technique to dose carboplatin, with a target AUC of 5–6 for previously untreated patients.

Adjuvant chemotherapy should begin as soon as feasible, usually within 2–4 weeks from surgery. Limited data suggest that a delay of greater than approximately 1 month in instituting chemotherapy may be associated with an inferior outcome [137, 138].

10.3 Intraperitoneal Chemotherapy

For optimal cytoreduction (<1 cm of residual disease) a combination of IV and intraperitoneal (IP) chemotherapy (IV/IP therapy) can also be considered. However, patients with suboptimal cytoreduction (≥1 cm of residual disease) are not candidates for IP therapy due to limited penetration of chemotherapy into larger tumours.

Random findings evaluating standard IV therapy with IV/IP treatment following primary cytoreductive surgery backs up intravenous/intraperitoneal (IV/IP) chemotherapy.

GOG 104, GOG 114, and GOG172 are three notable trials that used a mix of IV and IP chemotherapy and compared it to IV-only chemotherapy control arms [139–141]. Cisplatin (100 mg/m^2) was the most commonly used IP chemotherapy drug, which was given every 3 weeks for 6 cycles. Overall, IP chemotherapy completion rates were lower than IV chemotherapy completion rates, i.e., 42% vs. 83%, respectively. High catheter-related complication rates, as well as severe haematological and gastrointestinal events, were cited for the discrepancy. IP chemotherapy patients had a median progression-free survival of 24–28 months, which was better than IV chemotherapy patients, who had a PFS of 11–22 months. Overall survival was also higher in the IP chemotherapy group, with a median of 49–66 months compared to 41–52 months in the IV group. Amongst all phase 3 GOG trials in advanced ovarian cancer found GOG-172 to have the superior median survival, 65.6 months in the IP group. IP cisplatin with paclitaxel showed a survival benefit after 10 years in the GOG172 long-term follow-up study.

GOG 252 compared intravenous carboplatin and paclitaxel to two IP regimens, the first of which contained IP carboplatin and another IP cisplatin and paclitaxel. IP cisplatin was administered at a dose of 75 mg/m^2, which was lower than the dose used in the earlier trial, GOG 172. In all three arms, bevacizumab was used. There was no difference in PFS between the three treatment arms in this trial [142]. Nevertheless, it was advised that IP chemotherapy could still be used in some patients with no substantial residual disease, but the original GOG-172 dose as well as schedule is to be considered. Furthermore, unlike prior trials, all GOG-252 regimens included bevacizumab, which may have compensated for the effects of intraperitoneal chemotherapy.

There is also a benefit seen in the survival using IP cisplatin in patients with DNA repair deficiency. In a secondary analysis of GOG 172 trial Lesnock et al. determined that aberrant BRCA1 expression improved survival from 47 to 84 months when treated with IP cisplatin [143]. Table 3 summarizes major randomized trials.

10.4 Hyperthermic Intraperitoneal Chemotherapy (HIPEC)

Recently delivering intraperitoneal cisplatin at high temperature (41–43 °C) through special tubing's (HIPEC) have come into practise. This approach results in:

1. Direct damage to cancer cells by impairing DNA repair
2. Enhancement of the cytotoxicity and penetration of chemotherapy
3. Inhibition of angiogenesis
4. Improvement in denaturation of proteins
5. Great tolerance without additional adverse effect
6. Kill the floating tumour cells and prevent them from getting entrapped in the resection sites

Intraoperative intraperitoneal chemotherapy, as opposed to postoperative intraperitoneal therapy, may allow for improved peritoneal perfusion because adhesions have not yet developed. In prospective trials, HIPEC protocols typically perfused chemotherapy for 60–90 min (depending on the dose and drug administered), with the solution heated to a 41–43 °C intraperitoneal temperature.

Metanalyses has shown that combination of CRS and HIPEC enhances the prognosis of ovarian cancer significantly causing not only improved OS but also PFS [144]. However, in recent years, some studies demonstrated that the HIPEC did not show any improvement in OS compared with the therapy without the HIPEC [145, 146]. HIPEC has also shown promising result in patients undergoing interval debulking surgery. Result of M06OVH-OVHIPEC trial showed that among patients with stage III epithelial ovarian cancer, the addition of HIPEC to IDS resulted in longer PFS and OS than surgery alone and did not result in higher rates of side effects [147].

In patients with stage III disease treated with NACT, the NCCN Guidelines now include an option to consider HIPEC at the time of IDS; however, with primary debulking surgery, HIPEC is not recommended based on preliminary results from a randomized clinical study revealing that HIPEC did not improve PFS or OS in a patient population with optimal cytoreduction (less than 1 cm residual) after PDS [127].

Table 3 Randomized trials of IV versus IP chemotherapy in patients with advanced epithelial ovarian cancer

Trial	Year of trial	Arms	Overall survival (months) (IV/IP) months	*P* value
GOG 104 Alberts et al. [139]	1996	IP cisplatin and IV cyclophosphamide *versus* IV cisplatin and cyclophosphamide	41/49	0.03
GOG 114 Markman et al. [140]	2001	IV carboplatin IP cisplatin and IV paclitaxel *versus* IV cisplatin and IV paclitaxel	52/63	0.057
GOG 172 Armstrong et al. [141]	2006	IV paclitaxel IP cisplatin day 2 and IP paclitaxel *versus* IV paclitaxel and IV cisplatin	49.7/65.6	0.03
GOG 252 Walker et al. [142]	2019	IV carboplatin Paclitaxel weekly IV plus bevacizumab *versus* Paclitaxel weekly plus carboplatin IP on day 1 every 21 days for cycles 1–6 Plus bevacizumab *versus* Paclitaxel IV on day 1 Plus cisplatin IP on day 2 Plus, IV on day 8 Every 21 days for cycles 1–6 Plus bevacizumab	98.8/104.8/not reached for IP cisplatin	

10.5 Dose-Dense Therapy

Dose-dense therapy is based on the hypothesis that if the interval between the chemotherapy cycle is reduced, there is a more significant reduction in tumour burden than dose escalation. The primary analysis of the JGOG 3016 trial showed that a dose-dense weekly paclitaxel and 3-weekly carboplatin regimen significantly improved PFS (28 months vs. 17.2 months) and OS (72.1% vs. 65.1% at 3 years) compared with the conventional regimen as first-line chemotherapy for patients with advanced ovarian cancer. The outcomes at a median follow-up period of 76.8 months also showed better survival in the dose-dense group.

The GOG 262 experiment was designed similarly to the JGOG 3016 trial, with the exception that patients could be administer IV bevacizumab 15 mg/kg every 3 weeks in both arms.

In this study there was a significant difference in PFS between the dose-dense and 21-day groups in women not receiving bevacizumab (14.2 months vs. 10.3 months, $p = 0.03$); nonetheless, in women receiving bevacizumab, there was no difference in PFS (14.9 months vs. 14.7 months, $p = 0.60$) [149].

The ICON 8 trial aimed to replicate the JGOG findings in European women. Stage IC–IV epithelial ovarian carcinoma patients were randomly assigned to one of three groups in this phase 3 trial: CarboplatinAUC5/6 and paclitaxel 175 mg/m^2 every 3 weeks in Group 1: Group 3 (carboplatin AUC2 and 80 mg/m^2 paclitaxel weekly): Group 2 (carboplatin AUC5/6 every 3 weeks and 80 mg/m^2 paclitaxel weekly). The results of the primary progression-free survival analysis demonstrated that dose-dense therapy may be provided successfully as first-line therapy, although without a substantial improvement in the PFS [150]. A different regimen of weekly carboplatin (AUC 2 mg/mL/min) and weekly paclitaxel (60 mg/m^2) was compared to carboplatin (AUC 6 mg/mL/min, delivered every 3 weeks) and paclitaxel (175 mg/m^2) in the Italian MITO-7 experiment. The weekly regimen did not increase PFS when compared to the traditional regimen (18.8 months vs. 16.5 months; $p = 0.18$), but it was linked to a higher quality of life and fewer adverse effects [151]. Results of the phase III studies are summarized in Table 4.

Table 4 Phase III trials comparing dose-dense therapy with conventional therapy

Trial	Population	Arms/number	Outcomes (months)	*P* value
JGOG 3016 [148]	Stage II–IV ovarian cancer first line	3 weekly Carboplatin AUC6 Paclitaxel 180 mg/m^2 (319) *versus*	PFS: 17.5 versus 28.2	0.0037
		Weekly Paclitaxel (80 mg/m^2) plus 3 weekly Carboplatin AUC6 (312)	OS: 62 versus 100.2	0.039
GOG 262 [149]	Stage III and IV incompletely resected	3 Weekly Carboplatin AUC5/6 Paclitaxel 175 mg/m^2 (346) *versus*	PFS (Those who did not receive Bevacizumab) 14 versus 14.7	0.18
		Weekly Paclitaxel (80 mg/m^2) plus 3 weekly Carboplatin AUC5/6 (346) 84% patients opted to receive bevacizumab in both arms	10.3 versus 14.2 (In patients receiving Bevacizumab)	0.03
ICON 8 [150]	Stage IC–IV first line	Group 1: 3 Weekly Carboplatin AUC5/6 Paclitaxel 175 mg/m^2 (522) *versus*	PFS 17.7 versus	*P* value
		Group 2: Weekly Paclitaxel (80 mg/m^2) plus 3 weekly Carboplatin AUC5/6 (523)	20.8 versus	Group 2 versus group 1:0.35
		Group 3: weekly Carboplatin AUC 2 and Paclitaxel (80 mg/m^2)	21	Group 3 versus group 1 1:0.51
MITO 7 [151]	Stage IC–IV first line	3 Weekly Carboplatin AUC 6 Paclitaxel 175 mg/m^2 versus weekly Paclitaxel (60 mg/m^2) plus 3 weekly Carboplatin	17.3 versus 18.3	0.66

11 Molecular Targeted Therapies

Anti-VEGF (Vascular Endothelial Growth Factor) monoclonal antibodies and PARP (poly-ADP-ribose polymerase) inhibitors are presently approved and are the most effective targeted drugs for epithelial ovarian cancer.

Bevacizumab is a monoclonal antibody against vascular endothelial growth factor-A that is increasingly routinely utilized (VEGF-A). GOG 218 and ICON 7 are two large Phase III randomized trials that looked into its role in the first-line setting. The GOG 218 trial comprised patients with stage III–IV ovarian cancer in three arms [152, 153]. The arms were 21-day cycles of IV carboplatin (AUC 6) and paclitaxel (175 mg/m^2) versus chemotherapy plus concurrent and maintenance bevacizumab (15 mg/kg, cycles 2–6) versus chemotherapy plus concurrent and maintenance bevacizumab (15 mg/kg, cycles 2–6) versus chemotherapy plus concurrent and maintenance bevacizumab (cycles 2–22). Macroscopic residual disease was required in patients with stage III illness. The median PFS in the control group was 12 months, whereas 18 months in the bevacizumab maintenance group after a median follow-up of 17.4 months. However, after a median follow-up of 102.9 months, no significant differences in disease-specific survival were observed among the groups. No survival benefit in the bevacizumab groups was observed after censoring patients who received bevacizumab at crossover or as second-line treatment [152, 153].

The ICON7 study, which involved patients with high-risk stage I, II, and III, IV ovarian cancer, had a similar approach. They were given either six cycles of chemotherapy alone or six cycles of chemotherapy with bevacizumab (7.5 mg/kg), followed by 12 cycles of bevacizumab maintenance every 3 weeks. The median PFS was 17.3 months in the control group versus 19 months in the bevacizumab group after a median follow-up of 19.4 months.

Long term follow-up at 48·9 months showed no overall survival benefit in both arms (44.6 months in chemotherapy versus 45.5 months in bevacizumab group). However, when a subgroup analysis of 502 patients with poor prognosis (stage III with >1 cm residual and stage IV) was made there was a significant difference in overall survival between women who received bevacizumab plus chemotherapy and those who received chemotherapy alone (39.3 months vs. 34.5 months). However, in non-high-risk patients, the mean survival time did not differ significantly between the two treatment groups with 49.7 months in the standard chemotherapy group vs. 48.4 month in the bevacizumab group [154].

Gastrointestinal perforation, surgery and wound-healing complications, and haemorrhage has been reported with the use of bevacizumab. Additional serious and sometimes fatal adverse effects include gastrointestinal fistulae, non-gastrointestinal fistulae, arterial thromboembolic events, proteinuria, venous thromboembolism, hypertension, and posterior reversible encephalopathy syndrome. Pain, hoarseness, and marrow suppression have also been documented [155].

PARP inhibitors hinder the enzyme poly-ADP ribose polymerase from repairing DNA single-strand breaks. They have been proven to considerably increase survival in patients with BRCA gene mutations. The medications are based on the idea that cells with a BRCA mutation have difficulties repairing DNA double-strand breaks through homologous DNA recombination (HR) and must rely on PARP activation to repair DNA damage. Synthetic lethality occurs when PARP inhibition causes cell death in these cells. Due to mutations in other HR repair genes or suppression of BRCA function due to DNA methylation, it is predicted that 30–50% of high-grade serous tumours are sensitive to PARP inhibitors [157].

PARP inhibitors were first developed as an upkeep therapy for patients who had a complete or partial response to platinum-based chemotherapy for recurrent disease and wanted to stay on it. Olaparib was approved by the FDA in December 2014 as a monotherapy for the treatment of ovarian cancer in patients with a germline BRCA mutation who have had at least three chemotherapy lines, based on promising evidence from a nonrandomized single-arm phase II trial [156].

Randomized phase III trial (SOLO3) was started to methodically assess the efficacy and safety of olaparib monotherapy compared with standard chemotherapy in the same population of patients; however, results are still pending. Recently, the phase III SOLO2/ENGOT Ov21 study evaluated olaparib as maintenance therapy in platinum-sensitive, relapsed ovarian cancer patients with a BRCA 1/2 mutation who received at least two lines of previous chemotherapy. Maintenance therapy with Olaparib (300 mg BD) significantly improved PFS when compared to placebo (19.1 months vs. 5.5 months). In view of these results, in August 2017, Olaparib was FDA-approved as maintenance treatment with recurrence in ovarian cancer following a complete or partial response to platinum-based chemotherapy, irrespective of BRCA status [158].

SOLO-1, PAOLA-1/ENGOT-OV25, PRIMA/ENGOT-OV26, and VELIA/GOG-3005159 are four phase III trials testing PARP inhibitors in the front-line situation. Olaparib demonstrated a significant improvement in PFS in the SOLO-1 trial. The median PFS for placebo was 13.8 months, while the median PFS for Olaparib has yet to be determined after a median follow-up of 41 months, and OS data are incomplete. Serious side effects were more common in the Olaparib group (21% vs. 12%), leading to treatment cessation in some patients [159, 160]. PARP inhibitors such as Olaparib, Niraparib, or Rucaparib now show a considerably broader spectrum of efficacy in high-grade tumours, which is broadly connected with "platinum-sensitivity". Olaparib and bevacizumab can be combined, according to phase I data, while it is unclear whether the two medications are additive.

PAOLA-1/ENGOT-OV25 is the first phase III trial to evaluate the efficacy and safety of a PARP inhibitor with bevacizumab as maintenance first-line therapy for advanced ovarian cancer, regardless of BRCA mutation status. PFS after follow-up of 22.7 months was significantly improved in the Olaparib arm whereas PFS of the other arm is immature [161]. Similar results were demonstrated for niraparib and veliparib in patients with newly diagnosed advanced ovarian cancer who responded to platinum-based chemotherapy in PRIMA/ENGOT-OV26/GOG-3012 and VELIA/GOG-3005 trial, respectively [162, 163].

Patients with stage II–IV disease with germline or somatic BRCA mutations who are in total or partial response after finishing primary treatment with surgery and chemotherapy should consider Olaparib as a maintenance therapy option, according to the NCCN. Maintenance Olaparib, on the other hand, is not suggested for patients who are on primary treatment and have progressive or stable disease [127].

12 Recurrent Ovarian Cancer

Despite optimal cytoreduction with aggressive surgery followed by chemotherapy majority (70%) of patients have recurrence within 2 years of treatment completion [164]. Around 50% of the recurrences occur at more than a year from the end of the first-line therapy and 25% of all recurrences occur at less than 6 months.

For the appropriate selection of a chemotherapeutic regimen at first relapse, patients are categorized according to treatment free interval (TFI) from last chemotherapy; patients with ≥12 months TFI have platinum sensitive disease, those with TFI <6 months have platinum resistant disease and are advised non platinum drugs as salvage therapy. Patients with TFI of 6–12 months have intermediate platinum sensitivity. Platinum based salvage therapy is used for these patients with TFI of >6 months. Patients, with disease progression while on therapy or less than 3 months platinum free interval, are defined as refractory disease.

13 Treatment Assessment

After completion of treatment, patients are re-evaluated every 2–4 months for first 2 years, then 3–6 months for the next 3 years followed by annual examination after 5 years. CA 125 levels can be used to monitor relapse if the levels were elevated prior to treatment. On each visit a complete physical examination including pelvic examination is done along with imaging as required. Increasing levels of CA-125 precede the signs and symptoms of recurrence by

3–5 months. In a study by Rustin et al. patients presumed to be in complete remission after primary therapy had CA-125 determinations every 3 months, but were blinded to the results [165]. When CA-125 values doubled outside the normal range, patients were randomized to have or not to have their physicians informed of the rising value. On final analysis there was no difference in overall survival nor any improvement found in quality of life by earlier treatment of recurrent disease. Thus, treatment based on rising CA-125 levels alone without evidence of recurrent disease clinically or on imaging does not lead to improved survival.

14 Secondary Cytoreductive Surgery for Recurrent Disease

Theoretically, surgery at the time of recurrence is beneficial because it reduces tumour burden and removes cancer with a low blood supply, increasing the efficacy of subsequent treatment. Although this strategy appears to be rational, published research has yielded inconsistent results.

The German/Swiss DESKTOP I trial enrolled patients with recurrent ovarian cancer who had secondary cytoreductive surgery and found that patients with carcinomatosis had a 19.9 months median survival versus 45.3 months for patients without disseminated disease [166]. In this trial, a score, the AGO score was developed to predict optimal cytoreduction in this recurrent patient group: good performance status (ECOG ≤ 1), complete debulking at first surgery, and less than 500 cc of ascites. The score was then tested in the DESKTOP II prospectively and 76% of the patients who fulfilled all three criteria had an optimal debulking to no residual disease [167].

The DESKTOP III trial, the GOG 213 trial, and the SOCceR trial randomized patients with potentially resectable platinum sensitive disease to secondary cytoreduction or no surgery. In the DESKTOP III trial, 407 patients with recurrent ovarian cancer and a first relapse after a 6-month or longer platinum-free interval were randomized between 2010 and 2014 to surgery (n = 206), followed by a chemotherapy, or immediate initiation of chemotherapy (n = 201). In both arms it was strongly recommended that chemotherapy consist of platinum-based combination therapy. Median OS was 53.7 months with and 46.0 months without surgery whereas median PFS was 18.4 months with surgery and 14.0 months without [168]. The survival benefit was highest and exclusively seen in the cohort with complete resection which indicated the importance of thorough patient selection process for secondary cytoreduction.

The GOG-213 trial had two main objectives: (1) to see if adding bevacizumab to paclitaxel and carboplatin treatment, as well as maintenance therapy, improved survival, and (2) to see if subsequent cytoreduction followed by chemotherapy improved survival.

Complete cytoreduction was achieved in 67% of the patients assigned to surgery. Platinum based chemotherapy with bevacizumab followed by bevacizumab maintenance was administered to 84% of the patients and was equally distributed between two groups. Comparison of the complete cytoreduction subpopulation (150 patients) with the no surgery group (245 patients) did not show a benefit with respect to overall survival (median OS, 56.0 months and 64.7 months, respectively), though there was a benefit with respect to progression-free survival (PFS 22.4 months and 16.2 months). The results of the trial revealed that secondary surgical cytoreduction followed by chemotherapy did not result in longer overall survival than chemotherapy alone [169].

It can be briefly said that the benefit of secondary cytoreduction is seen in properly selected patients.

In nearly all studies, patients with longer treatment-free intervals, isolated tumours, and those without ascites or carcinomatosis appear to benefit the most.

15 Chemotherapy for Recurrent Ovarian Cancer

15.1 Platinum-Sensitive Disease

Platinum sensitive patients are more likely to respond to retreatment with a chemotherapy regimen that contains a platinum agent. Combination chemotherapy is preferred to single-agent chemotherapy, as it is associated with better progression-free survival [170–172]. In parallel phase III trials ICON-4 and AGO-OVAR-2.2, women with platinum-sensitive ovarian cancer were randomized to platinum-based chemotherapy carboplatin alone; or cisplatin, doxorubicin and cyclophosphamide (CAP) with or without paclitaxel.

In both trials, a considerable number of patients had not previously received paclitaxel. When the studies were combined for analysis, it was discovered that the paclitaxel-containing medication had a considerable survival advantage. The absolute 2-year survival advantage was 7% with a 5-month improvement in median survival (29 months vs. 24 months), with a median follow-up of 42 months [173].

A phase III study conducted by the Gynaecologic Cancer Intergroup (GCIG) randomly assigned treatment with 21-day cycles of carboplatin alone or carboplatin plus gemcitabine. Compared with single-agent carboplatin, combined therapy resulted in an improved PFS (8.6 months vs. 5.8 months), although OS was not improved (18 months vs. 17.3 months, respectively). Patients receiving gemcitabine experienced an increase in serious (grade 3/4) hematologic toxicity and required granulocyte colony stimulating factors (G-CSF) more frequently (24% vs. 10%) [174].

Carboplatin and liposomal doxorubicin were compared to carboplatin and paclitaxel in a large GCIG trial (CALYPSO trial). A total of about 1000 patients were registered. For a median follow-up of 22 months, the PFS for the carboplatin and liposomal doxorubicin arm was statistically superior to the carboplatin and paclitaxel arm (11.3 months vs. 9.4 months, respectively). This trial showed that carboplatin with liposomal doxorubicin had a better PFS and therapeutic index than carboplatin and paclitaxel, and this regimen is now frequently used [175].

A subset of women may not be candidates for retreatment with platinum agents either due to a history of a hypersensitivity reaction or persistent toxicities from first-line therapy. Oral Etoposide, Topotecan, Pegylated liposomal doxorubicin, Gemcitabine, nab-paclitaxel, Trabectedin can be used in such situation.

15.2 Platinum-Resistant and Refractory Disease

Platinum-resistant and refractory disease carry the worst prognosis compared with platinum-sensitive disease. Chemotherapy options are non-platinum monotherapy with paclitaxel, docetaxel, pegylated liposomal doxorubicin (PLD), topotecan and gemcitabine. Overall response rates range from 10 to 35% in phase II studies with relatively short-lived responses of less than 8 months [176].

Sequential single-agent salvage chemotherapy is considered superior to multiagent chemotherapy as multiagent regimens increase toxicity without clear benefit. However, no preferred sequence of single agents is recommended. The choice of agent should be individualized depending on the history of prior treatment, residual toxicities, patient preferences in terms of toxicity and the availability, cost and convenience of treatments. Consideration should be given to adding molecular targeted therapy to chemotherapy in select patients. The patient should however be counselled regarding the lack of proven survival benefit, added toxicities and practical concerns such as potential cost.

15.3 Targeted Therapy in Recurrent Setting

The randomized Phase III OCEANS Trial [177] found bevacizumab to be effective in treating patients with platinum-sensitive recurrence.

Patients with detectable illness and a recurrence within 6 months of receiving first-line platinum-based therapy were randomized to carboplatin and gemcitabine plus either bevacizumab or placebo for 6–10 cycles. The treatment with bevacizumab or a placebo was then administered until the disease progressed. The PFS for the bevacizumab arm was significantly better than the placebo arm (12.4 months in the bevacizumab arm compared to 8.4 months in the placebo arm). The outcomes of this trial support the use of bevacizumab in selected patients with platinum-sensitive recurrent ovarian cancer, despite the lack of evidence on overall survival.

Another Multicenter Phase III Randomized Trial including second line chemotherapy either with or without bevacizumab in patients with platinum sensitive ovarian cancer previously treated with bevacizumab is the MITO16/MaNGO-OV2B study. The attending physicians gave carboplatin-based chemotherapy with either doxorubicin, gemcitabine, or paclitaxel to the patients in the control arm. The median PFS was 8.8 months in the chemotherapy-only group and 11.8 months in the bevacizumab-combination chemotherapy group after a median follow-up time of 20.3 months. In recurrent patients already treated with bevacizumab, they observed that rechallenge with platinum-based chemotherapy plus bevacizumab is a therapeutic option. Patients who received paclitaxel and carboplatin treatment in combination with bevacizumab had the longest PFS [178].

There have been research in the platinum resistant setting as well. AURELIA is a randomized trial in which women with platinum-resistant recurrent ovarian cancer were randomly assigned to receive monthly pegylated doxorubicin, weekly topotecan, or weekly paclitaxel with or without bevacizumab [179]. The PFS of the women in the experimental group was much longer (6.7 months vs. 3.4 months). Overall survival did not differ between the groups, which could be due to the fact that patients who did not receive bevacizumab initially could receive it during relapse. The weekly paclitaxel group had a highly significant overall survival improvement in subgroup analysis. This study backs the use of bevacizumab in combination with chemotherapy in patients with platinum-resistant ovarian cancer.

JGOG3023 study is an ongoing open-labelled, parallel-arm, randomized, phase II trial aimed to assess the efficacy and safety of chemotherapy with or without bevacizumab in patients with platinum-resistant recurrent epithelial ovarian cancer who were previously treated with bevacizumab for front-line or platinum-sensitive ovarian cancer.

In the recurrent situation, PARP inhibitors have been thoroughly investigated. The significant improvement in PFS seen in three randomized phase III trials—NOVA/ENGOT-OV16, SOLO-2/ENGOT-OV21, and ARIEL3—led to regulatory approval of niraparib, olaparib, and rucaparib as maintenance therapy for platinum-sensitive recurrent ovarian cancer, regardless of biomarker status [159, 180, 181].

PARP inhibitors have been reported as a viable treatment option in patients of platinum resistant ovarian cancer with germline BRCA mutation carriers [182]. However, in the recurrent setting, platinum sensitivity is the most reliable marker for sensitivity to PARP inhibitors. The Phase III trials on PARP inhibitors, usage and toxicity have been summarized in Tables 5, 6, and 7.

16 Hormonal Therapy

The role of hormone therapy in the treatment of ovarian cancer is not clear. Drugs that are potentially effective include anastrozole, letrozole, leuprorelin acetate, megestrol acetate and tamoxifen. However, information on the efficacy of these drugs for recurrent ovarian cancer come from phase II studies or retrospective studies, and the evidence level is not very high.

Table 5 Comparisons of phase III trials involving PARP inhibitors

Drug/phase	Population	Setting	Results
Olaparib maintenance Phase 3 Moore et al. (2018) (SOLO1) [160]	BRCA1, BRCA2 mutated	In first line post CR or PR to therapy	60% vs. 27% ($P < 0.001$)
PAOLA-1/ENGOT-OV25 [161] Phase III, Olaparib tablet with bevacizumab as first-line maintenance	Advanced (IIIA-IV) HG serous or endometrioid ovarian, fallopian tube, or peritoneal cancer.	CR or PR following first-line platinum based plus bevacizumab	PFS (on-going)
PRIMA/ENGOT-OV26 [162] Phase III, Niraparib tablet	Advanced HG serous or endometrioid ovarian, fallopian tube, or peritoneal cancer	CR or PR to first-line platinum based CT	mPFS 13.8% vs. 8.2% ($P < 0.0001$) HR 0.62
VELIA/GOG-3005 Phase III [163]	HG serous carcinoma of ovarian, fallopian tube, or primary peritoneal origin.	Arm 1: CP + PL then PL maintenance Arm 2: CP + V then PL maintenance Arm 3: CP + V then V maintenance	mPFS 20.5% vs. 23.5% vs. 17.3 %
Olaparib tablet Phase 3 Pujade-Lauraine (2017) (SOLO2) [158]	High-grade serous ovarian cancer with a BRCA1 or BRCA2 mutation	Platinum sensitive relapse	Median PFS was significantly longer with olaparib than with placebo: 19.1 months vs. 5.5 months
Niraparib maintenance Phase 3 Mirza (2016) [180]	Patients characterized as per germline BRCA and absent germline BRCA	Platinum-sensitive, recurrent ovarian cancer	21.0 months vs. 5.5 months in patients with gBRCA 12.9 months vs. 3.8 months in patients with non-gBRCA
Rucaparib maintenance Phase 3 Coleman (2017) (ARIEL3) [181]	Stratified as per BRCA and HRD presence or absence	Platinum-sensitive, recurrent, high-grade ovarian cancer	Patients with BRCA-mutant carcinoma: 16.6 vs. 5.4 months Patients with HRD carcinoma: 13.6 vs. 5.4 months The intention-to-treat population: 10.8 months vs. 5.4 months

Table 6 Common toxicities of PARP inhibitors

Drug	Olaparib	Rucaparib	Niraparib
Common side effects	Nausea (58–76%) Fatigue (29–66%) Vomiting (30–37%) Diarrhoea (21–33%) Dysgeusia (27%) Headache (20–25%)	Nausea 75%) Fatigue (69%) Vomiting (37%) Diarrhoea (32%) Dysgeusia (39%) LFT elevation (34%)	Nausea (74%) Fatigue (59%) LFT elevation (36%) Vomiting (34%) Headache (26%) Insomnia (24%) Hypertension (19%)
Grade 3 toxicities (CTCAE v5)	Anaemia (16–19%), neutropenia (5–9%)	Anaemia (19%), neutropenia (7%)	Thrombocytopenia (34%), anaemia (25%), neutropenia (20%)

Table 7 Current approval status of PARP inhibitors

Olaparib	Niraparib	Rucaparib
First-line maintenance therapy for *BRCA*-mutated advanced ovarian cancer		
Maintenance therapy for recurrent ovarian cancer regardless of *BRCA* mutation status	Maintenance therapy for recurrent ovarian cancer regardless of *BRCA* mutation status	Maintenance therapy for recurrent ovarian cancer regardless of *BRCA* mutation status
Fourth-line and beyond treatment for advanced ovarian cancer with germline *BRCA* mutations		Third-line and beyond treatment for advanced ovarian cancer with *BRCA* mutations

17 Summary

The current management of advanced EOC necessitates a multidisciplinary team approach, with the decision to proceed with surgery or chemotherapy depending on a comprehensive examination of clinical symptoms, imaging, pathology, and surgical skill availability. Individualization of therapy through the development of genomics-based data: Primary debulking surgery versus neoadjuvant chemotherapy is a contentious issue right now, and it is likely to become a reality in the near future.

Targeted drugs, which are said to have superior efficacy and less toxicity, are the future of ovarian cancer treatment. Folate receptors is one such promising option. Although folate receptor (FR) is not expressed in normal ovarian tissue, it is present in about 70% of primary epithelial ovarian malignancies and 80% of recurrent epithelial ovarian cancers [183].

The preliminary clinical evaluations of the first folate receptor-targeting agents farletuzumab and vintafolide provided critical evidence for FRα as a target for cancer treatment. However, neither demonstrated meaningful efficacy over chemotherapy alone when evaluated as part of combination regimens in advanced-stage, recurrent epithelial ovarian cancer in Phase III trials. In contrast, mirvetuximab soravtansine (IMGN853) which is an antibody drug conjugate has shown encouraging evidence of clinical activity in platinum-resistant disease, resulting in the initiation of Phase III monotherapy trial in this patient population (FORWARD I) [184]. Immunotherapy, CAR T cell therapy targeting mesothelin, another molecule expressed on ovarian cancer cells and vaccines are areas of active experimental evaluation and research. The future may see further characterization of therapy tailored to ovarian cancer histology and genetic makeup of the tumours. Thus, as we continue to understand and comprehend the complex biology of this disease, our approach will increase in precision and specificity in the management of ovarian cancer.

References

1. National Cancer Institute. Ovarian Cancer—Cancer Stat Facts (Internet). p. 1. seer.cancer.gov. 2018 [cited 2020 Aug 30]. Available from: https://seer.cancer.gov/statfacts/html/ovary.html
2. Sung H, Ferlay J, Siegel RL, Laversanne M, Soerjomataram I, Jemal A, Bray F. Global cancer statistics 2020: GLOBOCAN estimates of incidence and mortality worldwide for 36 cancers in 185 countries. CA Cancer J Clin. 2021;71(3):209–49.
3. Zhang Y, Luo G, Li M, Guo P, Xiao Y, Ji H, et al. Global patterns and trends in ovarian cancer incidence: age, period and birth cohort analysis. BMC Cancer. 2019;19(1):1–14.
4. National Cancer Registry Programme. Comparison of cancer incidence and patterns of all population based cancer registries. In: Three-year report of population based cancer registries 2012-2014. Bengaluru: Indian Council of Medical Research; 2016. p. 70–90.
5. Kotsopoulos J, Gronwald J, Karlan B, Rosen B, Huzarski T, Moller P, et al. Age-specific ovarian cancer risks among women with a BRCA1 or BRCA2 mutation. Gynecol Oncol. 2018;150(1):85–91.
6. Gates MA, Rosner BA, Hecht JL, Tworoger SS. Risk factors for epithelial ovarian cancer by histologic subtype. Am J Epidemiol. 2010;171(1):45–53.
7. Boyd. Specific keynote: hereditary ovarian cancer: what we know. Gynecol Oncol. 2003;88(1):s8–10.
8. Alsop K, Fereday S, Meldrum C, deFazio A, Catherine Emmanuel J, et al. BRCA mutation frequency and patterns of treatment response in BRCA

mutation-positive women with ovarian cancer: a report from the Australian Ovarian Cancer Study Group. J Clin Oncol. 2012;30(21):2654–63.

9. Hanley GE, McAlpine JN, Miller D, Huntsman D, Schrader KA, Blake Gilks C, et al. A population-based analysis of germline BRCA1 and BRCA2 testing among ovarian cancer patients in an era of histotype-specific approaches to ovarian cancer prevention. BMC Cancer. 2018;18(1):254.
10. Ricker C. From families syndromes to genes... the first clinical and genetic characterizations of hereditary syndromes predisposing to cancer: what was the beginning? Rev Méd Clín Las Condes. 2017;28(4):482–90.
11. Levy-Lahad E, Catane R, Eisenberg S, Kaufman B, Hornreich G, Lishinsky E, et al. Founder BRCA1 and BRCA2 mutations in Ashkenazi Jews in Israel: frequency and differential penetrance in ovarian cancer and in breast- ovarian cancer families. Am J Hum Genet. 1997;60(5):1059–67.
12. Scully R. Role of BRCA gene dysfunction in breast and ovarian cancer predisposition. Breast Cancer Res. 2000;2:324–30.
13. Collins N, McManus R, Wooster R, Mangion J, Seal S, Lakhani SR, et al. Consistent loss of the wild type allele in breast cancers from a family linked to the BRCA2 gene on chromosome 13q12-13. Oncogene. 1995;10(8):1673–5.
14. Nielsen FC, Van Overeem HT, Sørensen CS. Hereditary breast and ovarian cancer: new genes in confined pathways. Nat Rev Cancer. 2016;16(9):599–612.
15. Lakhani SR, Manek S, Penault-Llorca F, Flanagan A, Arnout L, Merrett S, et al. Pathology of ovarian cancers in BRCA1 and BRCA2 carriers. Clin Cancer Res. 2004;10(7):2473–81.
16. Jong M A-d, de Bock GH, van Asperen CJ, Mourits MJE, de Hullu JA, Kets CM. Germline BRCA1/2 mutation testing is indicated in every patient with epithelial ovarian cancer: a systematic review. Eur J Cancer. 2016;61:137–45.
17. Safra T, Ori Rogowski FMM. The effect of germ-line BRCA mutations on response to chemotherapy and outcome of recurrent ovarian cancer. Int J Gynecol Cancer. 2014;24(3):488–95.
18. Kim SI, Lee M, Kim HS, Chung HH, Kim JW, Park NH, et al. Effect of BRCA mutational status on survival outcome in advanced-stage high-grade serous ovarian cancer. J Ovarian Res. 2019;12(1):40.
19. Candido-dos-Reis FJ, Song H, Goode EL, Cunningham JM, Fridley BL, Larson MC, et al. Germline mutation in BRCA1 or BRCA2 and ten-year survival for women diagnosed with epithelial ovarian cancer. Clin Cancer Res. 2015;21(3):652–7.
20. King MC, Marks JHMJ. Breast and ovarian cancer risks due to inherited mutations in BRCA1 and BRCA2. Science. 2003;302(5645):643–6.
21. Antoniou A, Pharoah PDP, Narod S, Risch HA, Eyfjord JE, Hopper JL, et al. Average risks of breast and ovarian cancer associated with BRCA1 or BRCA2 mutations detected in case series unselected for family history: a combined analysis of 22 studies. Am J Hum Genet. 2003;72(5):1117–30.
22. Walsh S. The pathology of Lynch syndrome. Diagnostic Histopathol (Internet). 2015;21(4):161–4. https://doi.org/10.1016/j.mpdhp.2015.04.007.
23. Wang Y, Wang Y, Li J, Cragun J, Hatch K, Chambers SK, et al. Lynch syndrome related endometrial cancer: clinical significance beyond the endometrium equal contributors. J Hematol Oncol. 2013;6:22.
24. Burgess BT, JK. Defective DNA repair in hereditary ovarian cancers: implications for therapy. Am J Heal Pharm. 2018;75:e698–708.
25. Lancaster JM, Powell CB, Chen LM, Richardson DL. Society of gynecologic oncology statement on risk assessment for inherited gynecologic cancer predispositions. Gynecol Oncol. 2015;136:3–7.
26. Lynch HT, Snyder CL, Shaw TG, Heinen CD, Hitchins MP. Milestones of Lynch syndrome: 1895-2015. Nat Rev Cancer. 2015;15(3):181–94.
27. Rosenthal AN, Fraser LSM, Philpott S, Manchanda R, Burnell M, Badman P, et al. Evidence of stage shift in women diagnosed with ovarian cancer during Phase II of the United Kingdom Familial Ovarian Cancer Screening Study. J Clin Oncol. 2017;35:1411–20.
28. Jacobs IJ, Menon U, Ryan A, Gentry-Maharaj A, Burnell M, Kalsi JK, et al. Ovarian cancer screening and mortality in the UK Collaborative Trial of Ovarian Cancer Screening (UKCTOCS): a randomised controlled trial. Lancet. 2016;387(10022):945–56.
29. Kurman RJ, Shih IM. The origin and pathogenesis of epithelial ovarian cancer: a proposed unifying theory. Am J Surg Pathol. 2010;34(3):433–43.
30. Rebbeck TR, Lynch HT, Neuhausen SL, Narod SA, Van't Veer L, Garber JE, et al. Prophylactic oophorectomy in carriers of *BRCA1* or *BRCA2* mutations. N Engl J Med. 2002;346(21):1616–22.
31. Statement SC. Society of Gynecologic Oncologists Clinical Practice Committee Statement on Prophylactic Salpingo-oophorectomy. Gynecol Oncol. 2005;98:179–81.
32. Guidelines N. NCCN guidelines for risk management for women with BRCA mutations (Internet) [cited 2020 Sep 1]. Available from:https://www.facingourrisk.org/understanding-brca-and-hboc/information/riskmanagement/introduction/basics/nccn_guidelines_for_women_with_brca.php
33. Gupta S, Ahnen DJ, Chen L-M, Chung DC, Cooper G, Early DS, et al. NCCN Guidelines Version 3.2019 genetic/familial high-risk assessment: colorectal. NCCN; 2019.
34. Committee on Practice Bulletins—Gynecology and the Society of Gynecologic Oncology. ACOG Practice Bulletin No. 147: Lynch syndrome. Obstet Gynecol. 2014;124(5):1042–54.
35. World Health Organization, International Agency for Research on Cancer (IARC), WHO Classification of Tumours Editorial Board. WHO classification

of tumours: female genital tumours, vol. 4. 5th ed. Lyon: IARC; 2020.
36. Seidman JD, Horkayne-Szakaly I, Haiba M, Boice CR, Kurman RJ, Ronnett BM. The histologic type and stage distribution of ovarian carcinomas of surface epithelial origin. Int J Gynecol Pathol. 2004;23(1):41–4.
37. Seidman JD, Kurman RJ, Ronnett BM. Primary and metastatic mucinous adenocarcinomas in the ovaries. Am J Surg Pathol. 2003;27(7):985–93.
38. Prat J. Subclassification of ovarian cancer based on pathology and genetics. Eur J Cancer. 2009;45(Suppl. 1):427–8.
39. Kurman RJ, Shih IM. Pathogenesis of ovarian cancer: lessons from morphology and molecular biology and their clinical implications. Int J Gynecol Pathol. 2008;27(2):151–60.
40. Nezhat FR, Apostol R, Nezhat C, Pejovic T. New insights in the pathophysiology of ovarian cancer and implications for screening and prevention. Am J Obstet Gynecol. 2015;213(3):262–7.
41. Fathalla MF. Incessant ovulation—a factor in ovarian neoplasia? Lancet. 1971;2(7716):163.
42. Piek JMJ, Van Diest PJ, Zweemer RP, Jansen JW, Poort-Keesom RJJ, Menko FH, et al. Dysplastic changes in prophylactically removed Fallopian tubes of women predisposed to developing ovarian cancer. J Pathol. 2001;195(4):451–6.
43. Jarboe E, Folkins A, Nucci MR, Kindelberger D, Drapkin R, Miron A, et al. Serous carcinogenesis in the fallopian tube: a descriptive classification. Int J Gynecol Pathol. 2008;27(1):1–9.
44. Visvanathan K, Vang R, Shaw P, Gross A, Soslow R, Parkash V, et al. Diagnosis of serous tubal intraepithelial carcinoma based on morphologic and immunohistochemical features: a reproducibility study. Am J Surg Pathol. 2011;35(12):1766–75.
45. Finch A, Shaw P, Rosen B, Murphy J, Narod SA, Colgan TJ. Clinical and pathologic findings of prophylactic salpingo-oophorectomies in 159 BRCA1 and BRCA2 carriers. Gynecol Oncol. 2006;100(1):58–64.
46. Shaw PA, Rouzbahman M, Pizer ES, Pintilie M, Begley H. Candidate serous cancer precursors in fallopian tube epithelium of BRCA1/2 mutation carriers. Mod Pathol. 2009;22(9):1133–8.
47. Kindelberger DW, Lee Y, Miron A, Hirsch MS, Feltmate C, Medeiros F, et al. Intraepithelial carcinoma of the fimbria and pelvic serous carcinoma: evidence for a causal relationship. Am J Surg Pathol. 2007;31(2):161–9.
48. Labidi-Galy SI, Papp E, Hallberg D, Niknafs N, Adleff V, Noe M, et al. High grade serous ovarian carcinomas originate in the fallopian tube. Nat Commun. 2017;8(1):1–11.
49. Chen EY, Mehra K, Mehrad M, Ning G, Miron A, Mutter GL, Monte N, Quade BJ, McKeon FD, Yassin Y, Xian W, Crum CP. Secretory cell outgrowth, PAX2 and serous carcinogenesis in the fallopian tube. J Pathol. 2010;222:110–6.
50. Köbel M, Rahimi K, Rambau PF, Naugler C, Le Page C, Meunier L, et al. An immunohistochemical algorithm for ovarian carcinoma typing. Int J Gynecol Pathol. 2016;35(5):430–41.
51. Kriplani D, Patel M. Immunohistochemistry: a diagnostic aid in differentiating primary epithelial ovarian tumors and tumors metastatic to the ovary. South Asian J Cancer. 2013;2(4):254.
52. Kaspar HG, Crum CP. The utility of immunohistochemistry in the differential diagnosis of gynecologic disorders. Arch Pathol Lab Med. 2015;139(1):39–54.
53. Burleson KM, Casey RC, Skubitz KM, Pambuccian SE, Oegema TR, Skubitz APN. Ovarian carcinoma ascites spheroids adhere to extracellular matrix components and mesothelial cell monolayers. Gynecol Oncol. 2004;93(1):170–81.
54. Shield K, Riley C, Quinn MA, Rice GE, Ackland ML, Ahmed N. $\alpha 2\beta 1$ integrin affects metastatic potential of ovarian carcinoma spheroids by supporting disaggregation and proteolysis. J Carcinog. 2007;6:11.
55. Pease JC, Brewer M, Tirnauer JS. Spontaneous spheroid budding from monolayers: a potential contribution to ovarian cancer dissemination. Biol Open. 2012;1(7):622–8.
56. Meyers MA, Oliphant M, Berne AS, Feldberg MAM. The peritoneal ligaments and mesenteries: pathways of intraabdominal spread of disease. Radiology. 1987;163(3):593–604.
57. Tan DS, Agarwal R, Kaye SB. Mechanisms of transcoelomic metastasis in ovarian cancer. Lancet Oncol. 2006;7(11):925–34.
58. Lengyel E. Ovarian cancer development and metastasis. Am J Pathol. 2010;177(3):1053–64.
59. Farsinejad S, Cattabiani T, Muranen T, Iwanicki M. Ovarian cancer dissemination—a cell biologist's perspective. Cancers (Basel). 2019;11(12):1957.
60. Laval G, Marcelin-Benazech B, Guirimand F, Chauvenet L, Copel L, Durand A, et al. Recommendations for bowel obstruction with peritoneal carcinomatosis. J Pain Symptom Manage. 2014;48(1):75–91.
61. Miyoshi A, Miyatake T, Hara T, Tanaka A, Komura N, Komiya S, et al. Etiology of ascites and pleural effusion associated with ovarian tumors: literature review and case reports of three ovarian tumors presenting with massive ascites, but without peritoneal dissemination. Case Rep Obstet Gynecol. 2015;2015:1–5.
62. Sehouli J, Senyuva F, Fotopoulou C, Neumann U, Denkert C, Werner L, et al. Intra-abdominal tumor dissemination pattern and surgical outcome in 214 patients with primary ovarian cancer. J Surg Oncol. 2009;99(7):424–7.
63. Kleppe M, Kraima AC, Kruitwagen RFPM, Van Gorp T, Smit NN, Van Munsteren JC, et al. Understanding lymphatic drainage pathways of the ovaries to predict sites for sentinel nodes in ovarian cancer. Int J Gynecol Cancer. 2015;25(8):1405–14.

64. Burghardt E, Girardi F, Lahousen M, Tamussino K, Stettner H. Patterns of pelvic and paraaortic lymph node involvement in ovarian cancer. Gynecol Oncol. 1991;40(2):103–6.
65. Chen SS, Lee L. Incidence of para-aortic and pelvic lymph node metastases in epithelial carcinoma of the ovary. Gynecol Oncol. 1983;16(1):95–100.
66. Coffman LG, Burgos-Ojeda D, Wu R, Cho K, Bai S, Buckanovich RJ. New models of hematogenous ovarian cancer metastasis demonstrate preferential spread to the ovary and a requirement for the ovary for abdominal dissemination. Transl Res. 2016;175:92–102.e2.
67. Ng LW, Rubin SC, Hoskins WJ, Jones WB, Hakes TB, Markman M, et al. Aggressive chemosurgical debulking in patients with advanced ovarian cancer. Gynecol Oncol. 1990;38(3):358–63.
68. Iii WEW, Maxwell GL, Tian C, Carlson JW, Ozols RF, Rose PG, et al. Prognostic factors for stage III epithelial ovarian cancer: a Gynecologic Oncology Group Study. J Clin Oncol. 2007;25(24):3621–7.
69. Cervantes A. Prognostic factors in advanced ovarian cancer. Int J Gynecol Cancer. 1997;7:4–8.
70. Young RC, Walton LA, Ellenberg SS, Homesley HD, Wilbanks GD, Decker DG, et al. Adjuvant therapy in Stage I and Stage II epithelial ovarian cancer. N Engl J Med. 1990;322(15):1021–7.
71. Hoskins WJ, Bundy BN, Thigpen JT, Omura GA. The influence of cytoreductive surgery on recurrence-free interval and survival in small-volume Stage III epithelial ovarian cancer: a Gynecologic Oncology Group study. Gynecol Oncol. 1992;47(2):159–66.
72. Heintz APM, Odicino F, Maisonneuve P, et al. Carcinoma of the ovary. 26th Annual Report on the Results of Treatment in Gynaecological Cancer. Int J Gynaecol Obs. 2006;95(Suppl 1):S161–92.
73. Dembo AJ, Davy M, Stenwig AE, Berle EJ, Bush RS, Kjorstad K. Prognostic factors in patients with Stage I epithelial ovarian cancer. Obstet Gynecol. 1990;75(2):263–73.
74. Elattar A, Bryant A, Winter-Roach BA, Hatem M, Naik R. Optimal primary surgical treatment for advanced epithelial ovarian cancer. Cochrane Database Syst Rev. 2011;8:CD007565.
75. Hannibal CG, Vang R, Junge J, Kjaerbye-Thygesen A, Kurman RJ, Kjaer SK. A binary histologic grading system for ovarian serous carcinoma is an independent prognostic factor: a population-based study of 4317 women diagnosed in Denmark 1978-2006. Gynecol Oncol. 2012;125(3):655–60.
76. Hess V, A'Hern R, Nasiri N, King DM, Blake PR, Barton DPJ, et al. Mucinous epithelial ovarian cancer: a separate entity requiring specific treatment. J Clin Oncol. 2004;22(6):1040–4.
77. Alexandre J, Ray-Coquard I, Selle F, Floquet A, Cottu P, Weber B, et al. Mucinous advanced epithelial ovarian carcinoma: clinical presentation and sensitivity to platinum-paclitaxel-based chemotherapy, the GINECO experience. Ann Oncol. 2010;21(12):2377–81.
78. Fujiwara K, Shintani D, Nishikawa T. Clear-cell carcinoma of the ovary. Ann Oncol. 2016;27:50–2.
79. Winter WE, Maxwell GL, Tian C, Carlson JW, Ozols RF, Rose PG, et al. Prognostic factors for stage III epithelial ovarian cancer: a Gynecologic Oncology Group study. J Clin Oncol. 2007;25(24):3621–7.
80. Chan JK, Loizzi V, Lin YG, Osann K, Brewster WR, DiSaia PJ. Stages III and IV invasive epithelial ovarian carcinoma in younger versus older women: what prognostic factors are important? Obstet Gynecol. 2003;102(1):156–61.
81. Gronlund B, Høgdall C, Hansen HH, Engelholm SA. Performance status rather than age is the key prognostic factor in second-line treatment of elderly patients with epithelial ovarian carcinoma. Cancer. 2002;94(7):1961–7.
82. Akahira JI, Yoshikawa H, Shimizu Y, Tsunematsu R, Hirakawa T, Kuramoto H, et al. Prognostic factors of stage IV epithelial ovarian cancer: a multicenter retrospective study. Gynecol Oncol. 2001;81(3):398–403.
83. Berek JS, Kehoe ST, Kumar L, Friedlander M. Cancer of the ovary, fallopian tube, and peritoneum. Int J Gynecol Obstet. 2018;143:59–78.
84. Committee on Practice Bulletins—Gynecology. Practice Bulletin No. 174 Summary: evaluation and management of adnexal masses. Obstet Gynecol. 2016;128(5):1193–5.
85. Moss EL, Hollingworth J, Reynolds TM. The role of CA125 in clinical practice. J Clin Pathol. 2005;58(3):308–12.
86. Brown J, Frumovitz M. Mucinous tumors of the ovary: current thoughts on diagnosis and management. Curr Oncol Rep. 2014;16(6):389.
87. Jacobs I, Bast RC. The CA 125 tumour-associated antigen: a review of the literature. Hum Reprod. 1989;4(1):1–12.
88. Buamah PK, Rake MO, Drake SR, Skillen AW. Serum CA 12-5 concentrations and CA 12-5/CEA ratios in patients with epithelial ovarian cancer. J Surg Oncol. 2006;44(2):97–9.
89. Moore RG, Miller MC, Steinhoff MM, Skates SJ, Lu KH, Lambert-Messerlian G, et al. Serum HE4 levels are less frequently elevated than CA125 in women with benign gynecologic disorders. Am J Obstet Gynecol. 2012;206(4):351.e1–8.
90. Bourne TH, Campbell S, Reynolds KM, Whitehead MI, Hampson J, Royston P, et al. Screening for early familial ovarian cancer with transvaginal ultrasonography and colour blood flow imaging. Br Med J. 1993;306(6884):1025–9.
91. National Institute for Care and Health Excellence. Ovarian cancer: recognition and initial management, vol. 2011. NICE; 2017.
92. Jacobs I, Oram D, Fairbanks J, Turner J, Frost C, Grudzinskas JG. A risk of malignancy index incorporating CA 125, ultrasound and menopausal status for the accurate preoperative diagnosis of ovarian cancer. Br J Obstet Gynaecol. 1990;97(10):922–9.

93. Tingulstad S, Hagen B, Skjeldestad FE, Onsrud M, Kiserud T, Halvorsen T, et al. Evaluation of a risk of malignancy index based on serum CA125, ultrasound findings and menopausal status in the preoperative diagnosis of pelvic masses. Br J Obstet Gynaecol. 1996;103(8):826–31.
94. Moore RG, McMeekin DS, Brown AK, DiSilvestro P, Miller MC, Allard WJ, et al. A novel multiple marker bioassay utilizing HE4 and CA125 for the prediction of ovarian cancer in patients with a pelvic mass. Gynecol Oncol. 2009;112(1):40–6.
95. Kaijser J, Bourne T, Valentin L, Sayasneh A, Van Holsbeke C, Vergote I, et al. Improving strategies for diagnosing ovarian cancer: a summary of the International Ovarian Tumor Analysis (IOTA) studies. Ultrasound Obstet Gynecol. 2013;41(1):9–20.
96. Adusumilli S, Hussain HK, Caoili EM, Weadock WJ, Murray JP, Johnson TD, et al. MRI of sonographically indeterminate adnexal masses. Am J Roentgenol. 2006;187(3):732–40.
97. Iyer VR, Lee SI. MRI, CT, and PET/CT for ovarian cancer detection and adnexal lesion characterization. Am J Roentgenol. 2010;194(2):311–21.
98. Bristow RE, Duska LR, Lambrou NC, Fishman EK, O'Neill MJ, Trimble EL, et al. A model for predicting surgical outcome in patients with advanced ovarian carcinoma using computed tomography. Cancer. 2000;89(7):1532–40.
99. Hu TWY, Nie D, Gou JH, Li ZY. Predictive significance of preoperative CT findings for suboptimal cytoreduction in advanced ovarian cancer: a meta-analysis. Cancer Manag Res. 2018;10:2019–30.
100. Fenchel S, Grab D, Nuessle K, Kotzerke J, Rieber A, Kreienberg R, et al. Asymptomatic adnexal masses: correlation of FDG PET and histopathologic findings. Radiology. 2002;223(3):780–8.
101. Woodward PJ, Hosseinzadeh K, Saenger JS. Radiologic staging of ovarian carcinoma with pathologic correlation. Radiographics. 2004;24(1):225–46.
102. Khiewvan B, Torigian DA, Emamzadehfard S, Paydary K, Salavati A, Houshmand S, et al. An update on the role of PET/CT and PET/MRI in ovarian cancer. Eur J Nucl Med Mol Imaging. 2017;44(6):1079–91.
103. Ayhan A, Gultekin M, Yigit Celik N, Dursun P, Taskiran C, Aksan G, et al. Occult metastasis in early ovarian cancers: risk factors and associated prognosis. Am J Obstet Gynecol. 2007;196:81.e1–6.
104. Schueler T, Hermans F. The yield of surgical staging in presumed early stage ovarian cancer: benefits or doubts? Int J Gynecol Cancer. 1998;8(2):95–102.
105. Manvelyan V, Khemarangsan V, Huang K-G, Adlan A-S, Lee C-L. Port-site metastasis in laparoscopic gynecological oncology surgery: an overview. Gynecol Minim Invasive Ther. 2016;5(1):1–6. https://doi.org/10.1016/j.gmit.2015.06.009.
106. Angioli R, Plotti F, Palaia I, Calcagno M, Montera R, Cafà EV, et al. Update on lymphadenectomy in early and advanced ovarian cancer. Curr Opin Obstet Gynecol. 2008;20(1):34–9.
107. Benedetti P, Scambia G, Baiocchi G, Greggi S, Mancuso S. Technique and feasibility of radical para-aortic and pelvic lymphadenectomy for gynecologic malignancies: a prospective study. Int J Gynecol Cancer. 1991;1(3):133–40.
108. Bentivegna E, Gouy S, Maulard A, Pautier P, Leary A, Colombo N, et al. Fertility-sparing surgery in epithelial ovarian cancer: a systematic review of oncological issues. Ann Oncol. 2016;27(11):1994–2004.
109. McKenney JK, Balzer BL, Longacre TA. Lymph node involvement in ovarian serous tumors of low malignant potential (borderline tumors). Am J Surg Pathol. 2006;30(5):614–24.
110. du Bois A, Trillsch F, Mahner S, Heitz F, Harter P. Management of borderline ovarian tumors. Ann Oncol. 2016;27(Suppl 1):i20–2.
111. Colombo N, Sessa C, du Bois A, Ledermann J, McCluggage WG, McNeish I, Morice P, Pignata S, Ray-Coquard I, Vergote I, Baert T. ESMO–ESGO consensus conference recommendations on ovarian cancer: pathology and molecular biology, early and advanced stages, borderline tumours and recurrent disease. Ann Oncol. 2019;30(5):672–705.
112. Morice P. Borderline tumours of the ovary and fertility. Eur J Cancer. 2006;42(2):149–58.
113. Suh-Burgmann E. Long-term outcomes following conservative surgery for borderline tumor of the ovary: a large population-based study. Gynecol Oncol. 2006;103(3):841–7.
114. du Bois A, Ewald-Riegler N, De Gregorio N, Reuss A, Mahner S, Fotopoulou C, et al. Borderline tumours of the ovary: a cohort study of the Arbeitsgmeinschaft Gynäkologische Onkologie (AGO) Study Group. Eur J Cancer. 2013;49(8):1905–14.
115. Gómez-Hidalgo NR, Martinez-Cannon BA, Nick AM, Lu KH, Sood AK, Coleman RL, et al. Predictors of optimal cytoreduction in patients with newly diagnosed advanced-stage epithelial ovarian cancer: time to incorporate laparoscopic assessment into the standard of care. Gynecol Oncol. 2015;137(3):553–8.
116. Schorge JO, McCann C, Del Carmen MG. Surgical debulking of ovarian cancer: what difference does it make? Rev Obstet Gynecol. 2010;3(3):111–7.
117. Yang L, Zhang B, Xing G, Du J, Yang B, Yuan Q, Yang Y. Neoadjuvant chemotherapy versus primary debulking surgery in advanced epithelial ovarian cancer: a meta-analysis of peri-operative outcome. PLoS One. 2017;12(10):e0186725.
118. Chang SJ, Hodeib M, Chang J, Bristow RE. Survival impact of complete cytoreduction to no gross residual disease for advanced-stage ovarian cancer: a meta-analysis. Gynecol Oncol. 2013;130(3):493–8.
119. du Bois A, Reuss A, Harter P, Pujade-Lauraine E, Ray-Coquard I, Pfisterer J. Potential role of lymphadenectomy in advanced ovarian cancer: a combined exploratory analysis of three prospectively randomized phase III multicenter trials. J Clin Oncol. 2010;28(10):1733–9.

120. Harter P, Sehouli J, Lorusso D, Reuss A, Vergote I, Marth C, et al. LION: lymphadenectomy in ovarian neoplasms—a prospective randomized AGO study group led gynecologic cancer intergroup trial. J Clin Oncol. 2017;35(15 Suppl):5500.
121. Vergote I, Tropé CG, Amant F, Kristensen GB, Ehlen T, Johnson N, et al. Neoadjuvant chemotherapy or primary surgery in Stage IIIC or IV ovarian cancer. N Engl J Med. 2010;363(10):943–53.
122. Kehoe S, Hook J, Nankivell M, Jayson GC, Kitchener H, Lopes T, et al. Primary chemotherapy versus primary surgery for newly diagnosed advanced ovarian cancer (CHORUS): an open-label, randomised, controlled, non-inferiority trial. Lancet. 2015;386(9990):249–57.
123. Fagotti A, Vizzielli G, Ferrandina G, Fanfani F, Gallotta V, Chiantera V, et al. Survival analyses from a randomized trial of primary debulking surgery versus neoadjuvant chemotherapy for advanced epithelial ovarian cancer with high tumor load (SCORPION trial). J Clin Oncol. 2018;36(15 Suppl):5516.
124. Onda T, Satoh T, Saito T, Kasamatsu T, Nakanishi T, Nakamura K, Wakabayashi M, Takehara K, Saito M, Ushijima K, Kobayashi H. Comparison of treatment invasiveness between upfront debulking surgery versus interval debulking surgery following neoadjuvant chemotherapy for stage III/IV ovarian, tubal, and peritoneal cancers in a phase III randomised trial: Japan Clinical Oncology Group Study JCOG0602. Eur J Cancer. 2016;64:22–31.
125. Kumar Prof L, Hariprasad R, Kumar S, Bhatla N, Thulkar S, Vijayaraghavan M, Deo S, Shukla N, Singh R. Neoadjuvant chemotherapy (NACT) followed by interval debulking surgery versus upfront surgery followed by chemotherapy (CT) in advanced epithelial ovarian carcinoma (EOC): a prospective randomized study—interim results. J Clin Oncol. 2007;25(18 Suppl):5531.
126. Pölcher M, Mahner S, Ortmann O, Hilfrich J, Diedrich K, Breitbach GP, et al. Neoadjuvant chemotherapy with carboplatin and docetaxel in advanced ovarian cancer—a prospective multicenter phase II trial (PRIMOVAR). Oncol Rep. 2009;22(3):605–13.
127. Armstrong DK, Alvarez RD, Bakkum-Gamez JN, Barroilhet L, Behbakht K, Berchuck A, et al. Ovarian cancer, version 1.2019 featured updates to the nccn guidelines. J Natl Compr Cancer Netw. 2019;17(8):896–909.
128. Tropé C, Kaern J. Adjuvant chemotherapy for early-stage ovarian cancer: review of the literature. J Clin Oncol. 2007;25(20):2909–20.
129. Winter-Roach BA, Kitchener HC, Lawrie TA. Adjuvant (post-surgery) chemotherapy for early stage epithelial ovarian cancer. Cochrane Database Syst Rev. 2012;2012:CD004706.
130. Bell J, Brady MF, Young RC, Lage J, Walker JL, Look KY, et al. Randomized phase III trial of three versus six cycles of adjuvant carboplatin and paclitaxel in early stage epithelial ovarian carcinoma: a Gynecologic Oncology Group study. Gynecol Oncol. 2006 Sep;102(3):432–9.
131. McGuire WP, Hoskins WJ, Brady MF, Kucera PR, Partridge EE, Look KY, et al. Cyclophosphamide and cisplatin compared with paclitaxel and cisplatin in patients with Stage III and Stage IV ovarian cancer. N Engl J Med. 1996;334(1):1–6.
132. Piccart MJ, Bertelsen K, James K, Cassidy J, Mangioni C, Simonsen E, et al. Randomized intergroup trial of cisplatin-paclitaxel versus cisplatin-cyclophosphamide in women with advanced epithelial ovarian cancer: three-year results. J Natl Cancer Inst. 2000;92(9):699–708.
133. Kyrgiou M, Salanti G, Pavlidis N, Paraskevaidis E, Ioannidis JPA. Survival benefits with diverse chemotherapy regimens for ovarian cancer: meta-analysis of multiple treatments. J Natl Cancer Inst. 2006;98(22):1655–63.
134. Ozols RF, Bundy BN, Greer BE, Fowler JM, Clarke-Pearson D, Burger RA, et al. Phase III trial of carboplatin and paclitaxel compared with cisplatin and paclitaxel in patients with optimally resected stage III ovarian cancer: a Gynecologic Oncology Group study. J Clin Oncol. 2003;21(17):3194–200.
135. du Bois A, Lück HJ, Meier W, Adams HP, Möbus V, Costa S, et al. A randomized clinical trial of cisplatin/paclitaxel versus carboplatin/paclitaxel as first-line treatment of ovarian cancer. J Natl Cancer Inst. 2003;95(17):1320–30.
136. Bookman MA, Brady MF, McGuire WP, Harper PG, Alberts DS, Friedlander M, et al. Evaluation of new platinum-based treatment regimens in advanced-stage ovarian cancer: a Phase III Trial of the Gynecologic Cancer Intergroup. J Clin Oncol. 2009;27(9):1419–25.
137. Hofstetter G, Concin N, Braicu I, Chekerov R, Sehouli J, Cadron I, et al. The time interval from surgery to start of chemotherapy significantly impacts prognosis in patients with advanced serous ovarian carcinoma—analysis of patient data in the prospective OVCAD study. Gynecol Oncol. 2013;131(1):15–20.
138. Tewari KS, Java JJ, Eskander RN, Monk BJ, Burger RA. Early initiation of chemotherapy following complete resection of advanced ovarian cancer associated with improved survival: NRG Oncology/Gynecologic Oncology Group study. Ann Oncol. 2016;27(1):114–21.
139. Alberts DS, Liu PY, Hannigan EV, O'Toole R, Williams SD, Young JA, et al. Intraperitoneal cisplatin plus intravenous cyclophosphamide versus intravenous cisplatin plus intravenous cyclophosphamide for Stage III ovarian cancer. N Engl J Med. 1996;335(26):1950–5.
140. Markman M, Bundy BN, Alberts DS, Fowler JM, Clark-Pearson DL, Carson LF, et al. Phase III trial of standard-dose intravenous cisplatin plus paclitaxel versus moderately high-dose carboplatin followed by intravenous paclitaxel and intraperitoneal cisplatin in small-volume stage III ovarian

carcinoma: an intergroup study of the Gynecologic Oncology Group, Southwestern Oncology Group, and Eastern Cooperative Oncology Group. J Clin Oncol. 2001;19(4):1001–7.
141. Armstrong DK, Bundy B, Wenzel L, Huang HQ, Baergen R, Lele S, et al. Intraperitoneal cisplatin and paclitaxel in ovarian cancer. N Engl J Med. 2006;354(1):34–43.
142. Walker JL, Brady MF, Wenzel L, Fleming GF, Huang HQ, DiSilvestro PA, et al. Randomized trial of intravenous versus intraperitoneal chemotherapy plus bevacizumab in advanced ovarian carcinoma: an NRG Oncology/Gynecologic Oncology Group Study. J Clin Oncol. 2019;37(16):1380–90.
143. Lesnock JL, Darcy KM, Tian C, Deloia JA, Thrall MM, Zahn C, et al. BRCA1 expression and improved survival in ovarian cancer patients treated with intraperitoneal cisplatin and paclitaxel: a Gynecologic Oncology Group Study. Br J Cancer. 2013;108(6):1231–7.
144. Zhang G, Zhu Y, Liu C, Chao G, Cui R, Zhang Z. The prognosis impact of hyperthermic intraperitoneal chemotherapy (HIPEC) plus cytoreductive surgery (CRS) in advanced ovarian cancer: the meta-analysis. J Ovarian Res. 2019;12(1):33.
145. Baiocchi G, Ferreira FO, Mantoan H, da Costa AABA, Faloppa CC, Kumagai LY, et al. Hyperthermic intraperitoneal chemotherapy after secondary cytoreduction in epithelial ovarian cancer: a single-center comparative analysis. Ann Surg Oncol. 2016;23(4):1294–301.
146. Mendivil AA, Rettenmaier MA, Abaid LN, Brown JV, Mori KM, Lopez KL, et al. Consolidation hyperthermic intraperitoneal chemotherapy for the treatment of advanced stage ovarian carcinoma: a 3 year experience. Cancer Chemother Pharmacol. 2017;80(2):405–10.
147. van Driel WJ, Koole SN, Sikorska K, Schagen van Leeuwen JH, Schreuder HWR, Hermans RHM, et al. Hyperthermic intraperitoneal chemotherapy in ovarian cancer. N Engl J Med. 2018;378(3):230–40.
148. Katsumata N. Dose-dense approaches to ovarian cancer treatment. Curr Treat Options Oncol. 2015;16(5):21.
149. Chan JK, Brady MF, Penson RT, Huang H, Birrer MJ, Walker JL, et al. Weekly vs. every-3-week paclitaxel and carboplatin for ovarian cancer. N Engl J Med. 2016;374(8):738–48.
150. Clamp AR, James EC, McNeish IA, Dean A, Kim JW, O'Donnell DM, et al. Weekly dose-dense chemotherapy in first-line epithelial ovarian, fallopian tube, or primary peritoneal carcinoma treatment (ICON8): primary progression free survival analysis results from a GCIG phase 3 randomised controlled trial. Lancet. 2019;394(10214):2084–95.
151. Pignata S, Scambia G, Katsaros D, Gallo C, Pujade-Lauraine E, De Placido S, et al. Carboplatin plus paclitaxel once a week versus every 3 weeks in patients with advanced ovarian cancer (MITO-7): a randomised, multicentre, open-label, phase 3 trial. Lancet Oncol. 2014;15(4):396–405.
152. Tewari KS, Burger RA, Enserro D, Norquist BM, Swisher EM, Brady MF, et al. Final overall survival of a randomized trial of bevacizumab for primary treatment of ovarian cancer. J Clin Oncol. 2019;37(26):2317–28.
153. Burger RA, Brady MF, Bookman MA, Fleming GF, Monk BJ, Huang H, et al. Incorporation of bevacizumab in the primary treatment of ovarian cancer. Obstet Gynecol Surv. 2012;67(5):289–90.
154. Oza AM, Cook AD, Pfisterer J, Embleton A, Ledermann JA, Pujade-Lauraine E, et al. Standard chemotherapy with or without bevacizumab for women with newly diagnosed ovarian cancer (ICON7): overall survival results of a phase 3 randomised trial. Lancet Oncol. 2015;16(8):928–36.
155. Monk BJ, Minion LE, Coleman RL. Anti-angiogenic agents in ovarian cancer: past, present, and future. Ann Oncol. 2016;27:i33–9.
156. Pennington KP, Walsh T, Harrell MI, Lee MK, Pennil CC, Rendi MH, et al. Germline and somatic mutations in homologous recombination genes predict platinum response and survival in ovarian, fallopian tube, and peritoneal carcinomas. Clin Cancer Res. 2014;20(3):764–75.
157. Domchek SM, Aghajanian C, Shapira-Frommer R, Schmutzler RK, Audeh MW, Friedlander M, et al. Efficacy and safety of olaparib monotherapy in germline BRCA1/2 mutation carriers with advanced ovarian cancer and three or more lines of prior therapy. Gynecol Oncol. 2016;140(2):199–203.
158. Pujade-Lauraine E, Ledermann JA, Selle F, Gebski V, Penson RT, Oza AM, et al. Olaparib tablets as maintenance therapy in patients with platinum-sensitive, relapsed ovarian cancer and a BRCA1/2 mutation (SOLO2/ENGOT-Ov21): a double-blind, randomised, placebo-controlled, phase 3 trial. Lancet Oncol. 2017;18(9):1274–84.
159. Mirza MR, Coleman RL, González-Martín A, Moore KN, Colombo N, Ray-Coquard I, et al. The forefront of ovarian cancer therapy: update on PARP inhibitors. Ann Oncol. 2020;31(9):1148–59.
160. Moore K, Colombo N, Scambia G, Kim B-G, Oaknin A, Friedlander M, et al. Maintenance olaparib in patients with newly diagnosed advanced ovarian cancer. N Engl J Med. 2018;379(26):2495–505.
161. Fujiwara K, Harter P, Leary A, Perol D, Pignata S, González-Martín A, Petru E, van Nieuwenhuysen E, Colombo N, Mäenpää J, Selle F. Phase III PAOLA-1/ENGOT-ov25 trial: Olaparib plus bevacizumab (bev) as maintenance therapy in patients (pts) with newly diagnosed, advanced ovarian cancer (OC) treated with platinum-based chemotherapy (PCh) plus bev. Ann Oncol. 2019;30:ix191–2.
162. González-Martín A, Pothuri B, Vergote I, DePont CR, Graybill W, Mirza MR, McCormick C, Lorusso D, Hoskins P, Freyer G, Baumann K. Niraparib in patients with newly diagnosed advanced ovarian cancer. N Engl J Med. 2019;381(25):2391–402.

163. Coleman RL, Fleming GF, Brady MF, Swisher E, Steffensen KD, Friedlander M, Okamoto A, Moore K, Ben-Baruch N, Werner TL, Oaknin A. VELIA/GOG-3005: integration of veliparib (V) with front-line chemotherapy and maintenance in women with high-grade serous carcinoma of ovarian, fallopian tube, or primary peritoneal origin (HGSC). Ann Oncol. 2019;30:v895–6.
164. Ushijima K. Treatment for recurrent ovarian cancer—at first relapse. J Oncol. 2010;2010:497429.
165. Rustin GJ, van der Burg ME. A randomized trial in ovarian cancer (OC) of early treatment of relapse based on CA125 level alone versus delayed treatment based on conventional clinical indicators (MRC OV05/EORTC 55955 trials). J Clin Oncol. 2009;27(18 Suppl):1.
166. Harter P, Du BA, Hahmann M, Hasenburg A, Burges A, Loibl S, et al. Surgery in recurrent ovarian cancer: the Arbeitsgemeinschaft Gynaekologische Onkologie (AGO) DESKTOP OVAR trial. Ann Surg Oncol. 2006;13(12):1702–10.
167. Harter P, Sehouli J, Reuss A, Hasenburg A, Scambia G, Cibula D, et al. Prospective validation study of a predictive score for operability of recurrent ovarian cancer: the Multicenter Intergroup Study DESKTOP II. A project of the AGO Kommission OVAR, AGO Study Group, NOGGO, AGO-Austria, and MITO. Int J Gynecol Cancer. 2011;21(2):289–95.
168. du Bois A, Sehouli J, Vergote I, Ferron G, Reuss A, Meier W, et al. Randomized phase III study to evaluate the impact of secondary cytoreductive surgery in recurrent ovarian cancer: final analysis of AGO DESKTOP III/ENGOT-ov20. J Clin Oncol. 2020;38(15 Suppl):6000.
169. Coleman RL, Spirtos NM, Enserro D, Herzog TJ, Sabbatini P, Armstrong DK, et al. Secondary surgical cytoreduction for recurrent ovarian cancer. N Engl J Med. 2019;381(20):1929–39.
170. Cantù MG, Buda A, Parma G, Rossi R, Floriani I, Bonazzi C, et al. Randomized controlled trial of single-agent paclitaxel versus cyclophosphamide, doxorubicin, and cisplatin in patients with recurrent ovarian cancer who responded to first-line platinum-based regimens. J Clin Oncol. 2002;20(5):1232–7.
171. Markman M, Rothman R, Hakes T, Reichman B, Hoskins W, Rubin S, et al. Second-line platinum therapy in patients with ovarian cancer previously treated with cisplatin. J Clin Oncol. 1991;9(3):389–93.
172. Van der Burg MEL, Hoff AM, van Lent M, Rodenburg CJ, van Putten WLJ, Stoter G. Carboplatin and cyclophosphamide salvage therapy for ovarian cancer patients relapsing after cisplatin combination chemotherapy. Eur J Cancer Clin Oncol. 1991;27(3):248–50.
173. Icon and Ago Collaborators. Paclitaxel plus platinum-based chemotherapy versus conventional platinum-based chemotherapy in women with relapsed ovarian cancer: the ICON4/AGO-OVAR-2.2 trial. Lancet. 2003;361(9375):2099–106.
174. Pfisterer J, Plante M, Vergote I, du Bois A, Hirte H, Lacave AJ, et al. Gemcitabine plus carboplatin compared with carboplatin in patients with platinum-sensitive recurrent ovarian cancer: an intergroup trial of the AGO-OVAR, the NCIC CTG, and the EORTC GCG. J Clin Oncol. 2006;24(29):4699–707.
175. Pujade-Lauraine E, Wagner U, Aavall-Lundqvist E, Gebski V, Heywood M, Vasey PA, et al. Pegylated liposomal doxorubicin and carboplatin compared with paclitaxel and carboplatin for patients with platinum-sensitive ovarian cancer in late relapse. J Clin Oncol. 2010;28(20):3323–9.
176. Markman M, Bookman MA. Second-line treatment of ovarian cancer. Oncologist. 2000;5(1):26–35.
177. Aghajanian C, Blank SV, Goff BA, Judson PL, Teneriello MG, Husain A, et al. OCEANS: a randomized, double-blind, placebo-controlled phase III trial of chemotherapy with or without bevacizumab in patients with platinum-sensitive recurrent epithelial ovarian, primary peritoneal, or fallopian tube cancer. J Clin Oncol. 2012;30(17):2039–45.
178. Pignata S, Lorusso D, Joly F, Gallo C, Colombo N, Sessa C, et al. Chemotherapy plus or minus bevacizumab for platinum-sensitive ovarian cancer patients recurring after a bevacizumab containing first line treatment: the randomized phase 3 trial MITO16B-MaNGO OV2B-ENGOT OV17. J Clin Oncol. 2018;36(15 Suppl):5506.
179. Pujade-Lauraine E, Hilpert F, Weber B, Reuss A, Poveda A, Kristensen G, et al. Bevacizumab combined with chemotherapy for platinum-resistant recurrent ovarian cancer: the AURELIA open-label randomized phase III trial. J Clin Oncol. 2014;32(13):1302–8.
180. Mirza MR, Monk BJ, Herrstedt J, Oza AM, Mahner S, Redondo A, Fabbro M, Ledermann JA, Lorusso D, Vergote I, Ben-Baruch NE. Niraparib maintenance therapy in platinum-sensitive, recurrent ovarian cancer. N Engl J Med. 2016;375(22):2154–64.
181. Coleman RL, Oza AM, Lorusso D, Aghajanian C, Oaknin A, Dean A, Colombo N, Weberpals JI, Clamp A, Scambia G, Leary A. Rucaparib maintenance treatment for recurrent ovarian carcinoma after response to platinum therapy (ARIEL3): a randomised, double-blind, placebo-controlled, phase 3 trial. Lancet. 2017;390(10106):1949–61.
182. Baghmar S, Agarwal A, Gauda C, Qureshi S, Malik PS, Vaibhav V. PARP inhibitor in platinum resistant ovarian cancer: single center real world experience. Ann Oncol. 2019;30:ix81–2.
183. Elnakat H, Ratnam M. Distribution, functionality and gene regulation of folate receptor isoforms: implications in targeted therapy. Adv Drug Deliv Rev. 2004;56(8):1067–84.
184. Martin LP, Konner JA, Moore KN, Seward SM, Matulonis UA, Perez RP, Su Y, Berkenblit A, Ruiz-Soto R, Birrer MJ. Characterization of folate receptor alpha (FRα) expression in archival tumour and biopsy samples from relapsed epithelial ovarian cancer patients: a phase I expansion study of the FRα-targeting antibody-drug conjugate mirvetuximab soravtansine. Gynecol Oncol. 2017;147(2):402–7.

Malignant Germ Cell Tumours of the Ovary

Amal Chandra Kataki, Upasana Baruah, Munlima Hazarika, and Pallavi Ramachandra

Ovarian germ cell cancers are considered to be the most chemo sensitive amongst all ovarian cancers and have got a very good prognosis. They constitute around 20–25% of ovarian neoplasms, however, barely around 5% of them are cancerous. Unlike epithelial ovarian cancers, they affect a younger demographic, with over 70% of cases occurring between the ages of 10 and 30 [1, 2]. It is a rarity to find women with this cancer after 40 years of age. Being chemo sensitive tumours and along with rapid progress in chemotherapy delivery there has been an exponential improvement in survival in this rare group of patients with survival as high as 100% for early stage and 75% for advanced disease [3]. In this chapter we aim at briefly describing the pathogenesis and treatment of this rare group of cancer.

A. C. Kataki (✉) · U. Baruah · M. Hazarika
Department of Gynaecologic Oncology, Dr. Bhubaneswar Borooah Cancer Institute (A Unit of Tata Memorial Centre, Mumbai), Guwahati, Assam, India

P. Ramachandra
Department of Gynaecological Oncology, Kidwai Memorial Institute of Oncology, Bengaluru, Karnataka, India

1 Pathologenesis and Classification

The nomenclature germ cell cancer is self-explanatory implying the origin of these cancers being the germ cell of the ovary. The pathogenic event resulting in tumour formation can be traced back to the embryogenic period although majority manifest during puberty [4]. Migration of primordial germ cells is the key event in gonadal formation and this explains the sporadic occurrence of germ cell tumours in extragonadal sites such as mediastinum or retroperitoneum [5]. Primordial germ cell of the ovary has the inherent capability to give rise to varied cells of either of three embryological germ layers or extraembryonic tissues. This capacity for differentiation becomes limited as the cells differentiate, thus from totipotent cells, they become limited to being pluripotent and multipotent cells.

Dysgerminoma cells and the germ cell component of gonadoblastoma have the ability to be stimulated to pluripotency, whereas embryonal carcinoma cells are considered to be intrinsically pluripotent [6].

These tumours can be divided into those that differentiate primarily toward embryo-like neoplasms (teratomas as well as their subtypes, and dysgerminomas) and all those that make a distinction largely toward extraembryonic placenta-like cell populations, or a combination of both

A. C. Kataki, D. Barmon (eds.), *Fundamentals in Gynaecologic Malignancy*,
https://doi.org/10.1007/978-981-19-5860-1_17

(choriocarcinoma and yolk sac tumour), focusing on their resemblance to embryological tissues.

These tumours are associated with distinctive genetic changes. Ovarian dysgerminoma and other primitive germ cell tumours are characterized by a gain of DNA material on the short arm of chromosome 12 [7, 8]. In contrast immature teratoma lack 12p amplification and showed no consistent gains or losses. This difference is consistent with the hypothesis that immature ovarian teratomas have a different pathway of development compared to other primitive germ celltumours [9].

Germ cell tumours have been grouped into three categories in the most recent classification, namely primitive germ cell tumours, biphasic or triphasic teratoma and monodermal teratoma, and somatic-type tumours associated with dermoid cysts [10] (Table 1).

1.1 Dysgerminoma

It is the commonest malignant germ cell in the reproductive age group, but it represents only 1–2% of ovarian malignant tumours [11, 12]. Grossly tumours are characterized by their large, solid, fleshy lobulated grey tan appearance on cut section. Majority of patients present with unilateral solid tumours though in 5–15% women it may be bilateral [13]. Dysgerminomas have the propensity to arise in dysgenetic gonads. Therefore, whenever a premenarcheal girl presents with a pelvic mass, karyotyping should be done, especially if there is a strong suspicion of dyagerminoma [14]. Histologically they have features similar to seminoma of testes. On microscopic examination the tumours have a distinctive appearance comprising of large and monotonous tumour cells, separated by fibrous septae and inflammatory infiltrate, mainly lymphocytes (Fig. 1). Occasionally there may be presence of HCG positive syncytiotrophoblasts which may be reflected by mild elevation of serum HCG. However, they are strongly associated with marked elevation serum LDH [15]. IHC markers characterizing dysgerminoma from other germ cells include positive staining for PLAP, CD-117, and D2–40 and negative staining for CD30 and AFP [16, 17].

Table 1 Classification of germ cell tumours of the ovary

GERM CELL TUMOUR OVARY CLASSIFICATION

PRIMITIVE GERM CELL TUMOURS	BIPHASIC/TRIPHASIC TERATOMA	MONODERMAL TERATOMA AND SOMATIC-TYPE TUMOURS ASSOCIATED WITH BIPHASIC OR TRIPHASIC TERATOMA
A. Dysgerminoma B. Yolk sac tumour C. Embryonal carcinoma D. Polyembryoma E. Nongestational choriocarcinoma F. Mixed germ cell 1. Diffuse embryoma variant	A. Immature teratoma B. Mature teratoma 1. Solid 2. Cystic (dermoid cyst) 3. Fetiform teratoma (homunculus)	A. Thyroid group B. Carcinoid group C. Central nervous system tumour group D. Carcinoma group E. Melanocytic group F. Sarcoma group G. Sebaceous tumour group H. Pituitary-type tumour group I. Retinal anlage tumour group J. Others

1.2 Immature Teratoma

Immature teratoma represents the second most common malignant germ cell tumour of the ovary [18]. It comprises of tissue derived from all the three germ layers and presence of immature neuroectodermal tissue is essential for classification as immature teratoma. Low serum AFP levels may occur. On gross appearance it is large, solid, and fleshy, with evidence of areas comprising necrotic, cystic, and haemorrhagic component. Few areas may show bone, cartilage, hair and cysts filled with seromucinous, colloid or fatty material. Microscopically both mature and immature elements are present (Fig. 2). Amongst the immature elements, neuroectodermal tissue is essential for diagnosis and grading of immature teratoma. If the immature element is less than 1 low power field (40×) under microscope it is categorised as grade 1 whereas presence in 1–3 and more than 3 low power field is categorised as grade 2 and 3 respectively [10]. Immature teratomas are mostly diagnosed morphologically, and there is no unique IHC marker. However, SOX-2, SALL-4, glypican, and CD99 may stain positive in neuroectoderm. In "enteroblastic" glands, SALL-4 and AFP staining can be observed [16, 19].

1.3 Yolk Sac Tumour

Yolk sac tumours develop from undifferentiated and multipotent embryonic carcinomas that have been selectively differentiated into endodermal extra embryonic vitelline structures (yolk sac). After dysgerminoma and teratoma, this is the third most prevalent malignant germ cell tumour of the ovary, as per studies. Most individuals have elevated AFP and CA-125 levels in their blood. It is usually invariably unilateral, big, and has solid and cystic areas, as well as bleeding and necrosis. The majority of tumours are larger than 10 cm in diameter and include cystic areas filled with gelatinous material. Tumours of the yolk sac can have a variety of histologic features. The most prevalent microscopic pattern is reticular or microcystic, which is defined by small honeycomb gaps walled by a single layer of tumour cells that may focally acquire a "signet-ring like" morphology (Fig. 3). The endodermal sinus (festoon) pattern has the characteristic Schiller–Duval bodies that are represented by a central capillary surrounded by connective tissue and a peripheral layer of columnar cells (Fig. 4). Approximately, 65% of yolk sac tumours contain Schiller–Duval Bodies [10]. Broad spectrum cytokeratin is positive for YST, but CK7 and

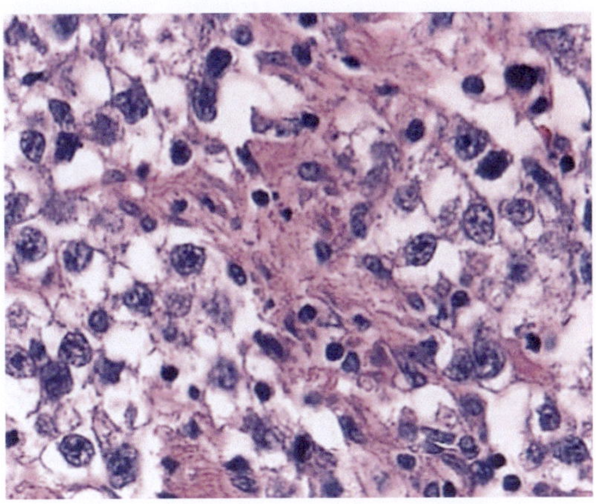

Fig. 1 Dysgerminoma characterized by large and monotonous tumour cells separated by fibrous septa

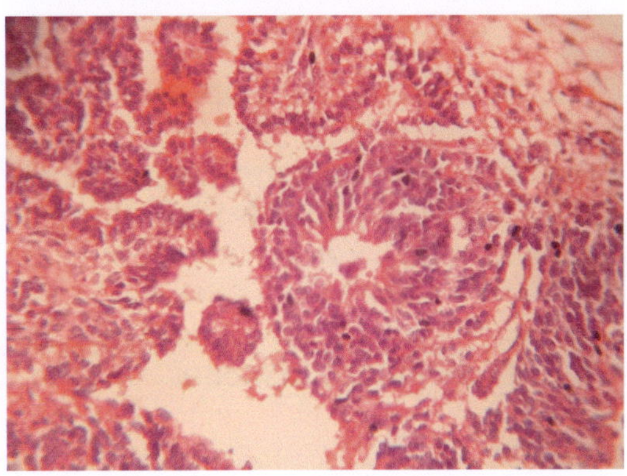

Fig. 2 Immature teratoma showing neuroepithelium

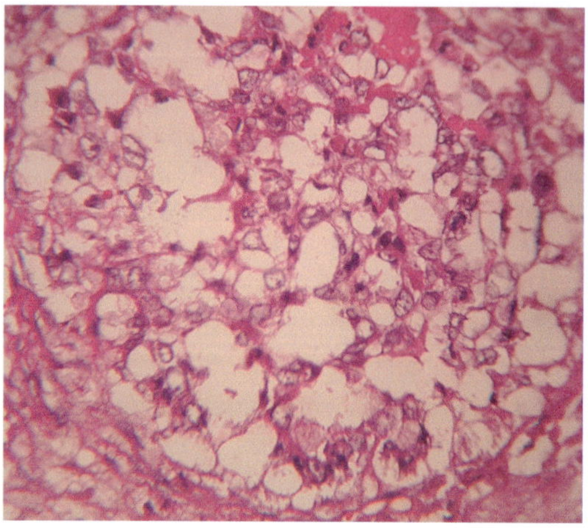

Fig. 3 Yolk sac tumour microcystic pattern

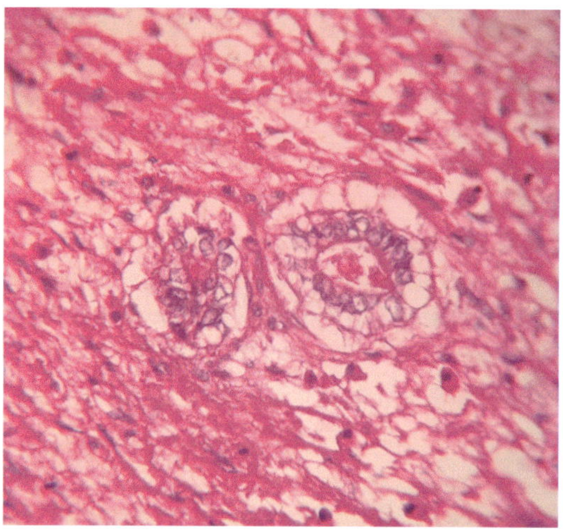

Fig. 4 Yolk sac tumour Schillar–Duval bodies

EMA are frequently negative. Glypican-3 and SALL-4 are frequently diffusely positive, with AFP being focally positive [20].

1.4 Embryonal Carcinoma

Embryonal carcinoma is characterized by the presence of the sheetlike proliferations of primitive cells and the absence of significant amounts of differentiated tissues derived from the three germ layers, particularly neuroepithelium. It is rare and when present, ovarian embryonal carcinoma is usually

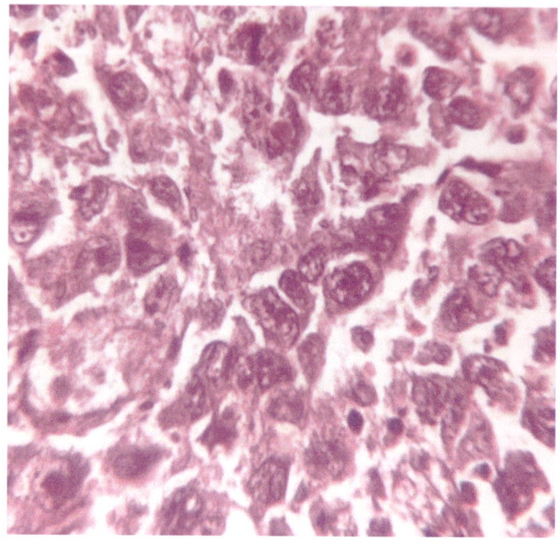

Fig. 5 Embryonal carcinoma with mitosis and pleomorphism

associated with yolk sac tumour in a mixed germ cell tumour. Mitotic figures and apoptotic bodies are numerous (Fig. 5). Syncytiotrophoblast cells are present in most cases. It is considered to be the progenitor of numerous other germ cell tumours since it is made up of undifferentiated cells which produce both hCG and AFP. Due to oestrogen secretion, certain individuals may experience signs and symptoms such as irregular vaginal bleeding, precocious puberty, amenorrhea, or mild hirsutism [10, 21]. Gonadal dysgenesis has been seen to cause it on rare occasions [10]. The tumour cells are typically positive for wide spectrum of IHC markers such as cytokeratin (AE1/AE3), CD30, OCT4, SALL4, and glypican 3 [10, 22, 23].

1.5 Non-gestational Choriocarcinoma

Non-gestational ovarian choriocarcinoma is exceedingly rare and occur in less than 1% of patient. Pure variety is uncommon and presence of other germ cell tumours such as immature teratoma, endodermal sinus tumour, embryonal carcinoma, and dysgerminoma is more frequent. It has a worse prognosis compared to gestational choriocarcinoma [24].

Considering trophoblastic cells have a natural ability to penetrate and destroy artery walls, the metastasis is predominantly haemorrhagic [24, 25]. On histomorphology, differentiating non-gestational choriocarcinoma with gestational choriocarcinoma is impossible until there is confirmation of pregnancy or another germ cell malignancy. The prognosis of gestational as well as non-gestational choriocarcinoma is established by DNA polymorphism analysis utilizing two or three relevant VNTR loci from tumour and the patient for paternal sequence identification [26]. The tumour is usually big, with a solid or solid and cystic cut surface, and haemorrhage and necrosis are prevalent. Microscopically, mononucleate trophoblastic cells and syncytiotrophoblastic cells are organized in a plexiform pattern, which is frequently accompanied with haemorrhage [10].

1.6 Polyembryoma

Ovarian polyembryoma is a very unusual germ cell tumour that contains embryoid entities that look very similar to embryos morphologically. Ovarian polyembryoma is identified with common malignant germ cell components such as dysgerminoma, endodermal sinus tumour, embryonal carcinoma, and predominantly immature teratoma [27].

1.7 Mixed Germ Cell Tumour

A combination of dysgerminoma and endodermal sinus tumour is the most prevalent mixed germ cell tumour, representing one-third over all cases. In decreasing order of frequency, choriocarcinoma and immature teratoma are amongst the others. They can rarely be combined with ovarian sex cord stromal tumours [28].

2 Presentation and Investigation

Ovarian germ cell tumours grow rapidly, however, most patients present with disease confined to single ovary [29]. Bilateral involvement may occur which may or may not be due to metastasis. Enlargement of the other ovary may be due to benign cystic teratoma, dysgerminoma, or a tumour with components of dysgerminoma. Patients typically present with abdominal enlargement due to the mass itself or presence of ascites. As the tumours have rapid growth approximately patients may present with acute abdomen due to rupture, haemorrhage, or torsion of the ovarian tumour [30]. Less commonly there may be evidence of precocious puberty or abnormal vaginal bleeding which may be related to hCG production [31]. Initial evaluation of a patient is a thorough history and physical examination. Presence of enlarged solid ovarian mass with heterogenous echotexture is diagnostic of germ cell tumour (Fig. 6). There may be associated ascites in advanced disease.

To help identify women with GCTs, alpha-fetoprotein and human chorionic gonadotrophin (hCG) serum levels should be examined if imaging suggests a malignant germ cell tumour. The current Royal College of Obstetricians and Gynaecologists Green-top Guideline for ovarian masses in premenopausal women advises determination of serum lactic dehydrogenase (LDH), AFP, and hCG in all women aged under 40 years [2]. To rule out distant metastases, a CT scan of the abdomen and pelvis, and then an X-ray of the chest, is advised. Karyotyping is advised if dysgenetic gonads are anticipated based on physical findings and the history of primary amenorrhea.

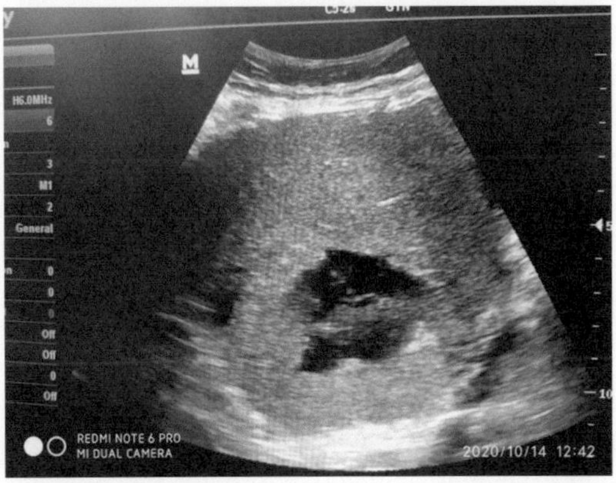

Fig. 6 USG showing enlarged solid ovarian mass with heterogenous echotexture

3 Surgical Management

Studies have shown that although germ cell tumours are large, approximately 60% are confined to the ovary [3, 32–34]. Surgical intervention is usually required for adnexal masses measuring 2 cm or more in premenarchal girls or complex masses measuring 8 cm or more in premenopausal patients [35]. Any patient with a complex adnexal mass who is suspected of having an early-stage germ cell tumour should be surgically staged. According to the current criteria provided by the International Federation of Gynaecology and Obstetrics (FIGO), they are staged similarly to epithelial ovarian tumours [36]. In addition, considering the disease's sensitivity to chemotherapy, fertility-sparing cytoreductive surgery is considered to be an effective first-line therapeutic option for patients with advanced stage cancer. In individuals with significant disease, where early debulking is not an option due to poor general health or clinical findings indicating an elevated risk of surgical morbidity, NACT followed by interval fertility sparing surgery may be an acceptable option [37].

Like epithelial ovarian cancer, the involved ovary should be removed and sent for frozen section. If malignancy is confirmed on frozen section, full surgical staging should be performed which includes peritoneal washings, infracolic omentectomy, biopsies of the diaphragmatic peritoneum, paracolic gutters, and pelvic peritoneum. In case of laparoscopic surgery, care must be taken to deliver the specimen intact using an endobag. However, unlike epithelial ovarian cancer the role of comprehensive surgical staging with retroperitoneal pelvic and paraaortic lymphadenectomy is not clear. Study by Billmere et al. has shown that paediatric ovarian malignant germ cell tumour (stages I–IV) has excellent survival with conservative surgical resection and platinum-based chemotherapy. In the paediatric age group, they suggested a more conservative surgical staging approach that included removing the affected ovary, palpating the retroperitoneal lymph nodes, and only excising firm or enlarged nodes, as well as any suspicious lesions in the abdomen and pelvis, rather than a complete lymphadenectomy [38]. Similar findings have also been reported by other studies which also included adult population [39–42].

Cystectomy is not recommended unless benign cystic teratoma is detected in the opposite ovary which may occur in 10% of cases [43, 44]. Biopsy of opposite ovary may result in future infertility resulting from adhesions or ovarian failure [45]. However, if the contralateral ovary appears abnormally enlarged, a biopsy or ovarian cystectomy should be performed. In the case of dysgerminoma, biopsy may be considered, because occult metastasis occurs in a small percentage of patients [46].

In the case of bilateral malignant ovarian germ cell tumours there are no data regarding the ability of chemotherapy to cure the tumour. In such cases, preservation of even a small part of the ovary is very likely to result in residual disease. Studies of gonadal preservation in case of bilateral involvement has shown a high rate of recurrence [47, 48]. The decision to preserve an involved ovary is difficult and must be made carefully considering patients' wishes. In the instance of bilateral ovarian involvement, uterine preservation may be considered following counselling for assisted reproduction with donor oocyte later on in life. Women who have done childbearing or who have gonadal dysgenesis, staging with bilateral salpingo-oophorectomy and hysterectomy is advised.

3.1 Second Look Laparotomy

The role of second-look surgery for ovarian germ cell tumour has been investigated in several studies, including the GOG trials. In the most of patients, the outcomes of the research did not justify the use of a second look procedure [3, 49–51]. Considering the potential of growing teratoma syndrome, patients with incompletely resected illness upon diagnosis, particularly those including teratomatous features, may benefit from growing teratoma syndrome [52–55].

3.2 The Role of Salvage Surgery

A small proportion of patients have chemorefractory disease and thus will not be candidates for salvage chemotherapy. Based on the experience from testicular germ cell malignancies, there is a large evidence base for the role of salvage surgery. Studies have shown a survival benefit with salvage surgery, particularly for immature teratoma [56–58].

4 Chemotherapy

Chemotherapy for malignant germ cell tumours of the ovary has been mostly drawn from the research on testicular cancer [59]. Except for individuals with stage IA grade 1 immature teratoma and stage IA and IB dysgerminoma, all patients should get adjuvant chemotherapy. According to studies, the BEP protocol is associated with a disease-free survival rate ranging from 79 to 96% and is indicated as the choice for the adjuvant therapy [60, 61] (Table 2). Acute and late-onset pulmonary toxicity, an increased chance of developing hematologic malignancies, and a danger of long-term renal and neurotoxicity from cisplatin are some of the toxicities associated with BEP. In patients who are unable to receive bleomycin, etoposide and carboplatin (EP) may be considered [62].

Table 2 BEP regimen for germ cell tumour ovary

Bleomycin etoposide cisplatin(BEP) regimen
• Bleomycin 30 U/mg IV bolus on days 1, 8, 15
• Etoposide 100 mg/m^2/day IV on days 1–5
• Cisplatin 20 mg/m^2/day IV on days 1–5

This regimen is administered for 3–4 cycles at 21-days intervals

4.1 Chemotherapy for Relapsed Disease

Around 20% of advanced germ cell tumours would become drug resistant or recur at a later stage [60]. BEP is the preferred treatment for people who have never had chemotherapy before. The salvage therapy regimen is determined by the past chemotherapy and the period between chemotherapy and relapse. Treatment failures can be classified as platinum sensitive or platinum resistant, akin to testicular cancer, considering the time between chemotherapy and relapse [63].

Platinum sensitive recurrence is characterized as a relapse that develops more than 4 weeks post-chemotherapy. Salvage chemotherapy regimens include ifosfamide and platinum, with or without paclitaxel, and are based on those being used testicular germ cell tumours. After initial BEP, the most widely utilized regimens are VeIP and TIP [64, 65]. Second-line treatment with VeIP/VIP produces a 36–56% complete response (CR) in testicular tumours, and TIP has a high CR rate about 70% [66]. VAC, AC, PVB, and VIP regimens have been phased out in favour of the newer regimens, despite the fact that they have been proven to be beneficial in the past. PVB and POMB-ACE have proven successful as salvage chemotherapy after previous irradiation and chemotherapy in a limited number of patients [67].

Maintaining with testicular cancer treatment approach, high dose chemotherapy (HDCT) with stem cell support may be regarded as a third-line therapeutic approach for patients who are experiencing an incomplete response or relapse after second-line conventional-dose chemotherapy, though evidence of such an approach in MOGCT is lacking [68, 69].

When a marker-negative complete response is not achieved after first-line treatment or when a good response is not reached following salvage treatment, testicular cancer is considered platinum refractory [70]. It is deemed unfavourable if patient's relapse within 4 weeks of finishing cisplatin chemotherapy. After cisplatin-based combinations and high-dose chemotherapy fail, treatment choices are restricted. With objective responses of 10–37%, several traditional single-agents such as paclitaxel, gemcitabine, oxaliplatin, oral etoposide, ifosfamide, and temozolomide were administered, but full responses and long-term remissions were rare [71, 72]. Due to their young age, lack of comorbidities, and maintained organ functioning, platinum-refractory patients are commonly eligible for additional combination chemotherapy treatments despite rigorous pre-treatment.

One of the most effective therapies to date is a triple-combination of gemcitabine, oxaliplatin, and paclitaxel, which could result in long-term remissions in 11% of patients when paired with later resection of residual masses [73]. For individuals who have failed first-line systemic treatment, salvage high-dose chemotherapy followed by autologous stem cell transplantation is a viable therapeutic option [74]. The benefit of dose-intensified treatment, on the other hand, is less evident for patients who have failed conventional dosage salvage treatment.

5 Prognosis and Post-treatment Issues

The long-term prognosis of malignant ovarian germ cell tumours is much better than epithelial ovarian cancer. The 5-year survival in almost 98% in stage IA disease [75]. However, survival depends on the age at presentation, stage, histology, and resectability of the tumour. In premenarchal girls and women more than 45 years, it is associated with a bad prognosis [76].

Tumours bigger than 10–15 cm diameter, age younger than 20 years, and microscopic characteristics such as numerous mitoses, anaplasia, as well as a medullary pattern have all been linked to a higher risk of recurrence in dysgerminoma [35].

Non-dysgerminomatous tumours with either metastasis beyond the lung, lymph nodes, and peritoneum or those with an AFP level of more than 10,000 ng/mL, hCG more than 50,000 mIU/mL, LDH more than ten times upper limit of normal are considered poor-risk groups and these patients may potentially benefit from more intensive chemotherapy [76–79].

Premature ovarian failure may result from chemotherapy; however, most women who receive platinum-based therapy for 3–4 cycles recover normal ovarian function and preserved fertility [80, 81]. However, premature menopause has been reported in women who received chemotherapy as children, adolescents, or young adults [82]. Many recommend gonadotropin-releasing hormone agonists (GnRHa) for ovarian function protection during chemotherapy, though its efficacy is still controversial [83, 84]. The decision concerning the use of assisted reproductive techniques before initiation of chemotherapy should be individualized and balanced against the delay in starting therapy. A significant late sequalae of chemotherapy is the development of secondary malignancies, both solid tumours and leukaemia and the risk is dose-related. Etoposide is considered as the main factor with the incidence of leukaemia being 0.5% with cumulative etoposide dose less than 2000 mg/m^2 and 5% with dose 2000 mg/m^2 and above [85]. Regardless of the risk of secondary leukaemia, risk–benefit assessments have reported benefits of etoposide-containing chemotherapy regimens in advanced MOGCTs.

6 Follow-up

Approximately, 75% of GCT relapses occur during the first year of treatment; one of the most prevalent regions is the peritoneal cavity, with retroperitoneal lymph nodes occurring lower frequently. The upper abdomen (55–70%) and also the pelvis (30–45%) are the most common recurrence sites [86]. Dysgerminoma could occur in 5–10% of women whose contralateral ovary has been retained over the next 2 years [87]. The most common and effective imaging procedures used to assess the response of chemotherapy in patients with detectable illness are a CT scan of the abdomen, pelvis, and chest (in patient with suspected lung metastases) and pelvic ultrasound. Inferring from seminoma testes' expertise PET-CT should be investigated in individuals who have bulky residual masses larger than 3 cm following treatment for more than 4 weeks [88]. If the PET–CT scans are positive or there is a hint of progressing disease on the images, histologic confirmation of residual disease is preferred before starting salvage therapy. The frequency of patient follow-up is determined by the tumour's histology. Physical examinations and serum indicators (if initially elevated) must be performed in 2–3 months during the first year of treatment, then 3–4 months during the second year of treatment and, then in 6 months from 3 to 5 year of treatment, and thereafter annually for 5 years for patients with Dysgerminoma. For women with non-dysgerminomatous germ cell tumours, physical examination and serum markers should be performed every 2 months during year 1–2, every 4–6 months during year 3, every 6 months during year 4–5, then annually after 5 years. CECT abdomen and pelvis must be undertaken after 3–4 months in the first year of treatment, every 4 to 6 months in the second year of treatment, every 6–12 months in the third to fifth year of treatment, and as clinically recommended beyond 5 years of treatment. During 1–2 year a chest X-ray can also be conducted [89, 90].

7 Conclusion

The current first-line chemotherapy cures the majority of advanced MOGCTs. However, 20–30% of individuals will face a relapse, necessitating second-line treatment. The best first-line therapy for salvage remains uncertain due to a paucity of randomized research. It is debatable if sequential high-dose chemotherapy (HDCT) or the conventional-dose chemotherapy (CDCT) would be the best treatment option for patients who progress following first-line treatment. In the future, the question might be answered by the ongoing TIGER trial which will establish which technique is most effective and safe.

References

1. Tewari K, Cappuccini F, Disaia PJ, Berman ML, Manetta A, Kohler MF. Malignant germ cell tumors of the ovary. Obstet Gynecol. 2000;95(1):128–33.
2. Royal College of Obstetricians and Gynaecologists. Management of female malignant ovarian germ cell tumours. Sci Impact Pap no 52; 2016. p. 1–10.
3. Gershenson DM. Management of ovarian germ cell tumors. J Clin Oncol. 2007;25(20):2938–43.
4. Looijenga LHJ, Zafarna G, Grygalewicz B, Summersgill B, et al. Role of gain of 12p in germ cell tumour development. APMIS. 2003;111(1):161–73.
5. Chaganti RSK, Rodriguez E, Mathew S. Origin of adult male mediastinal germ-cell tumours. Lancet. 1994;343(8906):1130–2.
6. Roth LM, Talerman A. Recent advances in the pathology and classification of ovarian germ cell tumors. Int J Gynecol Pathol. 2006;25(4):305–20.
7. Cossu-Rocca P, Zhang S, Roth LM, Eble JN, Zheng W, Abdul Karim FW, et al. Chromosome 12p abnormalities in dysgerminoma of the ovary: a FISH analysis. Mod Pathol. 2006;19(4):611–5.
8. Van Nieuwenhuysen E, Busschaert P, Neven P, Han SN, Moerman P, Liontos M, et al. The genetic landscape of 87 ovarian germ cell tumors. Gynecol Oncol. 2018;151(1):61–8.
9. King ME, DiGiovanni LM, Yung J-F, Clarke-Pearson DL. Immature teratoma of the ovary grade 3, with karyotype analysis. Int J Gynecol Pathol. 1990;9(2):178–84.
10. World Health Organization, International Agency for Research on Cancer (IARC), WHO Classification of Tumours Editorial Board. WHO classification of tumours: female genital tumours, vol. 4. 5th ed. Lyon: IARC; 2020.
11. Chen Y, Luo Y, Han C, Tian W, Yang W, Wang Y, et al. Ovarian dysgerminoma in pregnancy: a case report and literature review. Cancer Biol Ther. 2018;19(8):649–58.
12. Michael KK, Wampler K, Underwood J, Hansen C. Ovarian dysgerminoma: a case study. J Diagn Med Sonogr. 2015;31(5):327–30.
13. Zogbi L, Gonçalves CV, Tejada VF, Martins D, Karam F, Machado dos Santos S, et al. Treatment of bilateral ovarian dysgerminoma with 11-year follow-up: a case report. Ann Med Surg. 2018;33:50–2.
14. Schellhas HF. Malignant potential of the dysgenetic gonad: Part I. Obstet Gynecol. 1974;44(2):298–309.
15. Schwartz PE, Morris JM. Serum lactic dehydrogenase: A tumor marker for dysgerminoma. Obstet Gynecol. 1988;72(3):511–5.
16. Trinh DT, Shibata K, Hirosawa T, Umezu T, Mizuno M, Kajiyama H, et al. Diagnostic utility of CD117, CD133, SALL4, OCT4, TCL1 and glypican-3 in malignant germ cell tumors of the ovary. J Obstet Gynaecol Res. 2012;38(5):841–8.
17. Rabban JT, Zaloudek CJ. A practical approach to immunohistochemical diagnosis of ovarian germ cell tumours and sex cord-stromal tumours. Histopathology. 2013;62(1):71–88.
18. Smith HO, Berwick M, Verschraegen CF, Wiggins C, Lansing L, Muller CY, et al. Incidence and survival rates for female malignant germ cell tumors. Obstet Gynecol. 2006;107(5):1075–85.

19. Cao D, Guo S, Allan RW, Molberg KH, Peng Y. SALL4 is a novel sensitive and specific marker of ovarian primitive germ cell tumors and is particularly useful in distinguishing yolk sac tumor from clear cell carcinoma. Am J Surg Pathol. 2009;33(6):894–904.
20. Kaur B. Pathology of malignant ovarian germ cell tumours. Diagn Histopathol. 2020;26(6):289–97.
21. Kurman RJ, Norris HJ. Embryonal carcinoma of the ovary. A clinicopathologic entity distinct from endodermal sinus tumor resembling embryonal carcinoma of the adult testis. Cancer. 1976;38(6):2420–33.
22. Lau SK, Weiss LM, Chu PG. D2-40 immunohistochemistry in the differential diagnosis of seminoma and embryonal carcinoma: a comparative immunohistochemical study with KIT (CD117) and CD30. Mod Pathol. 2007;20(3):320–5.
23. Cheng L. Establishing a germ cell origin for metastatic tumors using OCT4 immunohistochemistry. Cancer. 2004;101(9):2006–10.
24. Rao KVLN, Konar S, Gangadharan J, Vikas V, Sampath S. A pure non-gestational ovarian choriocarcinoma with delayed solitary brain metastases: case report and review of the literature. J Neurosci Rural Pract. 2015;6(4):578–81.
25. Goswami D, Sharma K, Zutshi V, Tempe A, Nigam S. Nongestational pure ovarian choriocarcinoma with contralateral teratoma. Gynecol Oncol. 2001;80(2):262–6.
26. Tsujioka H, Hamada H, Miyakawa T, Hachisuga T, Kawarabayashi T. A pure nongestational choriocarcinoma of the ovary diagnosed with DNA polymorphism analysis. Gynecol Oncol. 2003;89(3):540–2.
27. Takemori M, Nishimura R, Yamasaki M, Kawabe Y, Hasegawa K. Ovarian mixed germ cell tumor composed of polyembryoma and immature teratoma. Gynecol Oncol. 1998;69(3):260–3.
28. Goyal LD, Kaur S, Kawatra K. Malignant mixed germ cell tumour of ovary—an unusual combination and review of literature. J Ovarian Res. 2014;7(1):1–4.
29. Zamani N, Rezaei Poor M, Ghasemian Dizajmehr S, Alizadeh S, Modares GM. Fertility sparing surgery in malignant ovarian germ cell tumor (MOGCT): 15 years experiences. BMC Womens Health. 2021;21(1):1–7.
30. Pectasides D, Pectasides E, Kassanos D. Germ cell tumors of the ovary. Cancer Treat Rev. 2008;34:427–41.
31. Rana AN, Humad H, Muhammad Asif A, Ghannam D, Nadeem N. Germ cell tumor presenting with precocious puberty in a girl in United Arab Emirates. Dubai Med J. 2020;3(1):32–6.
32. Jorge S, Jones NL, Chen L, Hou JY, Tergas AI, Burke WM, et al. Characteristics, treatment and outcomes of women with immature ovarian teratoma, 1998–2012. Gynecol Oncol. 2016;142(2):261–6.
33. Kurman RJ, Norris HJ. Endodermal sinus tumor of the ovary. A clinical and pathologic analysis of 71 cases. Cancer. 1976;38(6):2404–19.
34. Jimerson GK, Woodruff JD. Ovarian extraembryonal teratoma. I. Endodermal sinus tumor. Am J Obstet Gynecol. 1977;127(1):73–9.
35. Berek JS, HackerNF HT. Gynecologic Oncology. 6th ed. Philadelphia: Lippincott Williams & Wilkins; 2015. p. 518p.
36. Prat J, Belhadj H, Berek J, Bermudez A, Bhatla N, Cain J, et al. Figo's staging classification for cancer of the ovary, fallopian tube, and peritoneum: abridged republication. J Gynecol Oncol. 2015;26(2):87–9.
37. Li J, Wu X. Current strategy for the treatment of ovarian germ cell tumors: role of extensive surgery. Curr Treat Options in Oncol. 2016;17(8):44.
38. Billmire DF, Vinocur C, Rescorla F, Cushing B, London W, Schlatter M, et al. Outcome and staging evaluation in malignant germ cell tumors of the ovary in children and adolescents: an intergroup study. J Pediatr Surg. 2004;39(3):424–9.
39. Qin B, Xu W, Li Y. Are omentectomy and lymphadenectomy necessary in patients with apparently early-stage malignant ovarian germ cell tumors? Int J Gynecol Cancer. 2019;29(2):398–403.
40. Mahdi H, Swensen RE, Hanna R, Kumar S, Ali-Fehmi R, Semaan A, et al. Prognostic impact of lymphadenectomy in clinically early stage malignant germ cell tumour of the ovary. Br J Cancer. 2011;105:493–7.
41. Göbel U, Schneider DT, Calaminus G, Haas RJ, Schmidt P, Harms D. Germ-cell tumors in childhood and adolescence. Ann Oncol. 2000;11(3):263–71.
42. Baranzelli MC, Bouffet E, Quintana E, Portas M, Thyss A, Patte C. Non-seminomatous ovarian germ cell tumours in children. Eur J Cancer. 2000;36(3):376–83.
43. Low JJH, Ilancheran A, Ng JS. Malignant ovarian germ-cell tumours. Best Pract Res Clin Obstet Gynaecol. 2012;26(3):347–55.
44. Low JJH, Perrin LC, Crandon AJ, Hacker NF. Conservative surgery to preserve ovarian function in patients with malignant ovarian germ cell tumors: a review of 74 cases. Cancer. 2000;89(2):391–8.
45. Buttram VC, Vaquero C. Post-ovarian wedge resection adhesive disease. Fertil Steril. 1975;26(9):874–6.
46. Schwartz PE, Chambers SK, Chambers JT, Kohorn E, McIntosh S. Ovarian germ cell malignancies: the Yale University experience. Gynecol Oncol. 1992;45(1):26–31.
47. Gomes PJ, Rustin GJS. Attempted preservation of one gonad in patients with bilateral germ cell tumours. Clin Oncol. 1996;8(6):397–9.
48. Zhao T, Liu Y, Jiang H, Zhang H, Lu Y. Management of bilateral malignant ovarian germ cell tumors: experience of a single institute. Mol Clin Oncol. 2016;5(2):383–7.
49. Williams SD, Blessing JA, DiSaia PJ, Major FJ, Ball HG, Liao SY. Second-look laparotomy in ovarian germ cell tumors: the gynecologic oncology group experience. Gynecol Oncol. 1994;52(3):287–91.
50. Williams S, Blessing JA, Liao SY, Ball H, Hanjani P. Adjuvant therapy of ovarian germ cell tumors with cisplatin, etoposide, and bleomycin: a trial of the gynecologic oncology group. J Clin Oncol. 1994;12(4):701–6.

51. Gershenson DM, Copeland LJ, Del Junco G, Edwards CL, Wharton JT, Rutledge FN. Second-look laparotomy in the management of malignant germ cell tumors of the ovary. Obstet Gynecol. 1986;67(6):789–93.
52. Logothetis CJ, Samuels ML, Trindade A, Johnson DE. The growing teratoma syndrome. Cancer. 1982;50(8):1629–35.
53. Willis GW, Hajdu SI. Histologically benign teratoid metastasis of testicular embryonal carcinoma: report of five cases. Am J Clin Pathol. 1973;59(3):338–43.
54. Merrin C, BaumBenigngartner G, Wajsman Z. Benign transformation of testicular carcinoma by chemotherapy. Lancet. 1975;305(7897):43–4.
55. Amsalem H, Nadjari M, Prus D, Hiller N, Benshushan A. Growing teratoma syndrome vs. chemotherapeutic retroconversion: case report and review of the literature. Gynecol Oncol. 2004;92(1):357–60.
56. Munkarah A, Gershenson DM, Levenback C, Silva EG, Messing MJ, Morris M, et al. Salvage surgery for chemorefractory ovarian germ cell tumors. Gynecol Oncol. 1994;55(2):217–23.
57. Rezk Y, Sheinfeld J, Chi DS. Prolonged survival following salvage surgery for chemorefractory ovarian immature teratoma: a case report and review of the literature. Gynecol Oncol. 2005;96(3):883–7.
58. Wu X, Han LY, Xu X, Li Z. Recurrent immature teratoma of the ovary: a case report of radical secondary cytoreduction with replacement of the aortic bifurcation. Gynecol Oncol. 2004;95(3):746–9.
59. Uccello M, Boussios S, Samartzis EP, Moschetta M. Systemic anti-cancer treatment in malignant ovarian germ cell tumours (MOGCTs): current management and promising approaches. Ann Transl Med. 2020;8(24):1713.
60. Dimopoulos MA, Papadimitriou C, Hamilos G, Efstathiou E, Vlahos G, Rodolakis A, et al. Treatment of ovarian germ cell tumors with a 3-day bleomycin, etoposide, and cisplatin regimen: a prospective multicenter study. Gynecol Oncol. 2004;95(3):695–700.
61. Horwich A, Sleijfer DT, Fosså SD, Kaye SB, Oliver RT, Cullen MH, Mead GM, Wit RD, De Mulder PH, Dearnaley DPCP. Randomized trial of bleomycin, etoposide, and cisplatin compared with bleomycin, etoposide, and carboplatin in good-prognosis metastatic nonseminomatous germ cell cancer: a multi-institutional Medical Research Council/European Organization for Research and. J Clin Oncol. 1997;15(5):1844–52.
62. Simone CG, Markham MJ, Dizon DS. Chemotherapy in ovarian germ cell tumors: a systematic review. Gynecol Oncol. 2016;141(3):602–7.
63. Parkinson CA, Hatcher HM, Earl HM, Ajithkumar TV. Multidisciplinary management of malignant ovarian germ cell tumours. Gynecol Oncol. 2011;121(3):625–36.
64. Loehrer PJ, Gonin R, Nichols CR, Weathers T, Einhorn LH. Vinblastine plus ifosfamide plus cisplatin as initial salvage therapy in recurrent germ cell tumor. J Clin Oncol. 1998;16(7):2500–4.
65. McCaffrey JA, Mazumdar M, Bajorin DF, Bosl GJ, Vlamis V, Motzer RJ. Ifosfamide- and cisplatin-containing chemotherapy as first-line salvage therapy in germ cell tumors: response and survival. J Clin Oncol. 1997;15(7):2559–63.
66. Mead GM, Cullen MH, Huddart R, Harper P, Rustin GJS, Cook PA, et al. A phase II trial of TIP (paclitaxel, ifosfamide and cisplatin) given as second-line (post-BEP) salvage chemotherapy for patients with metastatic germ cell cancer: a medical research council trial. Br J Cancer. 2005;93(2):178–84.
67. Bower M, Newlands ES, Holden L, Rustin GJS, Begent RHJ. Treatment of men with metastatic non-seminomatous germ cell tumours with cyclical POMB/ACE chemotherapy. Ann Oncol. 1997;8(5):477–83.
68. Broun ER, Nichols CR, Gize G, Cornetta K, Hromas RA, Schacht B, et al. Tandem high dose chemotherapy with autologous bone marrow transplantation for initial relapse of testicular germ cell cancer. Cancer. 1997;79(8):1605–10. [cited 2020 Nov 17]. Available from: https://pubmed.ncbi.nlm.nih.gov/19822531/
69. De Giorgi U, Richard S, Badoglio M, Kanfer E, Bourrhis JH, Nicolas-Virelizier E, et al. Salvage high-dose chemotherapy in female patients with relapsed/refractory germ-cell tumors: a retrospective analysis of the European Group for Blood and Marrow Transplantation (EBMT). Ann Oncol. 2017;28(8):1910–6.
70. Schmoll HJ, Jordan K, Huddart R, Pes MPL, Horwich A, Fizazi K, et al. Testicular seminoma: ESMO clinical practice guidelines for diagnosis, treatment and follow-up. Ann Oncol. 2010;21(Suppl. 5):140–6.
71. Porcu P, Bhatia S, Sharma M, Einhorn LH. Results of treatment after relapse from high-dose chemotherapy in germ cell tumors. J Clin Oncol. 2000;18(6):1181–6.
72. Kollmannsberger C, Honecker F, Bokemeyer C. Pharmacotherapy of relapsed metastatic testicular cancer. Expert Opin Pharmacother. 2008;9(13):2259–72.
73. Bokemeyer C, Oechsle K, Honecker F, Mayer F, Hartmann JT, Waller CF, et al. Combination chemotherapy with gemcitabine, oxaliplatin, and paclitaxel in patients with cisplatin-refractory or multiply relapsed germ-cell tumors: A study of the German Testicular Cancer Study Group. Ann Oncol. 2008;19(3):448–53.
74. Lorch A, Neubauer A, Hackenthal M, Dieing A, Hartmann JT, Rick O, et al. High-dose chemotherapy (HDCT) as second-salvage treatment in patients with multiple relapsed or refractory germ-cell tumors. Ann Oncol. 2009;21(4):820–5.
75. Guo H, Chen H, Wang W, Chen L. Clinicopathological features, prognostic factors, survival trends, and treatment of malignant ovarian germ cell tumors: A SEER Database Analysis. Oncol Res Treat. 2021;44(4):145–53.
76. Meisel JL, Woo KM, Sudarsan N, Eng J, Patil S, Jacobsen EP, et al. Development of a risk stratification system to guide treatment for female germ cell tumors. Gynecol Oncol. 2015;138(3):566.

77. De La Motte RT, Pautier P, Rey A, Duvillard P, Kerbrat P, Troalen F, et al. Prognostic factors in women treated for ovarian yolk sac tumour: a retrospective analysis of 84 cases. Eur J Cancer. 2011;47(2):175–82.
78. Solheim O, Gershenson DM, Tropé CG, Rokkones E, Sun CC, Weedon-Fekjaer H, et al. Prognostic factors in malignant ovarian germ cell tumours (the surveillance, epidemiology and end results experience 1978-2010). Eur J Cancer. 2014;50(11):1942–50.
79. Murugaesu N, Schmid P, Dancey G, Agarwal R, Holden L, McNeish I, et al. Malignant ovarian germ cell tumors: identification of novel prognostic markers and long-term outcome after multimodality treatment. J Clin Oncol. 2006;24(30):4862–6.
80. Gershenson DM, Miller AM, Champion VL, Monahan PO, Zhao Q, Cella D, et al. Reproductive and sexual function after platinum-based chemotherapy in long-term ovarian germ cell tumor survivors: a Gynecologic Oncology Group Study. J Clin Oncol. 2007;25(19):2792–7.
81. Maltaris T, Boehm D, Dittrich R, Seufert R, Koelbl H. Reproduction beyond cancer: a message of hope for young women. Gynecol Oncol. 2006;103(3):1109–21.
82. Sklar CA, Mertens AC, Mitby P, Whitton J, Stovall M, Kasper C, et al. Premature menopause in survivors of childhood cancer: a report from the childhood cancer survivor study. J Natl Cancer Inst. 2006;98(13):890–6.
83. Oktay K, Harvey BE, Partridge AH, Quinn GP, Reinecke J, Taylor HS, et al. Fertility preservation in patients with cancer: ASCO Clinical Practice Guideline Update. J Clin Oncol. 2018;36(19):1994–2001. [cited 2022 Jan 27]. Available from: https://pubmed.ncbi.nlm.nih.gov/29620997/
84. Demeestere I, Brice P, Peccatori FA, Kentos A, Dupuis J, Zachee P, et al. No evidence for the benefit of gonadotropin-releasing hormone agonist in preserving ovarian function and fertility in lymphoma survivors treated with chemotherapy: final long-term report of a prospective randomized trial. J Clin Oncol. 2016;34(22):2568–74.
85. Pedersen-Bjergaard J, Daugaard G, Hansen SW, Philip P, Larsen SO, Rørth M. Increased risk of myelodysplasia and leukaemia after etoposide, cisplatin, and bleomycin for germ-cell tumours. Lancet. 1991;338(8763):359–63.
86. Colombo N, Peiretti M, Castiglione M. Non-epithelial ovarian cancer: ESMO clinical recommendations for diagnosis, treatment and follow-up. Ann Oncol. 2009;20(Suppl. 4):iv24–6.
87. Behtash N, Zarchi MK. Dysgerminoma in three patients with Swyer syndrome. World J Surg Oncol. 2007;23(5):71.
88. Bilen MA, Hariri H, Leon C, Guo CC, Kuban DA, Pisters LL, et al. Positive FDG-PET/CT scans of a residual seminoma after chemotherapy and radiotherapy: case report and review of the literature. Clin Genitourin Cancer. 2014;12:e147–50.
89. Salani R, Khanna N, Frimer M, Bristow RE, Chen L, may. An update on post-treatment surveillance and diagnosis of recurrence in women with gynecologic malignancies: Society of Gynecologic Oncology (SGO) recommendations. Gynecol Oncol. 2017;146(1):3–10. [cited 2022 Jan 27]. Available from: https://pubmed.ncbi.nlm.nih.gov/28372871/
90. NCCN.org. NCCN Clinical Practice Guidelines in Oncology (NCCN Guidelines®) NCCN Guidelines for Patients® [cited 2022 Jan 27]; Available from: www.nccn.org/patients

Stromal Tumour of Ovary

Upasana Baruah, Santosh Menon,
Amal Chandra Kataki, and Debabrata Barmon

1 Introduction

Ovarian sex cord-stromal tumours (SCSTs) comprise both benign and malignant tumours. The majority are benign or of low malignant potential and have a long-term favourable prognosis but, a subset of these may have an aggressive course. Few of these tumours have the potential to produce a variety of steroid hormones with their consequent clinical manifestations. Therefore, adequate knowledge of the pathogenesis and clinical manifestation of these tumours is a prerequisite in diagnosing and managing these tumours. These are rare neoplasms that primarily present before 40 years of age. Adult granulosa cell tumours, however, typically present later, at around 50–55 years [1].

Being rare, there is paucity of data on these tumours as compared to epithelial ovarian cancers. Neoplastic transformation of mesenchymal and mesonephric elements of the ovary is the putative precursor of these tumours. Granulosa and Sertoli cells are homologous and are derived from the sex cord cells, whereas the pluripotent mesenchymal cells are the precursors of theca cells, leydig cells, and fibroblasts [2].

Recent studies have delineated the key genetic events associated with these tumours and have provided valuable insight into their pathogenesis. Also, certain syndromes associated with SCST, namely Peutz-Jeghers Syndrome, Ollier disease, Maffucci syndrome, and DICER1 syndrome have been characterized in recent years.

Peutz-Jeghers Syndrome is caused by autosomal dominant germline mutations in the STK 11 gene on chromosome 19. It is characterized by the pigmentation of the lips, buccal mucosa, hamartomatous polys in GI tract and may include benign and malignant tumours of various organs [3, 4]. *Ollier disease and Maffucci syndrome are rare inherited disorders characterized by enchondroma. Both are frequently associated with Juvenile granulosa cell tumours* [5, 6]. *Whereas Ollier disease is associated with multiple enchondromas at multiple sites, in Maffucci syndrome, these are associated with multiple soft tissue haemangiomata. Isocitrate dehydrogenase gene mutations are present in enchondroma in both Ollier disease and Maffucci syndrome* [7]. *DICER1 syndrome results from germline mutations in the DICER1 gene, which plays a fundamental role in processing microRNA to their mature forms and are associated with familial pleuro-pulmonary blastoma, ovarian Sertoli–*

U. Baruah (✉) · A. C. Kataki · D. Barmon
Department of Gynaecologic Oncology,
Dr. Bhubaneswar Borooah Cancer Institute
(A Unit of Tata Memorial Centre, Mumbai),
Guwahati, Assam, India
e-mail: dydiracademic@bbci.tmc.gov.in

S. Menon
Tata Memorial Centre, Mumbai,
Mumbai, Maharashtra, India

A. C. Kataki, D. Barmon (eds.), *Fundamentals in Gynaecologic Malignancy*,
https://doi.org/10.1007/978-981-19-5860-1_18

Table 1 Classification of sex cord-stromal tumours

Pure stromal tumours	Pure sex cord tumours	Mixed sex cord-stromal tumours
Fibroma NOS Cellular fibroma ThecomaNOS Thecoma luteinised Fibrosarcoma NOS Sclerosing stromal tumour Signet-ring stromal tumour Microcystic stromal tumour Leydig cell tumour NOS Steroid cell tumour NOS Steroid cell tumour, malignant	Adult granulosa cell tumour Juvenile granulosa cell tumour Sertoli cell tumour NOS Sex cord tumour with annular tubules	Sertoli–Leydig cell tumours • Well-differentiated • Moderately differentiated with heterologous elements • Poorly differentiated with heterologous elements • Retiform with heterologous elements Sex cord-stromal tumours NOS, NOS: Not otherwise specified

Leydig cell tumour, benign thyroid pathologies, and other tumours [8, 9].

Studies showing changes at a genomic level in ovarian sex cord-stromal tumours have primarily been restricted to adult granulosa cell tumours as they are the most common type of SCST [10]. Approximately 5–20% of granulosa cell tumours are aneuploid but this is not associated with the prognosis of the disease [10]. Approximately 30% of juvenile granulosa cell tumours contain the GSP oncogene's somatic mutation, while 60% are associated with mutation in the AKT gene [11, 12]. In adult granulosa cell tumours, a somatic mutation in the FOXL2 is found in almost all cases [13]. However, the role of molecular events on the stage, behaviour, and prognosis of adult granulosa cell tumours remains undetermined.

Ovarian SCCT are grouped into pure stromal, pure sex cord, and mixed sex cord-stromal tumours according to The World Health Organization (WHO) classification (Table 1) [14].

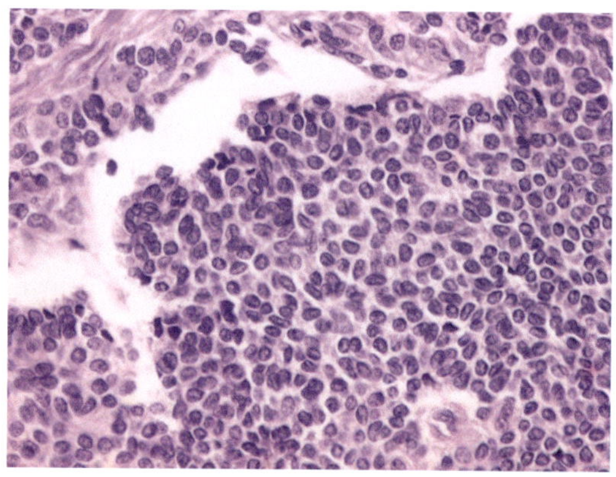

Fig. 1 Granulosa cell tumour, Adult: The tumour is composed of ovoid cells with pale nuclei and prominent nuclear grooves. (H and E ×200). The inhibin stain marks the tumour cells strongly (Indirect immunoperoxidase)

1.1 Pure Sex Cord Tumours

1.1.1 Granulosa Cell Tumours of the Ovary (GCT)

Granulosa cells comprise 70% of malignant / malignant potential sex cord stromal tumours of the ovary [15]. They originate from granulosa cells of preovulatory follicle and secrete oestrogen, inhibin, and Mullerian inhibiting substance. Inhibin B is the predominant form of inhibin secreted by granulosa cell tumours and has been reported to reflect disease status more accurately than inhibin A or total inhibin [16]. Delayed tumour recurrence and slow growth is characteristic of this disease. Oestrogen secretion may result in inappropriate pre-pubertal or postmenopausal estrogenization, causing precocious puberty and postmenopausal bleeding. Endometrial cancer may be present in 5–20% of cases [17].

Two subtypes of granulosa cells have been described based on clinical and histopathological characteristics, the juvenile and the adult form. The adult form is much more common and accounts for 95% of GCT [18].

Adult type (Fig. 1): Most patients present with abnormal vaginal bleeding, abdominal distention, and abdominal pain. Breast tenderness may be present due to hyperestrogenism. They are low grade and have a low clinical stage at presentation but have the potential for late recurrence. The median time of recurrence is 5 years after surgical treatment of the primary tumour. Still, numerous cases of recurrence are reported in the literature even after 20–30 years of initial diagnosis [19]. The majority are diagnosed with stage I disease with a 10-year survival rate of more than 80% [20, 21]. Grossly the tumours are usually between 5 and 15 cm, and more than 95% are unilateral. The cut surfaces are typically solid and cystic with fluid or blood-filled cysts separated by solid, yellow to white, soft to firm tissue. Microscopically they are characterized by diffuse, insular, trabecular, corded, nodular, follicular, and sarcomatoid patterns. The diffuse pattern is most common which is characterized by densely cellular sheets of cells with scant cytoplasm with small blue cell tumour appearance. The characteristic feature of tumour cells is the presence of longitudinal nuclear grooves/indentations with pale nuclei. The insular pattern has discrete nests usually surrounded by a conspicuous stroma. The microfollicular pattern is characterized by numerous small cavities (Call–Exner bodies) that contain eosinophilic fluid, degenerating nuclei, hyalinised basement membrane material, or rarely basophilic fluid. The macrofollicular pattern is characterized by cysts lined by well-differentiated granulosa cells. Water silk (moire silk), gyriform, or diffuse (sarcomatoid) patterns are uncommon [22].

Juvenile type (Fig. 2): Over 80% of juvenile granulosa cell tumours occur in the first two decades. Ten percent of cases present during pregnancy [23]. There may be clinical evidence of precocious puberty. Rarely a patient may present with virilization due to androgen secretion. Pain, dysuria, constipation, increasing abdominal girth are other symptoms. Acute abdominal symptoms from tumour rupture and hemoperitoneum occur in 10% of cases [24–26]. Although the adult form has a long latent period, the juvenile counterpart behaves aggressively if advanced. Recurrence is generally within 3 years of the initial diagnosis. The appearances of juvenile form are similar to the adult form with a solid and cystic appearance and presence of haemorrhagic fluid. Microscopically, the cells of juvenile granulosa cell tumours have rounded, hyperchromatic nuclei, with moderate to abundant eosinophilic or vacuolated (luteinized) cytoplasm. In contrast, the adult form has a more regular arrangement and pale grooved nuclei [27].

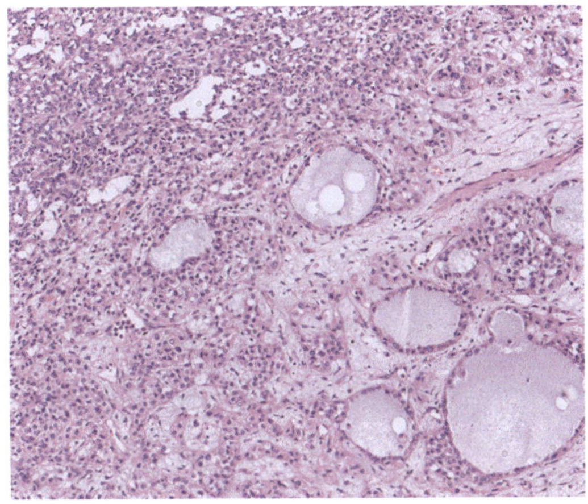

Fig. 2 Juvenile granulosa cell tumour showing the characteristic follicle-like spaces and sheets of monomorphic ovoid cells with scant to moderate eosinophilic cytoplasm. These cells seldom show nuclear groove which are seen in adult type granulosa cell tumour

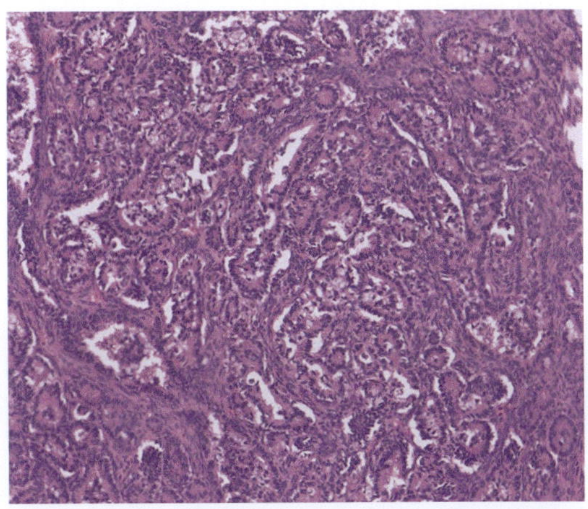

Fig. 3 Sertoli cell tumour, well differentiated: Tumour has a predominant tubular pattern and arrangement of cells with lumen. The individual cells appear pink eosinophilic, with inconspicuous mitosis.(H and E ×100)

1.1.2 Sertoli Cell Tumours

Sertoli cell tumours are rare and are present in women of reproductive age and sometimes in children (Fig. 3). They are hormonally active in approximately 40–60% of cases, and majority have estrogenic activity. Occasionally androgenic secretion may be present. The presence of isochromosome 1q is the sole chromosomal abnormality present in these tumours. Occasionally, it occurs in patients with Peutz–Jeghers syndrome. Most Sertoli cell tumours are stage I, unilateral and clinically benign, but higher stage is also documented which have adverse outcomes [28, 29].

1.1.3 Sex Cord-Stromal Tumours with Annular Tubules

Sex cord-stromal tumours with annular tubules develop in young patients with a mean age of 22 years. It can be either sporadic or associated with Peutz–Jeghers syndrome. When associated with Peutz–Jeghers syndrome (36%), the tumour is usually very small, benign, bilateral, or multifocal. On the other hand, sporadic cases are generally unilateral, large, and may have malignant potential [30, 31].

1.2 Pure Stromal Tumours

Fibromas commonly present after 40 years. They are the most common sex cord-stromal tumours and represents 4% of all ovarian neoplasms (Fig. 4) [32]. They are solid, benign, hormonally inactive tumours that arise from spindle-shaped stromal cells that form collagen. Fibromas are commonly unilateral; however, bilateral cases may occur. Sometimes, they are associated with nevoid basal cell carcinoma syndrome (Gorlin syndrome) [33]. It is asymptomatic when the lesion is small but can cause ovarian torsion as the size increases. It causes the classic Meigs' syndrome (hydrothorax, ascites, and fibroma), which typically disappears after surgery [34].

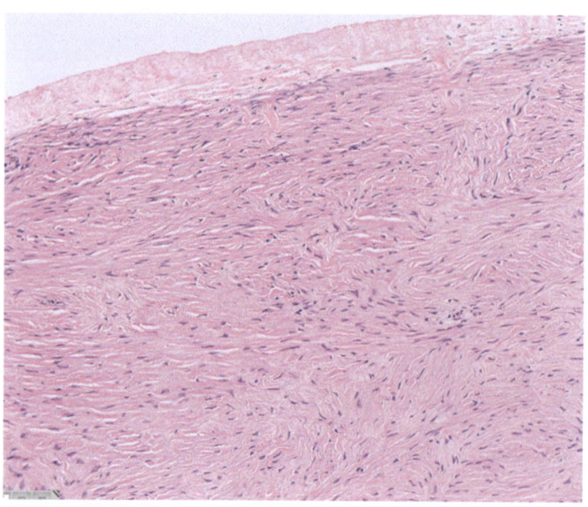

Fig. 4 Fibroma: Bland appearing spindle cells with pink eosinophilic cytoplasm in short fascicles, having a fibroblastic appearance comprise the Fibroma. The ovarian capsule is seen ensheathing the ovarian fibroma (H and E ×100)

Cellular fibromas have low malignant potential, exhibit mild nuclear atypia, and have more than four mitotic figures per 10 high-powered fields [35]. Clinically they cannot be differentiated from fibroma, but they tend to be larger with necrosis and haemorrhage [35].

Ovarian fibrosarcoma is a very rare malignant sex cord-stromal tumour. They are common in postmenopausal women and present as large masses associated with necrosis and haemorrhage. Histologically they comprise spindle-shaped cells with moderate to severe atypia and high mitotic counts. Immunohistochemistry is non-specific but Ki-67 index is high. Tumour may also be positive for Vimentin, inhibin A, SMA, oestrogen receptor, and progesterone receptor [36, 37].

Thecomas account for 0.5–1% of all primary ovarian tumours and mainly occurs in postmenopausal women [38]. They are considered benign neoplasms and are composed of lipid-laden stromal cells that resemble theca cells, encircling the ovarian follicles. They exhibit estrogenic activity in most cases. Affected women experience oestrogen-related symptoms such as postmenopausal or abnormal uterine bleeding, endometrial hyperplasia, and endometrial carcinoma (reported in 20% of cases) [39]. The term "luteinized thecomas", is used if there is an association with sclerosing peritonitis. Even though associated with sclerosing peritonitis luteinized thecoma is hormonally inert tumour and present at an average age of 28 years [40]. Sclerosing peritonitis also known as abdominal cocoon syndrome is characterized by small bowel loops entirely encapsulated by a fibrocollagenous membrane in the centre of the abdomen, and it may very rarely manifest as complete mechanical bowel obstruction [41].

Sclerosing stromal tumours are benign, unilateral, and mostly occur in young women under 30 years of age. They are hormonally inactive tumours, however, few hormonally active tumours have been documented in the literature [31, 42]. Menstrual irregularities and/or pelvic pain are common manifestations. Microscopically they are heterogeneous and contrasts with the relative homogeneity of other stromal tumours like thecoma and fibroma. Cellular psuedolobules, prominent interlobular fibrosis, marked vascularity and dual cell population, collagen-producing spindle cells, and lipid containing round or ovoid cells are characteristics of these tumours [43].

Steroid cell tumours are very rare and comprise 0.1% of all ovarian tumours [44]. Formally, the term "stromal luteoma" was used for a small steroid cell tumour limited to the ovarian cortex but has been removed in recent classifications. Histologically they are composed exclusively of cells resembling steroid-secreting cells without Reinke crystals. In contrast, intracytoplasmatic Reinke crystals are present in Leydig cell tumours. Reinke crystals are rod-like cytoplasmic inclusions that are present in Leydig cells of the testes with unknown functions. The majority are androgenic, and patients exhibit virilizing symptoms in 50% of cases, however, occasionally, these tumours may demonstrate estrogenic manifestations, hypercortisolism, and progestational changes [45]. Leydig tumours usually occur in older women, and hyperandrogenicity is evident in majority of these patients. Whereas Leydig cell tumours are benign, clinically malignant behaviour occurs in 25–40% of the patients of steroid cell tumour [45–47].

1.3 Mixed Sex Cord-Stromal Tumours

Sertoli–Leydig cell tumour is very rare and often encountered in women younger than 40 years. The majority are stage I at diagnosis. Histologically it is characterized by testicular structures (Sertoli and Leydig cells) that can produce androgens, but all are not active functionally. Depending on the presence of varied histological elements which comprise presence of mitotic activity and atypia, tubular versus solid differentiation or evidence of sarcomatoid pattern they are categorized into either well, intermediate or poorly differentiated tumours. It is more common for heterologous elements like chondroid, leiomyogenic, rhabdomyogenic, gastrointestinal or carcinoid differentiation to be associated with intermediate and poorly differentiated subtypes but association with well-differentiated tumours is not rare [48, 49]. Patients present with abdominal pain or androgenic symptoms such as oligomenorrhea, amenorrhea, and hirsutism. Virilization and clitoromegaly may be present. Patients may also manifest symptoms due to excess oestrogen secretion such as abnormal uterine bleeding and postmenopausal bleeding. They are typically unilateral tumours, with only 1% occurring bilaterally [49].

2 Diagnosis and Management

A sex cord-stromal tumour is suspected when an adnexal mass with endocrine effects is present. When suspected, levels of inhibin, estradiol, testosterone, and AFP should be measured. Endometrial sampling should be performed when associated with abnormal uterine bleeding or thickened endometrium in postmenopausal women, as endometrial hyperplasia or carcinoma may be associated with some of these tumours.

The initial workup should include a thorough history with careful attention to family history of possible tumour predisposition. Physical examination should be done with particular attention to the presence of precocious puberty, delayed menarche, hyperpigmented macules, or thyroid nodules that are suggestive of Peutz-Jeghers and DICER1 syndrome. Apart from endocrine manifestations, large tumours may rupture, resulting in an acute presentation with hemoperitoneum.

The radiologic appearances of these tumours vary depending on their morphologies. The initial imaging modality to evaluate these tumours is ultrasound, where a large mass with a heterogenous appearance is commonly seen. Adult granulosa cell tumours can appear as solid masses with haemorrhagic or fibrotic changes, multilocular cystic lesions, or completely cystic tumours [50, 51]. Typical appearance is demonstrated in fibromas which have a solid hypoechoic and homogenously isodense feature and a distinctive trait of hypointensity on T1-weighed images, strong hypointensity on T2-weighted images, and delayed enhancement following IV contrast [52]. Leydig cell tumours are usually small, and only clues might be morphologic changes within the ovary, especially on MRI and transvaginal ultrasound with colour Doppler [50]. Sclerosing stromal tumours frequently manifest on ultrasound as unilateral tumours comprising star-shaped hypoechoic areas enclosed by solid areas and on MRI, the pseudolobular solid areas exhibit a spoke-wheel pattern [53].

3 Surgical Management

Unilateral salpingo-oophorectomy is adequate therapy for a benign tumour but for older patients, hysterectomy and bilateral salpingo-oophorectomy is appropriate. Ovarian cystectomy may be considered if complete excision is possible and the patient desires preservation of the ovary. However, for patients with thecoma in the menopausal transition/postmenopausal women a total hysterectomy with bilateral salpingo-oophorectomy should be done as due to estrogenic effects, a synchronous endometrial neoplasm may be present [54].

Malignant SCST of the ovary is surgically staged and follow the same principles of epithelial ovarian cancer staging. However, only pelvic and paraaortic sampling should be carried out because lymph node metastases are rare with these tumours [55, 56]. Although hysterectomy and bilateral salpingo-oophorectomy are components of surgical staging fertility preservation is an acceptable option for young patients with tumours confined to the ovary. However, the contralateral ovary should be carefully inspected, and biopsy is done only if any abnormality is detected. If a hysterectomy is not performed, endometrial sampling should be performed to rule out coexistent endometrial malignancy in the setting of an oestrogen-secreting SCST, particularly granulosa cell tumours.

Due to the rarity of these tumours definitive diagnosis is often not made preoperatively or intraoperatively. Being rare neoplasms, even expert gynaecologic pathologists may not provide a definite diagnosis based on intraoperative frozen section examination. Hence, the surgeon will need to make an intraoperative decision based on imperfect histologic information, intraoperative findings, and the patient's preferences. This is also complicated by the fact that epithelial neoplasms, particularly endometrioid carcinoma, can mimic SCST. Therefore, patients who undergo conservative surgery, the potential need for further surgery should be discussed preoperatively.

4 Adjuvant Treatment

Due to the rarity of these tumours and lack of randomized controlled trials, there is no uniform recommendation for postoperative adjuvant therapy. Although adjuvant chemotherapy has been associated with more prolonged disease-free survival among those with advanced granulosa cell tumours, there is no evidence supporting an overall survival benefit. Also, there is no consensus regarding the use of chemotherapy for stage IC disease. In a study by Wang et al., adjuvant chemotherapy failed to improve disease-free interval (DFI) for stage IC [57]. The number of cycles of chemotherapy also did not add to improved DFI in this study. The MITO-9 study, which was a retrospective multi-institutional review of patients with GCT, demonstrated similar results [58]. Studies on juvenile GCTs have shown that adjuvant chemotherapy results in prolonged DFI and is usually recommended for stage IC disease and a high mitotic index (≥20 per 10 high power fields) [59–61]. It is also recommended with more advanced stage. It is, however, difficult to extrapolate these results to adult granulosa cell tumours, which have a lower proliferative rate and greater risk of late recurrences than the juvenile type.

Despite the lack of overall survival benefit, postoperative chemotherapy is recommended for patients with resected stage IC to IV disease as there is potential for long-term survival in patients with advanced disease. Both European Society of Gynaecological Oncology (ESGO) and the European Society for Pediatric Oncology (SIOPE) recommends expectant management for stage IC1 juvenile GCTs and three to four cycles of cisplatin-based chemotherapy for stage IC2 and IC3 adult GCTs [62]. As per NCCN guidelines for stage IC and higher disease, adjuvant chemotherapy is recommended, but observation is also considered as an acceptable strategy in patients with IC disease [63].

For well-differentiated SLCT, stage I tumours, surgery alone is sufficient. However, tumours containing either heterologous elements or retiform patterns or poorly differentiated SLCT have high recurrence rate, and adjuvant therapy is recommended. In contrast to other SCST, such as ovarian GCTs, SLCT tends to relapse early, with a relapse rate of 95% within 5 years [64].

The most commonly used regimens are bleomycin, cisplatin, plus etoposide (BEP), as used for testicular and ovarian germ cell tumours [65]. Paclitaxel plus carboplatin is also recommended as adjuvant therapy. For younger, BEP is preferred, while paclitaxel plus carboplatin is preferred for patients over 40 years old due to toxicity concerns with the BEP regimen. GOG 264 and SCST-01 are ongoing trials comparing the two regimens, and the results may guide the optimal first-line regimen in this rare disease.

4.1 Role of Endocrine Therapy

Hormonal therapy has been suggested primarily for granulosa cell tumours. Evidence suggests mutation of FOXL2 results in unrepressed expression of CYP17 and production of steroids, dysregulation of cell cycle, and apoptosis. There is increased aromatization and excess oestrogen secretion by the ovary [66]. Evidence supporting use of hormonal therapy is derived from a meta-analysis studying the response to various hormonal therapy in recurrent GCT comprising 31 eligible women. The results of the analysis had shown an overall response of 71% out of which 25% had complete response. Aromatase inhibitors (AIs) have the maximal response when compared to eight other hormonal therapies used [67]. Data on response rate of both AI and non-AI was published by a review in 2018 where meta-analysis of 50 patients with 9 different non-AIs (included GnRH, megestrol, medroxyprogesterone acetate, DES or in combination) and 25 patients with AI were analysed. An overall response (complete, partial, and stable disease) of 66% was evident in the non-AI users as compared to 76% in AI users. Given the favourable side effect profile, the authors concluded that AI might be an alternative to chemotherapy [68]. Contradictory evidence comes from the PARAGON trial which evaluated the efficacy of anastrozole in a varied cohort of gynaecological malignancies including a small subset of 41 women with recurrent GCTs. This phase 2 trial had a very low response rate to anastrozole as compared to previous findings and reiterated the superiority of prospective studies over retrospective findings and emphasized on the need to re-evaluate the utility of AI over chemotherapy [69]. Other drugs under evaluation are androgen receptor signalling inhibitor, enzalutamide, progesterone antagonist onapristone, nonsteroidal inhibitor orteronel, and the anti-fungal ketoconazole.

5 Posttreatment Surveillance

NCCN guidelines recommend reviewing symptoms and physical examination at 6–12 monthly interval based on the clinical stage [63]. It is estimated that in around 30–45% of patients recurrence occur in the pelvis [70]. Imaging cannot replace physical evaluation and complete evaluation after completion of treatment should include not only a thorough physical examination, appropriate imaging as indicated by physical findings and tumour marker if it was elevated initially. Monitoring multiple markers rather than a single marker appears to be superior for the detection of macroscopic disease. Computed tomography or other imaging is usually indicated for the evaluation of patients with symptoms or elevation in a serum tumour marker level.

6 Recurrent Disease

Recurrent disease has a poor prognosis and is mostly treated with chemotherapy. Multifocal recurrent disease and residual tumour after surgery are associated with diminished disease-free and overall survival. Limited data from recurrent GCT suggests that surgical treatment may afford a survival advantage if recurrence appears resectable [71, 72]. For patients who are not candidates for surgery due to the extent of disease, poor performance status, or those who experience multiple recurrences, chemotherapy alone is generally suggested. BEP regimen and paclitaxel plus carboplatin are the most commonly used platinum-based regimens for recurrent disease based on their response as adjuvant therapy. Paclitaxel plus carboplatin is preferred if BEP was used previously. In the instances where there is no response to platinum-based regimen consideration should be given to other agents which have shown efficacy in second line scenario. Paclitaxel is one of the drugs to be considered which has shown appreciable response rate of 29% in a study undertaken by GOG (GOG 187) where 31 women with previous history of chemotherapy had obtained a median progression free survival of 10 months and overall survival of around 73 months [73]. Another evidence in favour of paclitaxel comes from the ALIENOR/ENGOT-ov7 study where randomization was done to ether weekly paclitaxel or in combination with bevacizumab in 60 women who had developed recurrence after receiving at least one platinum-based chemotherapy regimen. Median PFS was 14.7 months with single-agent paclitaxel and 14.9 months with combination therapy. The trial concluded that adding bevacizumab to weekly paclitaxel did not improve clinical benefit. However, in this study, it was found that median PFS with weekly paclitaxel was longer than historical data for three weekly paclitaxel (10.0 months) and compared favourably with other chemotherapy regimens or anastrozole in the single-arm PARAGON trial (8.6 months) [74]. Other chemotherapeutic regimens with reported therapeutic efficacy include doxorubicin, carboplatin plus etoposide, cisplatin, vinblastine, plus bleomycin (PVB or VBP) and cyclophosphamide, doxorubicin, plus cisplatin (CAP). Limited data indicate that treatment of recurrent disease with aromatase inhibitors, tamoxifen, progesterone alone, or a combination of tamoxifen and progesterone can result in long-term clinical responses.

7 Summary and Conclusion

Surgery is the most effective therapeutic approach for the management of both primary and relapsed SCST. Conserving the contralateral ovary and the uterus is possible in patients who wish to preserve fertility, but the feasibility depends on tumour histology and stage. Presently the consensus for delivering postoperative chemotherapy is limited to patients in advanced stage of their disease or when complete resection of disease is not feasible as there is weak evidence of the efficacy in adjuvant setting and also due to the side effects associated with it. Hormonal therapy appears promising for relapsed tumours, but further assessment is needed. Identifying therapeutic targets and developing targeted therapeutic agents for managing aggressive and recurrent tumours is a challenging task due to the rarity of these tumours. Because available effective therapies for patients with metastatic disease are limited, genomic profiling may be pursued to identify common mutations targetable by novel agents in clinical trials.

References

1. Schultz KAP, Harris AK, Schneider DT, Young RH, Brown J, Gershenson DM, et al. Ovarian sex cord-stromal tumors. J Oncol Pract. 2016;12(10):940.
2. Chen VW, Ruiz B, Killeen JL, Coté TR, Wu XC, Correa CN, et al. Pathology and classification of ovarian tumors. Cancer. 2003;97(S10):2631–42.

3. Hemminki A, Markie D, Tomlinson I, Avizienyte E, Roth S, Loukola A, et al. A serine/threonine kinase gene defective in Peutz-Jeghers syndrome. Nature. 1998;391(6663):184–7.
4. Yoo LI, Chung DC, Yuan J. LKB1—a master tumour suppressor of the small intestine and beyond. Nat Rev Cancer. 2002;2(7):529–35.
5. Tamini HK, Bolen JW. Enchondromatosis (Ollier's disease) and ovarian juvenile granulosa cell tumor: a case report and review of the literature. Cancer. 1984;53(7):120.
6. Pansuriya TC, Kroon HM, Bovée JV. Enchondromatosis: insights on the different subtypes. Int J Clin Exp Pathol. 2010;3(6):557.
7. Amary MF, Damato S, Halai D, Eskandarpour M, Berisha F, Bonar F, et al. Ollier disease and Maffucci syndrome are caused by somatic mosaic mutations of IDH1 and IDH2. Nat Genet. 2011;43(12):1262–5.
8. Conlon N, Schultheis AM, Piscuoglio S, Silva A, Guerra E, Tornos C, et al. A survey of DICER1 hotspot mutations in ovarian and testicular sex cord-stromal tumors. Mod Pathol. 2015;28(12):1603–12.
9. Wang Y, Chen J, Yang W, Mo F, Senz J, Yap D, et al. The oncogenic roles of DICER1 RNase IIIb domain mutations in ovarian Sertoli-Leydig cell tumors. Neoplasia. 2015;17(8):650–60.
10. Fuller PJ, Leung D, Chu S. Genetics and genomics of ovarian sex cord-stromal tumors. Clin Genet. 2017;91:285–91.
11. Kalfa N, Ecochard A, Patte C, Duvillard P, Audran F, Pienkowski C, et al. Activating mutations of the stimulatory G protein in juvenile ovarian granulosa cell tumors: a new prognostic factor? J Clin Endocrinol Metab. 2006;91(5):1842–7.
12. Auguste A, Bessière L, Todeschini AL, Caburet S, Sarnacki S, Prat J, et al. Molecular analyses of juvenile granulosa cell tumors bearing AKT1 mutations provide insights into tumor biology and therapeutic leads. Hum Mol Genet. 2015;24(23):6687–98.
13. Kalfa N, Philibert P, Patte C, Ecochard A, Duvillard P, Baldet P, et al. Extinction of FOXL2 expression in aggressive ovarian granulosa cell tumors in children. Fertil Steril. 2007;87(4):896–901.
14. WHO Classification of Tumours of Ovary. Female genital tumours. 5th ed. London: IARC Press; 2020.
15. Levin G, Zigron R, Haj-Yahya R, Matan LS, Rottenstreich A. Granulosa cell tumor of ovary: a systematic review of recent evidence. Eur J Obstet Gynecol Reprod Biol. 2018;225:57–61.
16. Mom CH, Engelen MJA, Willemse PHB, Gietema JA, ten Hoor KA, de Vries EGE, van der Zee AGJ. Granulosa cell tumors of the ovary: the clinical value of serum inhibin a and B levels in a large single center cohort. Gynecol Oncol. 2007;105(2):365–72.
17. Bacalbasa N, Stoica C, Popa I, Mirea G, Balescu I. Endometrial carcinoma associated with ovarian granulosa cell tumors - a case report. Anticancer Res. 2015;35(10):5547–50.
18. Colombo N, Parma G, Zanagnolo V, Insinga A. Management of ovarian stromal cell tumors. J Clin Oncol. 2007;25(20):2944–51.
19. Hines JF, Khalifa MA, Moore JL, Fine KP, Lage JM, Barnes WA. Recurrent granulosa cell tumor of the ovary 37 years after initial diagnosis: a case report and review of the literature. Gynecol Oncol. 1996;60(3):484–8.
20. Björkholm E, Silfverswärd C. Prognostic factors in granulosa-cell tumors. Gynecol Oncol. 1981;11(3):261–74.
21. Stenwig JT, Hazekamp JT, Beecham JB. Granulosa cell tumors of the ovary. A clinicopathological study of 118 cases with long-term follow-up. Gynecol Oncol. 1979;7(2):136–52.
22. Young RH. Ovarian sex cord-stromal tumours and their mimics. Pathology. 2018;50(1):5–15.
23. Ye Y, Lv C, Xu S, Chen Y, Qian R, Wang P, et al. Juvenile granulosa cell tumors of the ovary. Am J Clin Pathol. 2020;154:635–44.
24. Wang Y, Wang W, Xu C, Huang X, Zhong L, Kang X, et al. Childhood ovarian juvenile granulosa cell tumor: a retrospective study with 3 cases including clinical features, pathologic results, and therapies. J Pediatr Hematol Oncol. 2011;33(3):241–5.
25. Fleming NA, de Nanassy J, Lawrence S, Black AY. Juvenile granulosa and theca cell tumor of the ovary as a rare cause of precocious puberty: case report and review of literature. J Pediatr Adolesc Gynecol. 2010;23(4):145.
26. Kalfa N, Méduri G, Philibert P, Boizet-Bonhoure CPB, Thibaut E, Pienkowski P, Jaubert F, Mishrahi M, Sultan C. Unusual virilization in girls with juvenile granulosa cell tumors of the ovary is related to intratumoral aromatase deficiency. Horm Res Paediatr. 2010;74(2):83–91.
27. Parikshaa G, Ariba Z, Pranab D, Nalini G, Manish SV, et al. Juvenile granulosa cell tumor of the ovary: a comprehensive clinicopathologic analysis of 15 cases. Ann Diagn Pathol. 2021;52(1):25.
28. Oliva E, Alvarez T, Young RH. Sertoli cell tumors of the ovary: a clinicopathologic and immunohistochemical study of 54 cases. Am J Surg Pathol. 2005;29(2):143–56.
29. Lee SH, Koh YW, Roh HJ, Cha HJ, Kwon YS. Ovarian microcystic stromal tumor: a novel extracolonic tumor in familial adenomatous polyposis. Genes Chromosomes Cancer. 2015;54(6):353–60.
30. Nosov V, Park S, Rao J, Memarzadeh S. Non-Peutz-Jeghers syndrome associated ovarian sex cord tumor with annular tubules: a case report. Fertil Steril. 2009;92(4):1497.e5–8.
31. Al Harbi R, McNeish IA, El-Bahrawy M. Ovarian sex cord-stromal tumors: an update on clinical features, molecular changes, and management. BMJ Spec J. 2021;31:161–8.
32. Yen P, Khong K, Lamba R, Corwin MT, Gerscovich EO. Ovarian fibromas and Fibrothecomas. J Ultrasound Med. 2013;32(1):13–8.

33. Fujii K, Miyashita T. Gorlin syndrome (nevoid basal cell carcinoma syndrome): update and literature review. Pediatr Int. 2014;56(5):667–74.
34. Montoriol PF, Mons A, Da Ines D, Bourdel D, Tixier N, Garcier JM. Fibrous tumours of the ovary: aetiologies and MRI features. Clin Radiol. 2013;68(12):1276–83.
35. Adad SJ, Laterza VL, Dos Santos CDT, Ladeia AAL, Saldanha JC, Da Silva CS, et al. Cellular fibroma of the ovary with multiloculated macroscopic characteristics: case report. Case Rep Med. 2012;2012:283948.
36. Sun TT, Cheng NH, Cao DY, Peng P. Ovarian fibrosarcoma: a single-institution experience and a review of the literature. J Ovarian Res. 2020;13(1):1–8.
37. García Jiménez A, Castellví J, Pérez Benavente A, de Corcuera D, Frutos I, Ramón y Cajal S. Ovarian fibrosarcoma: clinicopathologic considerations about the intraoperative and post-surgical procedures. Case Rep Med. 2009;2009:1–4.
38. Chen H, Liu Y, Shen L, Jiang M, Yang Z, Fang G. Ovarian thecoma-fibroma groups: clinical and sonographic features with pathological comparison. J Ovarian Res. 2016;9(1):1–7.
39. Deavers MT, Oliva E, Nucci MR. Sex cord-stromal tumors of the ovary. In: Gynecologic pathology. London: Elsevier; 2009. p. 445–500.
40. De A, Mukhopadhyay S, Nandi A, Das I. Sclerosing peritonitis with unilateral ovarian luteinized thecoma in a post-menopausal woman: a case report. J Midlife Health. 2014;5(4):198.
41. Saqib SU, Pal I. Sclerosing peritonitis presenting as complete mechanical bowel obstruction: a case report. J Med Case Reports. 2019;13(1):1–4.
42. Tanaka YO, Tsunoda H, Kitagawa Y, Ueno T, Yoshikawa H, Saida Y. Functioning ovarian tumors: direct and indirect findings at MR imaging. Radiographics. 2004;24(Suppl 1):S147–66.
43. Khanna M, Khanna A, Manjari M. Sclerosing stromal tumor of ovary: a case report. Case Rep Pathol. 2012;2012(5):442–4.
44. Patil V, VemiReddy P, Taqdees A, Arakeri S. Steroid cell tumor of the ovary—a rare case report and review of literature. Int J Appl Basic Med Res. 2019;9(3):185.
45. Horta M, Cunha TM. Sex cord-stromal tumors of the ovary: a comprehensive review and update for radiologists. Diagn Interv Radiol. 2015;21(4):277.
46. Faten H, Dorra G, Slim C, Wajdi S, Nadia C, Kais C, et al. Ovarian steroid cell tumor (not otherwise specified): a case report of ovarian hyperandrogenism. Case Rep Oncol Med. 2020;2020:1–6.
47. Jiang W, Tao X, Fang F, Zhang S, Xu C. Benign and malignant ovarian steroid cell tumors, not otherwise specified: case studies, comparison, and review of the literature. J Ovarian Res. 2013;6(1):1–5.
48. Abu-Zaid A, Azzam A, Alghuneim LA, Metawee MT, Amin T, Al-Hussain TO. Poorly differentiated ovarian sertoli-leydig cell tumor in a 16-year-old single woman: a case report and literature review. Case Rep Obstet Gynecol. 2013;2013:1–6.
49. Durmuş Y, Kılıç Ç, Çakır C, Yüksel D, Boran N, Karalök A, Gökhan Boyraz ATT. Sertoli-Leydig cell tumor of the ovary: analysis of a single institution database and review of the literature. J Obstet Gynaecol Res. 2019;45(7):1311–8.
50. Jung SE, Rha SE, Lee JM, Park SY, Oh SN, Cho KS, et al. CT and MRI findings of sex cord–stromal tumor of the ovary. Am J Roentgenol. 2005;185(1):207–15.
51. Outwater EK, Wagner BJ, Mannion C, McLarney JK, Kim B. From the archives of the AFIP: sex cord-stromal and steroid cell tumors of the ovary. Radiographics. 1998;18(6):1523–46.
52. Troiano RN, Lazzarini KM, Scoutt LM, Lange RC, Flynn SD, McCarthy S. Fibroma and fibrothecoma of the ovary: MR imaging findings. Radiology. 1997;204(3):795–8.
53. Javadi S, Ganeshan DM, Jensen CT, Iyer RB, Bhosale PR. Comprehensive review of imaging features of sex cord-stromal tumors of the ovary. Abdom Radiol. 2021;46(4):1519–29.
54. Björkholm E, Silfverswärd C. Theca-cell tumors clinical features and prognosis. Acta Oncol (Madr). 1980;19(4):241–4.
55. Thrall MM, Paley P, Pizer E, Garcia R, Goff BA. Patterns of spread and recurrence of sex cord-stromal tumors of the ovary. Gynecol Oncol. 2011;122(2):242–5.
56. Brown J, Sood AK, Deavers MT, Milojevic L, Gershenson DM. Patterns of metastasis in sex cord-stromal tumors of the ovary: can routine staging lymphadenectomy be omitted? Gynecol Oncol. 2009;113(1):86–90.
57. Wang D, Xiang Y, Wu M, Shen K, Yang J, Huang H, et al. Is adjuvant chemotherapy beneficial for patients with FIGO stage IC adult granulosa cell tumor of the ovary? J Ovarian Res. 2018;11(1):1–7.
58. Mangili G, Ottolina J, Cormio G, Loizzi V, De Iaco P, Pellegrini DA, et al. Adjuvant chemotherapy does not improve disease-free survival in FIGO stage IC ovarian granulosa cell tumors: the MITO-9 study. Gynecol Oncol. 2016;143(2):276–80.
59. Schneider DT, Calaminus G, Wessalowksi R, Pathmanathan R, Selle B, Sternschulte W, et al. Ovarian sex cord-stromal tumors in children and adolescents. J Clin Oncol. 2003;21:2357–63.
60. Biscotti CV, Hart WR. Juvenile granulosa cell tumors of the ovary. Arch Pathol Lab Med. 1989;113(1):40–6.
61. Calaminus G, Wessalowski R, Harms D, Göbel U. Juvenile granulosa cell tumors of the ovary in children and adolescents: results from 33 patients registered in a prospective cooperative study. Gynecol Oncol. 1997;65(3):447–52.
62. Sessa C, Schneider DT, Planchamp F, Baust K, Braicu EI, Concin N, et al. ESGO–SIOPE guidelines for the management of adolescents and young adults with non-epithelial ovarian cancers. Lancet Oncol. 2020;21:e360–8.

63. Ovarian cancer including fallopian tube cancer and primary peritoneal cancer. NCCN Guidelines Version 3. 2021.
64. Litta P, Saccardi C, Conte L, Codroma A, Angioni S, Mioni R. Sertoli-Leydig cell tumors: current status of surgical management: literature review and proposal of treatment. Gynecol Endocrinol. 2013;29:412–7.
65. Schumer ST, Cannistra SA. Granulosa cell tumor of the ovary. J Clin Oncol. 2003;21:1180–9.
66. Li J, Chu R, Chen Z, Meng J, Yao S, Song K, et al. Progress in the management of ovarian granulosa cell tumor: a review. Acta Obstet Gynecol Scand. 2021;100:1771–8.
67. Van Meurs HS, Van Lonkhuijzen LRCW, Limpens J, Van Der Velden J, Buist MR. Hormone therapy in ovarian granulosa cell tumors: a systematic review. Gynecol Oncol. 2014;134:196–205.
68. Yang AD, Curtin J, Muggia F. Ovarian adult-type granulosa cell tumor: focusing on endocrine-based therapies. Int J Endocr. Oncologia. 2018;5(2):IJE08.
69. Banerjee SN, Tang M, O'Connell RL, Sjoquist K, Clamp AR, Millan D, et al. A phase 2 study of anastrozole in patients with oestrogen receptor and/progesterone receptor positive recurrent/metastatic granulosa cell tumours/sex-cord stromal tumours of the ovary: the PARAGON/ANZGOG 0903 trial. Gynecol Oncol. 2021;163(1):72–8.
70. Salani R, Backes FJ, Fung Kee Fung M, Holschneider CH, Parker LP, Bristow RE, et al. Posttreatment surveillance and diagnosis of recurrence in women with gynecologic malignancies: Society of Gynecologic Oncologists recommendations. Am J Obstet Gynecol. 2011;204:466–78.
71. Malmström H, Högberg T, Risberg B, Simonsen E. Granulosa cell tumors of the ovary: prognostic factors and outcome. Gynecol Oncol. 1994;52(1):50–5.
72. Mangili G, Sigismondi C, Frigerio L, Candiani M, Savarese A, Giorda G, et al. Recurrent granulosa cell tumors (GCTs) of the ovary: a MITO-9 retrospective study. Gynecol Oncol. 2013;130(1):38–42.
73. Burton ER, Brady M, Homesley HD, Rose PG, Nakamura T, Kesterson JP, et al. A phase II study of paclitaxel for the treatment of ovarian stromal tumors: an NRG oncology/gynecologic oncology group study. Gynecol Oncol. 2016;140(1):48–52.
74. Ray-Coquard I, Harter P, Lorusso D, Dalban C, Vergote I, Fujiwara K, et al. Effect of weekly paclitaxel with or without Bevacizumab on progression-free rate among patients with relapsed ovarian sex cord-stromal tumors: the ALIENOR/ENGOT-ov7 randomized clinical trial. JAMA Oncol. 2020;6(12):1923–30.

Secondary Ovarian Tumour

Sharda Patra, Abraham Peedicayil, and Amal Chandra Kataki

1 Introduction

Secondary ovarian tumours (SOT) comprise 10–25% of all ovarian malignancies [1]. Most common sites of primary tumour identified so far are from the stomach, colon, rectum, breast, endometrium, and appendix [2] (Table 1). Tumour metastasizing to ovary are termed as Krukenberg's tumour (KT), based on the presence of more than 10% mucin filled signet ring cells [3]. Earlier the terms KT and secondary ovarian tumours were used interchangeably, but now it has been recognized that all SOTs are not KT. Only 30–40% of all SOTs are Krukenberg tumours [4] and the commonest primary tumour is signet ring adenocarcinoma of pylorus of the stomach. In the usual scenarios of presentation, detection of secondary ovarian tumour precedes the detection of primary tumour. Thus, its diagnosis poses a challenge both to the gynaecologic oncologist and pathologist. A correct pathological diagnosis is also important for its timely and complete man-

Table 1 Primary tumours metastasizing to ovaries—Krukenberg and Non-Krukenberg

Primary tumours metastasizing to ovary	
Krukenberg metastasis (primary adenocarcinoma with signet ring metastasis)	Non-Krukenberg metastasis
Non-gynaecological primary tumour	*Non-gynaecological primary tumour*
Stomach (pylorus—most common)	Melanoma
Colorectal cancer	Lymphoma
Appendix	Carcinoid
Pancreaticobiliary tract, including gallbladder	Pulmonary and mediastinal tumours
Small bowel	Extragenital sarcomas
Breast	*Peritoneal tumours metastatic to the ovaries*
Lung	Peritoneal mesotheliomas
Urinary bladder	Intra-abdominal desmoplastic small round cell tumour
Gynaecological primary tumour	*Gynaecological primary tumour*
Contralateral ovary	Fallopian tube carcinoma
Endometrium	Endometrial carcinoma
Cervix	Vulvar and vaginal tumours

S. Patra (✉)
Department of O&G, Lady Hardinge Medical College, New Delhi, India
e-mail: sharda.patra@lhmc-hosp.gov.in

A. Peedicayil
Sultan Qaboos Comprehensive Cancer Center, Muscat, Oman

A. C. Kataki
Department of Gynaecologic Oncology, Dr. Bhubaneswar Borooah Cancer Institute (A Unit of Tata Memorial Centre, Mumbai), Guwahati, Assam, India

A. C. Kataki, D. Barmon (eds.), *Fundamentals in Gynaecologic Malignancy*,
https://doi.org/10.1007/978-981-19-5860-1_19

agement and structured counseling of the patient and her relatives. The risk factors and prognostication vary depending on the type of primary tumour and the stage of detection of SOT. Usually, the presence of SOTs is known to have a dismal prognosis.

2 Epidemiology

Frequency of detection of type of primary varies with the following variables: [5].

- Geographical variation: People of Asian ethnicity are more prone to the occurrence of risk factors of SOT as compared to caucasians [1, 2].
- Age of the women: Primary gastro-intestinal tract (GI) tumours are seen more in older age group as compared to non-GI tumours. Breast tumours as primary are seen at much younger age [2, 4].
- Method of diagnosis used and expertise of the pathologist.

3 Pathogenesis

The spread of a tumour from primary cancer site to secondary site, i.e., ovary, may occur via one of three routes; lymphogenous, hematogenous, or transcelomic [6]. The predilection to a particular route of spread depends on the primary tumour as in colonic cancer, which spreads via hematogenous route in contrast to lymphogenous route spread that is seen in gastric cancer. The rich lymphatic supply in the stomach enables spread of gastric cancer to ovaries at a very early stage [7, 8]. Transcoelomic spread does not play a major role in SOT and is more predominantly found in primary ovarian tumour [9].

Another theory of preferential spread of cancer from primary organ to ovary can be explained by the concept of "Metastatic Organotropism." [10] Multiple hypothesis behind these include:

- Attraction of tumour cells to a specific organ.
- Survival of cancer cells in a specific site.
- Adhesion of cells to endothelium of specific organ.
- Extravasation of tumour cells into a specific organ.
- Loss of specific miRNA.

4 Symptoms and Signs

Majority of women present in advanced stage of tumour. The symptoms range from being nonspecific in majority to postmenopausal bleeding [7, 11] (Table 2). The differential diagnosis of GI malignancy with ovarian metastasis is given in Table 3.

4.1 Diagnosis

In most cases, the diagnosis of secondary ovarian tumour precedes the detection of primary tumour. Thorough history and complete physical examination hold the most important place in reaching an accurate diagnosis. The other diagnostic modalities are:

- Baseline blood and biochemical analysis including tumour markers.
- Imaging methods.

Table 2 Symptoms and signs in secondary ovarian tumour

Clinical presentation	
Symptoms	Signs
• Nonspecific (70%)	• Poor general condition
• Abdominal pain (42%).	• Cachexia
• Postmenopausal bleeding (18%)	• Supraclavicular lymph node enlargement
• Abdominal distension (15%)	• Ascites
• Weight loss in 6%	• Mass felt per-abdomen
• Abnormal menstrual bleeding, virilization or hirsutism in cancers causing luteinization of ovarian stroma	• Bleeding per vaginum
	• Bleeding per rectum

Table 3 Differential diagnosis of common GI primary tumours metastasizing to ovary

Types	Gastric carcinoma	Intestinal carcinoma	Appendiceal cancer
Tumour type	With signet ring histology—Krukenberg	80% of the primaries originating in rectum or sigmoid colon	Low-grade mucinous appendix tumours
Clinical presentation	Adenexal mass, Ascitis, GI symptoms predominant Pathology in stomach in endoscopy	Predominant GI symptoms with adenexal mass Pathology in sigmoid/rectum in endoscopy	Adenexal mass with dilated appendix, pseudomyxoma peritonei
Age	45 years Usually premenopausal	Any age	35–45
Ovarian involvement	Bilateral (80%)	Bilateral (>50%) Even Unilateral	Bilateral
Size	Predominantly solid masses	Large solid or cystic masses	Multicystic, >10 cm may reach up to about 15–20 cm in diameter
Gross	Firm, white, round masses that may reach considerable sizes		Multicystic appearance with mucoid material is common
D/D	Sertoli–Leydig tumours, clear cell carcinoma mucinous carcinoid	Endometrioid carcinoma and mucinous adenocarcinoma	

- Endoscopy: both upper GI and lower GI tract.
- Histopathology and immunohistochemistry.
- Genomics.

5 Tumour Markers

CA125 is not sensitive for detection of SOT although it is seen to be elevated in 70% of cases [11, 12]. CA125/CEA ratio is important especially in cases of differentiation of primary ovarian tumour from colorectal cancer metastasis [13]. Overall, there is no role of epithelial tumour markers in diagnosis of SOT. Pre-operative values can only be of help in following the progress of treatment.

6 Imaging

Ultrasound with or without color Doppler is usually the first modality used for the diagnosis of adnexal masses. A few ultrasonographic features can help in differentiating primary from SOT (Image: 1). Specific features seen are as follows: [14].

- Bilateral solid lesions, usually less than 10 cm.
- Solid lesions are more predominantly seen in breast and stomach primaries.
- Irregular echogenic soft tissue pattern with areas of cystic degeneration seen at later stages when the primary tumour is colorectal.

SOTs are more commonly found to be bilateral than primary ovarian cancers. CT scan with contrast of chest, whole abdomen, and pelvis is the most important diagnostic test in SOT with sensitivity of 82%. Other modalities like FDG-PET are not recommended as routine imaging owing to its limitations of detecting cancers less than 1 cm size and low FDG uptake by cells of breast, GI, and renal cancer [15]. However, none of the imaging methods can definitely differentiate secondary from primary ovarian tumour.

7 Endoscopy

Endoscopy is recommended especially in cases with signs suggestive of GI tract involvement, elevated tumour markers (especially serum CEA, CA19.9) or imaging or histopathology pointing towards the same. It is a useful modality as it can help in detection of GI primary in the least invasive manner by providing histopathological specimen [16].

8 Histopathology

Features suggestive of SOT on gross examination are: [17].

- The size of SOT's is in a majority, less than 10 cm. Breast cancer metastases tend to be smaller in size as compared to those from colon cancer.
- Usually they are bilateral in around 69% cases [2]. Breast, gastric, and appendix metastasis tends to be bilateral and colorectal cancers as unilateral in majority.
- Nodular growth pattern.
- Presence of tumour on the surface of the ovary.

8.1 Histology

The histological pattern is similar to the site of primary tumour. Most commonly found is the mucinous adenocarcinoma, which in 45% cases may be mis-diagnosed as primary ovarian tumour [2]. Features suggestive of secondary metastasis are: [17].

- Infiltrative growth pattern with stromal dysplasia.
- Invasion of superficial ovarian cortex.
- Hilar or lymphovascular invasion.

Specific histological patterns seen and their sites of primary are as follows: [5].

- Signet ring cells—Gastric cancer.
- Invasive ductal cancer cells—Breast cancer.
- Adenocarcinoma—Endometrial cancer.
- Squamous cell cancer—Cervical cancer.
- *Immunohistochemistry (IHC) with Special stains*

Immunohistochemistry should always be performed along with histopathological evaluation as it provides additional information. Immunophenotype in primary and secondary ovarian tumour are depicted in Table 4 [18].

Table 4 Various IHC markers in primary and secondary ovarian cancer

Type of tumour	Positive IHC	Negative IHC
Primary		
Serous	CK7, CA125, HAM56, PAX 8	CK20
Mucinous	CK7, CEA, HAM56, PAX 8, CK20, MUC5AC	CA125
Endometrioid	CK7, CA125, HAM54, PAX 8, ER, PR	CK20, CEA
Secondary		
Colorectum	CK20, CEA, CDX2	CK7, CA125, HAM56, MUC5AC
Appendix	CK20, CEA, MUC5AC	CK7, CA125
Stomach	CK7, CK20, MUC5AC	CA125, HAM56
Breast	GCDFP15, GATA3, ER, PR, Mammoglobin	CA125, WT1, Vimentin
Pancreas	CK7, CK20, MUC5AC, CEA, CA19–9	CA125, HAM56, DPC4
Renal	Vimentin, AE1/AE3, CD10, RCC, PAX8	CK7, CK20,34βe12
Cervical	p16, CEA, HPV	ER, PR

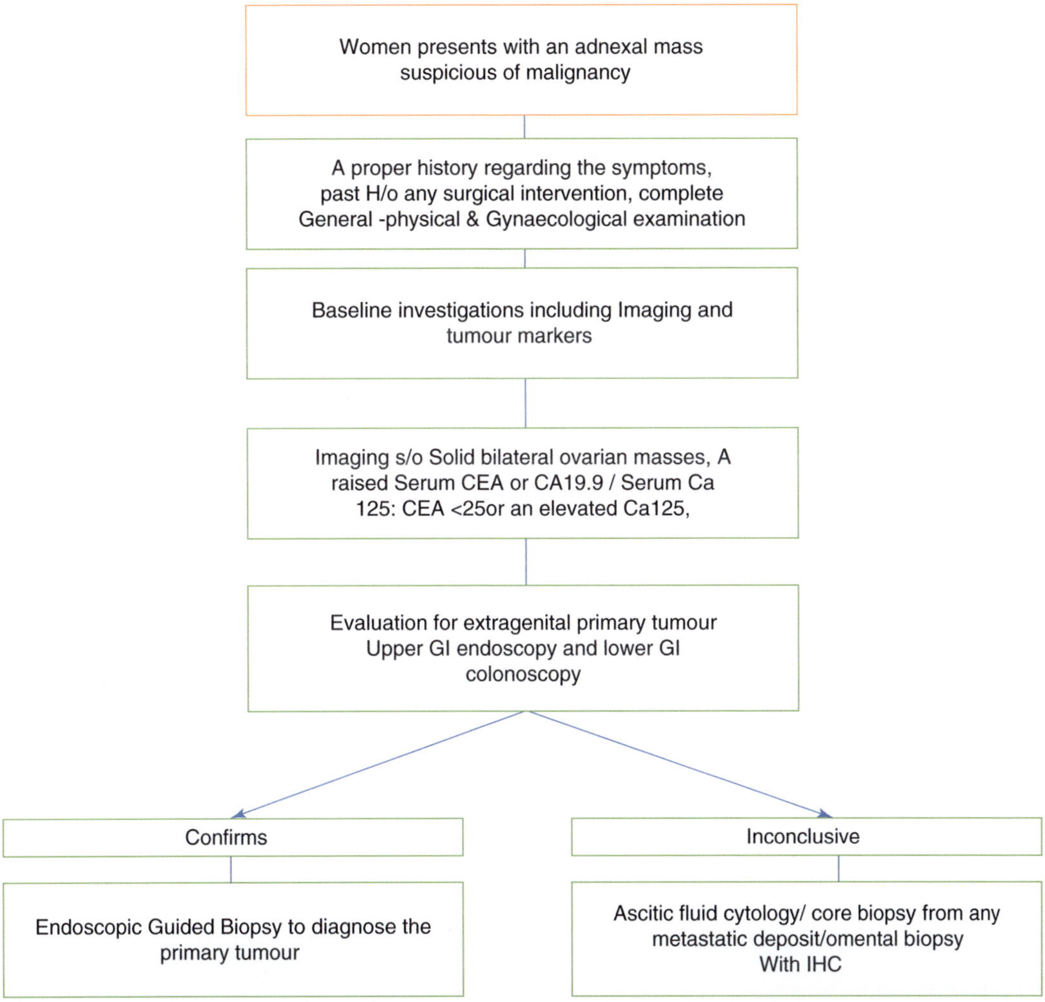

Fig. 1 Algorithmic approach to women with metastatic ovarian masses. Based on clinical, biochemical and imaging

8.2 Genomics

Gene expression profiling is an effective approach in identifying primary ovarian tumour from SOT, especially in cases with equivocal histopathological and IHC findings. Expression of m RNA or mi RNA can be detected with the help of reverse transcriptase PCR analysis or oligonucleotide microarray technology [19, 20].

The algorithmic work up of women with metastatic ovarian cancer based on clinical parameters and IHC is given in Figs. 1 and 2.

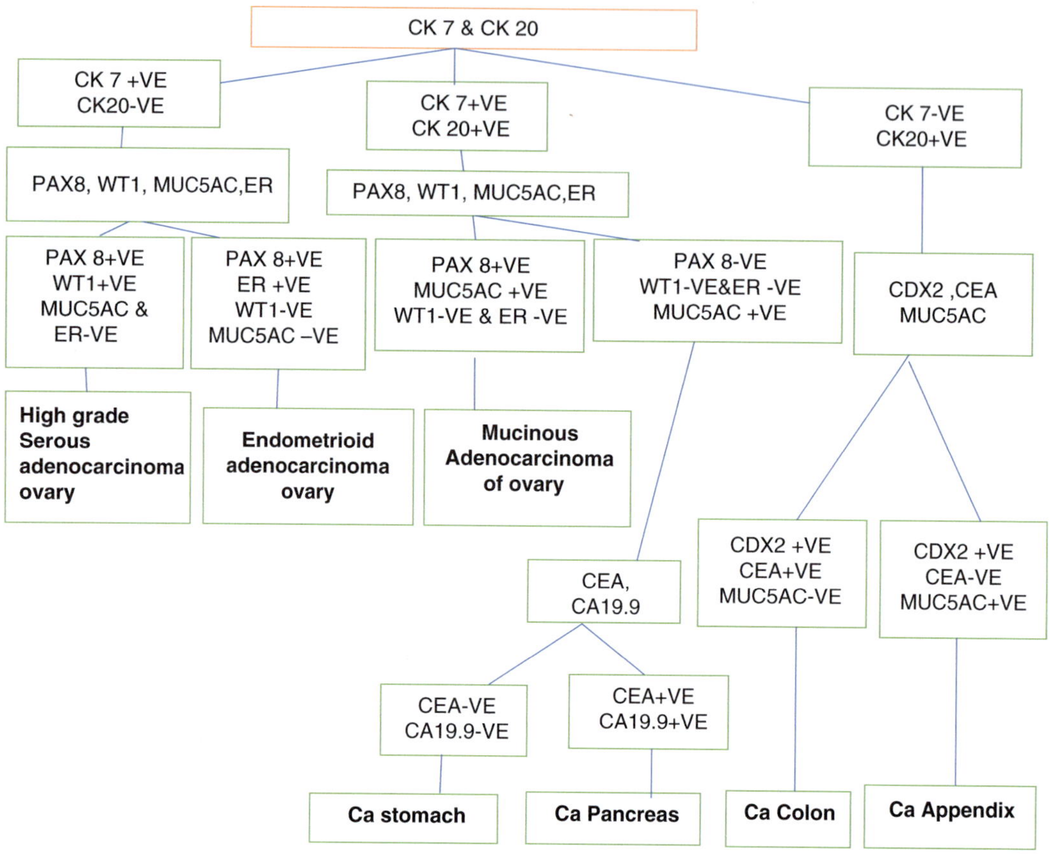

Fig. 2 Algorithmic approach to diagnose primary tumour in women with metastatic ovarian masses. Based on immune histochemistry markers

9 Treatment

Owing to the rarity of diagnosis of SOTs and its variable prognosis, there exists no uniform guidelines in the management of these tumours. Management primarily relies on the primary tumour identified and its stage. Treatment should be individualized according to the diagnosis. These cases should be discussed in a multidisciplinary team meeting. Role of cytoreductive surgery and adjuvant chemotherapy is not very clear due to lack of randomized prospective control trials and their use has to be individualized.

9.1 Role of Cytoreductive Surgery

There exist no prospective trials highlighting the advantage of cytoreductive surgery in all cases of SOT. The benefit has been found in cases as follows: [21, 22].

- Metastatic Colorectal cancer.
- Cancers with good performance status.
- Cancers with possibility of almost complete residual disease-free status.

Whenever found to be of benefit, bilateral oophorectomy is performed owing to the possibility of presence of metachronous metastasis in absence of obvious involvement of one of the ovaries.

No benefit has been seen in cases of gastric cancer as they primarily have a poorer prognosis. There has been no role of mastectomy in women with SOT with breast cancer as the primary tumour. Extent of cytoreductive surgery as in primary ovarian tumour defines the prognosis and survival rate, with better prognosis if residual disease post-surgery is less than 2 cm.

9.2 Role of Adjuvant Chemotherapy

Following cytoreductive surgery, the use of adjuvant chemotherapy has a role in improving overall survival of the patient. Various studies have compared the mode of administration of chemotherapy, i.e., intravenous or intraperitoneal and have found variable results [23, 24]. 5-flourouracin and leucovorin are the drugs of choice which have been found to increase progression free survival for the patients with no obvious improvement seen in overall survival [25].

9.3 Prognostic Factors

Prognostic factors are as follows that affect the 5-years survival rate of a women with SOT: [11, 26, 27].

- Age: Women presenting with SOT are usually younger than those presenting with primary epithelial ovarian cancer. In one study, it was found that 55% of women had age less than 36 years and had primary tumour of gastric origin. Advanced age at presentation is associated with poor prognosis.
- Type of primary tumour- Pancreatic and small intestine primaries are known to be associated with poor prognosis. Similarly, metastatic colon cancer has better prognosis than gastric cancer.
- Pre-operative CA125 levels.
- Pre-operative size of secondary ovarian tumour.
- Unilateral or bilateral.
- Presence of peritoneal dissemination.
- Extent of cytoreductive surgery.
- Presence of SMAD Family member-4 and Lysine methyl transferase 2D (KMT2D) are associated with poor prognosis.

10 Conclusion

It is a challenging task for the clinician to differentiate secondary ovarian tumours from primary ovarian malignancy. Although survival rate of these cancers has shown improvement over the years, still overall result and performance of these cancers are disappointing. Lack of randomized prospective trials make the treatment of SOT also challenging with no definite guidelines. Team effort comprising of a gynecologist, surgeon, and oncologists are required for efficient and effective management of these obnoxious tumours.

References

1. Lee SJ, Bae JH, Lee AW, et al. Clinical characteristics of metastatic tumors of the ovaries. J Korean Med Sci. 2009;24(1):114–9.
2. de Wall YR, Thomas CM, Oei AL, et al. Secondary ovarian malignancies: frequency, origin and characteristics. Int J Gynecol Cancer. 2009;19(7):1160–5.
3. Kiyokawa T, Young RH, Scully RE. Krukenberg tumors of the ovary: a clinicopathological analysis of 120 cases with emphasis on their variable pathological manifestations. Am J Pathol. 2006;30(3):277–99.
4. Young RH. From Krukenberg to today. The ever-present problem posed by metastatic tumor in the ovary: part 1. Historical perspective, general principles, mucinous tumors including the Krukenberg tumor. Adv Anat Pathol. 2006;13(5):205–27.
5. Kondi-Pafiti A, Kairi-Vasilator E, Lavazzo C, et al. Metastatic neoplasm of the ovaries: a clinicopathological study of 97 cases. Arch Gynecol Obstet. 2011;284(5):1283–8.
6. Shah B, Tang W, Karn S. An up to date understanding of the Krukenberg tumor. Mech Adv Reprod Sci. 2016;4:31–6.
7. Moore RG, Chung M, Granai CO, et al. Incidence of metastasis to the ovaries from non-genital tract primary tumors. Gynecol Oncol. 2004;93(1):87–91.
8. Yamanshi Y, Koshiyama M, Ohnaka M, et al. Pathways of metastasis from primary organ to the ovaries. Obstet Gynecol. 2011;2011:612817.
9. Tan DS, Agarwal R, Kaye SB. Mechanism of transcelomic metastasis in ovarian cancer. Lancet Oncol. 2006;7(11):925–34.
10. Kall SL, Koblinski E. Metastatic cancer. Clinical and biological perspectives. Genes that mediate metastasis organotropism. Austin: Landes Bioscience; 2013.
11. Kikkawa F, Shibata K, Ino K, et al. Preoperative findings in non-gynecological carcinoma metastasizing to the ovaries. Gynecol Obstet. 2002;54(4):221–7.

12. Pepin K, de Carman M, Brown A, et al. CA125 and epithelial ovarian cancer: role in screening, diagnosis and surveillance. Am J Hematol Oncol. 2014;10(6):22–9.
13. Yeslema CA, Kenemens P, Wobbess T, et al. Use of serum tumor markers in the differential diagnosis between ovarian and colorectal metastasis. Tumor Biol. 1992;13(1–2):18–26.
14. Ahmed SA, El Taieb HA. Variations in radiological features between primary and secondary ovarian malignancies. Egypt J Radiol Nucl Med. 2018;49:828–37.
15. Park HL, Yoole R, O JH, et al. F18 FDG-PET/CT findings of metastatic ovarian tumors from gastrointestinal tract origin. J Cancer Res Clin Oncol. 2015;141(10):1871–8.
16. Varadhachary GR. Carcinoma of unknown primary origin. Gastrointest Cancer Res. 2007;1(6):229–35.
17. Kurman RJ, International Agency for Research on Cancer, WHO. WHO classification of tumors of female reproductive organs. World Health Organization classification of tumors. 4th ed. Lyson: International Agency for Research on Cancer.
18. Kubecek O, Laco J, Spacek J, et al. The pathogenesis, diagnosis and management of metastatic tumors to the ovary: a comprehensive review. Clin Exp Metastasis. 2017;34:295–307.
19. Greco F, Lennington WJ, Spigel JR, et al. Poorly differentiated neoplasms of unknown primary sites: diagnostic usefulness of a molecular cancer classifier assay. Mol Diagn Ther. 2015;19(2):91–7.
20. Meiri E, Mueller WC, Rosenwald S, et al. A second-generation micro-RNA bases assay for diagnosing tumors or tissue origin. Oncologist. 2012;17(6):801–12.
21. Rayson D, Bouttel E, Whiston F, et al. Outcome after ovarian/adnexal mastectomy in metastatic colorectal carcinoma. J Surg Oncol. 2000;75(3):186–92.
22. Mc Cormick CC, Giuntoli RL 2nd, Gardner GJ, et al. The role of cytoreductive surgery for colon cancer metastatic to ovary. Gynecol Oncol. 2007;105(3):791–5.
23. Cheong JH, Hyung WJ, Chen J, et al. Survival benefit of mastectomy for Krukenberg's tumor from gastric cancer. Gynecol Oncol. 2004;94(2):477–82.
24. Lu LC, Shao YY, Hsu CH, et al. Mastectomy of Krukenberg's tumor may be associated with survival benefits in patients with metastatic gastric cancer. Anticancer Res. 2012;32(8):3397–401.
25. Porteir G, Elias D, Bouche O, et al. Multicenter randomized trial of adjuvant fluorouracil and folinic acid compared with surgery alone after resection of colorectal liver metastasis: FFCD ACHBTH AURC 9002 trials. J Clin Oncol. 2006;24(31):4976–82.
26. Miller BE, Pittman B, Wan JY, et al. Colon cancer with metastasis to the ovary at the time of initial diagnosis. Gynecol Oncol. 1997;66(3):368–71.
27. Ganesh K, Shah RH. Clinical and genetic determinants of ovarian metastasis from colorectal cancer. Cancer. 2017;123(7):1134–43.

Fallopian Tube Carcinoma

Megha Nandwani, Debabrata Barmon,
and Amal Chandra Kataki

1 Introduction

Fallopian tube carcinoma occurrence is a rarity. The reported incidence of the same in literature is less than 0.5% of all gynaecological malignancies. It is often seen to occur along with epithelial ovarian cancer and recent studies have also reported that the origin of epithelial ovarian carcinomas to be from fallopian tube cells. The risk factors, staging, and management of fallopian tube cancers are similar to epithelial ovarian tumours and the prognosis also seems to be in comparison to their ovarian counterpart.

2 Pathogenesis

The origin of fallopian tube cancers are from mullerian epithelium. Due to genetic predisposition and environmental factors, this epithelium undergoes dysplasia due to DNA damage and TP53 mutations leading to the formation of cancer precursor cells that are called as p53 signatures.

M. Nandwani (✉)
Department of Gynaecologic Oncology, Dharamshila Narayana Superspeciality Hospital, New Delhi, India

D. Barmon · A. C. Kataki
Department of Gynaecologic Oncology,
Dr. Bhubaneswar Borooah Cancer Institute
(A Unit of Tata Memorial Centre, Mumbai),
Guwahati, Assam, India
e-mail: dydiracademic@bbci.tmc.gov.in

The initiation of this p53 mutations are as a result of repeated ovulation and environmental stress that leads to damage of the secretory epithelium of the fallopian tube causing intracellular inflammation. When the process is repeated, it finally leads to the formation of progenitor cells that evade apoptosis and gives rise to p53 signatures.

These p53 signatures when undergo further dysplastic changes lead to formation of serous tubal intraepithelial carcinoma (STIC) and when they disrupt the basement membrane leads to formation of invasive serous carcinoma [1, 2]. These changes are seen to occur more commonly in patients with BRCA1/2 mutations.

With the advent of new techniques in pathology, it has been seen that Sectioning and Extensive Examination of the Fimbria (SEE-FIM) protocol has helped in diagnosing STIC lesions which in the future would have developed into high grade serous carcinomas of the tube and ovaries. The SEEFIM protocol is especially used in patients with germline positivity who underwent risk reducing salpingo-oopherectomy [3].

The most common type of fallopian tube carcinoma (FTC) is secondary from other primary tumours in the body like from ovary, endometrium, colon, and appendix. The primary tumour that is commonly seen in fallopian tubes is adenocarcinoma (Figs. 1 and 2). Leiomyosarcoma, transitional cell carcinoma are rare variants of FTC.

A. C. Kataki, D. Barmon (eds.), *Fundamentals in Gynaecologic Malignancy*,
https://doi.org/10.1007/978-981-19-5860-1_20

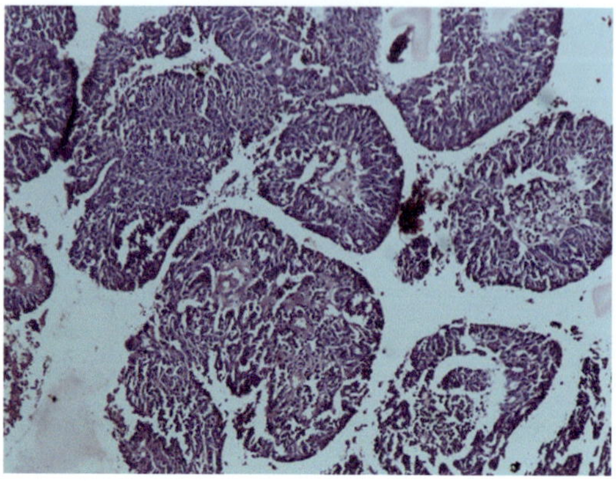

Fig. 1 Low power view (10×) of moderately differentiated papillary adenocarcinoma in the lumen of the fallopian tube

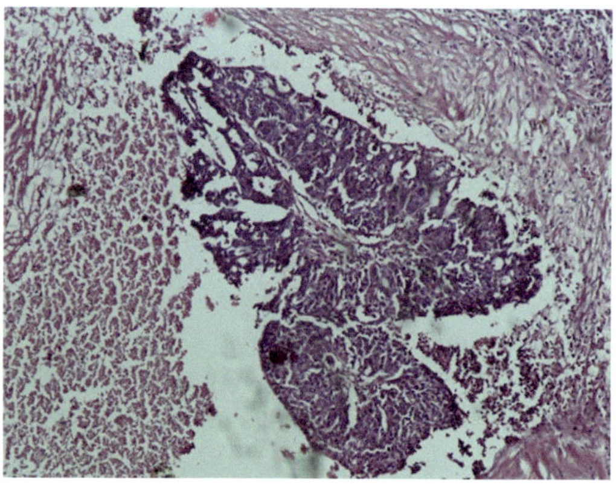

Fig. 2 Papillary adenocarcinoma of fallopian tube (High power view)

3 Clinical Features and Diagnosis

The symptoms of fallopian tube carcinoma are not specific and similar to those of ovarian carcinoma. FTC occur more commonly in nulliparous, postmenopausal women. Patients often present with pain abdomen, distension, loss of weight, loss of appetite, bowel and bladder symptoms, and white discharge per vagina.

Hydrops tubae profluens, that is characterized by colicky lower abdominal pain and is relieved by intermittent profuse watery vaginal discharge, occurs in few cases.

The Latzko triad [4] is often seen in fallopian tube carcinoma that includes watery vaginal discharge or hydrops tubae profluens, pelvic pain, and pelvic mass.

The diagnosis is made after investigating the patient and on imaging but confirmation is after biopsy report.

In the year 1959, Hu [5] gave a pathologic criteria to help in the diagnosis of fallopian tube malignancy that included:

- On gross inspection—the main tumour is in the fallopian tube.
- On microscopic examination, the mucosa is involved and shows a papillary pattern.
- If the tubal wall is involved extensively, transition between benign and malignant epithelium should be demonstrable.

In 1978, Sedlis et al. [6] gave the modification for Hu criteria of fallopian tube cancer that includes:

- The tumour arises from endosalpinx.
- The histologic pattern reproduces the epithelium of tubal mucosa.
- There is transition from benign to malignant epithelium.
- Ovary and endometrium are either normal (Fig. 3) or with a tumour that is smaller than the tumour in the tube.

CECT whole abdomen will guide on the spread of the disease, ultrasound whole abdomen is one of the initial investigations, MRI abdomen

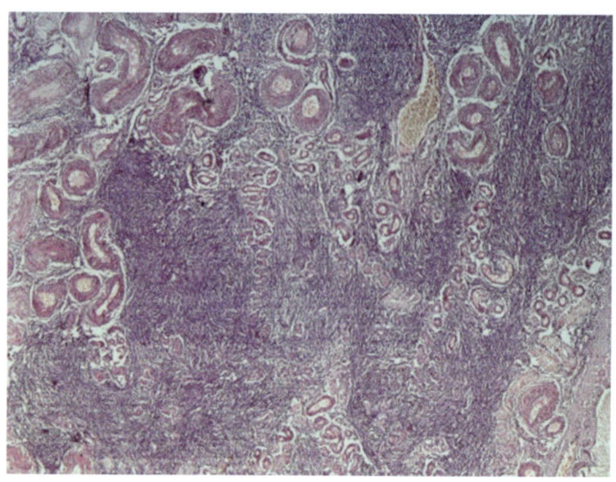

Fig. 3 Section of left ovary showing unremarkable stroma

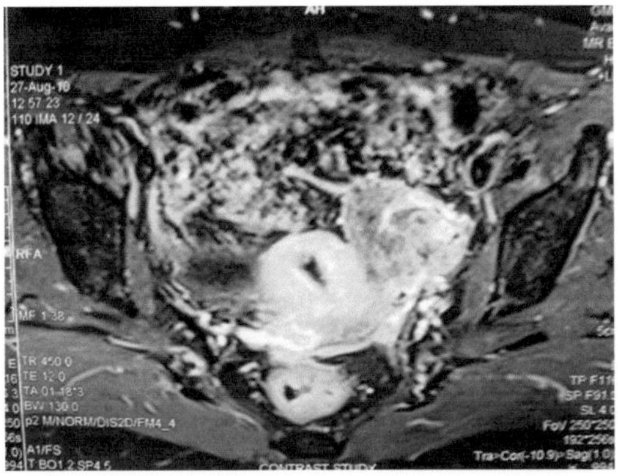

Fig. 4 MRI study showing the left adnexal mass (On HPE: Fallopian Tube Carcinoma)

(Fig. 4) may be helpful and few cases may require PET CT scan.

Ca 125 is also raised in FTC and helpful in monitoring treatment and follow-up.

Wethington et al. [7] in 2008 studied the comparison between ovarian and fallopian tube cancer among patients based on the SEER database and reported that fallopian tube cancers presented at an earlier stage as compared to their ovarian counterparts and also have a better survival as compared to ovarian cancer when presented at an advanced stage. The median age of diagnosis of both these tumours is 64 years.

Over the years, the diagnosis of fallopian tube carcinoma has almost increased four-fold in the USA. This can be attributed to better understanding of the pathology and improved diagnostic techniques [8].

4 Staging

The staging of fallopian tube carcinoma is similar to ovarian and peritoneal cancers and the updated staging for the same was given by FIGO in 2014.

5 Patterns of Spread

The pattern of spread of fallopian tube cancer follows that of ovarian cancer.

Transcoelomic spread is the most common mode of spread where tumour cells are disseminated by the process of exfoliation of cells.

Other modes of spread include lymphatic and hematogenous.

6 Prevention and Treatment

Prevention is always better than cure and it has been seen that women having germline mutation positivity of BRCA1/2 have increased incidence of fallopian tube cancer [9]. Also, since now the pathogenesis of this carcinoma is better understood, it is recommended by the Society of Gyneacologic Oncology that women belonging to the age group of 35–40 years should consider undergoing a risk reducing bilateral salpingo-oophorectomy (RR-BSO) [10]. If women at that age are not willing to undergo a surgical menopause, they should undergo bilateral salpingectomy and bilateral oophorectomy once they are ready for the same [10]. It is also observed that women with mutations of BRIP1, RAD51C, and RAD51D are at an increased risk of FTC and thus NCCN guidelines recommend women with these mutations to consider undergoing a RR-BSO at the age of 45–50 years. It is also recommended that whenever a woman undergoes any pelvic surgery like hysterectomy, bilateral salpingectomy should be considered in order to reduce the risk of fallopian tube and ovarian malignancy [11].

The treatment of fallopian tube carcinoma primarily involves surgery and platinum based chemotherapy. The newer drugs for treatment of these cancers include targeted therapy like bevacizumab and PARP {poly (adenosine diphosphate [ADP]-ribose) polymerase} inhibitors and immunotherapy.

The treatment approach toward FTC is similar to ovarian and primary peritoneal malignancies due to the similarity in their clinical behavior. There are no specific guidelines for management of fallopian tube carcinoma.

NCCN recommends that ovarian carcinomas including fallopian tube and peritoneal cancers be managed by a gynaecologic oncologist as the optimal debulking surgery is crucial in the treatment of these cancers [12]. The timing of cytoreductive surgery can be either at the beginning of treatment or after three to four cycles of neo-adjuvant chemotherapy. ASCO has recommended to offer primary cytoreductive surgery whenever feasible. However, in women when optimal debulking is not possible it is recommended to go for neo-adjuvant chemotherapy first and then to plan for interval debulking surgery [13]. Many studies in the past have been conducted which show similar survival results when primary debulking surgery was compared to neoadjuvant chemotherapy followed by interval debulking surgery and thus indicating no clear benefit of one approach over the other [14, 15].

The main chemotherapeutic agents used in FTC include carboplatin and paclitaxel. The traditional route of administering these drugs are intravenous, every three weekly for six cycles [16, 17]. The intraperitoneal route of administering these drugs has also been tried and has shown survival advantages whenever optimal debulking surgery was performed [18, 19]. In the ICON 8 trial, dose dense weekly intravenous chemotherapy regimen was compared to the three weekly protocol and that showed no survival advantage in particular [20].

The newer approaches for treatment of fallopian tube cancers include agents like bevacizumab (anti-VEGF monoclonal antibody). Various trials have tested the efficacy of bevacizumab in recurrent high grade serous epithelial ovarian cancers and have shown improved progression free survival outcomes with no benefit in the overall survival [21, 22].

The GOG 213 was the trial that showed improved overall survival with the addition of bevacizumab maintenance therapy in platinum sensitive epithelial ovarian cancer [23]. And, on the basis of GOG 218 trial results, the FDA has approved bevacizumab as one of the first line drugs in maintenance therapy for high grade serous epithelial ovarian carcinomas [24].

PARP inhibitors are also one of the novel treatments that are under research. FDA has approved olaparib, rucaparib, and niraparib agents for the treatment of epithelial ovarian cancers in patients with germline or somatic BRCA mutations, the patients with at least a partial response to platinum based chemotherapy can receive any of these three drugs as maintenance therapy in case of recurrence [25–27].

Many trials are going on to study the role of PARP inhibitors as first line maintenance therapy in patients with epithelial ovarian cancers irrespective of their mutation status. These trials include the PAOLA-1 trial, PRIMA trial and also the GOG3005 trial which is studying the role of veliparib.

Another recent approach whose role is yet to be defined is HIPEC that is hyperthermic intraperitoneal chemotherapy. Many studies have shown improved progression free survival with the use of HIPEC in first line and recurrent settings but the overall survival did not show any significant improvement [28].

Immunotherapy with pembrolizumab which is a programmed cell death protein [PD]-1 inhibitor is under research as it has shown some promise in tumours with microsatellite instability (MSI) and MSI is a rare phenomenon in ovarian cancers. Research is going on to find the appropriate immunotherapy agent for the treatment of epithelial ovarian and fallopian tube cancers.

7 Conclusion

Fallopian tube cancers are a rare occurrence and no defined guidelines are present for its management. Due to its clinical behavior and similar pathogenesis with high grade serous epithelial ovarian and peritoneal malignancies, it is staged and treated on similar lines.

References

1. Levanon K, Crum C, Drapkin R. New insights into the pathogenesis of serous ovarian cancer and its clinical impact. J Clin Oncol. 2008;26(32):5284–93. https://doi.org/10.1200/JCO.2008.18.1107.
2. Tone AA. Taking the tube: from normal fallopian tube epithelium to ovarian high-grade serous carcinoma. Clin Obstet Gynecol. 2017;60:697–710.

3. Medeiros F, Muto MG, Lee Y, et al. The tubal fimbria is a preferred site for early adenocarcinoma in women with familial ovarian cancer syndrome. Am J Surg Pathol. 2006;30:230–6.
4. Lau H-Y, Chen Y-J, Yen M-S, Chen R-F, Yeh S-O, Twu N-F. Primary fallopian tube carcinoma: a clinicopathologic analysis and literature review. J Chin Med Assoc. 2013;76:1–19.
5. Hu CY, Taymor ML, Hertig AT. Primary carcinoma of the fallopian tube. Am J Obstet Gynecol. 1950;59:58.
6. Sedlis A. Carcinoma of the fallopian tube. Surg Clin N Am. 1978;58:25–30.
7. Wethington SL, Herzog TJ, Seshan VE, et al. Improved survival for fallopian tube cancer: a comparison of clinical characteristics and outcome for primary fallopian tube and ovarian cancer. Cancer. 2008;113:3298–306.
8. Liao CI, Chow S, Chen LM, et al. Trends in the incidence of serous fallopian tube, ovarian, and peritoneal cancer in the US. Gynecol Oncol. 2018;149:318–23.
9. Vicus D, Finch A, Cass I, et al. Prevalence of BRCA1 and BRCA2 germ line mutations among women with carcinoma of the fallopian tube. Gynecol Oncol. 2010;118:299–302.
10. Walker JL, Powell CB, Chen LM, et al. Society of Gynecologic Oncology recommendations for the prevention of ovarian cancer. Cancer. 2015;121:2108–20.
11. Daly MB, Pilarski R, Berry M, et al. NCCN guidelines insights: genetic/familial high-risk assessment: breast and ovarian, version 2.2017. J Natl Compr Canc Netw. 2017;15:9–20.
12. National Comprehensive Cancer Network: ovarian cancer including fallopian tube cancer and primary peritoneal cancer. NCCN clinical practice guidelines in Oncology 2021; Version 1.2021.
13. Wright AA, Bohlke K, Armstrong DK, et al. Neoadjuvant chemotherapy for newly diagnosed, advanced ovarian cancer: society of gynecologic oncology and American Society of clinical oncology clinical practice guideline. J Clin Oncol. 2016;34:3460–73.
14. Vergote IB, De Wever I, Decloedt J, et al. Neoadjuvant chemotherapy versus primary debulking surgery in advanced ovarian cancer. Semin Oncol. 2000;27:31–6.
15. Kehoe S, Hook J, Nankivell M, et al. Primary chemotherapy versus primary surgery for newly diagnosed advanced ovarian cancer (CHORUS): an open-label, randomised, controlled, non-inferiority trial. Lancet. 2015;386:249–57.
16. International Collaborative Ovarian Neoplasm Group. Paclitaxel plus carboplatin versus standard chemotherapy with either single-agent carboplatin or cyclophosphamide, doxorubicin, and cisplatin in women with ovarian cancer: the ICON3 randomised trial. Lancet. 2002;360:505–15.
17. Ozols RF, Bundy BN, Greer BE, et al. Phase III trial of carboplatin and paclitaxel compared with cisplatin and paclitaxel in patients with optimally resected stage III ovarian cancer: a gynecologic oncology group study. J Clin Oncol. 2003;21:3194–200.
18. Armstrong DK, Bundy B, Wenzel L, et al. Intraperitoneal cisplatin and paclitaxel in ovarian cancer. N Engl J Med. 2006;354:34–43.
19. Trimble EL, Christian MC. Intraperitoneal chemotherapy for women with advanced epithelial ovarian carcinoma. Gynecol Oncol. 2006;100:3–4.
20. Clamp A, Harrell MI, Dean A, et al. ICON 8: a GCIG phase III randomised trial evaluating weekly dose-dense chemotherapy integration in first-line epithelial ovarian/fallopian tube/primary peritoneal carcinoma (EOC) treatment: results of primary progression-free survival (PFS) analysis. Ann Oncol. 2017;28(Suppl. 5):abstract 929O_PR.
21. Aghajanian C, Blank SV, Goff BA, et al. OCEANS: a randomized, double-blind, placebo-controlled phase III trial of chemotherapy with or without bevacizumab in patients with platinum-sensitive recurrent epithelial ovarian, primary peritoneal, or fallopian tube cancer. J Clin Oncol. 2012;30:2039–45.
22. Pujade-Lauraine E, Hilpert F, Weber B, et al. Bevacizumab combined with chemotherapy for platinum-resistant recurrent ovarian cancer: the AURELIA open-label randomized phase III trial. J Clin Oncol. 2014;32:1302–8.
23. Coleman RL, Brady MF, Herzog TJ, et al. Bevacizumab and paclitaxel-carboplatin chemotherapy and secondary cytoreduction in recurrent, platinum-sensitive ovarian cancer (NRG oncology/gynecologic oncology group study GOG-0213): a multicentre, open-label, randomised, phase 3 trial. Lancet Oncol. 2017;18:779–91.
24. Burger RA, Brady MF, Bookman MA, et al. Incorporation of bevacizumab in the primary treatment of ovarian cancer. N Engl J Med. 2011;365:2473–83.
25. Mirza MR, Monk BJ, Herrstedt J, et al. Niraparib maintenance therapy in platinum-sensitive, recurrent ovarian cancer. N Engl J Med. 2016;375:2154–64.
26. Coleman RL, Oza AM, Lorusso D, et al. Rucaparib maintenance treatment for recurrent ovarian carcinoma after response to platinum therapy (ARIEL3): a randomised, double-blind, placebo-controlled, phase 3 trial. Lancet. 2017;390:1949–61.
27. Ledermann J, Harter P, Gourley C, et al. Olaparib maintenance therapy in platinum-sensitive relapsed ovarian cancer. N Engl J Med. 2012;366:1382–92.
28. van Driel WJ, Koole SN, Sikorska K, et al. Hyperthermic intraperitoneal chemotherapy in ovarian cancer. N Engl J Med. 2018;378:230–40.

Carcinoma Vulva

Dimpy Begum, Pariseema Dave,
Amal Chandra Kataki, Debabrata Barmon,
and Apurba Kumar Kalita

1 Introduction

Carcinoma of vulva is one of the rare malignancies of females, accounting for only 2–5% of all gynaecological malignancy. Earlier it was known as a disease of postmenopausal women, but due to the high prevalence of HPV infection age of incidence has decreased over the years [1, 2].

The total number of new cases in 2020 (world) was 44,240 and age standardize ratio was 0.9. The total number of deaths (worldwide) was 17424 [3].

D. Begum (✉) · A. C. Kataki · D. Barmon
Department of Gynaecologic Oncology,
Dr. Bhubaneswar Borooah Cancer Institute
(A Unit of Tata Memorial Centre, Mumbai),
Guwahati, Assam, India
e-mail: dydiracademic@bbci.tmc.gov.in

P. Dave
Department of Gynaecological Oncology,
Gujarat Cancer and Research Institute,
Ahmedabad, Gujarat, India
e-mail: pariseema.dave@gcriindia.org

A. K. Kalita
Department of Radiation Oncology, Dr. B Borooah
Cancer Institute, Guwahati, Assam, India

2 Surgical Anatomy

The vulva consists of female external genital organs which include clitoris, labia majora, labia minora vaginal vestibule perineal body with skin, and all subcutaneous tissue. Anteriorly mons pubis is the element containing hair and lies over the pubic symphysis and posteriorly anus is the limit.

2.1 Vascular Supply

The vulva receives its vascular supply mainly from the internal pudendal artery, superficial and deep pudendal arteries. The internal pudendal artery is a branch of anterior division of the internal iliac artery while superficial and deep pudendal arteries are branches of the femoral artery. The internal pudendal artery gives rise to lateral and medial branches when it passes through the ischiorectal fossa. After reaching the infero-medial edge of the gluteus maximus muscle lateral branches supply the skin over this area. The medial branches of internal pudendal artery supply the skin over the perianal area in addition to the skin over the infero-medial edge of the gluteus maximus muscle. The superficial external pudendal artery gives ascending and descending branches and they supply the anterior part of genitalia and anastomose with the cutaneous branch of the deep external pudendal artery.

A. C. Kataki, D. Barmon (eds.), *Fundamentals in Gynaecologic Malignancy*,
https://doi.org/10.1007/978-981-19-5860-1_21

2.2 Lymphatic Drainage

The study of the lymphatics in the vulva is of utmost importance for the surgical treatment planning of vulvar carcinoma.

The vulva has a rich lymphatic supply with a dense interconnecting network.

2.2.1 Local Channels

The lymphatics from both sides of vulva freely intercommunicate. Because of these existing communications midline lesions and lesions within 1 cm of the midline can drain bilaterally.

Lymphatic channels from each side of anterior half of the labia majora intercommunicate with the lymphatics of opposite side in the mons pubic area and drains directly to superficial inguinal lymph nodes.

Posterior half of the labia majora directly drains to superficial inguinal nodes. Lymphatic channels from clitoris and labia minora communicate with each side and drains into superficial inguinal nodes.

2.2.2 Draining Nodes

The primary draining nodes of vulval lymphatics are inguinal nodes, which can be divided into superficial and deep nodal groups. There are around 10–20 superficial nodes that can be grouped into superior and inferior groups. All of the superficial lymph nodes in the inguinal region are located deep within the subcutaneous fat and connective tissue.

In relation to the femoral vessels, the deep inguinal lymph nodes are located deep in the cribriform fascia. The uppermost one is situated on the femoral septum proper and is called the node of Rosenmuller or Cloquet.

The external iliac lymph nodes receive drainage from the deep inguinal lymph nodes via perforations in the femoral septum of Cloquet. Superficial inguinal lymph nodes drains into the deep inguinal lymph nodes through the cribriform fascia or through direct channels to the external iliac lymph nodes (Figs. 1 and 2). From the external iliac they go to the common iliac and then to the para-aortic nodes.

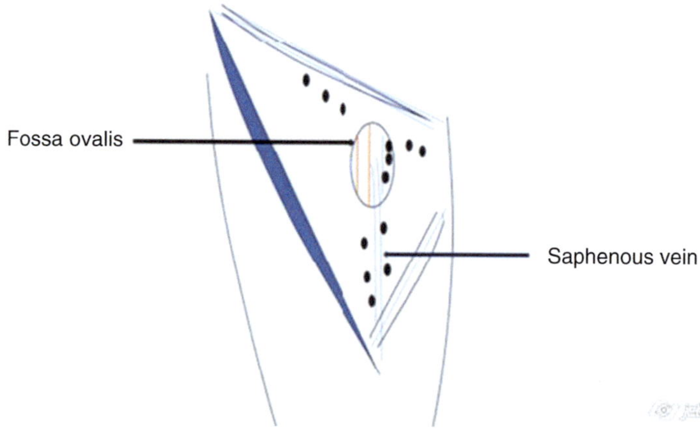

Fig. 1 Arrangement of lymph nodes in femoral triangle

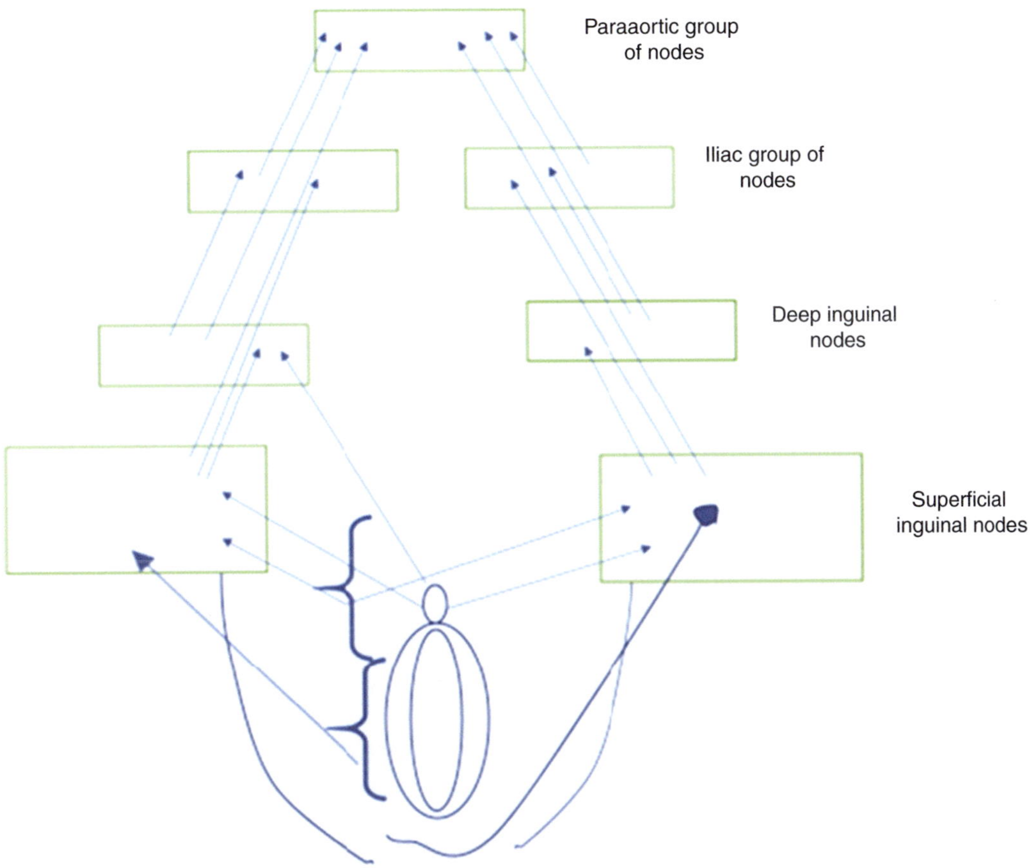

Fig. 2 Schematic representation of lymphatic drainage of vulva

3 Premalignant Diseases of Vulva

The nomenclature of vulval intraepithelial neoplasia (VIN) has changed from its initial nomenclature of VIN 1,2 and differentiated VIN to LSIL, HSIL and differentiated VIN. In 1986 ISSVD divided premalignant lesion into VIN1, 2&3 and differentiated VIN [4–6] (Table 1). This nomenclature was changed to Flat condylomata or HPV effect, VIN the usual type (VIN warty, VIN, basaloid, VIN, mixed) and VIN differentiated type. In LAST 2012 nomenclature was again changed to LSIL, HSIL, and Differentiated VIN (dVIN).

The term squamous vulvar intraepithelial neoplasia (VIN) implies to a premalignant skin disorder of vulva. Usually patient gives a history of long duration of severe pruritus. It may be also associated with psychosexual dysfunction. VIN includes a variety of clinical and histological forms and is separated into two different subgroups usual VIN and differentiated VIN, by International Society for the Study of Vulvar Disease (ISSVD) 2004. Persistent infection with high-risk Human papillomavirus (HPV) is known to be a causative agent of usual VIN, and differentiated type VIN is seen to be associated with lichen sclerosis.

Table 1 Adapted from: Hoang et al. [4] Bornstein et al. [5] Sideri et al. [6] (LAST-lower anogenital ISSVD 1986

ISSVD 1986	ISSVD 2004	LAST 2012
VIN1	Flat condylomata or HPV effect	LSIL
VIN2&3	VIN, the usual type 1. VIN warty 2. VIN, basaloid 3. VIN, mixed	HSIL
DIFFERENTIATED VIN	VIN, differentiated type	Differentiated VIN, dVIN

The two types of VIN are different in etiology, clinical features, morphology, biology, and malignant potential. The WHO classification, which includes the three subtypes VIN 1, 2, and 3, is still extensively used, however, VIN 1 is no longer considered.

A usual type of VIN (uVIN) may be warty basaloid or mixed. They are more common and associated with HPV infection. uVIN is commonly seen in younger age group. HPV deoxyribonucleic acid (DNA) mostly type 16 is present in up to 90% of classical VIN. Classical VIN has multifocality and is related to multicentric involvement of the vagina and cervix. Usual VIN progresses to cancer in 3–10% of treated patients.

Treatment—Topical imiquimod, cidofovir, indole-3 carbinol, and surgery are the main treatment options. Cidofovir cream is currently not licensed for use in uVIN.

Differentiated VIN (dVIN) is less common than uVIN. The exact cause is unknown, however, it has the most malignant potential and accounts for less than 5% of vulva preneoplastic lesions. It has a significantly higher rate of squamous vulvar carcinoma progression and a shortened time to disease progression. It also has a high rate of recurrence than HSIL. In less than 2% cases it is associated with persistent HPV infection. It is characteristically seen in postmenopausal women and in association with lichen sclerosis. The ideal treatment of choice is excision of the lesion. A free margin of 0.5–1 cm is recommended to allow proper evaluation and to rule out occult invasion [7, 8].

Non-randomized studies have suggested that good control of lichen sclerosis and lichen planus can be achieved with Clobetasol 17-propionate 0.05%, which is an ultra-potent topical steroid, and it reduces the risk of squamous cell carcinoma progression [9–11].

Non-pharmacological management should be also advised to the patients. These include avoiding irritants like soap, detergent, and scratching of the affected area.

3.1 Diagnosing Premalignant Disease of the Vulva

There is no standard screening program exist to detect vulvar carcinoma or its precursor lesions till date. However, Shakun et al. [12] described a scoring system to find out premalignant lesions of vulva. They proposed a detailed history taking and physical examination by inspecting the vulva with naked eye and under bright light by using a colposcope. 5% acetic acid was applied to vulva for 3 min and vulva was inspected for any acetowhite areas both under naked eye and under vulvoscopic examination. After that 1% aqueous solution of Toluidine blue was applied to the area and it was allowed to stay for 3 min. Then colposcopy examination of cervix and vagina was performed. After that dye is removed using 1% acetic acid and areas of toluidine blue retention were observed. After washing off toluidine blue with acetic acid hyperkeratosis was seen as areas retaining pale blue stain. A detailed examination of vulva is done by naked eye and under magnification and was looked for number and distribution of lesion, ulcer, elevated area (surface topography), hyperkeratosis, pigment change, extension over urethra, anal canal, and vagina. Then they formulated a scoring system and a score of 6 was given including the 6 factors that were found to be associated with high grade lesion which were duration more than 6 months, surface elevation, hyperkeratosis, induration, positive toluidine blue staining, and asymmetrical distribution of the lesion. Significant association with high grade lesion was found when the score was 3 or more.

4 Aetiology of Vulval Carcinoma

The exact etiology of vulval cancer is not known but it is seen to be associated with the following factors:

1. HPV infection- HPV 6 and 11 are most common HPV associated with vulvar condyloma accuminata and is later associated with the development of malignant disease of vulva. Other HPV serotype associated with vulval cancer are 16,18,33,52.
2. Smoking-It hampers T cell mediated immunity.
3. HIV-Chronic immunosuppression is associated with development of invasive vulvar cancer.
4. Other factors-Like premalignant diseases of vulva.

5 Modes of Spread

Vulvar cancers metastasize in the following ways:

1. Local growth and extension into nearby organs.
2. Lymphatic embolization to regional inguinal lymph nodes, and.
3. Hematogenous spread to distant sites, e.g., to lung, bone, and liver.

Metastasis to inguinal nodes can be predicted by the presence of multiple risk factors such as tumour diameter, higher histologic grade, depth of stromal invasion, and lymph- vascular space invasion [13]. Following are the important clinical observations regarding nodal metastases in vulval carcinoma:

(a) Inguinal nodes are the most common site of lymphatic metastasis.
(b) In-transit metastases within the vulvar epithelium and deep tissues are very rare and it indicate that most initial lymphatic metastases are by embolization.
(c) Metastasis to the contralateral groin or deep pelvic nodes are usually not seen in the absence of ipsilateral groin metastases.
(d) Nodal involvement occurs in a systematic way from the superficial inguinal to the deep inguinal and then to the pelvic nodes [13].

Lymphatic spread is strongly associated with lesion size. When size of the tumour is less than 2 cm in diameter metastasis is present in 20–30% of tumours and metastasis is seen around 44% of cases when tumour is more than 2 cm in size [14]. Lymph node involvement also co-relate with the depth of invasion. Usually tumours with less than 1-mm depth of invasion have less than1% risk of nodal spread [15, 16].

6 Clinical Presentation

Symptoms

1. Vulval pruritus is the most common symptom which is usually of long duration.
2. Vulval ulcer- Patients who ignore pruritus for a long duration present with proliferative growth or vulval ulcer.
3. Other symptoms- Though not common but patient may present with a mass over the inguinal area. In late stages patient may come with the complaints of bleeding also from ulcerated vulval area (Fig. 3).

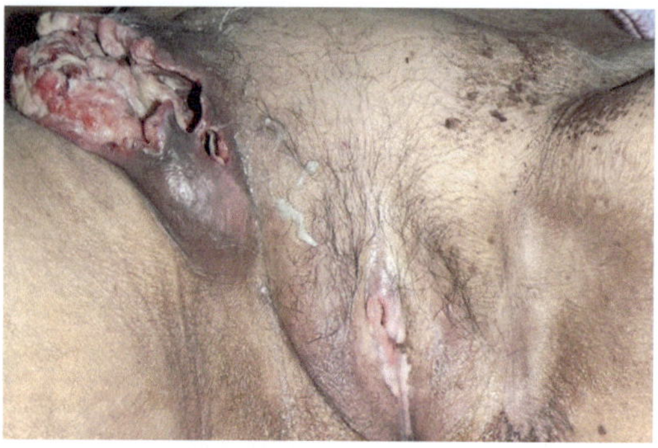

Fig. 3 Patient presenting with ulcerated inguinofemoral lymph node

7 Evaluation

7.1 Biopsy

Incisional biopsy is the recommendation of choice. It may be punch biopsy or wedge biopsy. Biopsy should be done from the area where there is a transition from normal to abnormal tissue is present. Adequate depth of the biopsy is necessary to differentiate between superficial and deep invasion of more than 1 mm.

Excisional biopsy is to be avoided always because of the following

- It often limits the option for conservative treatment.
- In case of a small lesion, the area heals well so later more definitive treatment of the area is not possible.
- And often once the surgery is done and local symptom is relieved patient refuses to undergo additional definite surgery.

Ideally, pre- and post-biopsy diagram of the area to be done. Key's biopsy forceps may be used for taking a biopsy.

7.2 Pre-Operative Investigation

1. Clinical examination for gross nodal enlargement should be done along with radiological imaging such as CT scan of the pelvis to evaluate pelvic nodal involvement.
2. Colposcopy and cervical pap smear.
3. FNAC/or core biopsy of the palpable groin nodes. It should be done as it alters the primary treatment modality. The treatment modality of involved node is always debulking of the node.
4. PET CT is indicated when a distant metastasis is suspected.

8 Staging

Since 1988, vulvar carcinoma has been surgically staged, and the final diagnosis is established from the histopathological reports of the vulvar and lymph node specimens. The FIGO staging of vulvar carcinoma is used which was revised in 2009 by the FIGO Committee on Gynaecologic Oncology [17] (Table 2). This system is applicable for most of the malignancies arising from the vulva, except melanoma.

Table 2 FIGO 2009 staging of vulval carcinoma

Stage I	Tumour confined to the vulva
IA	Lesion ≤2 cm in size, confined to the vulva or perineum and with stromal invasion ≤1.0 mm, no nodal metastasis
IB	Lesions >2 cm in size or with stromal invasion >1.0 mm, confined to the vulva or perineum, with negative nodes
Stage II	Tumour of any size with extension to adjacent perineal structures (lower third of urethra, lower third of vagina, anus) with negative nodes
Stage III	Tumour of any size with or without extension to adjacent perineal structures (lower third of urethra, lower third of vagina, anus) with positive inguinofemoral nodes
IIIA	(a) With 1 lymph node metastasis (≥5 mm), or (b) With 1–2 lymph node metastasis(es) (<5 mm)
IIIB	(a) With 2 or more lymph node metastases (≥5 mm), or (b) With 3 or more lymph node metastases (<5 mm)
IIIC	With positive nodes with extracapsular spread
Stage IV	Tumour invades other regional (upper 2/3 urethra, upper 2/3 vagina) or distant structures Tumour invades any of the following:

Table 2 continued

IVA	(a) upper urethral and/or vaginal mucosa, bladder mucosa, rectal mucosa, or fixed to pelvic bone, or (b)fixed or ulcerated inguinofemoral lymph nodes
IVB	Any distant metastasis including pelvic lymph nodes

8.1 New FIGO Staging of Vulval Carcinoma

Recently, FIGO society revised the vulval cancer staging in 2021 [18] with a goal of simplification. This staging system actively collaborated with the United States National Cancer Database to analyze prospectively collected data on carcinoma of the vulva. Recently, FIGO society revised the vulval cancer staging in 2021 [18] (Table 3) with a goal of simplification. This staging system actively collaborated with the United States National Cancer Database to analyze prospectively collected data on carcinoma of the vulva.

Important modifications done in this staging are:

1. Lymph node positivity should correspond to the micro-metastasis and macro-metastasis criteria as used in cervical cancer staging.
2. Individual tumour cells (ITC) will not count toward lymph node metastasis.
3. Cross-sectional imaging results to be included in the staging of vulvar cancer similar to cervical cancer.
4. This staging applies to all morphological types of vulvar cancer, not just the most common squamous cell carcinoma. The only exception is melanoma of the vulva.
5. It is strongly recommended to record the HPV status of vulvar cancer (HPV related or HPV independent). This is assessed by p16 blocking type immunoreactivity and/or HPV positive molecular test.

Table 3 FIGO 2021 staging for carcinoma vulva

Stage	Description
Stage I	Tumour confined to the vulva IA Tumour size ≤2 cm and stromal invasion ≤1 mm[a] IB Tumour size >2 cm or stromal invasion >1 mm[a]
Stage II	Tumour of any size with extension to lower one-third of the urethra, lower one-third of the vagina, lower one-third of the anus with negative nodes
Stage III	Tumour of any size with extension to upper part of adjacent perineal structures, or with any number of nonfixed, nonulcerated lymph node
IIIA	Tumour of any size with disease extension to upper two-thirds of the urethra, upper two-thirds of the vagina, bladder mucosa, rectal mucosa, or regional lymph node metastases ≤5 mm
IIIB	Regional[b] lymph node metastases >5 mm
IIIC	Regional[b] lymph node metastases with extracapsular spread
Stage IV	Tumour of any size fixed to bone, or fixed, ulcerated lymph node metastases, or distant metastases
IVA	Disease fixed to pelvic bone, or fixed or ulcerated regional[b] lymph node metastases
IVB	Distant metastases

[a] Depth of invasion is measured from the basement membrane of the deepest, adjacent, dysplastic, tumour-free rete ridge (or nearest dysplastic rete peg) to the deepest point of invasion
[b] Regional refers to inguinal and femoral lymph nodes

9 Pathology

During evaluating a histopathological specimen, the following points are to be noted:

1. Type of carcinoma- Squamous cell carcinoma may be nonkeratinizing, keratinizing, basaloid, and warty condylomata. Less common types are acantholytic SCC, SCC with tumour giant cells and spindle cell squamous carcinoma, SCC with sarcoma-like stroma.
2. Specimen lesion size- Size of tumour is important for staging purpose as size is related to lymph vascular invasion.

3. Grading-Grading of squamous cell carcinoma are G1, G2, and G3. Grading depends upon extent of keratinization, intercellular bridges, and cellular pleomorphism. Higher the grade poorer is the survival.
4. Depth of invasion- It is a good indicator to know the likelihood of regional lymph node involvement.
5. Lymphovascular invasion- It plays a major role in spread of vulval cancer and predicts regional lymph node involvement.
6. Clearance margin-1 cm tumour free margin is recommended.
7. Lymph node status- It is the single most important factor for determining prognosis of the disease.

10 Management

It may be surgical or radiotherapy:

(a) Surgical management includes management of primary site, nodal management, and management of complications.
(b) Radiotherapy may be given as primary, adjuvant, neoadjuvant, and in palliative modality.

10.1 Surgical Management

10.1.1 Primary Lesion

Surgery is the mainstay of the treatment of vulval carcinoma in all stages but in advanced stage IV disease, surgery is limited to palliate symptoms only.

The initial vulval surgery has changed from single en-block butterfly incision by Taussig and Way to newer three incisional surgery. The three incisional surgery has earned its place because of lesser wound breakdown rate. A triple incision technique for radical vulvectomy with bilateral inguino-femoral lymphadenectomy from three separate incisions were first introduced by Byron and colleagues. It helped to overcome the extensive butterfly resection that was used earlier [19].

Surgery for vulval primary can be as follows:

- Radical vulvectomy,
- Radical hemi vulvectomy, and.
- Wide local radical excision.

Over the years, the terms such as simple vulvectomy and radical vulvectomy were used by various surgeons. Hence, ISSVD in 2020 [20] has given new terminology by defining extent of surgery in each case to standardize the nomenclature. The newly defined nomenclature divided vulva and inguino femoral lymphadenectomy surgery into superficial and deep.

Superficial vulvectomy is removal of the most superficial layer with a variable amount of dermis and subcutaneous tissue. Removal of vulval tissue up to aponeurosis of urogenital diaphragm or pubic bone is termed as deep vulvectomy.

Superficial inguinofemoral lymph node dissection term is used when nodes are removed located near the inguinal ligament and around the upper part of the great saphenous vein and its branch. Whereas deep inguinofemoral lymph node dissection is removal of the deep femoral lymph nodes located in the subfascial space between or along the femoral vessels.

Stage IA—Wide local excision is defined as the removal of vulval skin with a thin layer of subcutaneous fat under the tumour with a margin of 1–2 cm.

Stage IB, II, III (selected) unifocal lesion—modified radical vulvectomy or radical local excision. Excision of primary tumour till an inferior layer of urogenital margin with a free margin of 1–2 cm. Consideration is given to spare vital structure like urethra clitoris and anal sphincter. The lower one-third of the urethra can be removed without causing any incontinence.

Locally advanced disease or multifocal disease

1. Radical vulvectomy where the entire vulva down to the layer of the deep fascia of the thigh, periosteum of the pubis, and the inferior layer of the urogenital diaphragm with a tumour free margin of 1–2 cm is removed.

2. Total pelvic exenteration—In advanced primary or relapsed vulvar carcinoma it is a therapeutic option which can offer median- to long-term survival for many patients. Although, spread to regional lymph nodes and complete resection is the most important prognostic factor [21].

For the covering of large vulvo-vaginal defect different kinds of flaps can be used. The aims of reconstructive surgery are the anatomical restoration of the external female genitalia, preservation of the normal body image, sexual function, micturition, and defecation [15].

Commonly used flaps for vulvar reconstruction are myo-cutaneous flaps and fascio-cutaneous flaps:

1. Fasciocutaneous flap—In this flap skin, subcutaneous fat, and underlying fascia are included, e.g., V-Y flap, lotus petal flap.
2. Myocutaneous flap—This type of flap consists of muscle which is supplied by a neurovascular bundle, e.g., Gracilis, Gluteus maximus, Tensor fascia latae, vertical rectus abdominals abdominal flap (VRAM), and anterolateral thigh flap (ALT).

It is the most commonly used technique to close small vulval defects where primary closure is not possible. The flaps are designed on the presence of a dense vascular network near the vaginal orifice. Therefore, it can be easily transposed to cover the defect area. These flaps resemble the petal of lotus [22] (Fig. 4). They are easy and fast to raise with excellent healing properties. This flap is based on the blood supply from internal pudendal vessels (Fig. 5). The width of the flap should be equal to the width of the defect.

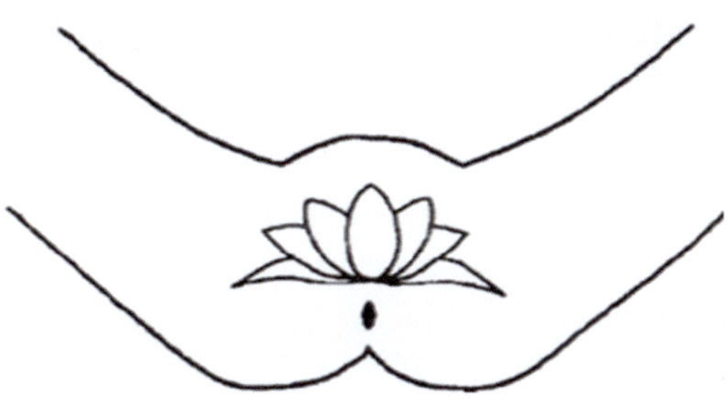

Fig. 4 Diagrammatic representation of Lotus petal flap

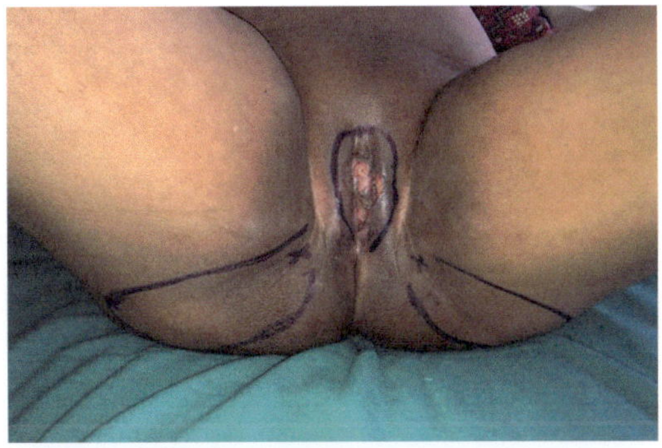

Fig. 5 Localization of Internal pudendal vessel

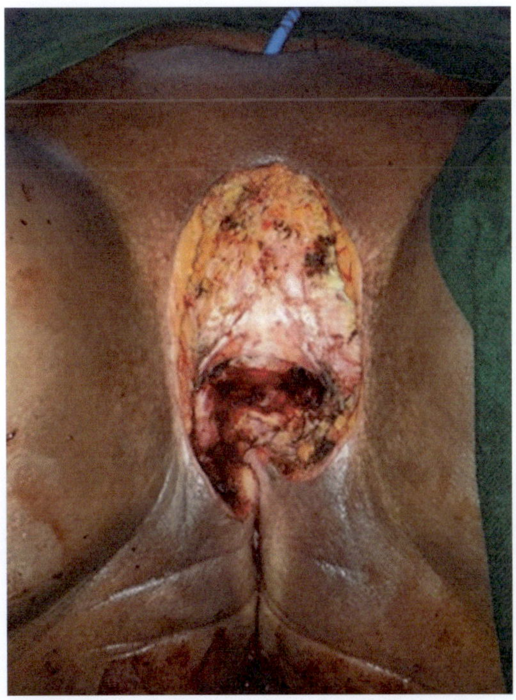

Fig. 6 Defect after excision of tumour

These flaps are simple to perform and have good cosmesis (Figs. 6 and 7).

It is based on medial circumflex artery, which is a branch of deep femoral artery. It has advantage of rotating 90 and 180 degree and can be used to fill groin and vulval defects.

It is used to fill defect in groin and vulval area and is commonly used for vaginal reconstruction at pelvic exenterative surgery. It can be based on superior and inferior epigastric vessels.

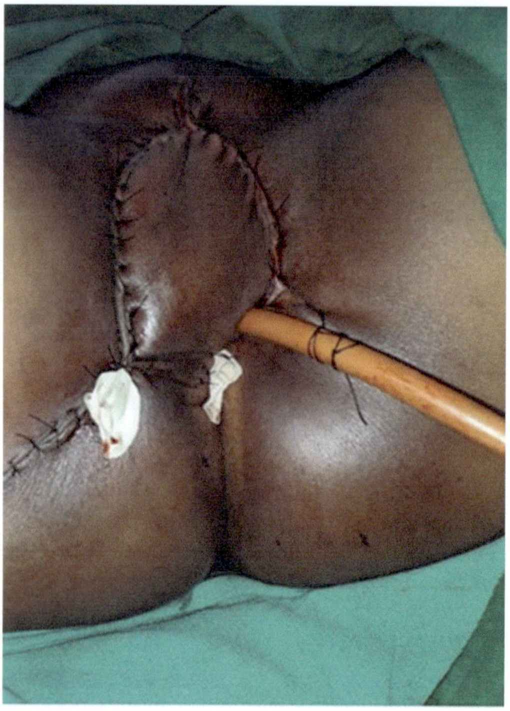

Fig. 7 Final lotus petal flap repair

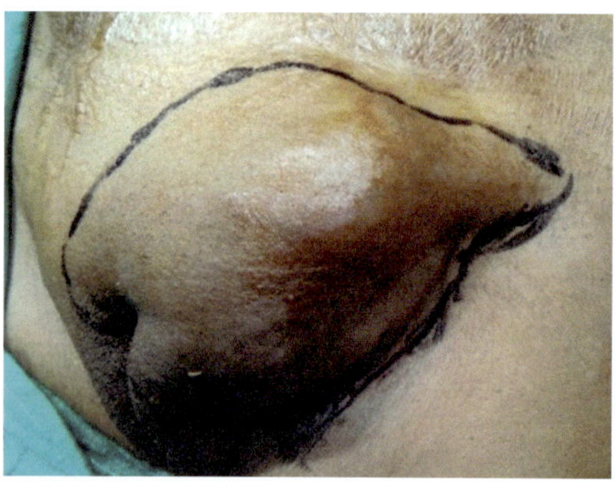

Fig. 8 Residual groin node post irradiation

Disadvantage of this flap is that it requires abdominal incision.

Usually used after surgery as a filling defect in post-irradiated groin nodal dissection (Figs. 8 and 9). Disadvantage of this flap is that it causes knee instability.

Antero lateral thigh flap (Fig. 10) can also be used to cover groin node defect.

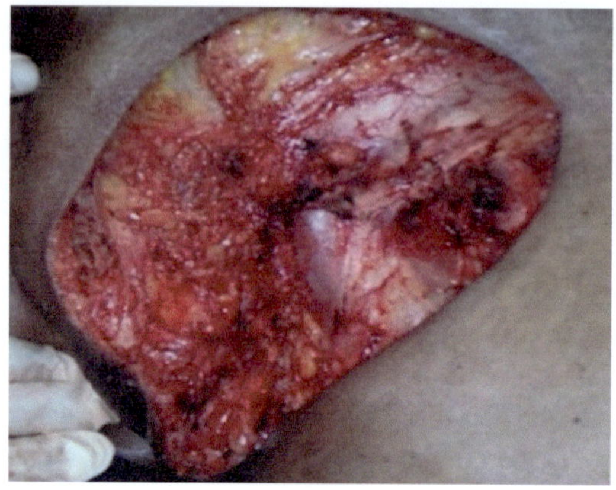

Fig. 9 Excision of the residual node post-irradiation

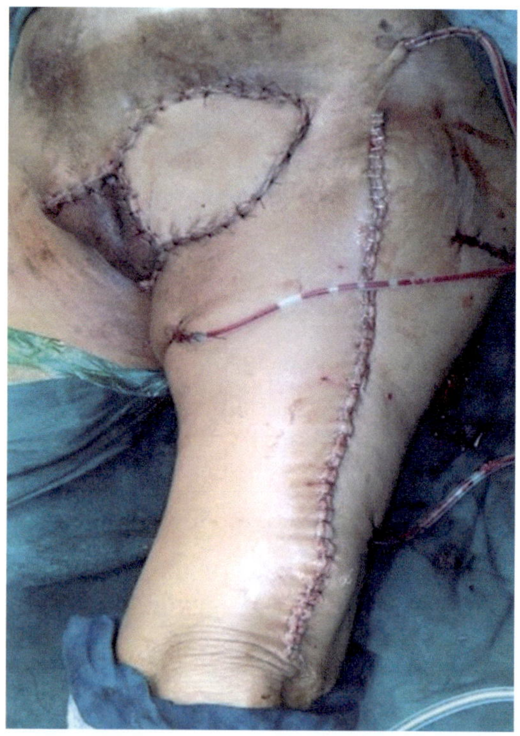

Fig. 10 Anteriolateral thigh flap repair of groin nodal area after post-radiation resection

10.1.2 Nodal Management

The nodal management can be done as follows:

1. Inguinofemoral lymphadenectomy.
2. Sentinel lymph node biopsy.

The anatomy and description regarding superficial and deep inguinofemoral lymphadenectomy already been discussed above.

Indications of inguinofemoral lymphadenectomy:

(a) Unilateral inguinofemoral lymphadenectomy can be done when the tumour is >2 cm from midline.
(b) Bilateral inguinofemoral lymphadenectomy to be done when the lesion is midline/medial.
(c) In all *T1 Tumours with stromal invasion >1 mm.
(d) In all **T2 and ***T3 lesions.

* T1 Tumour category of TNM staging is corresponds to stage I of FIGO classification of vulval cancer.

** T2 Corresponds to stage II of FIGO classification of vulval cancer.

*** T3 Corresponds to stage IVa of FIGO classification of vulval cancer.

Incision—Inguinal lymph nodes in the femoral triangle can be approached by following the ways of incisions:

1. Incision 2 cm below and in medial two third of a line joining parallel to inguinal ligament extending from anterior superior iliac spine to pubic tubercle. Drawing of femoral triangle anatomy before giving incision as shown in Fig. 11 is often useful.
2. Incision designed as an ellipse at least 4 cm wide extending from the anterior superior iliac [23] spine to the base of the femoral triangle.
3. Vertical lazy S incision or also known as hockey stick incision- It is associated with higher morbidity [24] but has the advantage of extending towards the abdomen to do pelvic lymphadenectomy.

Raising skin flap and removing nodes-The dissection is carried through subcutaneous tissue over to the superficial fascia. Dissection is carried out up to 1 cm above the inguinal ligament. The skin flaps are to be handled carefully to keep vascularity intact which can reduce postoperative flap necrosis. The superficial inguinal nodes are removed en-bloc after proper exposure of saphenous vein. Deep inguinal nodes are accessed by exposing the areolar tissue near femoral vessels deep to fascia lata. The dissection is carried out till medial border of sartorius and medially to lateral border of adductor longus.

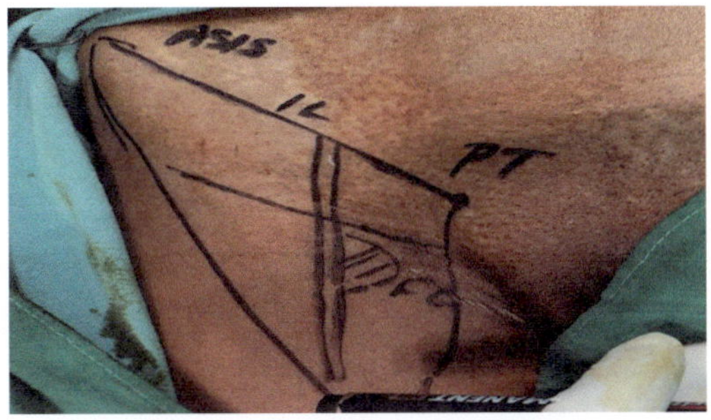

Fig. 11 Drawing the line of incision and femoral anatomy before inguinal lymph node dissection

Controversy among surgeons prevails regarding the preservation or sacrifice of the saphenous vein due to the lack of sufficient evidence.

A meta-analysis of four studies of patients undergoing inguinal lymphadenectomy with saphenous vein preservation has concluded that in comparison to individuals who underwent a radical inguinal lymphadenectomy, there was a decreased rate of wound necrosis (OR 0.34, 95% CI 0.19–0.59) and lymphedema (OR 0.24, 95% CI 0.11–0.53) in saphenous vein preservation group. Similarly, the meta-analysis also found that the saphenous vein preservation group had a decreased rate of acute cellulitis (OR 0.4, 95% CI 0.16–0.96) [25].

Closure of inguinal wound-The skin incision can be closed with absorbable sutures or with staples. A closed suction drain is to be placed. Drain should be removed when output is less than 25 mL/day.

Complications

1. Wound dehiscence.
2. Cellulitis.
3. Lymphocyst- Occurs in 40% of cases [26].
4. Lymphedema- Occurs in 62% Of cases. 50% of cases occurred in within 3 months and while 85% patient experienced in 12 months [27].

5. Recurrent lymphangitis, urinary stress incontinence, introital stenosis, femoral hernia, pubic osteomyelitis, and rectovaginal or retroperitoneal fistulae are late complications.

Methods to decrease postoperative morbidity

1. VEIL- Tobias-Machado et al. [28] found that VEIL group had a 20% complication rate compared to a 70% complication rate in patients who received a traditional open lymphadenectomy.

   Other techniques like preservation of fascia lata, omental flap pediculoplasty, and myocutaneous flap [29] techniques shown to demonstrate post-operative morbidity.
2. Sentinel lymph node biopsy.

Due to a higher rate of complications of inguinal lymph node dissection it has become standard for vulval cancer surgery when indicated.

Sentinel lymph nodes are the first draining lymph node of a tumour identified by dye tracing techniques. Morton and colleagues for the first time had given the modern concept of SLN by demonstrating in patients with cutaneous melanoma and subsequently described in patients with vulvar cancer [30, 31].

GROINS V and GOG 173 trials strongly support that, SLNB should be offered to eligible women with vulvar cancer when facilities are available.

The Groningen International Study on Sentinel Nodes in Vulvar Cancer (GROINSS-V) trial used a prospective, observational design, enrolling 403 evaluable women with tumours ≤4 cm who underwent SLNB alone. At 5 years, the rate of isolated inguinal node recurrence was 2.5% for sentinel node-negative individuals and 8% for sentinel node-positive patients. The authors found that, while sentinel node-negative individuals have a good prognosis, the significant rate of local recurrence in these patients is alarming [32].

GOG 173 is a randomized phase III trial which included 452 women who underwent the planned procedures, and 418 had at least one sentinel lymph node identified. 132 node- positive women, with 11 (8.3%) with false-negative nodes were included in the study. 23% of the true-positive cases were detected by immunohistochemical analysis of the sentinel lymph node. Sensitivity detected was 91.7% (90% lower confidence bound, 86.7%) and false-negative predictive value (1-negative predictive value) was 3.7% (90% upper confidence bound, 6.1%). When the size of the tumour was less than 4 cm size, the false-negative predictive value was 2.0% (90% upper confidence bound, 4.5%). As per this trial sentinel lymph node biopsy is an acceptable alternative to inguinal femoral lymphadenectomy in selected women with vulvar squamous cell carcinoma [33].

Isosulfan blue (Fig. 12), blue-violet, or methylene blue, or a radioactive tracer called technetium-99m (99mTc) with lymphoscintigraphy are dyes that can be used. Combined blue dye and 99m Tc has the highest rate of detection of the sentinel lymph node [34].

For pathological examination- As frozen sectioning of lymph nodes during surgery can result in tissue loss, paraffin-embedded tissue analysis is recommended.

SLND is indicated in unifocal disease with depth of invasion >1 mm, with a tumour size of <4 cm in vivo where perilesional injection is possible. Tumour should not encroach on the urethra, anus, or vagina and there should not be clinical or radiological evidence of involved nodes.

When SLN is the positive additional treatment of the area either in the form of unilateral lymphadenectomy or bilateral lymphadenectomy (when indicated) or radiotherapy to the area needed as

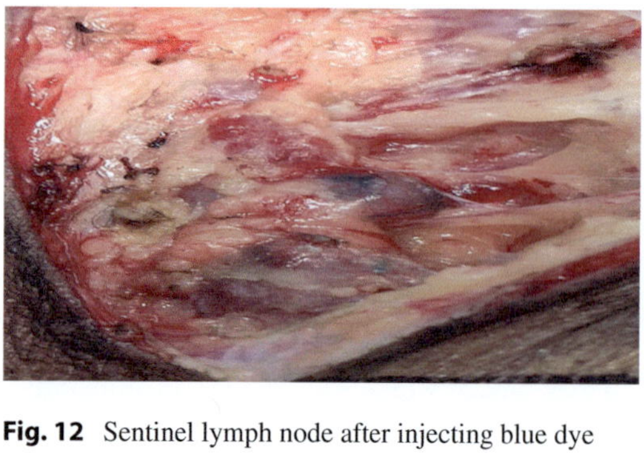

Fig. 12 Sentinel lymph node after injecting blue dye

there is significant increase in risk of spread of disease to other nodes.

SLN management should be done according to following recommendations [35]:

1. It should be done by experts after proper training only in lesion were indicated with radioisotope.
2. Preoperative lymphoscintigraphy is recommended.
3. Bilateral SLND should be performed if the tumours involve the midline. The detection of a unilateral SLN in these cancers should be considered "method failure," and inguinofemoral lymphadenectomy of the contralateral groin (no sentinel identified) should be considered [4].
4. Intraoperative frozen section can be done.
5. Ultra-staging should be done when node is negative on H&E stain. Sections for ultra-staging should be done at 200 μm apart.
6. When SLN is positive then inguinofemoral lymphadenectomy is the treatment of choice.

Woelber et al. [36] have shown that in SLND negative cases inguinofemoral lymphadenectomy can be safely omitted. The Groningen International Study on Sentinel nodes in Vulvar cancer (GROINSS-V)-II Conducted a prospective phase II multicentric trial to find a safe alternative to inguinofemoral lymphadenectomy in vulval cancer. They compare radiotherapy to inguinofemoral lymphadenectomy with micrometastasis cases in terms of isolated groin recurrence in 24 months. The trial was conducted from 2005 to 2016 and 1535 patients were included. Unifocal macro invasive squamous cell carcinoma of the vulva less than 4 cm in size with preoperative radiological imaging of groins showed no suspicious groin nodes or if found suspicious metastasis was rule out with FNAC were included in the trial. Sentinel lymph node biopsy done by routine hematoxylin and eosin stain and ultra-staging. In 322 patients showed sentinel lymph node positivity. In June 2010, with 91 SN-positive patients included, the stopping rule was activated because the isolated groin recurrence rate in this group went above our predefined threshold. Among ten patients with an isolated groin recurrence, nine had SN metastases 2 mm and/or extracapsular spread.

The protocol was amended and patient with sentinel node positivity with SN macro metastases (> 2mm) underwent inguinofemoral lymphadenectomy and patients with SN micro metastases (≤2 mm) received inguinofemoral radiotherapy at a dose of 50 Gy in 25–28 fractions of 1.8–2 Gy, five fractions/week. Out of 160 micro-metastasis positive sentinel lymph node, 126 received radiotherapy. They had an ipsilateral groin recurrence rate of 1.6% at 2 years. Out of 162 patients having macro metastasis positive sentinel lymph node recurrence rate at 2 years was 22% in radiotherapy group and 6.9% in inguinofemoral lymphadenectomy group. Morbidity with radiotherapy group was less compared to surgical group. Therefore, inguinofemoral radiotherapy is a safe alternative in micro-metastasis with less morbidity [37].

Management of pelvic nodes

- Pelvic nodes are also affected in 20–30% of the patient with inguinofemoral lymph node metastasis.

Pelvic radiotherapy is superior to surgery regarding overall survival [38].

11 Radiotherapy (RT)

In vulval carcinoma, radiotherapy can be used as an adjuvant, primary or as palliative treatment modality.

Indication adjuvant radiotherapy are as follows:

- More than one positive lymph node.
- One node if Extracapsular spread is present.
- Margin positive cases when repeat surgery for revision of margin cannot be done.
- Histopathologically Negative margin <2 mm, where repeat surgery not advisable [35].
- Close margin <8 mm histopathologically.

The adjuvant treatment to the pelvis is recommended to a patient with a positive inguinofemoral lymph node. In the adjuvant setting, the radiotherapy dose to the nodal area range from 45 to 50 Gy in 1.8–2 Gy per fraction followed by a boost to the primary area to an added dose of 60 Gy. Traditionally the radiotherapy is delivered using conventional 2D techniques in supine frog-leg position to reduce toxicity to the groin skin folds. More conformal techniques such as 3D CRT and IMRT with proper IGRT protocol are used nowadays to minimize radiation dose to the surrounding normal structures.

Faul et al. [39] studied 62 patients retrospectively with close and positive margin. In this study adjuvant radiotherapy vs. observation was done. 58% recurrence occurred in the observed group and 16% recurrence in the radiotherapy group. They concluded that adjuvant radiation therapy significantly reduced local recurrence rates and may improve overall survival in this group of patients.

11.1 Adjuvant Chemotherapy or Chemoradiation

The role of chemotherapy or chemoradiation in vulvar cancer in the adjuvant setting is not established yet. Bellati et al. [40] 2005, Han et al. [41] 2000, and Moore et al. [42] 2005 have studied regarding the role of chemotherapy in vulval carcinoma.

Bellati et al. [40] included 14 patients and treated with single-agent cisplatin after radical surgery for advanced vulvar cancer in an adjuvant setting. These patients did not receive radiotherapy and only patients with two or more affected inguinofemoral lymph nodes were included. This treatment led to a 3-year progression-free survival of 71% and an overall survival of 86%. Due to the small number of patients in this trial the trial is not recommended to use in clinical settings.

Han et al. [41] recruited 54 patients and compared adjuvant chemoradiation vs. radiotherapy alone in the adjuvant setting and showed an improvement in chemoradiation arm. However, a statistically significant result was not found.

The AGO-CaRE-1 study is a retrospective multicenter study in vulvar cancer, included 1249 cases. The included 447 (35.8%) patients had one or two nodes positive. They reported that adjuvant radiotherapy was linked to a better prognosis in node-positive individuals, which might help alleviate worries about adjuvant treatment. But outcome even after adjuvant radiotherapy in node positive patients is poor compared with node-negative patients. 3 year PFS was 35.2% in node-positive versus 75.2% in node-negative cases. They concluded that adjuvant chemoradiation could be a possible strategy to improve therapy because it is superior to radiotherapy alone in other squamous cell carcinomas.

11.2 Radiotherapy as a Primary Modality in Treating Vulval Carcinoma vs. Neoadjuvant Radiotherapy

Surgery is the treatment of choice in all stages of vulval carcinoma but in advanced stage vulval cancer when patients not suitable for surgery, primary radiotherapy can be used as a treatment modality [35]. In radical setting prophylactic nodal areas should be irradiated to 45–50 Gy and boost to the primary and nodal disease to a dose of 60–66 Gy in 1.8–2 Gy per fraction. The technique being the same as in adjuvant setting.

It has the advantage of improving organ preservation and decrease surgical morbidity.

Neoadjuvant chemoradiation followed by surgery vs. definite chemoradiation.

A study was conducted by Natesan et al. [43] to see the patterns of care and the survival impact of primary radiation and preoperative radiation therapy with surgery in patients of locally advanced vulvar cancer. They included around 2046 women from 2004 to 2012 diagnosed and treated for vulval carcinoma. They found that primary nonsurgical management of vulvar cancer with RT modality, had poor overall survival compared with preoperative RT with surgery (At 3 years, 41.7% vs. 57.1%, respectively, with significant P value). Concurrent chemotherapy improved OS of primary RT when more than 55 Gy was used compared to CRT + S (hazards ratio, 1.107; 95% confidence interval, 0.919–1.334; $P = 0.234$) [43].

11.3 Palliative Radiotherapy

Patients with very advanced disease not suitable for surgery are offered palliative radiotherapy to relief various symptoms. Commonly prescribed dose schedules are 30 Gy in 10 fractions or 20 Gy in 5 fractions.

12 Recurrent Vulval Carcinoma

The most common site of occurrence of recurrent disease is the vulva and most of the recurrence occur within 2 years [44].

The site of recurrence in vulva may be:

1. Primary tumour site recurrence (up to and 2 cm within vulvectomy scar). Survival after this recurrence is poor 3-year survival is only 15.4%.
2. Remote vulval recurrence (>2 cm from the primary site of tumour)—It has a good prognosis.

3-year survival is 66.7%.

3. Skin bridge recurrence is associated with poor survival.

Local vulval recurrence is responsive to surgical resection.

Interstitial brachytherapy can be used to treat local recurrence.

Distant recurrence is usually difficult to manage. Chemotherapy can be an option to treat in those cases with agents such as cisplatin, cyclophosphamide, mitomycin, and methotrexate.

An epidermal growth factor receptor inhibitor, e.g., erlotinib, can also be used as targeted therapy [44]. Clinical benefit rate was 67.5% with 11 (27.5%) partial responses (PR), 16 (40.0%) stable disease (SD), and 7 (17.5%) progressive disease. Duration of responses were short. All pre- and post-treatment biopsies showed EGFR staining of more than 2+ [45].

13 Follow-Up

People diagnosed and treated with vulval carcinoma should be seen for a physical examination:

1. Every 3 months for 2 years.
2. Then every 6 months for 3–5 years.
3. Then yearly after that.

14 Prognosis

The most important prognostic factors that affect recurrence risk and disease-specific mortality are:

1. Nodal status particularly the number of positive nodes.
2. Size of the largest metastasis.
3. The presence or absence of extracapsular extension [40].

Two-year survivals for vulvar cancer patient with positive groin lymph node is 68%, and with positive pelvic lymph node is 23%. The 5 years survival of stage I is 95%, in stage II is 75–85%, in stage III it is 55% whereas it decrease to 5–20% in stage IV disease.

15 Paget's Disease of Vulva

Extramammary Paget's disease is a rare form of superficial skin cancer. The most common site of involvement is vulva. It is mainly seen in postmenopausal white women. Around 15% of women with vulvar Paget's disease have underlying primary adenocarcinoma, usually arising within apocrine glands or the underlying Bartholin's glands. The Wilkinson and Brown etiologic classification of vulvar Paget's disease divides Paget's disease into two groups: cutaneous and non-cutaneous origin. The most common types of non-cutaneous Paget's disease are associated with colorectal adenocarcinoma or bladder urothelial carcinoma.

Cutaneous Paget's disease is most commonly a primary intraepithelial neoplasm, and in such cases, the intraepithelial Paget's disease may have an associated invasive Paget's disease.

Clinically they present with complaint of white and red scaly areas on the vulva which may be itchy and painful. Treatment is surgical excision, Mohs micrographic surgery being the preferred technique which offers the most reliable margin control, adequate tissue preservation, and has the lowest recurrence rates (16–28%) [46, 47].

Other treatment modalities include-Topical medication, such as imiquimod (self-applied cream); radiotherapy; chemotherapy; photodynamic laser therapy; or a combination of these modalities of treatment. Recurrences are common.

Currently, there is no evidence to compare each modality of treatment in terms of prolonging survival, improving QoL, delaying progression or recurrence, or minimizing toxicity [48].

16 Melanoma

It is the second most common vulvar carcinoma. Relapse rates are high and co-relate with the depth of invasion. The tumour may be nodular, ulcerated, or elevated.

Although tumours are pigmented a non-pigmented melanoma can be seen also. Historically, vulvar malignant melanomas have been subclassified histopathologically into three categories: superficial spreading malignant melanoma, mucosal lentiginous melanoma, and nodular melanoma. Mucosal lentiginous melanoma which is also known as mucosal/acral lentiginous melanoma [49].

Surgery is the primary treatment modality.

17 Bartholin's Gland Carcinoma

It is a rare malignancy accounting approx. 5% of all vulval tumours. Usually diagnosed in late stages.

Histological type may be adenocarcinoma, squamous cell carcinoma, and transitional cell carcinoma.

The main treatment modality is surgery. Usually, surgery needed deep dissection in ischiorectal fossa and inguinofemoral lymph node dissection is recommended [50].

Primary carcinoma of the Bartholin's gland are usually diagnosed at a more advanced stage, but they have similar oncologic outcomes and survival rates compared to patients with non-Bartholin's gland related vulvar carcinoma [51].

18 Basal Cell Carcinoma

A rare variant of vulval carcinoma. They only metastasize to node when large and invasive in nature. Local excision is recommended and inguinofemoral lymph node dissection can be omitted in this tumour.

19 Verrucous Carcinoma

A variant of squamous cell carcinoma with an excellent prognosis. Usually present with exophytic growth and should be differentiated from giant condyloma. There is no need for inguinofemoral lymph node dissection in this type of cancer.

References

1. Kang YJ, Smith M, Barlow E, Coffey K, Hacker N, Canfell K. Vulvar cancer in high-income countries: increasing burden of disease. Int J Cancer. 2017;141:2174–86.
2. Butt JL, Botha MH. Vulvar cancer is not a disease of the elderly: treatment and outcome at a tertiary referral center in South Africa. S Afr Med J. 2017;107:1000–4.
3. Sung H, Ferlay J, Siegel RL, Laversanne M, Soerjomataram I, Jemal A, Bray F. Global cancer statistics 2020: GLOBOCAN estimates of incidence and mortality worldwide for 36 cancers in 185 countries. CA Cancer J Clin. 2021;71:209–49. https://doi.org/10.3322/caac.21660.
4. Hoang LN, Park KJ, Soslow RA, Murali R. Squamous precursor lesions of the vulva: current classification and diagnostic challenges. Pathology. 2016;48:291–302.
5. Bornstein J, Bogliatto F, Haefner HK, et al. The 2015 International Society for the Study of Vulvovaginal disease (ISSVD) terminology of vulvar squamous intraepithelial lesions. Obstet Gynecol. 2016;127:264–8.
6. Sideri M, Jones RW, Wilkinson EJ, et al. Squamous vulvar intraepithelial neoplasia: 2004 modified ter-

minology, ISSVD vulvar oncology subcommittee. J Reprod Med. 2005;50:807–10.
7. Allbritton JI. Vulvar neoplasms, benign and malignant. Obstet Gynecol Clin North Am. 2017;44:339–52.
8. Eva LJ, Ganesan R, Chan KK, Honest H, Luesley DM. Differentiated-type vulvar intraepithelial neoplasia has a high-risk association with vulvar squamous cell carcinoma. Int J Gynecol Cancer. 2009;19:741–4.
9. Cooper SM, Gao XH, Powell JJ, Wojnarowska F. Does treatment of vulvar lichen sclerosus influence its prognosis? Arch Dermatol. 2004;140(6):702–6.
10. Renaud-Vilmer C, Cavelier- Balloy B, Porcher R, Dubertret L. Vulvar lichen sclerosus: effect of long-term topical application of a potent steroid on the course of the disease. Arch Dermatol. 2004;140(6):709–12.
11. Lee A, Bradford J, Fischer G. Long-term management of adult vulvar lichen sclerosus: a prospective cohort study of 507 women. JAMA Dermatol. 2015;151(10):1061–7.
12. Tyagi S, Tripathi R, Batra S. Clinical scoring system to detect malignant and premalignant vulval lesions. J Obstet Gynecol. 2014;64:41–6. https://doi.org/10.1007/s13224-013-0458-3.
13. Gonzalez Bosquet J, Magrina JF, Magtibay PM, et al. Patterns of inguinal groin metastases in squamous cell carcinoma of the vulva. Gynecol Oncol. 2007;105(3):742–6.
14. De Hullu JA, van der Avoort IA, Oonk MH, van der Zee AG. Management of vulvar cancers. Eur J Surg Oncol. 2006;32:825–31. https://doi.org/10.1016/j.ejso.2006.03.035.
15. Joura EA, Losch A, Haider-Angeler MG, Breitenecker G, Leodolter S. Trends in vulvar neoplasia. Increasing incidence of vulvar intraepithelial neoplasia and squamous cell carcinoma of the vulva in young women. J Reprod Med. 2000;45:613–5.
16. Levenback CF, Ali S, Coleman RL, Gold MA, Fowler JM, Judson PL, Bell MC, De Geest K, Spirtos NM, Potkul RK, Leitao MM Jr, Bakkum-Gamez JN, Rossi EC, Lentz SS, Burke JJ 2nd, Van Le L, Trimble CL. Lymphatic mapping and sentinel lymph node biopsy in women with squamous cell carcinoma of the vulva: a gynaecologic oncology group study. J Clin Oncol. 2012;30(31):3786–91. https://doi.org/10.1200/JCO.2011.41.2528.
17. Rogers LJ. Cuello MA cancer of the vulva. Int J Gynecol Obstet. 2018;143:4–13. https://doi.org/10.1002/ijgo.12609.
18. Olawaiye AB, Cotler J, Cuello MA, et al. FIGO staging for carcinoma of the vulva: 2021 revision. Int J Gynecol Obstet. 2021;155:43–7. https://doi.org/10.1002/ijgo.13880.
19. Byron S, Lamb E, Yonemoto R, Kase S. Radical inguinal node dissection in the treatment of cancer. Surg Gynecol Obstet. 1962;114:401–8.
20. Micheletti L, Haefner H, Zalewski K, MacLean A, Gomez Cherey F, Pereira C, Sluga C, Solé-Sedeno JM, Vargas-Hernandez VM, Preti M. The International Society for the Study of Vulvovaginal disease surgical oncological procedure definitions committee surgical terminology for vulvar cancer treatment. J Low Genit Tract Dis. 2020;24(1):62–8. https://doi.org/10.1097/LGT.0000000000000501.
21. Forner DM, Lampe B. Exenteration in the treatment of stage III/IV vulvar cancer. Gynecol Oncol. 2012;124(1):87–91. https://doi.org/10.1016/j.ygyno.2011.09.014.
22. Yii NW, Niranjan NS. Lotus petal flaps in vulvovaginal reconstruction. Br J Plast Surg. 1996;49(8):547–54. https://doi.org/10.1016/s0007-1226(96)90132-0.
23. Vordermark JS, Jones BM, Harrison DH. The trustees of British Association of Plastic Surgeons. Surgical approaches to block dissection of the inguinal lymph nodes. Br J Plast Surg. 1985;38(3):321–5.
24. Tonouchi H, Ohmori Y, Kobayashi M, Konishi N, Tanaka K, Mohri Y, et al. Operative morbidity associated with groSin dissections. Surg Today. 2004;34:413–8.
25. Abbas S, Seitz M. Systematic review and meta-analysis of the used surgical techniques to reduce leg lymphedema following radical inguinal nodes dissection. Surg Oncol. 2011;20:88–96.
26. Gaarenstroom KN, Kenter GG, Trimbos JB, Agous I, Amant F, Peters AA, Vergote I. Postoperative complications after vulvectomy and inguinofemoral lymphadenectomy using separate groin incisions. Int J Gynecol Cancer. 2003;13(4):522–7. https://doi.org/10.1046/j.1525-1438.2003.13304.x.
27. Ryan M, Stainton MC, Slaytor EK, Jaconelli C, Watts S, Mackenzie P. Aetiology and prevalence of lower limb lymphoedema following treatment for gynecological cancer. Aust N Z J Obstet Gynaecol. 2003;43(2):148–51. https://doi.org/10.1046/j.0004-8666.2003.00040.x.
28. Tobias-Machado M, Tavares A, Molina WR Jr, et al. Video endoscopic inguinal lymphadenectomy (VEIL): minimally invasive resection of inguinal lymph nodes. Int Braz J Urol. 2006;32:316–21.
29. Nirmal TJ, Gupta AK, Kumar S, et al. Tensor fascia lata flap reconstruction following groin dissection: is it worthwhile? World J Urol. 2011;29:555–9.
30. C Royal College of Obstetricians and Gynaecologists. Guidelines for the diagnosis and management of vulval carcinoma. London: RCOG; 2014.
31. Breslow A. Thickness, cross-sectional areas and depth of invasion in the prognosis of cutaneous melanoma. Ann Surg. 1970;172(5):902–8.
32. Te Grootenhuis NC, van der Zee AG, van Doorn HC, van der Velden J, Vergote I, Zanagnolo V, Baldwin PJ, Gaarenstroom KN, van Dorst EB, Trum JW, Slangen BF, Runnebaum IB, Tamussino K, Hermans RH, Provencher DM, de Bock GH, de Hullu JA, Oonk MH. Sentinel nodes in vulvar cancer: long-term follow-up of the GROningen INternational study on sentinel nodes in vulvar cancer (GROINSS-V) I. Gynecol Oncol. 2016;140(1):8–14. https://doi.org/10.1016/j.ygyno.2015.09.077.
33. Levenback CF, Ali S, Coleman RL, Gold MA, Fowler JM, Judson PL, Bell MC, De Geest K, Spirtos NM,

Potkul RK, Leitao MM Jr, Bakkum-Gamez JN, Rossi EC, Lentz SS, Burke JJ 2nd, Van Le L, Trimble CL. Lymphatic mapping and sentinel lymph node biopsy in women with squamous cell carcinoma of the vulva: a gynecologic oncology group study. J Clin Oncol. 2012;30(31):3786–91. https://doi.org/10.1200/JCO.2011.41.2528.
34. Meads C, Sutton AJ, Rosenthal AN, et al. Sentinel lymph node biopsy in vulval cancer: systematic review and meta-analysis. Br J Cancer. 2014;110(12):2837–46.
35. Morrison J, Baldwin P, Buckley L, Cogswell L, Edey K, Faruqi A, Ganesan R, Hall M, Hillaby K, Reed N, Rolland P, Fotopoulou C, British Gynaecological Cancer Society (BGCS). Vulval cancer guidelines: recommendations for practice. Eur J Obstet Gynecol Reprod Biol. 2020;252:502–52.
36. Woelber L, Eulenburg C, Grimm D, et al. The risk of contralateral non-sentinel metastasis in patients with primary vulvar cancer and unilaterally positive sentinel node. Ann Surg Oncol. 2016;23(8):2508–14.
37. Oonk M, Slomovitz B, Baldwin P, et al. Radiotherapy versus inguinofemoral lymphadenectomy as treatment for vulvar cancer patients with micro metastases in the sentinel node: results of GROINSS-VII. J Clin Oncol. 2021;39(32):3623–32. https://doi.org/10.1200/JCO.21.0000.
38. Homesley HD, Bundy BN, Sedlis A, Adcock L. Radiation therapy versus pelvic node resection for carcinoma of the vulva with positive groin nodes. Obstet Gynecol. 1986;68(6):733–40.
39. Faul CM, Mirmow D, Huang Q, Gerszten K, Day R, Jones MW. Adjuvant radiation for vulvar carcinoma: improved local control. Int J Radiat Oncol Biol Phys. 1997;38(2):381–9. https://doi.org/10.1016/s0360-3016(97)82500-x.
40. Bellati F, Angioli R, Manci N, Angelo Zullo M, Muzii L, Plotti F, et al. Single-agent cisplatin chemotherapy in surgically resected vulvar cancer patients with multiple inguinal lymph node metastases. Gynecol Oncol. 2005;96:227–31.
41. Han S, Kim D, Higgins S, Carcangiu M, Kacinski B. Chemoradiation as primary or adjuvant treatment for locally advanced carcinoma of the vulva. Int J Radiat Oncol Biol Phys. 2000;47:1235–44.
42. Moore DH, Ali S, Koh WJ, et al. A phase II trial of radiation therapy and weekly cisplatin chemotherapy for the treatment of locally-advanced squamous cell carcinoma of the vulva: a gynecologic oncology group study. Gynecol Oncol. 2012;124(3):529–33.
43. Natesan D, Hong JC, Foote J, Sosa JA, Havrilesky L, Chino J. Primary versus preoperative radiation for locally advanced vulvar cancer. Int J Gynecol Cancer. 2017;27(4):794–804. https://doi.org/10.1097/IGC.0000000000000938.
44. Gonzalez Bosquet J, Magrina JF, Gaffey TA, Hernandez JL, Webb MJ, Cliby WA, Podratz KC. Long-term survival and disease recurrence in patients with primary squamous cell carcinoma of the vulva. Gynecol Oncol. 2005;97(3):828–33. https://doi.org/10.1016/j.ygyno.2005.03.006.
45. Horowitz NS, Olawaiye AB, Borger DR, Growdon WB, Krasner CN, Matulonis UA, Liu JF, Lee J, Brard L, Dizon DS. Phase II trial of erlotinib in women with squamous cell carcinoma of the vulva. Gynecol Oncol. 2012;127(1):141–6. https://doi.org/10.1016/j.ygyno.2012.06.028.
46. Boehringer A, Leiter U, Metzler G, Moehrle M, Garbe C, et al. Extramammary Paget's disease: extended subclinical growth detected using three-dimensional histology in routine paraffin procedure and course of the disease. Dermatol Surg. 2011;37(10):1417–26. https://doi.org/10.1111/j.1524-4725.2011.02091.x.
47. Hendi A, Brodland D, Zitelli J. Extramammary Paget's disease: surgical treatment with Mohs micrographic surgery. J Am Acad Dermatol. 2004;51(5):767–73. https://doi.org/10.1016/j.jaad.2004.07.004.
48. Edey KA, Allan E, Murdoch JB, Cooper S, Bryant A. Interventions for the treatment of Paget's disease of the vulva. Cochrane Database Syst Rev. 2019;6:Cd009245. https://doi.org/10.1002/14651858.CD009245.pub3.
49. Benda JA, Platz CE, Anderson B. Malignant melanoma of the vulva: a clinicopathologic review of 16 cases. Int J Gynecol Pathol. 1986;5(3):202–16.
50. Leuchter RS, Hacker NF, Voet RL, Berek JS, Townsend DE, Lagasse LD. Primary carcinoma of the Bartholin gland: a report of 14 cases and review of the literature. Obstet Gynecol. 1982;60(3):361–8.
51. Bhalwal AB, Nick AM, Dos Reis R, Chen CL, Munsell MF, Ramalingam P, Salcedo MP, Ramirez PT, Sood AK, Schmeler KM. Carcinoma of the bartholin gland: a review of 33 cases. Int J Gynecol Cancer. 2016;26(4):785–9. https://doi.org/10.1097/IGC.0000000000000656.

Carcinoma Vagina

Dimpy Begum, Bijal Patel, Debabrata Barmon, and Amal Chandra Kataki

Primary vaginal cancer is one of the rare entities. It accounts for around 1–2% of all female genital tract malignancy [1]. Because most of these tumours have metastasized from another original site, diagnosis of primary vaginal cancer is uncommon. The majority of these metastases are due to primary in other reproductive organs including the cervix, endometrium, or ovaries, while metastasis from distant sites like the colon, breast, and pancreas has also been observed.

Primary vaginal cancer is defined as cancer that is found in vagina without any evidence, i.e. histopathological or clinical evidence of vulval or cervical cancer or a history of these two cancers in last 5 years [2].

D. Begum (✉) · D. Barmon · A. C. Kataki
Department of Gynaecologic Oncology, Dr. Bhubaneswar Borooah Cancer Institute (A Unit of Tata Memorial Centre, Mumbai), Guwahati, Assam, India

B. Patel
Department of Gynaecological Oncology, The Gujarat Cancer and Research Institute, Ahmedabad, Gujarat, India

1 Anatomy

The vagina is a fibromuscular organ with a length of around 3–4 in. It extends from cervix to the vestibular opening. The posterior vaginal wall is longer than anterior vaginal wall. The anterior, posterior, and lateral fornixes are formed due to invaginations between the vaginal mucosa and cervix. The vagina is composed of fibromuscular and elastic tissue with many mucosal folds. Vaginal wall consists of three layers named as inner non keratinizing squamous epithelium, middle lamina propria, and outer adventitial layers.

Lymphatics—The vaginal lymphatics lies underneath the submucosal and muscularis layer (Fig. 1).

The upper part of vagina drains primarily via cervical lymphatics. The lymphatics of the cervix drain the superior anterior region of the vagina to the interiliac and parametrial nodes, and the inferior gluteal, presacral, and anorectal nodes receive posterior upper vaginal lymphatics. The inguinal and femoral nodes, as well as the pelvic nodes, drain the inferior portion of the vagina.

Proximal part of vagina is supplied by the vaginal artery, which is a branch of uterine artery. The venous plexus runs parallel to the arteries, draining into the internal iliac vein. The vagina is innervated by the lumbar plexus and pudendal nerve, with branches from sacral roots 2–4, part of inferior hypogastric plexus (S2–S4).

A. C. Kataki, D. Barmon (eds.), *Fundamentals in Gynaecologic Malignancy*,
https://doi.org/10.1007/978-981-19-5860-1_22

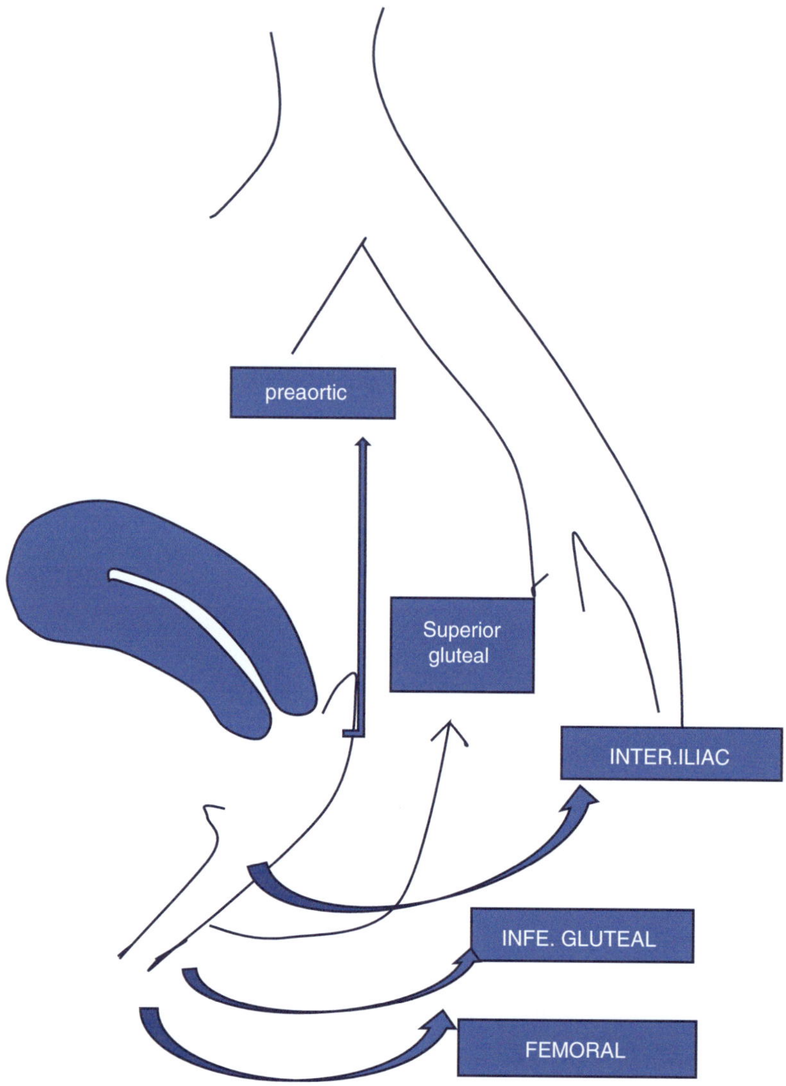

Fig. 1 Schematic presentation of lymphatic drainage of vagina

2 Premalignant Neoplasm of Vagina (VAIN)

The terminology of premalignant lesion of vagina has changed over the years. In 2014 WHO classification replaced three tier system (VAIN 1–3) to two tier system of LSIL and HSIL [3].

They are usually asymptomatic but detected in usual surveillance of cervical or vulval cancer.

The risk of HSIL progressing to invasive cancer has been estimated to be between 2%–12% [4]. In case of abnormal vaginal smear, colposcopy and visualization after applying acetic acid and Lugol's iodine should be done. Biopsy of suspicious lesion are to be done.

Treatment of premalignant lesion ranges from observation to surgical excision.

Biopsy proven LSIL lesion can be kept under follow-up and observation with smear and colposcopy [5].

HSIL lesions can be treated with laser ablation, surgical excision or topical, imiquimod application.

Individualization of treatment depends on type of lesion, number of lesion, and availability of treatment options. Surgical excision is ideal for lesion in upper third of vagina or in vault.

3 Malignant Neoplasm of Vagina

3.1 Epidemiology

Vaginal carcinoma is mostly seen in perimenopausal and post-menopausal age groups. It may be seen in young women if associated with HPV infection or metastasis to vagina.

Risk Factors—The common risk factors are HPV infection, immunocompromised status, previous history of cervical or vaginal cancer, multiple sexual partners, and early age of first intercourse.

HPV 16,33, 18 are the most common HPV associated with vaginal carcinoma [6].

Incidence—According to GLOBOCAN 2020 the total number of new cases was 17,908 and death due to ca vagina was 7995 [7].

A study carried out in rural India found that vaginal cancer comprised of 1.6% cancers in women, 3.3% gynaecological cancers between 1982 and 1987, 0.4% cancers in women, and 0.6% gynaecological cancers between 2008 and 2012. Only 7% women were of less than 50 years, 37% were of 50–60 years, 56% above 65 years [8].

The incidence of vaginal cancer increases with age with approximately 50% of patients over 70 years old and 20% over 80 years old [9].

3.2 Histological Types

Squamous cell carcinoma is the most common vaginal carcinoma which may be keratinizing, nonkeratinizing, basaloid, warty, or verrucous types**.** Verrucous type of SCC is less aggressive in nature and rarely metastasize. Squamous cell carcinoma accounts 90% of all vaginal carcinomas. They can be of G1—well differentiated, G2—moderately differentiated, and G3- poorly differentiated. Rest 10% are adenocarcinoma. Melanoma, Sarcoma, and lymphoma of vagina are extremely rare cancers.

3.3 Pattern of Spread

Vaginal cancer spread either by direct extension to adjacent organ, lymphatic spread to regional lymph node or hematogenous spread to distant organ.

3.4 Clinical Presentation

Vaginal bleeding is the most common presenting symptom [10]. Other symptoms are vaginal discharge or vaginal mass. Urinary symptoms or rectal symptoms are seen when disease has spread into this organ. The most common site of involvement is upper third of vagina.

3.5 Evaluation

A proper history taking with clinical examination is most important first step towards diagnosis.

Vaginal cancer is staged clinically. Vaginal carcinoma is to be diagnosed only after excluding cervical and vulval carcinoma.

During examination inguinal node palpation should be done and if enlarged then biopsy to be done along with biopsy of vaginal lesion. Biopsy is the gold standard of diagnosis.

Radiological investigation like CT and MRI can be done to know the extent of the disease and to guide management.

PET-CT scans have limited utility in the diagnosis of vaginal cancer. It has advantage of detecting nodal metastasis early [11].

4 Staging

FIGO 2009 staged vaginal cancer clinically that involved clinical examination and examination under anesthesia (Table 1). Although FIGO supports the use of modern imaging modalities to aid therapy, including computed tomography, magnetic resonance imaging (MRI), and positron emission tomography (PET), the imaging findings cannot be used to change or reassign the stage [5].

Table 1 FIGO staging of carcinoma vagina [5]

Stage	Description
Stage I	Carcinoma is limited to vaginal wall
Stage II	Carcinoma has involved the subvaginal tissue but has not extended to the pelvic wall
Stage III	Carcinoma extended to pelvic wall
Stage IV	Carcinoma has extended beyond the true pelvis or tumour invades bladder and/or rectal mucosa and/or direct extension beyond the true pelvis has involved the mucosa of the bladder Or rectum; bullous edema as such does not permit a case to be allotted to stage IV
Stage IVA	Tumour invades bladder and/or rectal mucosa and/or direct extension beyond the true pelvis
Stage IVB	Distant metastasis

5 Prognostic Factors

Stage of disease- It is also significant prognostic factor.

Size of the lesion.

Grades of differentiation-significant predictor of prognosis. Higher the grade poorer is the prognosis [12].

Lymph node involvement.

6 Treatment

Treatment options would be surgery, radiation, chemotherapy and palliative care depending on factors like tumour type, stage, size and location of tumour.

6.1 Surgery

Surgery has a limited role in management of vaginal carcinoma. It is indicated in lesion in upper third of vagina. Radical wide local excision with inguinofemoral node dissection can be done in well demarcated small and superficial type of lesions when lesions are confined to lower third of vagina.

Radical upper vaginectomy with pelvic lymphadenectomy along with radical hysterectomy is indicated in invasive upper vaginal cancer.

Pelvic exenteration surgery is indicated in case of previously irradiated patient where further radiation is not possible or in case of central recurrence after radiation treatment.

Palliative surgery, e.g., colostomy, etc. is indicated in palliative setting of rectovaginal fistula cases.

6.2 Radiotherapy

It is the treatment of choice. Radiation can be given in the form of external beam radiation (EBRT), brachytherapy (intracavitary or interstitial) or groin radiation depending on stage and performance status of patient. Patient is planned for RT in supine frog lagged position to decrease groin fold toxicities.

A total dose of 46 Gy for EBRT is recommended, with a brachytherapy dose of 25–30 Gy. For large lesions or those involving the rectovaginal septum, an EBRT boost to 64–70 Gy can be utilized instead of brachytherapy. 70gy is the ideal dose for a good response [13–15].

The stagewise RT is given below (Table 2) [16].

Table 2 Stagewise RT treatment

Stage	Type and dose of RT
Stage I	Vaginal brachytherapy alone or combined with EBRT
Stage II	EBRT to the primary and pelvic lymph nodes along with brachytherapy boost is recommended. If the parametria are involved, treatment should include parametrial boost
Stage III and IVA	EBRT to the primary and pelvic lymph nodes along with parametrial boost and brachytherapy boost, with concurrent chemotherapy is recommended

6.3 Chemoradiotherapy

In individuals with primary vaginal cancer, RTCT is linked to a longer survival time. Except for those with adenocarcinoma, tumour size 2 cm, or FIGO stage I, most patients with primary vaginal cancer should receive RTCT instead of RT alone [17].

7 Follow-Up

Once treatment is completed follow up is done 3 monthly for first 2 years then 6 monthly for next 3 years followed by annually thereafter.

8 Prognosis

The 5-year survival in stage I in carcinoma vagina is 73%, while in stage II it is 58%. This 5-year survival decreases to 25–58% in stage III and 0–40% in stage IV.

9 Recurrence

Pelvic recurrences are more common than distant recurrences. Locoregional recurrences and distant failures are noted within 2 years following treatment [18].

10 Vaginal Adeno Carcinoma

Primary vaginal adenocarcinoma may be DES related and non-DES related. Non-DES related carcinoma are extremely rare. Treatment is done as that of squamous cell carcinoma.

11 Vaginal Melanoma

Incidence of vaginal melanoma is very rare, and surgery is the mainstay of treatment.

References

1. Adhikari P, Vitjea P, Mount S. Premalignant and malignant leisons of vagina diagnosis. Histopathology. 2016;23:28–34.
2. Edge SB, Compton CC. The American joint committee on cancer: the 7th edition of AJCC cancer staging and manual and the future of TNM. Ann Surg Oncol. 2010;17:1471–4.
3. Reich O, Regauer S, Marth C, et al. Precancerous lesions of the cervix, vulva and vagina according to the 2014 WHO classification of tumors of the female genital tract. Geburtshilfe Frauenheilkd. 2015;75:1018–20.
4. Hodeib M, Cohen JG, Mehta S, et al. Recurrence and risk of progression to lower genital tract malignancy in women with high grade VAIN. Gynecol Oncol. 2016;141:507–10.
5. Adams TS, Cuello MA. Cancer of the vagina. Int J Gynecol Obstet. 2018;143:14–21. https://doi.org/10.1002/ijgo.12610.
6. Sinno AK, Saraiya M, Thompson TD, et al. Human papillomavirus genotype prevalence in invasive vaginal cancer from a registry-based population. Obstet Gynecol. 2014;123(4):817–21. https://doi.org/10.1097/AOG.0000000000000171.
7. Sung H, Ferlay J, Siegel RL, Laversanne M, Soerjomataram I, Jemal A, Bray F. Global cancer statistics 2020: GLOBOCAN estimates of incidence and mortality worldwide for 36 cancers in 185 countries. CA Cancer J Clin. 2021;71(3):209–49. https://doi.org/10.3322/caac.21660.
8. Chhabra S, Bandebuche S, Deshpande A. Vaginal cancer trends in women of low resources settings. J Univ Surg. 2016;4:3.
9. Creasman WT, Phillips JL, Menck HR. The National Cancer Data Base report on cancer of the vagina. Cancer. 1998;83(5):1033–40.
10. Shrivastava SB, Agrawal G, Mittal M, Mishra P. Management of vaginal cancer. Rev Recent Clin Trials. 2015;10(4):289–97.
11. Lamoreaux WT, Grigsby PW, Dehdashti F, et al. FDG-PET evaluation of vaginal carcinoma. Int J Radiat Oncol Biol Phys. 2005;62:733–7.
12. Prameela CG, Ravind R, Gurram BC, Sheejamol VS, Dinesh M. Prognostic factors in primary vaginal cancer: a single institute experience and review of literature. J Obstet Gynaecol India. 2016;66(5):363–71. https://doi.org/10.1007/s13224-015-0697-6.
13. Kirkbride P, Fyles A, Rawlings GA, et al. Carcinoma of the vagina–experience at the Princess Margaret hospital (1974–1989). Gynecol Oncol. 1995;56:435–43.
14. Lian J, Dundas G, Carlone M, Ghosh S, Pearcey R. Twenty-year review of radiotherapy for vaginal cancer: an institutional experience. Gynecol Oncol. 2008;111:298–306.

15. Perez CA, Grigsby PW, Garipagaoglu M, Mutch DG, Lockett MA. Factors affecting long-term outcome of irradiation in carcinoma of the vagina. Int J Radiat Oncol Biol Phys. 1999;44:37–45.
16. Dasari P, Vivekanandam S, Raghava KSA. Radiation for gynaecological malignancies. London: Intech Open; 2017. https://doi.org/10.5772/67202.
17. Zhou WL, Yue YY. Radiotherapy plus chemotherapy is associated with improved survival compared to radiotherapy alone in patients with primary vaginal carcinoma: a retrospective SEER study. Front Oncol. 2020;10:570933. https://doi.org/10.3389/fonc.2020.570933.
18. Pingley S, Shrivastava SK, Sarin R, Agarwal JP, Laskar S, Deshpande DD, Dinshaw KA. Primary carcinoma of the vagina: Tata memorial hospital experience. Int J Radiat Oncol Biol Phys. 2000;46(1):101–8. https://doi.org/10.1016/s0360-3016(99)00360-0.

Gestational Trophoblastic Disease

Dimpy Begum, Bhagyalaxmi Nayak,
Debabrata Barmon, and Amal Chandra Kataki

1 Introduction and Classification

Gestational trophoblastic disease (GTD) is a pregnancy-associated neoplastic condition [1]. It is uncommon but not a rare condition. The range of GTD includes hydatidiform mole, complete mole, partial mole, invasive mole, choriocarcinoma, placental site trophoblastic tumour (PSTT), and epithelioid trophoblastic tumours (ETT).

Persistent GTD refers to a condition that does not subside or become malignant after molar products evacuation and requires active treatment. All GTDs arise from extraembryonic structure tissue and are characterized by secretion of hCG.

Broadly GTD consists of a mixture of benign and malignant disorders and can be classified as follows.

Classification of GTD [2]:

1. Benign GTD—complete and partial hydatidiform mole.
2. Malignant GTD.
   (a) Non-metastatic—invasive mole and malignant choriocarcinoma.
   (b) Metastatic—malignant choriocarcinoma, placental site trophoblastic neoplasia (PSTT), and epithelioid trophoblastic tumours (ETT).In 2020 WHO has given a new classification of GTD [3]:

- *Tumour-Like Lesions.*
  - Exaggerated placental site reaction.
  - Placental site nodule and plaque.
- *Molar Pregnancies.*
  - Partial hydatidiform mole.
  - Complete hydatidiform mole.
  - Invasive and metastatic hydatidiform moles.
- *Gestational Trophoblastic Neoplasms.*
  - Epithelioid trophoblastic tumour (ETT).
  - Placental site trophoblastic tumour (PSTT).
  - Gestational choriocarcinoma.

Mixed trophoblastic tumour.GTD is one of the most curable gynaecologic malignancies because of the following reasons:

1. The proliferating trophoblast is extremely sensitive to certain chemotherapy drugs, such as methotrexate and actinomycin D.
2. The proliferation of various trophoblasts produces human chorionic gonadotropin (hCG). The concentration of hCG in urine or serum is directly related to the number of surviving tro-

D. Begum (✉) · D. Barmon · A. C. Kataki
Department of Gynaecologic Oncology,
Dr. Bhubaneswar Borooah Cancer Institute
(A Unit of Tata Memorial Centre, Mumbai),
Guwahati, Assam, India
e-mail: dydiracademic@bbci.tmc.gov.in

B. Nayak
Department of Gynaecological Oncology, Acharya
Harihar Cancer Hospital, Cuttack, Odisha, India

A. C. Kataki, D. Barmon (eds.), *Fundamentals in Gynaecologic Malignancy*,
https://doi.org/10.1007/978-981-19-5860-1_23

phoblasts. Therefore, hCG is a unique and sensitive marker for the treatment of GTD patients.

2 Epidemiology

The reported incidence of GTD in India is not consistent [4]. Some studies show significant differences in molar pregnancy rates worldwide [5]. The incidence in Indonesia, India, and Turkey is 12 per 1000 pregnancies. But in Japan and China it is 1–2 per 1000 pregnancies. In north America incidence is 0.5–1 per 1000 pregnancies. In Asia, the incidence of GTD is one in 250 pregnancies [6]. Although different studies showed different incidences across the world, but mostly the incidence is 1 in 1000 pregnancies [7].

Advanced maternal age more than 40 years and history of previous GTD are the most common risk factors [8]. The risk increases with the previous history of molar pregnancy. If a woman has been diagnosed with hydatidiform mole (HM) before, her risk of developing HM in a subsequent pregnancy is 1% and increases to 25% with more than one pregnancy with HM. The risk associated with maternal age is bimodal, and the risk increases for mothers under 20 and over 35 (especially mothers older than 45). More than 98% of women who fall pregnant after a molar conception will not develop another hydatidiform mole, and their pregnancies will not be at risk of other obstetric difficulties [9]. The association with the father's age is inconsistent. Numerous exposures for GTD have been studied, but no clear associations with smoking, drinking, diet, and oral contraceptives have been found [8].

3 Pathology

All GTDs arise from the placenta and it is a presentation of abnormal proliferation of villous and extravillous (interstitial) trophoblast counterparts.

3.1 Hydatidiform Mole (HM)

Hydatidiform mole is characterized by abnormal swelling and proliferation of placental cytotrophoblast and syncytiotrophoblast. There may be an abnormal foetus present or absent. A foetus is present in partial hydatidiform mole (PHM), and its absence denotes complete hydatidiform mole (CHM). Nonhydropic villi resemble 'cauliflower like' or 'club-shaped' vesicles, while complete hydatidiform moles resemble 'bunch of grapes' vesicles [10] (Fig. 1).

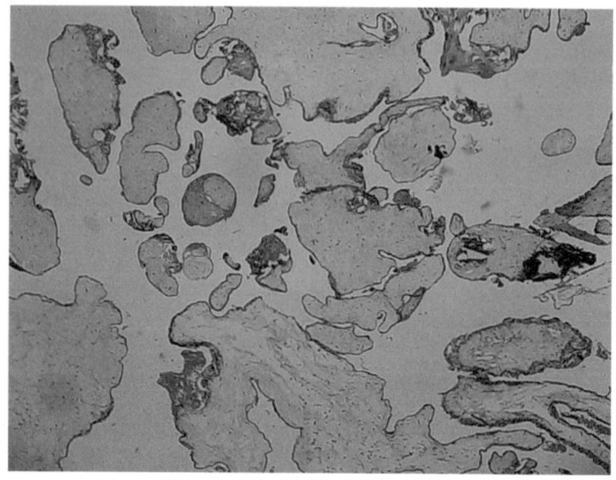

Fig. 1 Complete hydatidiform mole. (PC: Dr. Pakesh Baishya)

3.2 Invasive Moles (Chorioadenoma Destruens)

Invasive moles are malignant form of GTD, and they are defined when CHM infiltrates the myometrium and is associated with a continuous increase in human chorionic gonadotropin (hCG) after molar removal. Rarely PHM may also become an invasive mole. It can be distinguished from gestational choriocarcinoma by the presence of chorionic villi.

3.3 Placental Site Trophoblastic Tumour (PSTT)/Epithelioid Trophoblastic Tumour (ETT)

Trophoblastic tumours originate from the implantation site of the placenta. It is characterized by a simple infiltrating nest and sheets of the mesenchymal trophoblast cell layer. It is associated with less vascular invasion, haemorrhage, necrosis, and lower levels of hCG. Compared with choriocarcinoma, PSTT usually affects lymph nodes. On IHC it is positive for human placental lactogen.

A variant of PSTT is ETT, with similar clinical behaviour with a characteristic transparent hyaline-like matrix.

3.4 Choriocarcinoma

It is a malignant tumour that produces hCG. It may be gestational or non-gestation-related [11].

Choriocarcinomas are characterized by myometrial infiltration, specific trophoblastic proliferation and underdevelopment, unformed villi with haemorrhage and central necrosis (Fig. 2). Approximately 25% of cases occurs after miscarriages or ectopic pregnancies. Another 25% is related to the delivery term and preterm, and the remaining 50% are from HM. However, it is estimated that only 2–3% of HM will develop into CC.

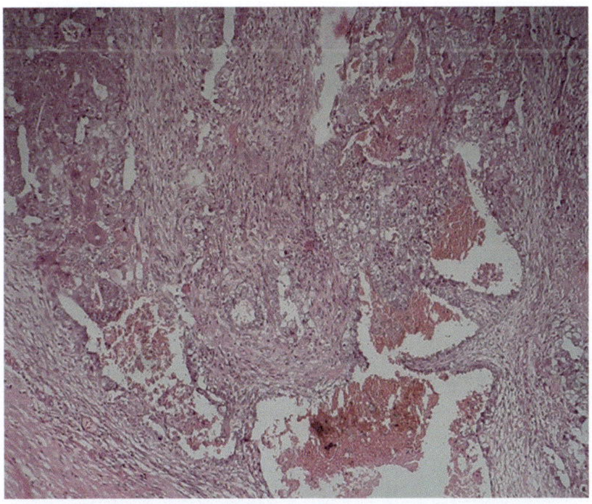

Fig. 2 Choriocarcinoma. (PC: Dr. Pakesh Baishya)

4 Molecular Biology

The chromosome composition of a complete mole is 46, XX. Both X chromosomes are paternal (double androgenic origin) [12].

The androgenic origin has been found to be the result of haploid paternal X sperm (23, X) replication and invasion of 'empty eggs' lacking functional maternal DNA which is shown in Fig. 3. However, the sperm mechanism (two haploid sperm passing through an 'empty egg cell') is also possible and may be the cause of 46, XX or 46, XY of paternal origin [13] (Fig. 4). Intact moles with single sperm are called 'homozygous' and the dispermic as 'heterozygous'. Complete and partial hydatidiform differ in pathogenesis and histologically which is shown in Table 1.

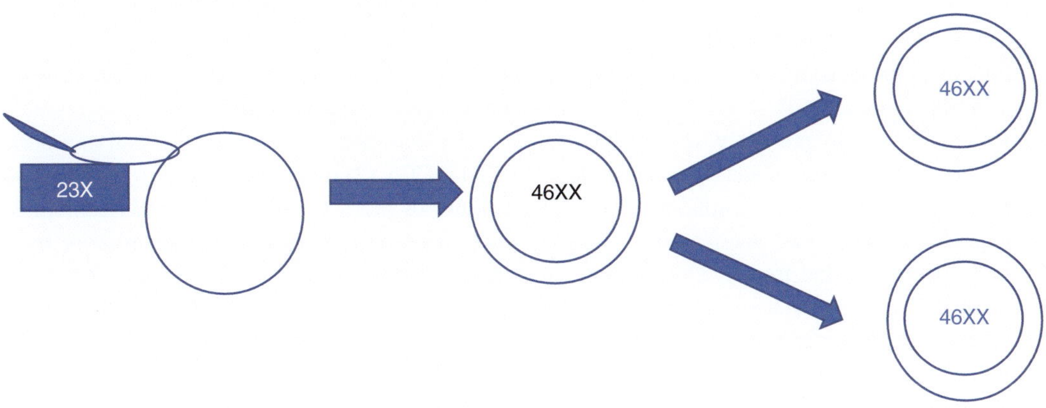

Fig. 3 Pathogenesis of complete mole by duplication of paternal chromosomal duplication after fertilizing inactivated gene containing ovum

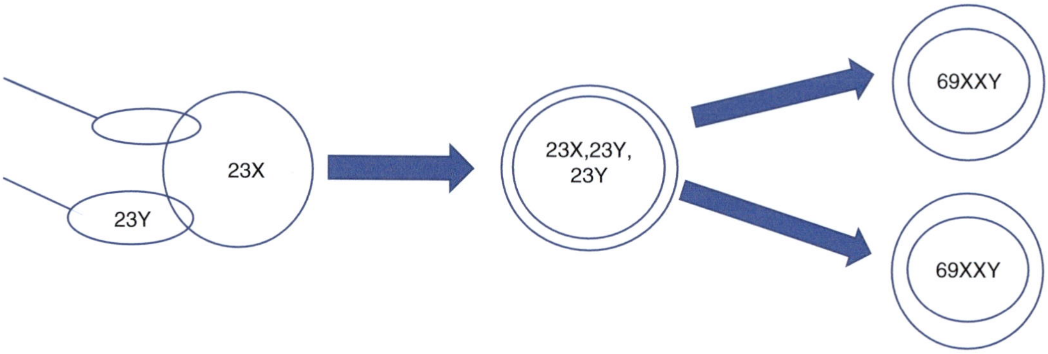

Fig. 4 Pathogenesis of partial mole by fertilization of normal ovum by two sperms either 23X or 23Y

Table 1 Differences between complete and partial mole

Features	Complete mole	Partial mole
Pathogenesis	Paternal origin	Have genetic material from both paternal and maternal side
Karyotype	46XX/46XY	69XXX/69XXY/69XYY
Embryonic material	Absent	Present
Trophoblastic proliferation	Diffuse	Focal
Villous scalloping	Absent	Present

5 Diagnosis

Symptoms and signs:

1. History of amenorrhea followed by vaginal bleeding is the most common presenting symptom in GTD.
2. Uterine size is usually more than gestational age. The molar tissues may separate from decidua and disrupt the maternal blood vessels, and collected blood distends the uterine cavity. This blood may undergo oxidation and liquefication, causing 'prune juice' like discharge per vaginum.
3. Patients may also present with hyperemesis gravidarum and toxaemia early in pregnancy.
4. Patients may also have complaints related to hyperthyroidism, e.g. tachycardia, weight loss, irritability, and tremor. Diagnosing and treating hyperthyroidism with a beta-adrenergic blocker is essential to prevent thyroid storm, which may occur during molar evacuation.
5. Respiratory distress—this may occur due to trophoblastic pulmonary embolization and patients may present with chest pain, dyspnoea, tachypnoea, tachycardia, and severe respiratory distress. These symptoms usually resolve 72 h after evacuation and proper supportive measure.
6. Theca lutein cyst >6 cm in diameter occurs due to excessive ovarian stimulation by β-hCG.
7. Persistence of lochia longer than usual.

5.1 Measurement of Serum hCG

hCG is a glycoprotein and has two non-covalently bound subunits, alpha and beta.

hCG has many forms: (1) intact heterodimeric hCG (hCG), (2) nicked hCG (hCG), (3) free beta subunit of hCG, (4) nicked free beta subunit of hCG (hCGbn), (5) hCG beta subunit core fragment (hCGbcf), (6) hyperglycosylated hCG (hCGH), and (7) sulphated hCG. Non-trophoblastic malignancies produce solely the free hCG subunit, which is a monomeric glycosylated version of hCG released by trophoblast neoplasms. In a variety of ways, GTD can create hCG molecules [14].

GTD patients are primarily monitored using assays that measure both hCG and β-hCG. The use of independent hCG and β-hCG assays makes it easier to distinguish between benign and malignant trophoblastic disorders. Relapse is diagnosed when there is a rise of hCH level after it has become undetectable whereas resistant disease is diagnosed when hCG levels remain elevated in spite of treatment.

Treatment failure or drug resistance is said to develop when three consecutive serum hCG values fall by less than 10% over 2 weeks or by one log hCG level over 2 weeks, or two consecutive hCG values rise, or if new metastases arise [15–17].

The phrase 'phantom hCG' is frequently misused to refer to any situation in which hCG is found in a non-pregnant person. The term implies the occurrence of a false positive hCG immunoassay caused by the presence of cross-reactive antibodies. Even when no actual hCG or trophoblastic tissue is present, patients with phantom hCG sometimes have a persistent mildly positive quantitative hCG test result. The most common cross-reactive substances that lead to 'ghost hCG' are heterophile antibodies. A negative urine hCG result at the same time as a positive serum hCG result from the same patient would be the most sensitive differentiating method to detect the condition.

5.2 FIGO criteria for diagnosing GTN after molar pregnancy are [18]:

1. hCG values of four or more that plateaued for at least 3 weeks (days 1, 7, 14, and 21),
2. hCG values that increased at least by 10% in 3 or more occasions over 2 weeks (days 1, 7, and 14),
3. Detection of features of choriocarcinoma histologically.

6 Role of Imaging

Diagnosis of GTN after molar pregnancy is done by measuring hCG titres and by use of FIGO diagnostic criteria [18]. Radiological imaging is used to assess the local extent of disease and monitor the patient's overall health. Imaging is also essential for detecting and treating problems, including uterine and pulmonary arteriovenous fistulas.

Ultrasonography: On ultrasonography complete hydatidiform mole has a 'snowstorm' appearance due to heterogeneous echogenic mass with several hypoechoic foci seen (Fig. 5). Theca lutein cyst may also be seen. The USG finding in invasive mole and choriocarcinoma is shown below (Figs. 6 and 7).

In the case of partial mole, USG findings are:

1. An empty gestational sac or one with amorphous echoes representing foetal parts.
2. Foetal demise, anomalies, or growth restriction.
3. Oligohydramnios.
4. An enlarged placenta size with 'Swiss cheese' appearance.

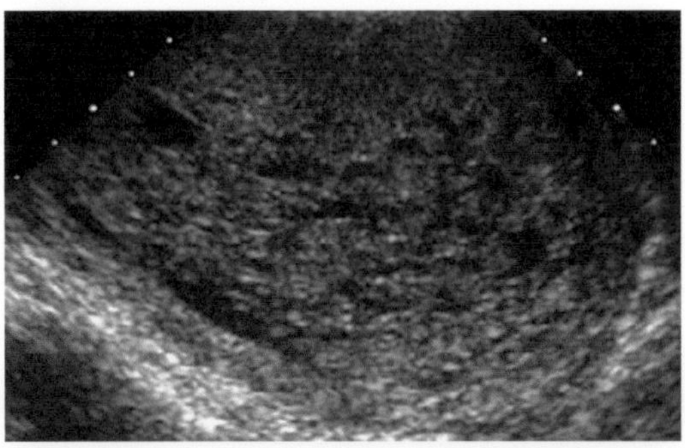

Fig. 5 USG finding of choriocarcinoma. (PC: Dr. Pavel Barmon)

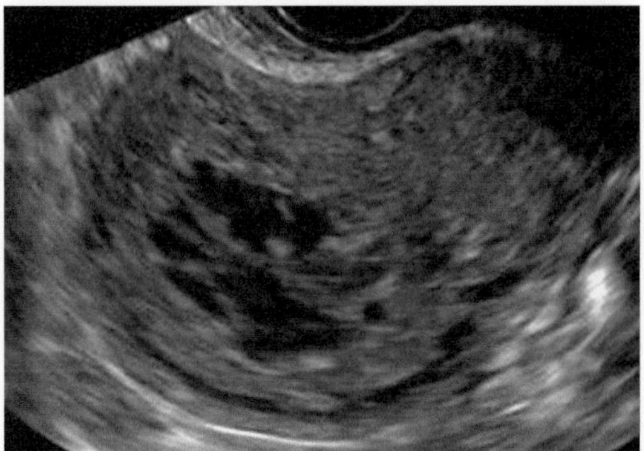

Fig. 6 TVS image of invasive mole. (PC: Dr. Pavel Barmon)

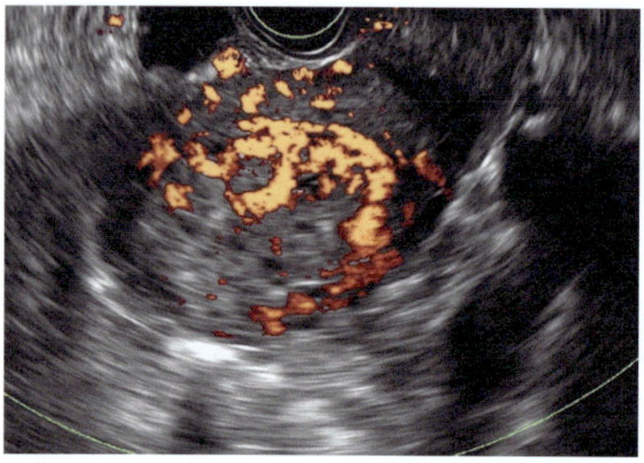

Fig. 7 Sagittal TVS image of increased vascularity in myometrium in a case of choriocarcinoma. (PC: Dr. Pavel Barmon)

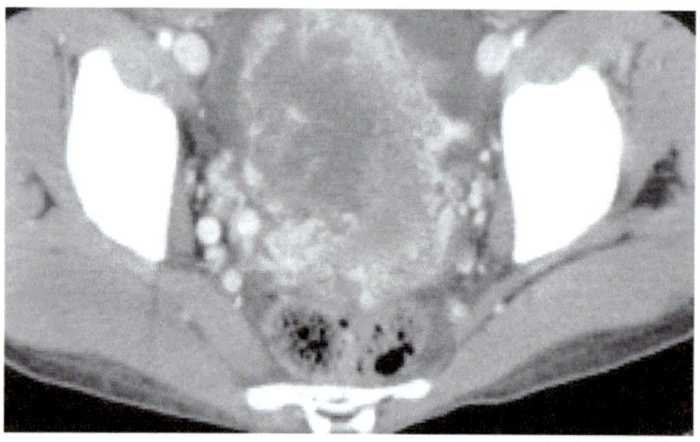

Fig. 8 Axial CT image of invasive choriocarcinoma extended to parametrium. (PC: Dr. Pavel Barmon)

Because of the increased incidence of postmolar GTN in CHM (18–29%) compared to PHM (5%), distinguishing between PHM and CHM has prognostic importance [19].

Computed tomography—It has limited use except in staging of GTN (Figs. 8 and 9). For detecting pulmonary metastasis chest CT scan is more sensitive than a chest X-ray. CT scan abdomen can also be done for a metastatic lesion in abdomen.

MRI—In GTN incidence of brain metastasis ranges from 3.4 to 8.8% [20].

In the case of pulmonary metastasis, brain MRI is done to look for brain metastasis.

PET-CT- (PET)/CT—In PET scan the metastatic sites appear as sites of increased metabolic activity. Its role in GTD is not well established as it does not have any advantage in tumour staging compared with conventional imaging [21].

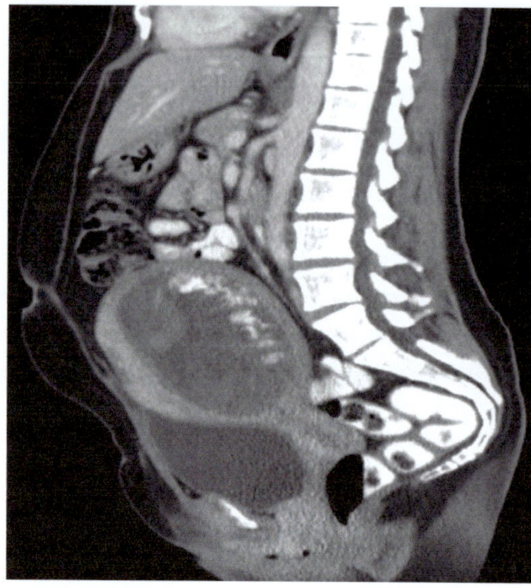

Fig. 9 Sagittal CT image of molar pregnancy. (PC: Dr. Pavel Barmon)

7 Metastasis in GTN

Four percent of patients after molar evacuation develop metastasis [22].

Metastasis is more common in GTN developing after non-molar pregnancy.

Pulmonary metastasis—At the presentation, 80% of patients of metastatic GTN present with lung metastasis. The usual presentation is cough, dyspnoea, chest pain, or haemoptysis. Typical radiological findings are alveolar snowstorm pattern, discrete rounded opacities, pleural effusion, or embolic pattern due to pulmonary artery occlusion.

Pulmonary artery hypertension may develop due to pulmonary artery occlusion.

Vaginal metastasis—It is seen in 30% of metastatic GTN. They are highly vascular and should not be biopsied. Sites are fornixes or suburethral area.

7.1 Hepatic Metastasis

Ten percent cases of metastatic GTN present with hepatic metastasis. Epigastric or right upper abdominal pain may be a presenting feature. They are friable and may rupture and cause bleeding.

7.2 Brain Metastasis

Ten percent of metastatic GTN present with brain and spinal cord metastasis. Almost all patients have pulmonary or vaginal metastasis. Neurological symptoms like nausea, vomiting, blurring of vision, and hemiparesis are presenting symptoms.

8 Staging and Risk Categorization

To date various scoring system for risk categorization has been developed for GTN [23–25].

In 1982 FIGO started staging based on spread into anatomical location. In 1983 a working group from WHO adopted 9 prognostic factors from Bagshawe's [23] scoring system. In 1992 the FIGO committee simplified 9 factors into 2. But in 2000 the FIGO committee changed the WHO score from 9 to 8 by removing the blood group, and they also changed the liver metastasis score from score 2 to 4.

In 2000 FIGO and WHO combined anatomic and WHO prognostic score for GTD staging which is described below [18]:

Stage I—When gestational trophoblastic tumours strictly confined to the uterus.

Stage II—Gestational trophoblastic tumours extending and involving adnexa or vagina but limited to the genital structures.

Stage III—Gestational trophoblastic tumours extending to the lungs, with or without genital tract involvement.

Stage IV—All other metastatic sites.

Before scoring a metastasis workup to be done as follows [18]:

1. Chest X-rays are appropriate for diagnosing lung metastases. It is used to count the number of metastases during the scoring of prognostic scoring.
2. Ultrasound/computed tomography scanning can be used for detecting liver metastasis.
3. MRI or CT scanning can be used for detection of brain metastasis.

8.1 Prognostic Scoring

Traditionally WHO divided GTN into low, medium, and high-risk groups, which was modified and divided into low-risk and high-risk group later on. Risk is defined as the risk of developing drug resistance and is determined by the WHO prognostic scoring system (Table 2).

Low-risk disease is diagnosed when score is less than or equal to 6 (≤6) and high-risk disease when score is more than 6 (>6).

While giving patient's diagnosis both staging and scoring are done and after denoting stage in Roman numerals score is given in Arabic numerals, which is separated by colon, i.e. stage I: 2, Stage III: 6.

9 Pretreatment Evaluation of GTN

1. Complete history taking is essential and it should include history of pregnancies, menstrual history including the last date of men-

Table 2 FIGO modified WHO prognostic scoring system [18]

	0	1	2	4
Age	<40	>40		
Antecedent pregnancy	Mole	Abortion	Term	–
Interval from index pregnancy, months	<4	4–6	7–12	>12
Pretreatment hCG mIU/mL	$<10^3$	$>10^3$–10^4	$>10^4$–10^5	$>10^5$
Largest tumour size including uterus, cm	–	3–4	≥5	–
Site of metastases including uterus	Lung	Spleen, kidney	GIT	Brain, liver
Number of metastases identified	–	1–4	5–8	>8
Previous failed chemotherapy	–	–	Single dose	Two or more drugs

struation, and use of oral contraceptive pills. If history of molar evacuation is present then date of evacuation, presence of bleeding, and any respiratory or central nervous system-related symptoms should be enquired.
2. Measurement of serum hCG levels.
3. Hepatic, renal thyroid function test.
4. Baseline peripheral WBC, CBC, and platelet counts.
5. Stool guaiac testing.
6. Chest X-ray pelvic USG—to confirm the absence of pregnancy, detect pelvic disease, retained products, and myometrial invasion.

Metastatic workup:

1. Chest CT, if chest X-ray is positive. If a chest X-ray is negative, it is not needed as micrometastasis does not affect the outcome.
2. USG/CT abdomen and pelvis.
3. MRI/CT brain.
4. CSF hCG level measurement.
5. Pathology review—histological confirmation of the diagnosis of GTN is not required for treatment. However, a biopsy of the metastatic site may be done if in doubt.

10 Treatment of Benign GTD

Suction and evacuation are the primary treatment of complete and partial moles.

Prophylactic Chemotherapy After Suction and Evacuation of Molar Pregnancy.

A Cochrane data review has done for prophylactic chemotherapy after suction and evacuation of molar pregnancy. They concluded that benefits from use of prophylactic chemotherapy is limited as all studies showing benefits either of low methodological values or has smaller sample size. In complete molar pregnancy where risk of malignant transformation to GTN is more, prophylactic chemotherapy may minimize the risk to progression. This method cannot currently be recommended because prophylactic chemotherapy may enhance medication resistance, delay GTN treatment, and expose women to hazardous adverse effects [26].

11 Treatment of Malignant GTN

Before starting treatment, proper workup and risk categorization of the disease is to be done. The primary management is chemotherapy which is different for low-risk and high-risk groups which are discussed below.

11.1 Low Risk

A simple evacuation of the uterus with judicious use of single-agent chemotherapy can cure low-risk GTN. Worldwide different chemotherapy regimen is followed, but the risk and benefits of each regimen are unclear.

Commonly Used Single Drug Regimens:

Methotrexate and actinomycin D are two drugs used commonly for single-drug regimens. The various regimens are shown in Table 3.

Alazzam et al. conducted a metaanalysis to analyse available data on the different treatment regimens of low-risk GTN and found six commonly used regimens. These were either single or combined regimens using methotrexate and dactinomycin. Methotrexate was used weekly, in a 5-day regimen, with folinic acid in an 8-day methotrexate-folinic acid regimen. Dactinomycin was used as in 'pulsed' dactinomycin, 5-day dactinomycin, and the combination therapy included use of both methotrexate and dactinomycin. They concluded that dactinomycin pulse therapy was superior to weekly methotrexate in terms of obtaining primary cure while posing a lower risk of toxicity [27, 28].

Another meta-analysis was performed to compare the regimen concluded that in low-risk GTN, Actinomycin D has a higher chance of achieving a primary cure rate with fewer chances of treatment failure than a methotrexate regimen. While comparing side effects between actinomycin D and methotrexate, there is no difference. But actinomycin D may have a higher

Table 3 Single-agent drug regimens

Regimen	Drug schedule	Response rate [27]
Methotrexate 5 day	MTX 0.4 mg/kg/day IV or IM for 5 days, not to exceed 25 mg/day Repeat cycle every 14 days	87–93%
Methotrexate 8-day alternate	MTX 1 mg/kg IM days 1, 3, 5, and 7 plus folinic acid 15 mg PO 30 h after each MTX dose on days 2, 4, 6, and 8 Repeat cycle every 14 days	74–90%
	MTX 100 mg/m² IVP, then 200 mg/m² in 500 mL D5W infused over 12 h on day 1 plus folinic acid 15 mg IM/PO q12h for 4 doses Initiate folinic acid 24 h after start of MTX Repeat cycle every 18 days or as needed	69–90%
Methotrexate weekly	MTX 30–50 mg/m² IM weekly	49–74
Actinomycin regimen 5-day act-D regimen	Act-D 10–13 µg/kg or 0.5-mg flat dose IV qd for 5 days Repeat cycle every 14 days	77–94
Actinomycin D pulsed	Actinomycin 1.25 mg/m² IV every 2 weeks	100

risk of severe adverse events than a methotrexate regimen [29].

Primary resistance develops in 10–30% of patients with low-risk GTN and is defined as either increase or plateau in two serial hCG values following single-agent treatment. hCG syndrome must be ruled out if hCG levels are low [30].

11.2 High-Risk Regimens

11.2.1 EMACO

EMACO chemotherapy, when used as primary treatment for metastatic high-risk GTN, has a remission rate of 72%, sustained remission rate of 80%, and survival rate of 86% [31, 32]. However, roughly 30–40% of women may develop resistance or recurrence following remission, necessitating salvage chemotherapy [33].

Day 1—Etoposide 100 mg/m² intravenous infusion over 30 min.

Actinomycin D 0.5 mg intravenous bolus.
Methotrexate 100 mg/m² intravenous bolus 200 mg/m² intravenous infusion over 12 h.

Day 2—Etoposide 100 mg/m² intravenous infusion over 30 min.

Actinomycin D 0.5 mg intravenous bolus.
Folinic acid rescue 15 mg intramuscularly or orally every 12 h for four doses (starting 24 h after beginning the methotrexate infusion).

Day 8—Vincristine 1 mg/m² intravenous bolus (maximum 2 mg).

Cyclophosphamide 600 mg/m² intravenous infusion over 30 min.

11.2.2 EMA-EP

Patients with high-risk GTN can achieve complete remission with the EMA/EP treatment in 88% of cases. In patients who have failed single-agent chemotherapy, EMA/EP is suggested as a first-line therapy. However, sufficient precautions should be taken to avoid and minimize EMA/EP haematological effects [32].

OTHER AGENTS are bleomycin, etoposide, cisplatin (BEP), Ifosfamide, carboplatin, etoposide (IEP), Etoposide, ifosfamide, cisplatin (VEP).

11.3 Ultra-High Risk

Patients having a FIGO score ≥12 are categorized as ultra-high-risk GTN. The 5-year overall survival (OS) of ultra-high-risk is around 67.9%. They have a poor prognosis compared to low-risk and high-risk GTN. Ultra-high-risk GTN following non-molar antecedent pregnancy, brain metastases, and previous multiagent chemotherapy failure needs more emphasis. Moreover, salvage surgery may improve the prognosis. Floxuridine-based multiagent chemotherapy is an effective regimen whose toxicities are manageable for ultra-high-risk GTN patients [16].

When normal chemotherapy is started in a patient with a large tumour, it can result in abrupt tumour collapse, severe bleeding, metabolic acidosis, myelosuppression, septicaemia, and multiple organ failure, all of which can lead to death. For this reason, the initial gentle use of chemotherapy as induction is an option. In induction chemotherapy etoposide and cisplatin are used. Dose of etoposide is 100 mg/m^2 on day 1 and day 2. Dose of cisplatin is 20 mg/m^2 on days 1 and 2. This regimen is repeated weekly for 1–3 weeks, before starting standard chemotherapy. In one study induction chemotherapy has shown to eliminate early deaths and in other studies showed promising results [34].

EP (etoposide and platinum)/EMA or another more intensive chemotherapy regimen than EMACO may provide a better response and outcome for patients with liver metastases, with or without brain metastases, or having a very high-risk score. A lengthier consolidation with four cycles of chemotherapy might be considered for such high-risk individuals [35].

Other salvage regimen are [18]:

- Etoposide, cisplatin, etoposide, methotrexate, and actinomycin D (EP-EMA).
- Paclitaxel, cisplatin/paclitaxel, etoposide (TP/TE).
- Methotrexate, bleomycin, etoposide (MBE).
- Etoposide, ifosfamide, and cisplatin or carboplatin (VIP/ICE).
- Bleomycin, etoposide, cisplatin (BEP).
- 5-fluorouracil, actinomycin D (FA)
- Floxuridine, actinomycin D, etoposide, vincristine (FAEV).
- Use of high-dose chemotherapy in association with autologous bone marrow or stem cell transplant.
- Use of immunotherapeutic agents like pembrolizumab.

Managing brain metastasis:

1. IV Methotrexate as methotrexate infusion to 1 g/m^2.
2. Intrathecal methotrexate dose is 12.5 mg.
3. Both IV and intrathecal methotrexate can be given during EMA-CO and EMA-EP regimen. They are administered during CO or EP phase of regimen.
4. Radiotherapy: whole brain RT or stereotactic RT.
5. Decompression surgery may sometimes be lifesaving when intracranial pressure is raised due to intracranial bleed.

12 Role of Surgery

1. Dilatation and evacuation is the mainstay of the evacuation of molar pregnancy in a patient desiring fertility. However, hysterectomy is another option for patients non-desirous of future fertility.

Hysterectomy may be used as primary treatment of unevacuated mole and management of GTD [36]. Hysterectomy reduces the number of cycles of chemotherapy needed in low-risk non-metastatic GTN patients [37]. However, acute blood loss is more than suction and evacuation.

Induction of labour and abdominal hysterotomy are rarely employed for the primary evacuation of hydatidiform moles due to higher morbidity and a high incidence of post-molar GTN [38].

In PSTT with non-metastatic disease, hysterectomy is curative in two-thirds of patients [39].

After a hysterectomy, the total risk of post-molar GTD drops to about 3.5%, compared to the expected 20% after a suction D&C [36].

Surgical intervention may be needed to control intractable bleeding or for stabilization of the patient for receiving chemotherapy in localized chemo-resistant disease. Secondary hysterectomy is indicated in localized drug-resistant cases.

Hysterectomy is also an indication for intractable bleeding p/v.

Theca lutein cyst—They may require several months to resolve. Surgical intervention is needed only in 3% of cases when there is torsion or rupture [40].

Other Surgeries- Thoracotomy is indicated when resistant pulmonary metastases are present. A craniotomy is indiacted for intracranial haemorrhagic and persistent drug-resistant metastasis.

13 Role of Radiotherapy

It has a limited role in the management of GTD. Brain RT and liver RT can be given to prevent haemorrhagic complications to this organ, 2000–4000 cGy in 10–20 equal fractions. Whole-brain radiation is given concurrently with combination chemotherapy, with reduced-field boosts given in selected patients.

The concurrent Chemotherapy-radiation therapy (CTRT) act as tumouricidal and haemostatic [41].

14 PSTT

PSTTs are a relatively rare GTD. They arise from the intermediate trophoblastic cell layer. Molecularly this tumour occurs due to alteration in intracellular signalling pathways, intercellular information transmission, and extracellular matrix. It is found that ERK, MAPK, mTOR signalling pathway, transcription factor NF-kB, Kiss-1, and GATA3 may play critical roles in the invasion and metastasis of PSTT [42].

PSTT is a disorder that affects women of childbearing age, who are on average 32 years old. PSTT can occur as a consequence of a full-term pregnancy, a premature birth, a hydatidiform mole, or choriocarcinoma. Duration of development from previous pregnancy may range from several months to several years.

But the most common time of occurrence is 1 year after the previous pregnancy. The main symptoms of PSTT include vaginal bleeding and amenorrhea. PSTT has an unusual clinical picture, which makes diagnosis difficult. After an interval of amenorrhea, patients frequently report with irregular vaginal bleeding or menorrhagia, as well as an enlarged uterus. Blood β-hCG usually normal or may be slightly increased and are not proportional to the tumour burden. This is in contrast to many GTDs, which contain a high level of β-hCG. Other forms of GTDs with low serum β-hCG levels, on the other hand, have been reported. Ultrasound findings are frequently unspecific. A mix of histology and IHC examinations is required for a clear diagnosis. Histologically PSTT is constituted of intermediate trophoblasts; cytotrophoblasts or chorionic villi are absent. The tumour cells show hPL strong positivity with weak positivity for hCG [43].

β-hCG is usually not raised in these tumours, and metastasis is usually late, but when metastasis occurs, the lung and brain are the commonest sites.

PSTT does not have a prognostic index score like GzTN.

The different poor prognosis factors of PSTT are:

The interval between antecedent pregnancy >2 years, deep infiltration, necrosis, mitotic index >5/10 under a microscope.

Patients with high risk are recommended to use multi-drug combined chemotherapy.

Patients in stage I can be treated with a straightforward hysterectomy, which can include or exclude pelvic nodal biopsy.

Hysterectomy with adjuvant chemotherapy is an ideal approach for FIGO stage II-IV patients [44].

If fertility preservation is necessary, conservative treatments such as uterine curettage, hysteroscopic resection, and chemotherapy may be considered, especially in a limited local lesion [45].

15 ETT

It is an unusual trophoblastic tumour. Usually, they are reported in the age group of 15–48 years. Abnormal vaginal bleeding is the most common presenting symptom.

The tumour often comprises a population of mononuclear cells that form nests and solid masses that mimic cells of the intermediate trophoblast of chorionic leaf. ETTs are well-demarcated, with a surrounding lymphocytic infiltrate. The tumour may also have typical extensive necrosis that creates a geographic pattern. This pattern is sometimes accompanied by dystrophic calcification [46].

The tumours are IHC positive for cytokeratin, epithelial membrane antigen, and inhibin. P63 is positive in the majority of ETTs and can be especially helpful when the differential diagnosis includes a placental trophoblastic tumour [47]. p63 expression is useful in the distinction of epithelioid trophoblastic and placental site trophoblastic tumours by profiling trophoblastic subpopulations [47].

hCG levels are usually raised.

ETTs do not respond to chemotherapy drugs used to treat other types of GTD.

Any GTD not responding to chemotherapy ETT must be ruled out first.

Hysterectomy is the treatment of choice. ETT is more aggressive in nature than PSTT.

16 Follow-Up

The normal follow-up routine for low-risk and high-risk GTN is as follows:

1. Molar pregnancy—after surgical treatment β-hCG is monitored weekly until 3 consecutive values are normal and then monthly for 6 months.
2. In GTN—during treatment β-hCG is monitored until 3 consecutive weekly values are normal. After that low-risk GTNs are followed with monthly β-hCG monitoring for 12 months, then 6 monthly for 1 year, and annually till 5 years.

   High-risk GTNs are followed with monthly β-hCG levels for 18 months, then 6 monthly for 2 years, and then annually till 5 years.

In case of complete molar pregnancy, if hCG level is normalized in 56 days of the pregnancy event, follow-up is indicated for 6 months from the date of suction and evacuation. But if β-hCG has failed to normalize within 56 days then follow-up is done for 6 months after the date of normalization of values.

Follow-up for partial molar pregnancy is till the hCG becomes normal on two samples, taken 4 weeks apart.

There is still a lack of consensus in the literature on how to follow up on PSST/ETT patients. PSTT/ETT patients should be observed for at least 5 years since they produce little hCG, grow slowly, and have late metastases [30].

17 Recurrent GTN

GTN is a highly chemo-sensitive tumour. But around 25% of tumours are resistant, relapse, or recur after initial treatment. As per FIGO 2020, re-staging is done for relapse, and a complete re-assessment of spread and previous chemotherapy response is used [18].

Second-line chemotherapy, with or without surgery, can be used to achieve remission after first-line treatment fails in low-risk GTN. Several secondary treatment regimens have been described, with varying success rates and toxicity profiles, including single-agent pulsed dactinomycin (where methotrexate has been used as first-line therapy); five-day dactinomycin etoposide and dactinomycin (EA); methotrexate, dactinomycin, and cyclophosphamide (MAC); and etoposide, methotrexate, and dactinomycin [48].

The most often utilized first-line therapy for high-risk GTN is EMA/CO, with platinum-etoposide combinations, particularly EMA/EP (etoposide, methotrexate, dactinomycin/etoposide, cisplatin), being preferred as salvage therapy. This resulted in a response rate of 75–80%. EMA/EP regimen is associated with significant hepatotoxicity and myelosuppression. According to some research, TE/TP (paclitaxel and etoposide alternated twice weekly with paclitaxel and cisplatin) is as effective as EMA-EP while being less hazardous [49].

Alternatives include BEP (bleomycin, etoposide, cisplatin), FAEV (floxuridine, dactinomycin, etoposide, vincristine), and FA (5-fluorouracil, dactinomycin).

However, it is unclear whether fluorouracil (5-FU), dactinomycin is as effective as EMA/EP and has fewer side effects [48].

Other regimens that can be used are MEA (methotrexate, etoposide, dactinomycin), MAC or methotrexate, dactinomycin, chlorambucil, FA (5-FU, dactinomycin) or FAV (5-FU, dactinomycin, vincristine), MEF (methotrexate, etoposide, 5-FU), EMA/EP (etoposide, methotrexate, dactinomycin/etoposide, cisplatin) whereby EMA and EP are alternated weekly, and CHAMOCA (methotrexate, dactinomycin, cyclophosphamide, doxorubicin, melphalan, hydroxyurea, vincristine).

The identification of isolated active disease areas susceptible to surgical excision benefits these individuals. Secondary hysterectomy and metastasectomy (pulmonary resection, craniotomy, and liver lobe resection) are important in chemo-resistant cases [50].

18 Contraception and Fertility Preservation

Patients are counselled not to conceive until all of their follow-up appointments have been completed. Contraception is correlated to hCG monitoring throughout follow-up, not to the chance of recurrence. For mole, oral contraceptive is recommended for 6 months. In low-risk cases advise is given to avoid pregnancy for 12 months, and in high-risk cases pregnancy is advised to be avoided for 18 months. The intrauterine device is not recommended, because of fear of perforating the uterus and irregular bleeding [51].

Oestrogen containing pills can be started after β-HCG becomes normal.

19 Subsequent Pregnancy

Women who had GTD or had a history of previously treated GTN usually have no problem with fertility. Around 83% of patients become pregnant after treatment with methotrexate or EMACO regimen [51]. Familial gestational trophoblastic disease has been seen to run in families and is due to genetic mutation at 19q13.4. Coexistent molar pregnancy with live foetus is a rare condition but caries risk to foetus and hence managed judiciously at high-risk centres.

But they have a risk of developing a GTD in a future pregnancy. The following are recommended for such cases:

1. Sonographic evaluation is recommended in early pregnancy.
2. At delivery, the placenta or products of conception are to be sent for pathological evaluation.
3. Serum β-hCG measurement at 6 weeks postpartum.

20 Secondary Malignancies

There is an increased risk of secondary malignancies like leukaemia, colon cancer, melanoma, and breast cancer.

This increased risk is attributed to etoposide use.

But a study done at Charing Cross Hospital in 2006 for cases from 1958 to 2000 concluded that following chemotherapy either MTX-FA or EMA-CO, the cancer risks for patients who were cured of gestational trophoblastic tumours with current chemotherapy appear to be similar to those of the general population, with no overall increased risk of malignancy. However, based on small patient numbers, there was evidence of an elevated risk of leukaemia after EMA-CO and some indication of other site-specific higher risks. Except for MTX-FA, all effective therapies raised the likelihood of early menopause [52].

21 Conclusion

GTNs are a group of the curable malignancies. In India actual incidences are not known. So multicentred studies are required in India to determine the true incidence and overall outcome of gestational trophoblastic diseases that will help in understanding the burden of disease and to produce the optimal outcome.

References

1. Lurain JR. Gestational trophoblastic disease: epidemiology, pathology, clinical presentation and diagnosis of gestational trophoblastic disease, and management of hydatidiform mole. Am J Obstet Gynecol. 2010;203(6):531–9.
2. Seckl MJ, Sebire NJ, Berkowitz RS. Gestational trophoblastic disease. Lancet. 2010;376(9742):717–29.
3. WHO. Reprinted from International Agency for Research on Cancer. WHO classification of female genital tumours. 5th ed. Lyon: IARC; 2020. p. 309–22.
4. Lakra P, et al. Outcome of gestational trophoblastic disease in a Rural Tertiary Center of Haryana, India. Int J Reprod Contracept Obstet Gynecol. 2016;6(1):271–5. https://doi.org/10.18203/2320-1770.ijrcog20164673.
5. Steigrad SJ. Epidemiology of gestational trophoblastic diseases. Best Pract Res Clin Obstet Gynaecol. 2003;17(6):837–47.
6. Shi YF, Li JQ, Zheng W, Chen XJ, Chen XJ, Qiao YH, et al. Survey of gestational trophoblastic disease incidence among 3.6 million pregnancies in China. Zhonghua Fu Chan Ke Za Zhi. 2005;40(2):76–8.
7. Hancock BW, Seckl MJ, Berkowitz RS. Gestational trophoblastic disease. 4th ed; 2015. http://test.registraid.com/gtd-book.html. Accessed 2 May 2018.
8. Sebire NJ, Fisher RA, Foskett M, Rees H, Seckl MJ, Newlands ES. Risk of recurrent hydatidiform mole and subsequent pregnancy outcome following complete or partial hydatidiform molar pregnancy. BJOG. 2003;110(1):22–6.
9. Altieri A, Franceschi S, Ferlay J, et al. Epidemiology and aetiology of gestational trophoblastic diseases. Lancet Oncol. 2003;4(11):670–8.
10. Baljeet Kaur FRCPath (Consultant Cellular Pathologist), Pathology of gestational trophoblastic disease(GTD). https://www.sciencedirect.com/science/journal/15216934.
11. Naniwadekar MR, Desai SR, Kshirsagar NS, Angarkar NN, Dombale VD, Jagtap SV. Pure choriocarcinoma of ovary diagnosed by fine needle aspiration cytology. Indian J Pathol Microbiol. 2009;52:417–20.
12. Kajii T, Ohama K. Androgenetic origin of hydatidiform mole. Nature. 1977;268(5621):633–4. https://doi.org/10.1038/268633a0.
13. Lawler SD, Fisher RA, Dent J. A prospective genetic study of complete and partial hydatidiform moles. Am J Obstet Gynecol. 1991;164:1270–7.
14. https://www.imperial.nhs.uk/~/media/website/services/cancer-services/gestational-trophoblastic-disease/gtd-clinic-guide-for-clinicians.pdf?la=en.
15. Covens A, Fialici VL, Burger RA, Osborne R, Chen MD. Phase II trial of pulse dactinomycin as salvage therapy for failed low-risk gestational trophoblastic neoplasia. Cancer. 2006;107(6):1280–6.
16. Homesley HD, Hancock BW. Chapter 13: treatment of non-metastatic gestational trophoblastic disease. In: Gestational trophoblastic disease. 3rd ed. Orange, CT: ISSTD: International Society for the Study of Trophoblastic Diseases; 2009. p. 366–79.
17. McGrath S, Short D, Harvey R, Schmid P, Savage PM, Seckl MJ. The management and outcome of women with post-hydatidiform mole 'low-risk' gestational trophoblastic neoplasia, but hCG levels in excess of 100 000 IU/L^{-1}. Br J Cancer. 2010;102(5):810–4.
18. Ngan HY, Seckl MJ, Berkowitz RS, Xiang Y, Golfier F, Sekharan PK, Lurain JR, Massuger L. Update on the diagnosis and management of gestational trophoblastic disease. Int J Gynecol Obstet. 2018;143:79–85. https://doi.org/10.1002/ijgo.12615.
19. Carey L, Nash BM, Wright DC. Molecular genetic studies of complete hydatidiform moles. Transl Pediatr. 2015;4(2):181–8. https://doi.org/10.3978/j.issn.2224-4336.2015.04.02.
20. Xiao C, Yang J, Zhao J, et al. Management and prognosis of patients with brain metastasis from gestational trophoblastic neoplasia: a 24-year experience in Peking union medical college hospital. BMC Cancer. 2015;15:318.
21. Lima LL, Parente RC, Maestá I, Amim Junior J, de Rezende Filho JF, Montenegro CA, Braga A. Clinical and radiological correlations in patients with gestational trophoblastic disease. Radiol Bras. 2016;49:241–50.
22. Berkowitz RS, Goldstein DP. Gynecologic oncology. 2. In: Knapp RC, Berkowitz RS, editors. The management of molar pregnancy and gestational trophoblastic tumors. New York: McGraw-Hill; 1993. p. 328–38.
23. Bagshawe KD. Risk and prognostic factors in trophoblastic neoplasia. Cancer. 1976;38:1373–85.
24. Hammond CB, Borchert LG, Tyrey L, Creaman WT, Parker RT. Treatment of metastatic trophoblastic disease: good and poor prognosis. Am J Obstet Gynecol. 1973;115(4):451–7.
25. WHO Scientific Group on Gestational Trophoblastic Diseases & World Health Organization. Gestational trophoblastic diseases: report of a WHO scientific group [meeting held in Geneva from 6 to 10 December 1982]. World Health Organization; 1983. https://apps.who.int/iris/handle/10665/39169
26. Wang Q, Fu J, Hu L, Fang F, Xie L, Chen H, He F, Wu T, Lawrie TA. Prophylactic chemotherapy for hydatidiform mole to prevent gestational trophoblastic neoplasia. Cochrane Database Syst Rev. 2017;9(9):CD007289. https://doi.org/10.1002/14651858. CD007289.pub3. PMID: 28892119; PMCID: PMC6483742
27. Alazzam M, Tidy J, Hancock BW, Osborne R. First line chemotherapy in low risk gestational trophoblastic neoplasia. Cochrane Database Syst Rev. 2009;(1):CD007102. https://doi.org/10.1002/14651858.CD007102.
28. Hao J, Zhou W, Zhang M, et al. Direct comparisons of efficacy and safety between actinomycin-D and methotrexate in women with low-risk gestational trophoblastic neoplasia: a meta-analysis of randomized and high-quality non-randomized studies. BMC

Cancer. 2021;21:1122. https://doi.org/10.1186/s12885-021-08849-7.
29. Lawrie TA, Alazzam M, Tidy J, Hancock BW, Osborne R. First-line chemotherapy in low-risk gestational trophoblastic neoplasia. Cochrane Database Syst Rev. 2016;2016(6):CD007102. CD007102.pub4. PMID: 27281496; PMCID: PMC6768658. https://doi.org/10.1002/14651858.
30. Santaballa A, García Y, Herrero A, et al. SEOM clinical guidelines in gestational trophoblastic disease (2017). Clin Transl Oncol. 2018;20(1):38–46. https://doi.org/10.1007/s12094-017-1793-0.
31. Cagayan MS. High-risk metastatic gestational trophoblastic neoplasia. Primary management with EMA-CO (etoposide, methotrexate, actinomycin D, cyclophosphamide and vincristine) chemotherapy. J Reprod Med. 2012;57(5–6):231–6.
32. Aminimoghaddam S, Nezhadisalami F, Anjidani S, Barzin TS. Outcome of treatment with EMA/EP (etoposide methotrexate and actinomycin-D/etoposide and cisplatin) regimen in gestational trophoblastic neoplasia. Med J Islam Repub Iran. 2018;32:36. PMID: 30159287; PMCID: PMC6108260. https://doi.org/10.14196/mjiri.32.36.
33. Goldstein DP, Berkowitz RS. Current management of gestational trophoblastic neoplasia. Hematol Oncol Clin N Am. 2012;26:111–31.
34. Bolze PA, Riedl C, Massardier J, et al. Mortality rate of gestational trophoblastic neoplasia with a FIGO score of ≥13. Am J Obstet Gynecol. 2016;214:390.e1–8.
35. Ahamed E, Short D, North B, Savage PM, Seckl MJ. Survival of women with gestational trophoblastic neoplasia and liver metastases: is it improving? J Reprod Med. 2012;57:262–9.
36. Zhao P, Lu Y, Huang W, et al. Total hysterectomy versus uterine evacuation for preventing post-molar gestational trophoblastic neoplasia in patients who are at least 40 years old: a systematic review and meta-analysis. BMC Cancer. 2019;19:13. https://doi.org/10.1186/s12885-018-5168-x.
37. Bolze PA, Mathe M, Hajri T, You B, Dabi Y, Schott AM, Patrier S, Massardier J, Golfier F. First-line hysterectomy for women with low-risk non-metastatic gestational trophoblastic neoplasia no longer wishing to conceive. Gynecol Oncol. 2018;150(2):282–7. Epub 2018 Jun 8. https://doi.org/10.1016/j.ygyno.2018.05.030.
38. Kaur B, Short D, Fisher RA, Savage PM, Seckl MJ, Sebire NJ. Atypical placental site nodule (APSN) and association with malignant gestational trophoblastic disease; a clinicopathologic study of 21 cases. Int J Gynecol Pathol. 2015;34:152–8.
39. Horowitz NS, Goldstein DP, Berkowitz RS. Placental site trophoblastic tumors and epithelioid trophoblastic tumors: biology, natural history, and treatment modalities. Gynecol Oncol. 2017;144:208–14. https://doi.org/10.1016/j.ygyno.2016.10.024.
40. Yadav RS, Shrestha S, Sharma S, Singh M, Bista KD, Ojha N. Partial invasive mole with bilateral torsion of theca lutein cysts. J Nepal Health Res Counc. 2017;15(37):298–300. https://doi.org/10.3126/jnhrc.v15i3.18861.
41. Soper JT. Role of surgery and radiation therapy in the management of gestational trophoblastic disease. Best Pract Res Clin Obstet Gynaecol. 2003;17:943–57.
42. Banet N, Gown AM, Shih IM, Kay Li Q, Roden RB, Nucci MR, et al. GATA-3 expression in trophoblastic tissues: an immunohistochemical study of 445 cases, including diagnostic utility. Am J Surg Pathol. 2015;39:101–8. https://doi.org/10.1097/PAS.0000000000000315.
43. Horn LC, Bilek K. Histologic classification and staging of gestational trophoblastic disease. Gen Diagn Pathol. 1997;143(2–3):87–101.
44. Alexander AL, Strohl AE, Maniar KP, Lurain JR. Placental site trophoblastic tumor: successful treatment of 13 cases. Gynecol Oncol Rep. 2020;32:100548. https://doi.org/10.1016/j.gore.2020.100548.
45. Zhao J, Lv WG, Feng FZ, et al. Placental site trophoblastic tumor: a review of 108 cases and their implications for prognosis and treatment. Gynecol Oncol. 2016;142:102–8.
46. Shih IM, Kumaran RJ. Epithelioid trophoblastic tumor: a neoplasm distinct from choriocarcinoma and placental site trophoblastic tumor simulating carcinoma. Am J Surg Pathol. 1998;22(11):1393–403.
47. Shih IM, Kumaran RJ. p63 expression useful in the distinction of epithelioid trophoblastic and placental site trophoblastic tumors by profiling trophoblastic subpopulations. Am J Surg Pathol. 2004;28(9):1177–83.
48. Alazzam M, Tidy J, Osborne R, Coleman R, Hancock BW, Lawrie TA. Chemotherapy for resistant or recurrent gestational trophoblastic neoplasia. Cochrane Database Syst Rev. 2016;12:CD008891. https://doi.org/10.1002/14651858.CD008891. pub3
49. Wang J, Short D, Sebire NJ, Lindsay I, Newlands ES, Schmid P, et al. Salvage chemotherapy of relapsed or high-risk gestational trophoblastic neoplasia (GTN) with paclitaxel/cisplatin alternating with paclitaxel/etoposide (TP/TE). Ann Oncol. 2008;19:1578–83. https://doi.org/10.1093/annonc/mdn181.
50. Doll KM, Soper JT. The role of surgery in the management of gestational trophoblastic neoplasia. Obstet Gynecol Surv. 2013;68:533–42. https://doi.org/10.1097/OGX.0b013e31829a82df.
51. Brown J, Naumann RW, Seckl MJ, Schink J. 15 years of progress in gestational trophoblastic disease: scoring, standardization, and salvage. Gynecol Oncol. 2017;144:200–7. https://doi.org/10.1016/j.ygyno.2016.08.330.
52. Savage P, Cooke R, O'Nions J, Krell J, Kwan A, Camarata M, Dancy G, Short D, Seckl MJ, Swerdlow A. Effects of single-agent and combination chemotherapy for gestational trophoblastic tumors on risks of second malignancy and early menopause. J Clin Oncol. 2015;33(5):472–8.

Gynaecological Cancer in Pregnancy

Debabrata Barmon and Amal Chandra Kataki

1 Introduction

Pregnancy-associated cancer (PAC) is usually defined as cancer diagnosed during pregnancy or within the first year after delivery. The most common cancers diagnosed in pregnancy will mirror those found in nonpregnant reproductive women. Any pregnancy complicated by cancer is a high-risk pregnancy and needs to be addressed by a multidisciplinary team, preferably in a specialised centre in order to improve obstetric outcome together with the most adequate cancer treatment. Patient counselling and decision making still remain an obstacle due to the rarity of the condition; however data is emerging from all over the world particularly the developed nations where the obstetrical registry is linked with the cancer registry. It remains a fact that unless these two registries are interlinked it is very difficult to estimate the real burden of the problem particularly in developing countries.

2 Epidemiology

Currently whatever data we have is mostly from the developed nations where there is a strong linkage between the obstetrical and oncological registries. As a whole, cancer in pregnancy is showing an upward trend all over the world mainly because of the fact that the incidence of cancer is increasing along with the increasing trend of maternal age. The incidence of pregnancy-associated cancer was reported to be about 1:1000–1:2000 pregnancies (50–100:100,000 pregnancies) [1, 2]; however the recent population-based data has shown the incidence of cancer diagnosed during pregnancy to be 17–25 per 100,000 [3–6] pregnancies and pregnancy-associated cancers at 81–140 per 100,000 pregnancies [5–8]. The risk increases significantly with age, from 60 per 100,000 for women younger than 30 years to 265 per 100,000 for women older than 40 years [9]. In a study by de Haan et al., comprising 1170 woman diagnosed with cancer during pregnancy, the most common invasive cancers in pregnancy were breast cancer (39%, $n = 462$), followed by cervical (13%, $n = 147$), lymphoma (10%, $n = 113$), ovarian (7%, $n = 88$), and leukaemia (6%, $n = 68$) [10]. For most research outcomes, it is not optimal to report results for the whole group, but for patients diagnosed during pregnancy and for those diagnosed postpartum, sep-

D. Barmon (✉) · A. C. Kataki
Department of Gynaecologic Oncology,
Dr. Bhubaneswar Borooah Cancer Institute
(A Unit of Tata Memorial Centre, Mumbai),
Guwahati, Assam, India
e-mail: dydiracademic@bbci.tmc.gov.in

A. C. Kataki, D. Barmon (eds.), *Fundamentals in Gynaecologic Malignancy*,
https://doi.org/10.1007/978-981-19-5860-1_24

arately. Each of the risk windows before (trimester I, II, III) and after delivery (0–6, 6–12, 12–24 months, 2–5, 5–10 years, etc.) represents different exposure levels to woman and foetus, as well as short- and long-term physiological effects of pregnancy. Recent data suggests the incidence of cervical cancer in pregnancy to be around 1.4–4.6 per 100,000 pregnancies and ovarian cancer 0.2–3.8 per 100,000; vulvar, vaginal and endometrial cancers are rare and very few cases are reported in the literature [5–9, 11–14].

3 Imaging Cancer in Pregnancy

Historically our knowledge about the effects of radiation on the foetus is based on the radiation disasters. Accurate radiological assessment of the disease and treatment response demands meticulous diagnostic imaging, which remains an important hurdle for the pregnant cancer patient as a balance between maternal benefit and foetal risk has to be taken care of. Radiation-induced teratogenesis and carcinogenesis are the two major risks involved, so careful selection of the best and safe imaging modality available to provide the optimum diagnostic information is of utmost importance while taking into consideration any potential risks to the mother and foetus. Multidisciplinary team involving radiologists and nuclear imaging physicians should be involved in the optimisation of diagnostic strategy following the "As low as reasonably achievable" (ALARA) principle. Staging algorithms with recommended imaging techniques for malignant disease in pregnancy are frequently precluded, due to concerns in relation to foetal exposure to ionising radiation and contrast medium. Significant risk for foetal damage is observed at a threshold cumulative dose of 100 mGy [15], any dose in excess of 100 mGy may lead to an all or nothing phenomenon during embryogenesis (Table 1).

Table 1 Relation between gestational age, radiation dose and teratogenicity

Gestational period	Effects	Estimated threshold dose
0–2 weeks	No effect	>100 mGy
<8 weeks	Death of embryo (all or nothing effect) Congenital anomalies (skeleton, eyes, genitals)	50–100 mGy 200 mGy
8–15 weeks	Growth retardation Severe mental retardation (high risk) Microcephaly Intellectual deficit	200–250 mGy 60–310 mGy 200 mGy 25 IQ point loss per grey
>16 weeks	Severe mental retardation (low risk)	250–280 mGy

The imaging modalities available for the diagnosis and staging of cancer are divided into (1) non-ionising imaging procedure like Grey-scale and Doppler Ultrasound (US) and Magnetic Resonance Imaging (MRI) and (2) ionising imaging procedures like Multi-Detector Computed Tomography (MDCT), Positron Emission Tomography (PET) and Nuclear Medicine studies; besides these the services of interventional radiology for tissue sampling and stenting may be required from time to time.

3.1 Non-Ionising Imaging Procedure

For determination of tumour size, extent of invasion and lymph node involvement in any trimester of pregnancy ultrasonography and MRI are preferred.

3.1.1 Grey-Scale, Doppler, Spectral and Contrast-Enhanced Ultrasound

The role of greyscale ultrasound in cancer staging is limited due to the inherent limitations of the modality, so focussed ultrasound examination to evaluate pleural effusions, liver lesions or biliary dilatation and evaluation of hydronephrosis may be beneficial. In pregnant cancer patients, subspeciality-targeted ultrasound examinations such as endobronchial ultrasound for evaluation of mediastinum, endoscopic ultrasound for local staging of oesophageal, pancreatic or rectal carcinoma, and transvaginal probes for the characterisation of ovarian masses are used. For evaluation of deep vein thrombosis (DVT) and other vascular studies doppler and spectral ultrasound may be used. Contrast-enhanced ultrasound (CEUS) is better to avoid during pregnancy.

The potential limitations of this modality are the experience of the operator and reduced sensitivity and specificity compared to cross-sectional techniques, particularly in obese patients. The U.S. Food and Drug Administration has recommended the spatial-peak temporal average intensity of [16] the ultrasound beam to be less than 720 mW/cm^2 in obstetric patients to reduce the theoretical risk of foetal tissue heating [17].

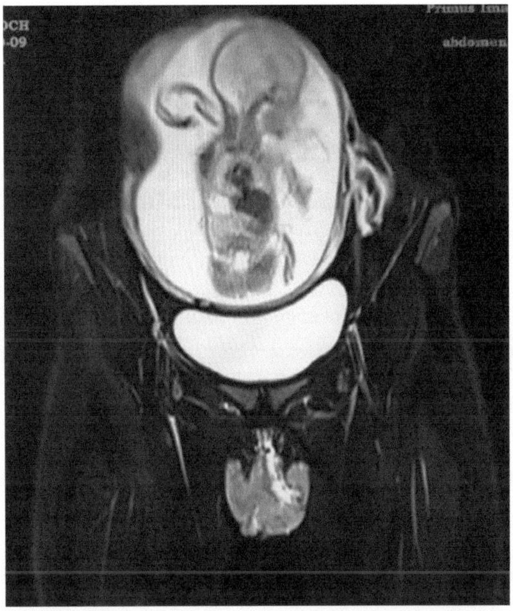

Fig. 1 MRI image showing vulvar growth with pregnancy

3.1.2 Magnetic Resonance Imaging (MRI)

Magnetic Resonance Imaging [MRI] is an operator independent modality with the ability to image deep soft tissue structures and is the safest modality for imaging cancer during pregnancy (Fig. 1). As of now no harmful foetal effects have been documented with the radiofrequency pulses used to acquire images from the 1.5 tesla MRI machines [18, 19].

The mandatory safety checklist prior to the MRI examination, e.g. cochlear and other non-compatible implants and renal function (GFR mL/min), should be evaluated prior to the examination; gadolinium chelates [Gd] can be administered if clinically justified when risks outweigh benefits [20]. No adverse foetal or neonatal outcomes have been reported following Gd exposure during pregnancy. Breast feeding should continue as normal following Gd administration.

A recent study has shown equal efficacy in the detection of nodal and distant metastasis, including bone metastasis, both in solid tumours and lymphomas between whole-body diffusion-weighted MRI (WB-DWI/MRI) and ^{18}F-FDG-PET/CT [21]. Therefore, WB-DWI/MRI could be a suitable alternative for staging and evaluation of tumour response following treatment in pregnant women with cancer [22].

3.2 Ionising Imaging Procedure

As radiation can affect the viability and development of the foetus, ionising imaging procedures should be avoided, if possible [10].

3.2.1 Multi-Detector Computed Tomography [MDCT]

The cooperation between the radiologist and physicist is of utmost importance whenever a MDCT is requested for imaging cancer in pregnancy. Appropriate precautions have to be taken to minimise the foetal exposure to ionising radiation as low as possible, and the principles of MDCT have to be followed as described in Table 2.

Table 2 Principles of MDCT during pregnancy

Obtain informed consent
Avoid exposure to ionising radiation if possible during pregnancy
Consider alternative imaging modalities [US or MRI]
Consultation with medical physics
Reduce the radiation dose to as low as reasonably achievable [ALARA]
The field of view should be limited and preferably exclude the foetus
A detailed history of allergy to contrast media, asthma and impaired renal function is required
Consider imaging in the left lateral decubitus position of 15 degree in pregnancy beyond 20 weeks
Iodinated contrast media can cross the placenta, so caution is advisable while using this, and should be used only if contrast material would provide important additional information or it could be withheld
No specific adverse effects related to contrast media exposure have been identified
Breast feeding can be continued as normal following contrast media administration in MDCT

3.2.2 Positron Emission Tomography [Pet] and Nuclear Scintigraphy

Radiation dose on the foetus from 18-FDG PET is low and adverse effects depend on the administered dose, foetal weight and the type of radiotracer used [21]. When 18FDG PET/CT scan is performed in a pregnant cancer patient, proper hydration and a bladder catheter should be used to reduce foetal radiation exposure. Procedures of sentinel node mapping using radioactive materials are contraindicated for cervical cancer; however it can be used for vulval cancer surgery during pregnancy. Use of indocyanine green is still in the experimental phase for use during pregnancy.

4 Impact of Cancer with Pregnancy in Laboratory Parameters

The changes occurring in the body due to pregnancy itself cause many alterations in the blood biochemical parameters. Few of the parameters are raised like serum alkaline phosphatase and serum LDH and few get lowered as the haematocrit values. Cancer associated with pregnancy can also cause decreased sensitivity and specificity of tumour markers [23]; pregnancy may cause physiological elevation of serum CA125, S. AFP, S beta HCG, S CA 15.3 thus reducing the role of tumour markers in the diagnosis of cancers during pregnancy [24, 25]. The decidua and granulosa cells produce S CA125 especially in the first and last trimester of pregnancy, the trophoblast secretes AFP and beta HCG, and hence the tumour markers assessment should be performed at least 2–10 weeks post-partum.

5 Treatment

The international cohort study showed us the improving acceptance of treatment and the outcome of cancer in pregnancy over the years [10]. The study has shown that for every 5 years beginning from 1996 to 2016, treatment acceptability increased by 10% (95% CI 5–15) and use of chemotherapy increased by 31% (95% CI 20–43). The resultant live birth rates also increased and preterm births decreased. Out of all the available modalities of treatment, surgery remains the mainstay of all the treatment protocols available with us as of now. The most favourable time of surgery is during the early part of second trimester as it reduces the risks of abortion and also gives ample space for the procedure.

During the procedure uterine handling should be minimal. Due to the physiological changes during pregnancy certain precautions during the preoperative, perioperative and postoperative period is needed. The anaesthesia of choice remains local or regional anaesthesia, but general anaesthesia may also be used during major oncological procedure with preferably left/right lateral tilt position. Perioperative monitoring should be very carefully done and any form of hypotension and hypoxia should be avoided as foetal cardiotocography monitoring is not possible during pelvic surgery. The transplacental transfer of anaesthetic drugs used should also be taken care of and used judiciously. The role of laparoscopy during pregnancy depends on the gestational age, expertise of the surgeon and the surgical procedure. When laparoscopy is planned we should ensure that the procedure is short and completed within 90–120 min, intra-abdominal pressure should be maintained between 10 and 13 mmHg and trocar entry should be done by open technique [26–28].

The role of chemotherapy in cancer with pregnancy should be balanced with the maternal benefit and foetal effects. Ideally any time beyond 14 weeks up to 35 weeks or 37 weeks in case of weekly regimens is considered safe; few of the chemotherapeutic drugs that can be used during pregnancy are platinum agents, taxanes, etoposide, bleomycin and anthracyclines. The dose is calculated based on the actual body weight of the pregnant patient and not on the prepregnant weight. Studies have shown that the rate of foetal malformations is comparable to the general population when chemotherapy is used beyond 14 weeks [29–35] and any exposure before 14 weeks leads to foetal malformation of 10–20% [36]. The use of targeted therapy during pregnancy is not recommended.

The role of radiation therapy during pregnancy with pelvic cancers is not possible unless foetal death is considered unavoidable in the process; it may also lead to malformations, growth disturbances and carcinogenic effects, so the role of proper counselling sessions with the patient and attendants is of paramount importance. Radiation therapy other than the pelvic areas may be considered as studies have shown healthy foetus following nonpelvic radiation therapy after proper precautions [37, 38].

Apart from these modalities of treatment psychosocial support is another important aspect in the care of these women. The care and support should start with the breaking of the bad news and should continue in the post-partum period [10]. Both the partners should be explained properly the implication on the pregnancy outcome and the effects on the offspring.

5.1 Management of Cervical Cancer in Pregnancy

Whenever management of cervical cancer in pregnancy is planned, multidisciplinary team approach focussing on the gestational age, stage, histology and desire for fertility should be considered. Gestational age remains the most important criteria for the management which may be immediate management whenever the gestational age is less than or equal to 22 weeks or expectant treatment in case of more than 22 weeks of gestation. However as of now we don't have any gold standard treatment protocol due to the scarcity of data or RCT. Based on the stage and gestational age at the time of diagnosis Halaska et al. devised a management algorithm which is represented in Tables 3, 4, and 5 [39].

Table 3 Management of cervical cancer stage IA2-IB1 (<2 cm) in pregnancy

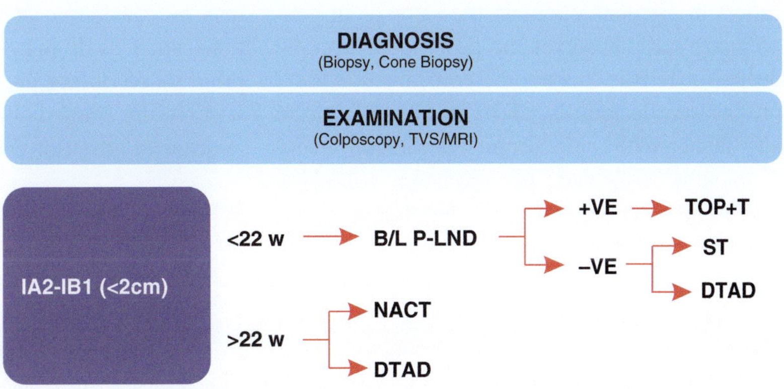

Table 4 Management of cervical cancer stage IB2 (≥2–<4 cm) in pregnancy

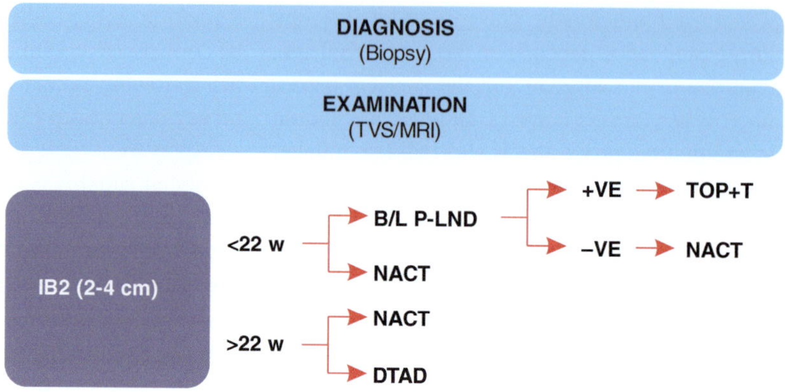

Table 5 Management of cervical cancer stage IB3 (≥4 cm)–IIA in pregnancy

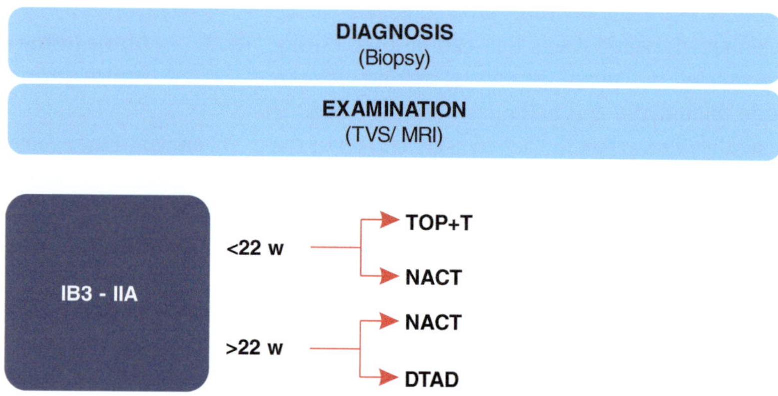

TVS transvaginal sonography, *MRI* magnetic resonance imaging, *PLND* pelvic lymph node dissection, *NAC* neoadjuvant chemotherapy, *TOP+T* termination of pregnancy and standard treatment, *ST* simple trachelectomy, *DTAD* delayed treatment after delivery

5.1.1 Role of Surgery for Cervical Cancer in Pregnancy with Desire for Fertility Preservation

The indications of surgical treatment for cervical cancer in pregnancy remain the same as in non-pregnant state; however the gestational age and desire for fertility need to be considered. All the pre-invasive lesions as CIN I to CIN III can be left alone with colposcopic evaluation every 3 months followed by excision following 6–8 weeks after delivery if needed. For stage I A disease conisation can be done preferably between 12 and 20 weeks [39], care should be taken regarding the depth of cone and ideally a coin-shaped cervical tissue is resected out under anaesthesia with a prophylactic cerclage considered. Any pregnancy less than 22 weeks can be offered radical hysterectomy with B/L PLND if fertility is not an issue, with a good oncological and obstetrical outcome [40]. When fertility is desired or gestational age is more than 22 weeks, nodal metastasis, neo-adjuvant chemotherapy may be considered [41]. Apart from this, conditions such as lymph nodal metastasis, disease progression during pregnancy and patient's wish will require immediate definitive treatment irrespective of gestational age [40].

5.1.2 Role of Neo-Adjuvant Chemotherapy for Cervical Cancer in Pregnancy with Desire for Fertility Preservation

This is generally used as an expectant treatment strategy beyond 22 weeks of gestation as it is believed to help in preventing the disease progression until foetal viability is achieved [42]. Cisplatin (50–100 mg/m^2) alone or in combination with paclitaxel (175 mg/m^2) every 3 weekly is the most commonly used regimen [40]. Neo-adjuvant chemotherapy during pregnancy can be given (1) in stage IA2, IB1, with node negative and tumour size less than 2 cm, to patients wishing to preserve pregnancy during the second trimester, (2) in stage IB2 (2–4 cm), NACT treatment can be given either to node-negative patients as before or after nodal assessment by lymphadenectomy and (3) in stages IB3-IIB, NACT is used until maturity and delivery as per the International Consensus Meeting on Gynaecological Cancers in Pregnancy [43].

5.1.3 Role of Surgery/Concomitant Chemoradiotherapy for Cervical Cancer in Pregnancy When Fertility Not Desired

In early operable disease surgery can be performed with the foetus in utero (Fig. 2) or after evacuation in later part of pregnancy. When the disease is not operable concomitant chemoradiotherapy can be planned with foetus in utero, preferably with early pregnancy and spontaneous abortion occurs within 4–6 weeks; otherwise first termination of pregnancy is carried out followed by concomitant chemoradiotherapy.

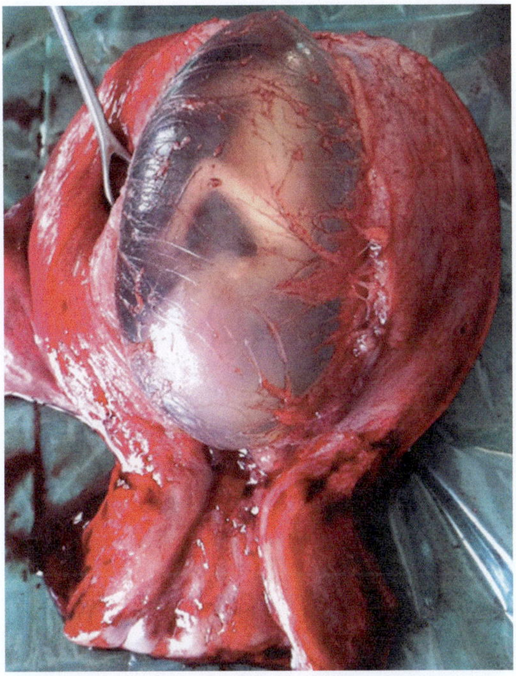

Fig. 2 Hysterectomy specimen of carcinoma uterine cervix. Stage IA2 with 16 weeks pregnancy

5.1.4 Obstetrical Management

Obstetrical management should be carried out in a well-equipped centre with good prenatal back up. Efforts should be made to continue the pregnancy up to 37 weeks and termination planned thereafter. When the size of the cervical lesion obstructs the birth passage, classical upper segment caesarean section is done under regional anaesthesia followed by radical hysterectomy under general anaesthesia. For patients where the disease is managed by local excision, vaginal delivery is preferred. Following normal delivery cancer-directed treatment can be started immediately and when caesarean section is done, cancer-directed treatment can be started after 7 days. During caesarean section ovaries should be marked with radio-opaque clips so that they can be spared during radiation therapy planning.

5.2 Management of Ovarian Cancer in Pregnancy

Ovarian cancer during pregnancy is the fifth most common cancer diagnosed during pregnancy and second to cervical cancer [44]. In contrast to the usual trend of majority being diagnosed at an advanced stage, almost 80% of ovarian cancer in pregnancy are diagnosed at an early stage [44] as incidental findings during routine imaging for pregnancy.

5.2.1 Role of Surgery for Ovarian Cancer in Pregnancy

For early-stage IA to IIA ovarian cancer, staging procedure by laparoscopic or open surgery along with pelvic and para-aortic nodal dissection is performed till 20 weeks of gestation [40].

However there are reports of conservative surgery during pregnancy followed by restaging after delivery. In advanced stage disease diagnosis is confirmed by image-guided tissue biopsy or laparoscopic assessment and biopsy followed by neoadjuvant chemotherapy after 14 weeks of pregnancy followed by completion surgery after delivery. In non-epithelial ovarian cancers which are generally diagnosed at an early stage, surgery remains the mainstay of treatment; however lymph node dissection is not recommended in these cases, only peritoneal staging is performed.

5.2.2 Role of Chemotherapy for Epithelial Ovarian Cancer in Pregnancy

In a systematic review published in 2012, using taxanes in ovarian cancer during the second and third trimester of pregnancy revealed that its use has no negative effect on organogenesis [45]. The standard chemotherapy regimen recommended in the treatment of EOC during pregnancy is paclitaxel plus carboplatin [40]. The dose is calculated based on the weight of the patient and not on the prepregnant weight. Although both cisplatin and carboplatin can be used during pregnancy however, carboplatin is preferred due to its reduced renal side effects. The side effects of chemotherapy are same as that of nonpregnant state and managed accordingly. Targeted therapy is nonindicated during pregnancy and intraperitoneal chemotherapy is also contraindicated during pregnancy. So to conclude paclitaxel and carboplatin during the second and third trimester up to 35 weeks or 37 weeks if given weekly seem safe for the treatment of EOC during pregnancy.

5.2.3 Role of Chemotherapy in Non-Epithelial Ovarian Cancer in Pregnancy

Germ cell and sex cord stromal tumours primarily constitute the non-epithelial group of ovarian cancers and as they are generally detected in early stage, surgical treatment is mostly offered; however few patients may present with advanced disease during pregnancy. Historically etoposide-platinum combination as BEP or EP was generally used during the second or third trimester, but off late reports of foetal teratogenic effects and growth restrictions even during the second and third trimester have been presented. Recent literatures including ESMO guidelines suggest the use of cisplatin (75 mg/m^2) and weekly paclitaxel (80 mg/m^2) after the first trimester in these patients [46, 47] with good outcomes.

5.3 Management of Vulval Cancer in Pregnancy

Surgery remains the mainstay of treatment for vulval cancer; however during pregnancy the vulval resection may lead to increased blood loss due to increased gestational blood flow, so care should be taken to reduce blood loss. Timing of the surgery is also important and it also depends on the extent of the disease. When groin nodes are involved then termination is preferred before 20 weeks of pregnancy or wait till maturity. When the gestational age is more than 20 weeks, then go for definitive treatment after delivery. The role of sentinel lymph node biopsy is limited with the use of technetium as short treatment protocol is followed and use of blue dye is not recommended during pregnancy. So in early stage when there is no role of radiotherapy, surgery can be performed anytime beyond 14 weeks; however when lymph node is involved and there is an indication for adjuvant radiotherapy then termination is must before 20 weeks or deliver the baby by caesarean section if near term and complete the adjuvant radiotherapy within 6–8 weeks.

5.4 Management of Vaginal Cancer in Pregnancy

There are no standardised treatment protocols for management of vaginal cancers in pregnancy due to the paucity of cases. Whatever knowledge we have to date is based on case reports; in fact very few cases have been reported in the literature. Surgery can be offered in small resectable lesions beyond 14 weeks and when surgery is not possible then depending on the gestational age pregnancy is either terminated or carried forward till foetal maturity and caesarean section offered followed by chemoradiotherapy.

6 Care of the Neonates and Paediatric Age Group

In view of the high-risk nature of the pregnancy, special care by the neonatologist is an essential aspect in the management of the newborn, as most of these newborn will be either preterm or small for gestational age infants. Babies of mothers receiving chemotherapy during their pregnancy need special attention, and they should be examined specifically looking for organ-specific side effects of the chemotherapeutic drugs used during pregnancy as cardiac evaluation by doing an echocardiography in the first week when the mother is administered anthracyclines. In case of platinum exposure assessing hearing functions is important [48]. Children who are exposed to anthracyclines or platinum during their antenatal period should undergo three yearly cardiac and hearing assessment respectively as a long-term follow-up protocol. Apart from these psychosocial supports is another important aspect as these children has a high probability of losing their mother in the following years at an early age, so they will definitely need special support to cope with it. So specialised medical surveillance and psychosocial family support should be taken care of in these children.

References

1. Nieminen U, Remes N. Malignancy during pregnancy. Acta Obstet Gynecol Scand. 1970;49(4):315–9.
2. Donegan WL. Cancer and pregnancy. Cancer J Clin. 1983;33(4):194–214.
3. Stensheim H, Moller B, Van Dijk T, Fossa SD. Cause-specific survival for women diagnosed with cancer during pregnancy or lactation: a registry-based cohort study. J Clin Oncol. 2009;27(1):45–51.
4. Haas JF. Pregnancy in association with a newly diagnosed cancer: a population-based epidemiologic assessment. Int J Cancer. 1984;34(2):229–35.
5. Eibye S, Kjær SK, Mellemkjær L. Incidence of pregnancy-associated cancer in Denmark, 1977–2006. Obstet Gynecol. 2013;122(3):608–17.
6. Andersson TM, Johansson AL, Fredriksson I, Lambe M. Cancer during pregnancy and the postpartum period: a population-based study. Cancer. 2015;121(12):2072–7.
7. Lee YY, Roberts CL, Dobbins T, Stavrou E, Black K, Morris J, Young J. Incidence and outcomes of pregnancy-associated cancer in Australia, 1994–2008: a population-based linkage study. BJOG. 2012;119(13):1572–82.
8. Smith LH, Danielsen B, Allen ME, Cress R. Cancer associated with obstetric delivery: results of linkage with the California cancer registry. Am J Obstet Gynecol. 2003;189(4):1128–35.
9. Parazzini F, Franchi M, Tavani A, Negri E, Peccatori FA. Frequency of pregnancy related cancer: a population based linkage study in Lombardy, Italy. Int J Gynecol Cancer. 2017;27(3):25.
10. de Haan J, Verheecke M, Van Calsteren K, Van Calster B, Shmakov RG, Gziri MM, Halaska MJ, Fruscio R, Lok CA, Boere IA, Zola P. Oncological management and obstetric and neonatal outcomes for women diagnosed with cancer during pregnancy: a 20-year international cohort study of 1170 patients. Lancet Oncol. 2018;19(3):337–46.
11. Cottreau CM, Dashevsky I, Andrade SE, Li DK, Nekhlyudov L, Raebel MA, Ritzwoller DP, Partridge AH, Pawloski PA, Toh S. Pregnancy-associated cancer: a US population-based study. J Womens Health. 2019;28(2):250–7.
12. Dalrymple JL, Gilbert WM, Leiserowitz GS, Cress R, Xing G, Danielsen B, Smith LH. Pregnancy-associated cervical cancer: obstetric outcomes. J Matern Fetal Neonatal Med. 2005;17(4):269–76.
13. Nazer A, Czuzoj-Shulman N, Oddy L, Abenhaim HA. Incidence of maternal and neonatal outcomes in pregnancies complicated by ovarian masses. Arch Gynecol Obstet. 2015;292(5):1069–74.
14. Leiserowitz GS, Xing G, Cress R, Brahmbhatt B, Dalrymple JL, Smith LH. Adnexal masses in pregnancy: how often are they malignant? Gynecol Oncol. 2006;101(2):315–21.
15. Valentin J. Biological effects after prenatal irradiation (embryo and fetus): ICRP publication 90 approved by the commission in October 2002. Ann ICRP. 2003;33(1–2):1–206.
16. Sachs HC. The transfer of drugs and therapeutics into human breast milk: an update on selected topics. Pediatrics. 2013;132(3):e796–809.
17. Barnett SB. Routine ultrasound scanning in first trimester: what are the risks? Semin Ultrasound CT MRI. 2002;23(5):387–91.
18. American College of Obstetricians and Gynecologists, Committee on Obstetric Practice. Committee opinion no. 656: guidelines for diagnostic imaging during pregnancy and lactation. Obstet Gynecol. 2016;127(2):75–80.
19. Chen MM, Coakley FV, Kaimal A, Laros RK. Guidelines for computed tomography and magnetic resonance imaging use during pregnancy and lactation. Obstet Gynecol. 2008;112(2):333–40.
20. De Santis M, Straface G, Cavaliere AF, Carducci B, Caruso A. Gadolinium periconceptional exposure: pregnancy and neonatal outcome. Acta Obstet Gynecol Scand. 2007;86(1):99–101.
21. Han SN, Amant F, Michielsen K, De Keyzer F, Fieuws S, Van Calsteren K, Dresen RC, Gziri MM, Vandecaveye V. Feasibility of whole-body diffusion-weighted MRI for detection of primary tumour, nodal and distant metastases in women with

cancer during pregnancy: a pilot study. Eur Radiol. 2018;28(5):1862–74.
22. Peccatori FA, Codacci-Pisanelli G, Del Grande M, et al. Whole body MRI for systemic staging of breast cancer in pregnant women. Breast. 2017;35:177–81.
23. Han SN, Lotgerink A, Gziri MM, Van Calsteren K, Hanssens M, Amant F. Physiologic variations of serum tumor markers in gynecological malignancies during pregnancy: a systematic review. BMC Med. 2012;10(1):86.
24. Sarandakou A, Protonotariou E, Rizos D. Tumor markers in biological fluids associated with pregnancy. Crit Rev Clin Lab Sci. 2007;44(2):151–78.
25. Moore RG, Miller MC, Eklund EE, Lu KH, Bast RC Jr, LambertMesserlian G. Serum levels of the ovarian cancer biomarker HE4 are decreased in pregnancy and increase with age. Am J Obstet Gynecol. 2012;206:349.e1–7.
26. Estadella J, Español P, Grandal B, Gine M, Parra J. Laparoscopy during pregnancy: case report and key points to improve laparoscopic management. Eur J Obstet Gynecol Reprod Biol. 2017;217:83–8.
27. Jackson H, Granger S, Price R, Rollins M, Earle D, Richardson W, Fanelli R. Diagnosis and laparoscopic treatment of surgical diseases during pregnancy: an evidence-based review. Surg Endosc. 2008;22(9):1917–27.
28. Ye P, Zhao N, Shu J, et al. Laparoscopy versus open surgery for adnexal masses in pregnancy: a meta-analytic review. Arch Gynecol Obstet. 2019;299(3):625–34.
29. Sood AK, Shahin MS, Sorosky JI. Paclitaxel and platinum chemotherapy for ovarian carcinoma during pregnancy. Gynecol Oncol. 2001;83(3):599–600.
30. Ngu SF, Ngan HY. Chemotherapy in pregnancy. Best Pract Res Clin Obstet Gynaecol. 2016;33:86–101.
31. Cardonick E, Iacobucci A. Use of chemotherapy during human pregnancy. Lancet Oncol. 2004;5(5):283–91.
32. Shachar SS, Gallagher K, McGuire K, Zagar TM, Faso A, Muss HB, Sweeting R, Anders CK. Multidisciplinary management of breast cancer during pregnancy. Oncologist. 2017;22(3):324.
33. Ricci C, Scambia G, De Vincenzo R. Locally advanced cervical cancer in pregnancy: overcoming the challenge. A case series and review of the literature. Int J Gynecol Cancer. 2016;26(8):15.
34. Mir O, Berveiller P, Goffinet F, Treluyer JM, Serreau R, Goldwasser F, Rouzier R. Taxanes for breast cancer during pregnancy: a systematic review. Ann Oncol. 2010;21(2):425–6.
35. Zheng X, Zhu Y, Zhao Y, Feng S, Zheng C. Taxanes in combination with platinum derivatives for the treatment of ovarian cancer during pregnancy: a literature review. Int J Clin Pharmacol Ther. 2017;55(9):753.
36. Weisz B, Meirow D, Schiff E, Lishner M. Impact and treatment of cancer during pregnancy. Expert Rev Anticancer Ther. 2004;4(5):889–902.
37. Kal HB, Struikmans H. Radiotherapy during pregnancy: fact and fiction. Lancet Oncol. 2005;6(5):328–33.
38. Vandenbroucke T, Verheecke M, Fumagalli M, Lok C, Amant F. Effects of cancer treatment during pregnancy on fetal and child development. Lancet Child Adolesc Health. 2017;1(4):302–10.
39. Köhler C, Oppelt P, Favero G, Morgenstern B, Runnebaum I, Tsunoda A, et al. How much platinum passes the placental barrier? Analysis of platinum applications in 21 patients with cervical cancer during pregnancy. Am J Obstet Gynecol. 2015;213(2):206.e1–5.
40. Amant F, Halaska MJ, Fumagalli M, Steffensen KD, Lok C, Van Calsteren K, Han SN, Mir O, Fruscio R, Uzan C, Maxwell C. Gynecologic cancers in pregnancy: guidelines of a second international consensus meeting. Int J Gynecol Cancer. 2014;24(3):54.
41. Vercellino GF, Koehler C, Erdemoglu E, Mangler M, Lanowska M, Malak AH, Schneider A, Chiantera V. Laparoscopic pelvic lymphadenectomy in 32 pregnant patients with cervical cancer: rationale, description of the technique, and outcome. Int J Gynecol Cancer. 2014;24(2):85.
42. Favero G, Chiantera V, Oleszczuk A, Gallotta V, Hertel H, Herrmann J, Marnitz S, Köhler C, Schneider A. Invasive cervical cancer during pregnancy: laparoscopic nodal evaluation before oncologic treatment delay. Gynecol Oncol. 2010;118(2):123–7.
43. Fruscio R, Villa A, Chiari S, Vergani P, Ceppi L, Dell'Orto F, Dell'Anna T, Chiappa V, Bonazzi CM, Milani R, Mangioni C. Delivery delay with neoadjuvant chemotherapy for cervical cancer patients during pregnancy: a series of nine cases and literature review. Gynecol Oncol. 2012;126(2):192–7.
44. Calsteren KV, Heyns L, Smet FD, Eycken LV, Gziri MM, Gemert WV, Halaska M, Vergote I, Ottevanger N, Amant F. Cancer during pregnancy: an analysis of 215 patients emphasizing the obstetrical and the neonatal outcomes. J Clin Oncol. 2010;28(4):683–9.
45. Zagouri F, Sergentanis TN, Chrysikos D, Filipits M, Bartsch R. Taxanes for ovarian cancer during pregnancy: a systematic review. Oncology. 2012;83(4):234–8.
46. Zagouri F, Dimitrakakis C, Marinopoulos S, Tsigginou A, Dimopoulos MA. Cancer in pregnancy: disentangling treatment modalities. ESMO Open. 2016;1(3):e000016.
47. Peccatori FA, Azim HA, Orecchia R, Hoekstra HJ, Pavlidis N, Kesic V, Pentheroudakis G. Cancer, pregnancy and fertility: ESMO clinical practice guidelines for diagnosis, treatment and follow-up. Ann Oncol. 2013;24:60–70.
48. Geijteman EC, Wensveen CW, Duvekot JJ, van Zuylen L. A child with severe hearing loss associated with maternal cisplatin treatment during pregnancy. Obstet Gynecol. 2014;124(2):454–6.

Role of MIS in Gynaecological Cancers

Apoorva Tak, Anupama Rajanbabu, Debabrata Barmon, and Amal Chandra Kataki

1 Introduction

The last two decades have witnessed a tremendous upsurge in minimally invasive surgery (MIS) procedures in gynaecologic oncology. Stepping-stones for use of laparoscopy in gynaecologic oncology were laid way back in the 1970s, when diagnostic laparoscopy was first used to assess adnexal masses.

In 1990, laparoscopic pelvic lymphadenectomy in cervical cancer was first described by Dennis Querleu [1]. In 1992, Nezhat et al. reported laparoscopic radical hysterectomy [2]. Since then numerous studies have been conducted validating the use of MIS in gynaecologic oncology.

With the ever-growing armamentarium of laparoscopic instruments, especially power resources and the robotic technology, that provides excellent dexterity of robotic arms and comfort of operating surgeon, MIS is in vogue.

Robotic surgery has emerged as the new standard for surgical staging of endometrial cancer in its early stages.

A. Tak (✉) · D. Barmon · A. C. Kataki
Department of Gynaecologic Oncology,
Dr. Bhubaneswar Borooah Cancer Institute
(A Unit of Tata Memorial Centre, Mumbai),
Guwahati, Assam, India
e-mail: drdiracademic@bbci.tmc.gov.in

A. Rajanbabu
Department of Gynaecologic Oncology, AIMS,
Kochi, India

Overall benefits of MIS include shorter hospital stay, early recovery, less blood loss, and better cosmesis. The landmark LACC trial published in 2018 [3] has altogether questioned the role of laparoscopy in cervical cancer.

As technology progresses, minimally invasive surgical procedures, next-generation robotic platforms with tactile input, and single-port surgery continue to evolve.

2 Principles of Laparoscopic Surgery

2.1 Preoperative Considerations

Changes in pulmonary function can also occur from increased intra-abdominal pressure and patient positioning, including reduced lung volumes, increased peak airway pressures, and decreased pulmonary compliance. In patients with significant pulmonary dysfunction, it is important to obtain preoperative pulmonary function testing, and often intraoperative arterial monitoring is helpful.

For cases with refractory hypoxemia, hypercapnia, or high airway pressures during laparoscopy, release of pneumoperitoneum with use of lower intra-abdominal pressures is practiced. Conversion to open is recommended for inadequate visualisation at lower pressures [4].

A. C. Kataki, D. Barmon (eds.), *Fundamentals in Gynaecologic Malignancy*,
https://doi.org/10.1007/978-981-19-5860-1_25

Gynaecologic oncology surgeries require VTE prophylaxis which can be in the form of low-dose unfractionated heparin, subcutaneous low molecular weight heparin, intermittent pneumatic compression stockings, graduated compression stockings, or a combination. Recent data has shown VTE incidence in patients undergoing minimally invasive surgery in gynaecologic oncology to be 0.65%, with no preoperative or postoperative VTE prophylaxis [5].

Positioning the patient for laparoscopic surgery should be chosen carefully. Patients are placed in the lithotomy position with the lower extremities in boot stirrups. There are four elements of lithotomy positioning: hip flexion should produce a trunk-to-thigh angle of approximately 170°; knee flexion should result in a thigh-to-calf angle of 90–120°; hip abduction should be of 90° or less; and minimal external hip rotation should exist. Excessive flexion at the hip can result in femoral nerve compression or stretching of the sciatic nerve; excessive hip abduction can result in obturator nerve injury, and external hip rotation can increase strain on the femoral, obturator, and sciatic nerves. Furthermore, common peroneal nerve injury, which can manifest as foot drop, results from prolonged flexion of the knee, compression along the lateral aspect of the leg, and excessive external rotation of the hip.

The arms should be tucked alongside the patient's body, both to allow for proper access for surgeon during surgery and to prevent brachial plexus nerve injury from excessive stretching of the outstretched arms. Gel pads along the patient's arm, especially covering the elbows and hands, can protect these vulnerable areas. To prevent the patient from slipping on the operative table in Trendelenburg position, shoulder blocks can be used; however one must be careful that they are placed directly over the acromioclavicular joint, and are only placed when the arms are tucked, in order to minimise risk of brachial plexus injury. Alternative to the shoulder blocks are anti-slide mechanisms such as gel or foam pads and surgical beanbags [6].

2.2 Abdominal Entry

Surgeons should consider each patient's medical history and characteristics and choose the appropriate method of entry that may be best for that patient.

In the closed entry technique pneumoperitoneum is created by Veress needle followed by the primary trocar entry at the level of the umbilicus. Supine position during the insertion of both the Veress needle and the primary trocar should be ensured and angle of the Veress needle insertion should be adjusted, 45° in non-obese to 90° in very obese women to avoid vessel injury.

Initial intra-abdominal pressures of 10 mmHg or less signifies correct intraperitoneal placement of the Veress needle. An adequate pneumoperitoneum is reached when the intra-abdominal pressure reaches 15 mmHg. Complication rates also increase sequentially with multiple insertion attempts. In patients with suspected periumbilical adhesions or after three failed insufflation attempts, an alternate method of entry should be considered. Insertion can be tried in left upper quadrant (LUQ), 3 cm below the left subcostal border in the midclavicular line, since the formation of adhesions in this area is rare. Also Veress should be introduced perpendicular to the skin and prior emptying of stomach by nasogastric suction should be ensured. Patients with previous splenic or gastric surgery, significant hepatosplenomegaly, portal hypertension, or gastropancreatic masses should be excluded from the LUQ entry technique [7].

In open or Hasson technique, a small incision is made at the level of the umbilicus, wide enough to dissect fascia and enter peritoneal cavity under direct vision. Sutures are placed on each side of the fascia, and the cannula with a blunt obturator is inserted. The sutures anchor the cannula in place and seal the abdominal wall incision, after which insufflation is started.

The direct trocar entry technique involves an umbilical skin incision wide enough to accommodate a trocar. The anterior abdominal wall is lifted by hand and the trocar is inserted directly into the peritoneal cavity. This method of entry is faster than any other mode of entry. Meta-analysis did demonstrate an advantage of this technique in reduced failed entry into the abdomen compared to the Veress needle. Additional advantages are avoidance of intestinal insufflation or gas embolism. In a review of 51 publications including 134,917 Veress/trocar, 21,547 open, and 16,739 direct entries, bowel injury rates were 0.04% (Veress), 0.11% (open), and 0.05% (direct), while vascular injury rates were 0.04%, 0.01%, and 0% respectively. In summary, there appears to be no evidence to demonstrate safety of one technique of laparoscopic entry over another [8].

The inferior epigastric vessels are the most common vascular trocar injury to occur during the placement of the lateral trocars. The inferior epigastric vessels are located medial to the exit of the round ligament into the abdominal wall.

The lateral trocars should be placed 3–4 cm lateral to the median umbilical ligament or lateral to the lateral margin of the rectus abdominus muscle. If the trocars are placed too laterally, they can endanger the deep circumflex epigastric artery. The trocars should be placed by inserting perpendicular to the skin surface, and under direct visualisation within the peritoneal cavity.

If injury to the inferior epigastric vessels occurs, the trocars should be left in place at first while the two bleeding ends of the vessels are sutured cephalad and caudad with through-and-through abdominal sutures, or a foley balloon can be used for tamponade.

2.3 Electrosurgery

2.3.1 Monopolar Electrosurgery

Its basic principle involves passage of current from generator through the active electrode, which spreads through the body tissues and comes out of the patient's body through the return electrode and returns back to the electrosurgical generator, which completes the circuit. Small surface area of the active electrode causes a high current density production at its tip and the resultant tissue effect. This density of electrons diminishes with an increase in distance from the electrode.

The most dreaded complication with monopolar electrosurgical techniques is arcing of the current resulting in severe undiagnosed injuries. They can also result in extensive diathermy burns if the return electrode is not properly applied. Monopolar electrosurgical techniques can interfere with pacemaker function and care should be taken to avoid them in such patients.

2.3.2 Bipolar Electrosurgery

In bipolar electrosurgical devices, the active and return electrode are formed by the two jaws of the instrument which are in close proximity to each other unlike monopolar in which current travels through patient body. As current passes between tips of the instrument, it only affects tissue grasped between the electrodes. Bipolar is relatively safe and more useful as compared to monopolar as it causes minimum collateral spread; reduced risk of interference with other devices and better coagulation.

The disadvantage of using conventional electrosurgery is that it cannot cut the tissue and requires more time to coagulate, therefore causing more charring and adherence of tissue. This may lead to tearing of adjacent vessel and more bleeding. These shortcomings were overcome by advanced new generation bipolar and ultrasonic electrosurgical devices.

Advanced bipolar devices combine the principle of thermo-fusion, with application of optimal mechanical pressure to ensure that the denatured protein forms a coagulum and a strong seal is achieved even in large vessel, up to a diameter of 7 mm. Advanced electrogenerators are available which sense tissue impedance and automatically stop the current flow when adequate sealing is achieved. This guards against prolonged device activation and decreases tissue charring and tissue adherence to the instrument. It also reduces lateral spread of current, which makes these devices extremely safe to use, especially in pelvic dissection.

2.3.3 Advanced MIS Devices

Both Enseal and Ligasure are advanced bipolar devices with tissue feedback mechanism.

Ligasure

The bipolar vessel sealing system (LigaSure) applies a precise amount of bipolar energy and pressure to fuse collagen and elastin within the vessel walls. This results in a permanent seal that can withstand three times the normal systolic pressure and seals vessels up to 7 mm. The sealing is achieved with minimal sticking and charring; thermal spread to adjacent tissues is approximately 2 mm.

EnSeal

This system provides vessel sealing by combining a compression mechanism with thermal energy control in a bipolar sealing device. The instrument is capable of achieving seal strengths up to seven times the normal systolic pressures on vessels up to 7 mm with a typical thermal spread of approximately 1 mm. The compression mechanism applies uniform pressure along the full length of the instrument jaw, achieving compression forces similar to those of a linear stapler. Compression is combined with controlled energy delivery utilising nanopolar thermostats to reach collagen denaturation temperatures in seconds, which are maintained at approximately 100 °C throughout the power delivery cycle. The device also has a cutting mechanism to allow one-step sealing and transection of vessels and soft tissues.

The ENSEAL Trio Tissue Sealing Device is indicated for bipolar coagulation and mechanical transection of tissue during laparoscopic and open procedures. It allows the surgeon to grasp, coagulate, and transect tissue with a single instrument.

One of the main differences between them is that Enseal is articulating. It can bend up to 66°. This is extremely helpful, especially for ipsilateral surgeons while sealing big vessels on the opposite site.

Ultrasonic cutting and coagulating device—The ultrasonic cutting and coagulating surgical devices (e.g. Harmonic Scalpel, Sonicision, and Thunderbeat) convert ultrasonic energy into mechanical energy at the functional end of the instrument. A piezoelectric crystal in the handpiece generates vibration at the tip of the active blade at 55,500 times per second over a variable excursion of 50 to 100 micrometres. This results in rupture of hydrogen bonds and produces heat, which leads to denaturation of proteins and, eventually, separation of tissue. These effects are reached at tissue temperatures of 60 to 80 °C, resulting in coagulum formation without the desiccation and charring caused by temperatures of 80 °C and higher associated with traditional electrosurgical methods. The Thunderbeat device also adds bipolar energy for a combination effect of both ultrasonic and bipolar energy. The Sonicision device is cordless, with the generator built into the handle. It was the first device to integrate both advanced bipolar energy and ultrasonically generated frictional heat energy in one instrument. There are two modes in the generator, level 1 seal (bipolar technology) for vessel sealing and level 2 seal and cut (ultrasonic technology) for precise dissection and cutting. It can seal vessels up to 7 mm in diameter.

The latest offering by Ethicon hailed as a major advancement to the Ultrasonic devices is Harmonic ACE+7 Shears. The makers claim that the median burst pressures in Advanced Haemostasis mode are much higher than other devices, and it can coagulate vessels up to 7 mm in diameter (FDA Approved).

Complications of Electrosurgery include [9, 10]:

- Defective insulation.
- Direct or capacitative coupling.
- Alternative site burns.
- Mistaken target application.
- Smoke generation, hampering visibility.
- Lateral thermal spread.

Trocar sites greater than 10 mm in size should have a fascial closure in order to prevent the occurrence of port site hernias. Additionally, failure to observe the omentum or bowel pushed into the intraperitoneal defect after trocar removal can cause hernias. Closure devices under direct vision are available to achieve the closure of both fascia and peritoneum at these narrow sites [11].

About 1% incidence of port site metastasis has been documented in the literature and is a potential concern for surgeons performing laparoscopic surgery in gynaecologic malignancies.

2.3.4 Special circumstances: Obesity

Various modifications are used for laparoscopy in morbidly obese patients.

To decrease the risk of injury from positioning, padded stirrups with extra padding around the ankles and knees or other pressure points are helpful. Insertion of Veress at steep angulation is safe due to the increased abdominal wall thickness and the location of the umbilicus 3 cm caudal to the aortic bifurcation.An extra-long Veress needle can be helpful, the skin incision can also be extended down to fascia, which can then be grasped and elevated prior to inserting a Veress needle, eliminating the passage of the needle through the subcutaneous tissue.Excess body weight causes reduced chest wall compliance. The increased abdominal pressure from a pneumoperitoneum and Trendelenburg position can raise intra-thoracic pressure and reduce functional residual capacity (FRC), resulting in an increase in respiratory resistance and impairment of arterial oxygenation. For a morbidly obese patient with central adipose tissue, the use of pressure control ventilation can improve the lung ventilation-perfusion ratio, generate higher instantaneous flow peaks, and may enable better alveolar recruitment. A tilt test should be performed once the patient is intubated and properly positioned. The patient can be placed in Trendelenburg position for 2–5 min while observing the patient's cardiac and respiratory status. A patient who is able to remain normotensive, maintaining inspiratory pressures at 30–40 mmHg during this test before and after insufflation is likely to do well during laparoscopy. A redundant rectosigmoid colon can be managed using a suture through the epiploicae to the anterior abdominal wall.

In MIS Laparoscopic or Robotic surgery exposure is the key factor for success of procedure. During deep pelvic surgeries, often redundant bowel and significant adipose makes retraction difficult. The T-Lift laparoscopic tissue and organ retraction system allows for stable, safe, and durable retraction.

3 Principles of Robotic Surgery

In 2005, the FDA authorised the Da Vinci Surgical System for use in gynaecology.

It is based on a computer-assisted management information system (MIS). An upgraded three-dimensional high-definition vision camera, instruments with endowrist to improve dexterity, and tremor cancelling software to sharpen precision in surgical dissection are all advantages of robotically assisted surgery. The advantages of robotic surgery in terms of technology and ergonomics were brought to overcome the challenges of traditional laparoscopy.

3.1 Parts of a Robot

3.1.1 Surgeon Console

It consists of three parts: two master controllers, footswitches, and a stereo viewer. The surgeon can easily sit at the console away from the patient's cart and does not have to scrub. They perform movements on the master controller, which are subsequently duplicated in real time on the surgical field by robotic hands and equipment. The stereo viewer provides the surgeon with a clear, magnified, three-dimensional image of the operative field. On each side of the footswitch panel are two groups of pedals, one for cautery and the other for camera control. A touchpad is also located on the armrest to operate and make system modifications such as telescope angle modulation, light intensity, and cautery settings. Surgeon can optimise settings for an ergonomic position to avoid muscle sprains.

3.1.2 Patient Cart

It is the robot's operating component, with four arms, three instrument arms, and one camera arm. These arms are capable of a wide range of complex movements.

3.1.3 The Vision Cart

An endoscope, cautery generators, a Firefly system, camera, recording system, and vision cart illuminator are all included in the vision cart. The video pictures are enlarged and in high definition. Endoscopes are offered in two configurations: 0° and 30°.

3.2 Docking of the Robot

All three components are digitally linked. The surgeon must first create a pneumoperitoneum and introduce the ports before proceeding with the surgery. Three to four 8 mm ports and one helper port are typical. The ports must be inserted perpendicular to the surface of the body. The markings on the ports should be on the inside of the abdominal wall. The theatre staff then 'docks' the robotic platform by positioning it precisely in relation to the patient. It is possible to dock on the side or in the centre. If a vaginal assistance is necessary during the surgery, side docking is suggested. Before docking, the patient must be in a steep Trendelenburg posture.

At the lower back, a sandbag or bolster can aid. Shoulder rests and chest strapping allow for a steep Trendelenburg position without the risk of the patient slipping upward. The OT table cannot be moved once the machine is docked. A scrubbed assistant at the bedside places the telescope into the second arm and aims the telescope towards the major anatomical location for surgery. All of the other robotic arms are automatically positioned. The bedside assistant surgeon connects cautery cables and inserts instruments into the ports under view [12].

At the surgeon's console, the chief surgeon sits comfortably. They have the ability to scroll and modify their ergonomic settings. In both master controller loops, a thumb and a finger are inserted. The instruments and their tips move in sync with the movements of the hands. The most widely used instruments in the first and third robotic arms, respectively, are a fenestrated bipolar grasper in the left hand and a hot shears scissors with monopolar energy in the right hand. The telescope will be mounted on the second arm. A tenaculum or force bipolar grasper can be held with the fourth arm. With the use of a toggle pedal, the third and fourth arms can be swapped out.

When the surgeon moves their head away from the console or the camera moves, the instruments remain in place. A hand clutch or a foot clutch can be used to adjust the arms to a more comfortable posture.

The camera is entirely at the control of the main surgeon, and it can be brought extremely close to the desired anatomical structure for a magnified view. This is particularly useful in difficult-to-reach areas such as the recto-vaginal plane, the Retzius space, the retroperitoneum, and the para-aortic region. The touch pad at the surgeon's console may control the level of illumination, cautery adjustments, telescope angulation, and Firefly. Instructions to the OT staff are given over a microphone at the surgeon's station during surgery.

It is critical to have an experienced table-side assistant and surgical personnel on hand to help speed up and reduce the cost of robotic procedures. Suction, retraction, uterine manipulation, and suture provision are all performed by the operating table assistant surgeon. The helper can change or clean an instrument whenever it is needed.

4 Role of Robotic Surgery in Gynaecologic Oncology

The surgical management of gynaecologic cancers has been permanently revolutionised thanks to robot-assisted surgery. Surgeons can undertake extensive and radical dissection to reach desired margins using 3-D imaging and magnification (up to 10 times) paired with wristed devices.

Endometrial cancer is the most common reason for using a robotic platform in gynaecologic oncology. For surgical staging of endometrial cancer, MIS has become the gold standard. In trials examining surgical methods in obese individuals, the benefits of robotic surgery have been shown. Robotic surgery was proven to have less blood loss than laparoscopic or laparotomy surgery. For robotic assistance, the percentage of conversion to laparotomy was 4.9, and for laparoscopic surgery, it was 9.9 [13].

Sentinel lymph node mapping combined with ultra-staging is quickly becoming the new standard for early endometrial cancer staging. Not only did this method increase upstaging by 18%, but it also reduced operative times and perioperative problems [14]. This is especially important in endometrial cancer patients, who frequently have obesity and other comorbidities. Despite the greater initial expenses of robotic surgery, long-term cost savings in the form of lower complication rates are undeniable.

In comparison to traditional laparoscopy, precision instrument control and 3-D HD stereoscopic vision allow for speedier surgical learning.

4.1 Benefits of Robotics Over Open Surgery

All of the advantages of minimally invasive surgery are included.

1. Recovery time is reduced.
2. A shorter stay in the hospital (1 day in many cases).
3. Minimal scars and little incisions.
4. Perioperative problems and postoperative ileus are less common.
5. Blood loss and transfusions are reduced.
6. Pain and discomfort are reduced.
7. In patients with a high BMI reduced number of complications was observed. When numerous aspects such as prolonged admission costs, including ICU stay, loss of working hours, and delay in adjuvant therapy in cancers are taken into account, overall cost in malignancies is reduced.

4.2 Benefits Over Traditional Laparoscopy

- Superior dexterity: The robotic tool outperforms the human hand in terms of dexterity and range of motion. The arms are capable of full 360-degree rotation. In contrast to usual straight sticklike movements in laparoscopy, the endowrist movement of the robotic instrument provides for improved precision in suture intensive operations. This enables the surgeon to perform operations that would be impossible without the use of a robot.
- Robotic-aided surgery has also been demonstrated to reduce surgeon tiredness and muscular strain, particularly during protracted surgeries and numerous surgeries in a single day. As the surgeon sits in an ergonomically comfortable posture at the console distant from the patient, this promotes precision and may reduce the frequency of medical errors.
- Access to difficult-to-reach locations: The robot's increased flexibility and precision allow the surgeon to access difficult-to-reach areas using a telescope that may be focused closer to the target tissue. In contrast, in laparoscopy, a human assistance holds an unstable camera.
- An operating surgeon has superior surgical autonomy and efficiency since he or she can control the camera and all three operative arms.
- A better visual field: The surgeon has a better vision of the operating region, which allows for more precise surgery. As a result, it makes it easier to remove endometriotic tissue and improve surgical margins in cancer patients.
- Learning curve: Robotic surgery has a shorter learning curve than traditional laparoscopic surgery.
- Fewer open surgery conversions.
- Blood loss and transfusions are reduced.
- Less pain and discomfort due to the tool tips' dexterity, which helps to minimise excessive leverage and force at the incision sites.
- A shorter stay in the hospital.
- Recovery time is reduced.
- Fewer problems, with the exception of surgeons with a limited volume (defined as 1–5 hysterectomies per year).
- With robotic aid, even in long and tough situations requiring a great deal of dissection and suturing, surgery is a joy. This is in contrast to the high level of stress and difficulty associated with laparoscopy.
- The capacity of the system to perform automated troubleshooting reduces the number of ancillary personnel required in the operation room. As a result, there are fewer interruptions to the surgeon.

4.3 Disadvantages of Robotic Surgery

- Surgery costs: The original installation, subsequent maintenance, and disposables costs are all too high. The expense of surgery is also increased by longer operative times. As a result, it might not be the first choice for minor gynaecological issues.
- Movement latency: In the event that a problem emerges during surgery, movement latency is a major worry. In such instances, the personnel should be educated in emergency undocking.
- Longer operation time when compared to laparoscopy, especially in the first few cases. This length quickly plateaus as the surgeon acquires experience.
- Unwieldy machine habits, as well as the requirement for additional personnel and training.
- Operating room efficiency can only be achieved with an experienced table-side assistant and surgical team who can potentially reduce the time and expense of robotic procedures.
- Lack of tactile feedback: This drawback is more than offset by the higher tissue details gained. Understanding the finer tissue texture may be aided by microscopic features and tissue motions.

If economic considerations are fulfilled, the robotic platform may become a more acceptable procedure among gynaecological surgeons. With market competition and system development, robotic costs will undoubtedly fall. In highly difficult surgeries requiring considerable dissection and optimal anatomic re-establishment, robotics has an advantage. V-Notes surgery is a significant advancement in robotic surgery.

5 Role of MIS in Endometrial Cancer

MIS has become the standard of care in management of endometrial cancer.

In 2009, the GOG undertook the LAP2 trial (laparoscopy vs. laparotomy for complete surgical staging of uterine cancer: gynaecologic oncology group study). It included 2616 patients and randomly assigned them to either laparotomy (920 patients) or laparoscopy (1696 patients) for endometrial cancer surgical staging. Twenty-six percent of the 1696 patients in the laparoscopy arm needed a laparotomy [15]. If lymph node dissection could not be completed laparoscopically, conversion to laparotomy was required; more than half of these conversions were due to poor exposure, 16% were due to metastasis, and 11% were due to haemorrhage.

The LAP 2 trial found significant improvements in QOL, pain levels, and early return to regular activities throughout the perioperative period. With similar overall survival the study concluded that surgical staging of uterine cancer by laparoscopy is a reasonable option.

LACE trial (laparoscopic approach to cancer of the endometrium) by Janda et al. also revealed improved QOL with fewer complications after TLH [16].

Obesity with associated comorbidities is usually found associated with endometrial cancer; it was shown in the study by Kohler et al. that lymph node yield was comparable in both laparotomy and laparoscopy arm [17].

According to a study by Scribner et al., laparoscopy was linked to a shorter hospital stay, fewer infection complications, and a lower incidence of ileus, with equivalent blood loss and lymph node yield, in patients more than 65 years of age [18].

Robotic surgery has emerged as the new way for surgical staging of apparent early-stage endometrial cancer. Except for lower blood loss and fewer conversions to laparotomy in robotic procedures, the majority of retrospective case series and two meta-analyses (eight and nine comparative studies, 1591 and 1640 total patients, respectively) have found parallels with laparoscopy in most areas [19].

Sentinel node evaluation is now part of standard of care in endometrial and cervical cancer, according to the National Comprehensive Cancer

Network's recommendations. Open and minimally invasive procedures for SLN testing are available both by laparoscopic and robotic approaches.

Sentinel node detection with MIS is preferable due to the increased magnification and illumination of the surgical field. Also as almost 57% of the cases have significant obesity, robotic surgery offers the best outcome. Adding sentinel lymph node biopsy to minimally invasive staging for apparent early-stage endometrial cancer saves operational hours and improves perioperative surgical outcomes, with morbidity comparable to hysterectomy alone.

Laparoscopic pelvic and para-aortic node dissection, both transperitoneal and extraperitoneal approaches, are being practised. While the transperitoneal approach has become the standard, the extraperitoneal approach may be useful especially in obese patients and for debulking of enlarged nodes.

It has been demonstrated that robotic and traditional laparoscopic surgery have superior results than laparotomy in terms of blood loss, blood transfusions, peri- and postoperative problems, wound infection, postoperative discomfort, faster recovery time, and shorter hospital stay. The three modalities also have similar pelvic and para-aortic lymph node counts, which are used to assess surgical quality. As a result, MIS is the method of choice for endometrial cancer staging.

6 Role of MIS in Vulval Cancer

The typical age of diagnosis for vulvar cancer is 68 years old, accounting for 4% of all gynaecological malignancies. The recent increase in incidence among young people has been attributed to an increase in HPV infection. Squamous cell carcinoma accounts for 90% of the cases. According to the SEER database, 5-year survival rates vary from 86% for localised disease (stages I/II), to 53% for regional or locally progressed disease (stages III/IVA), and just 19% for individuals with stage IVB disease [20].

Surgery for vulval cancers have come a long way, beginning from the single butterfly incision technique of radical vulvectomy and inguinofemoral dissection described by basset in 1912 to the less aggressive approach with separate incisions designed by Taussig. Today, this 'triple incision' technique involving wide local excision or modified radical vulvectomy with 1 cm tumour-free margin along with bilateral inguinofemoral lymphadenectomy is the standard approach to treat vulval cancer.

In stage IA, the groin dissection or sentinel lymph node (SLN) assessment can be skipped since the chance of metastasis is less than 1%. It is advised in IB/II disease because the probability of lymph nodes metastasis is more than 8% in stage IB and significantly higher in stage II.

Unilateral inguinofemoral lymphadenectomy and SLN biopsy are viable alternatives for primary vulvar tumours of 2–4 cm diameter, unilateral, positioned 2 cm from midline, and with clinically negative lymph nodes.

But groin dissection is associated with high postoperative complications such as wound infection, wound breakdown, chronic lymphoedema, lymphocyst formation, and skin flap necrosis. Almost 20–40% of patients have wound complications and 30–70% experience chronic lymphoedema [21].

In order to minimise these complications, minimally invasive techniques for dissection of inguinal lymph node such as sentinel lymph node biopsy and video-endoscopic inguinofemoral lymphadenectomy (VEIL) are being popularised.

VEIL is a novel minimally invasive technique and has shown to reduce the morbidity associated with open lymphadenectomy [22]. As the surgical incision is made away from inguinal folds, it decreases postoperative complications. Long-terms oncological outcomes are not yet available to draw any conclusion, but the reported literature to date seems promising.

Based on the insertion's site of the trocars, two types of endoscopic approaches have been described: (I) when trocars inserted at the lower limb level (VEIL-L, limb subcutaneous approach); (II) when trocars inserted at the level of abdomen (VEIL-H, hypogastric subcutaneous approach).

6.1 VEIL Procedure (Limb Subcutaneous Approach)

- Being a prolonged surgery it is better performed under GA or Epidural. A 1–1.5 cm incision is made, 2 cm below the level of apex of the femoral triangle for the camera port placement. Scarpa's fascia is identified and subscarpa's plane is created either by sharp dissection or blunt finger dissection to create adequate space for insertion of secondary ports.
- A right-hand 10 mm secondary port and left-hand 5 mm port with a 10 mm camera balloon port for a right-handed surgeon is fixed to the skin.
- Surgeon stands lateral to the patient's legs and pneumoperitoneum of 15–16 mm hg is created to dissect out the subscarpa plane.
- Dissection is performed laterally and medially to the borders of the femoral triangle once the subscarpa's plane has been dissected up to the level of the inguinal ligament and the external oblique aponeurosis has been seen. To avoid subcutaneous emphysema of the abdomen, CO_2 pressure should be decreased to 5–6 mmHg.
- Using harmonic scalpel in coagulation mode, small venous tributaries are divided and superficial nodes at the floor of the femoral triangle are dissected out. Deep fascia dissection is started at the apex of femoral triangle and all the fibrofatty lymphoareolar tissue with deep fascia is divided along the lateral and medial border of the triangle.
- 2–3 cm medial to the femoral triangle's apex, the saphenous vein is kept. When the deep fascia covering the femoral arteries is dissected, lymphatics flow parallel to the artery and vein. Postoperative lymphorrhea and lymphoedema might be worse by splitting these lymphatics. The femoral nerve is found and preserved on the artery's lateral side.
- The saphenofemoral junction is revealed when the fascia lata is opened, and the saphenous vein is separated from the fibro fatty tissue to protect the vein and limit the possibility of lymphoedema. If required, deep pelvic lymph node dissection can also be done.
- After removing surgical specimens in a bag and ensuring haemostasis, suction drains are placed bilaterally through lateral port and continued till 24-h output is less than 10–20 mL.

6.2 Robotic VEIL (R-VEIL)

The robot is positioned 45° to the left of the patient in this technique, and the helper sits opposite the robot on the right side of the patient. Three robotic ports (two 8-mm and one 10-mm) are employed, as well as one helper port. The robot uses the lateral port for suction or retraction, and the assistant uses it to apply clips. The primary tools are the bipolar Maryland and monopolar scissors.

The main advantages of robotic approach compared to laparoscopy are ease to the surgeon, 3-dimensional view with higher magnification, and higher degree of freedom with instruments. Currently, limited evidence is available in literature for this newer procedure [23].

7 Role of MIS in Ovarian Cancer

The risk of tumour rupture, upstaging disease, and port site metastasis limits the use of MIS in Ovarian cancer. Following are the various clinical scenarios where minimal invasive approach may be contemplated:

1. Assessing feasibility of upfront optimal surgical cytoreduction using laparoscopy.
2. Primary cytoreduction in early ovarian cancer.
3. Primary cytoreduction of advanced ovarian cancer.
4. Second look laparoscopy after primary treatment.
5. Assessment of the extent of diseases and operability in recurrent disease.

In the evaluation of disease for feasibility of optimal cytoreduction diagnostic laparoscopy can help to assess disease extent and operability and provide tissue for definitive histopathological diagnosis. The risk of port site metastasis was found to be high but this was not found to worsen the prognosis [24].

This evaluation is done using a FAGOTTI scoring system that assigns a score of 2 (positive/extensive) or 0 (absence/limited) to the following factors:

- Peritoneal carcinomatosis.
- Diaphragmatic disease.
- Mesenteric disease.
- Omental disease.
- Bowel infiltration.
- Stomach infiltration.
- Liver metastases.

A score of eight negates the possibility of optimal cytoreduction, and such patients are advised to proceed with NACT [25].

Nezhat et al. conducted one of the biggest series of 36 individuals to investigate the effect of laparoscopic examination in the staging and diagnosis of apparent early ovarian cancer. The study found that when conducted by gynaecologic oncologists with extensive laparoscopic experience, it appears to be viable and thorough without jeopardising life [26].

Though a number of retrospective and prospective studies have provided evidence for feasibility, lack of level I on long-term oncologic outcomes with laparoscopy and laparotomy, also difficult exposure of certain areas like posterior surface of diaphragm needed for cytoreduction, risk of port site recurrences and tumour rupture during surgery are the main limitations to the implementation of MIS in carcinoma ovary.

The use of a laparoscopic bag, controlled aspiration, and minimising the danger of rupture should be ensured to decrease the occurrence of tumour contamination of the abdominal cavity. With limited capacity to move tissues during laparoscopic surgery, peritoneal surface metastases are the most difficult to detect. According to the findings of Davidson et al., using MIS for IDS was safe and practical, with acceptable optimum cytoreduction rates [27].

Second-look laparoscopy after primary treatment of ovarian cancer was performed to confirm any residual disease. With the advent of advanced imaging, second-look laparotomies are not routinely practised now.

In 2019 Fagotti et al. published the International Mission Study: Minimally Invasive Surgery in Ovarian Neoplasm After Neoadjuvant chemotherapy, with the aim to identify the feasibility, extent, and outcome. Amongst the 127 women from five gynaecological centres that participated in the study, six (4.7%) patients had intraoperative complications and it was concluded that minimal invasive surgery can be considered in women with advanced ovarian cancer who undergo surgery after neoadjuvant chemotherapy. The study found a median progression-free survival of 23 months and a 5-year overall survival rate of 52% [28].

Melamed et al. compared 450 women who received minimally invasive cytoreduction to 2621 women who underwent laparotomy in 2017 and found no difference in overall survival or surgical outcomes between the two groups, even after controlling for a variety of possible confounders [29].

The Laparoscopic Cytoreduction After Neoadjuvant Chemotherapy (LANCE) trial is a non-inferiority phase III trial that compares minimally invasive surgery to laparotomy in women with advanced stage high-grade epithelial ovarian cancer who had a complete or partial response to three or four cycles of neoadjuvant chemotherapy and normalisation of CA-125.

It will randomly assign 580 patients in a 1:1 ratio to one of two research arms prior to surgery (by minimisation). Patients in Arm A (experimental arm) will receive minimally invasive surgery, whereas those in Arm B (reference arm) will have a laparotomy. The first 100 individuals will be recruited in a pilot study to see if it is feasible.

All remaining patients will be recruited in the Phase III section if it is proven viable and will be followed for a maximum of 2 years after the final patient is enrolled, or until the patient's 5-year follow-up phase is completed, whichever comes first [30].

Due to the lack of RCTs conclusive evidence regarding oncologic safety of MIS staging in early ovarian cancer is yet to be determined. Intraoperative tumour rupture is known to upstage the disease. While laparoscopic procedures ensure better visualisation with the ability to detect small lesions, on the other hand it can be difficult to thoroughly perform surgical staging owing to the technical challenges and varied locations of tumour implantation. Though data from various case series have shown comparable overall survival with MIS and open surgeries, until it is proved in prospective trials surgical staging of ovarian cancer using MIS remains under grey zone.

Similarly, larger prospective trials are needed to determine the safety of endoscopic surgery for advanced ovarian cancer, and two of them are currently underway (Minimally Invasive Interval Debulking Surgery in Ovarian Neoplasm: a Feasibility Study [MISSION] Trial NCT02324595 and Feasibility of Interval Debulking Surgery by Laparoscopy for Peritoneal Carcinosis in Chemosensitive Patients [CILOVE] Trial NCT019051).

8 Role of MIS in Cervical Cancer

Multiple retrospective articles have documented the feasibility, benefits, and oncologic safety of a minimally invasive technique for radical hysterectomy during the past 25 years.

However, two recent manuscripts published in the *New England Journal of Medicine* (NEJM) in October 2018 (the LACC trial and a large epidemiologic study involving women from cancer-accredited hospitals in the USA) showed that patients who underwent minimally invasive radical hysterectomy had higher rates of recurrence and death [18, 19]. Since then, a number of retrospective investigations have revealed similar findings, prompting revisions to the NCCN, ESGO, and ESMO recommendations [31].

Women with stage IA 1 cervical malignancies with lymph-vascular space invasion (LVSI) and those with stage IB1 tumours were both enrolled in the study. Squamous cell carcinoma was the most common histological subtype. The research was terminated early when an interim analysis revealed that the MIS study arm had a considerably higher death rate.

Cervix manipulation during surgery, spillage of cells after pelvic lymphadenectomy, and intra-abdominal CO_2 utilised in MIS operations are among the several hypotheses postulated for these unexpected results.

A small number of patients recruited in some centres and variations in surgical skill levels were the major limitations of the study. The LACC trial saw unusually high number of intra-abdominal recurrences after MIS which raises the possibility that cervical cancer cells might disseminate from the vagina to the abdomen and pelvis because of extensive cervical manipulation during MIS. To limit this, various surgical strategies have been proposed, including the avoidance of uterine manipulators and isolating the cervix by surgical closure of the vagina prior to laparoscopy.

For women with early-stage cervical cancer stage IA1 tumours with LVSI and stage IB1 cancers, the FIGO gynaecologic oncology committee advises open surgery as the 'gold standard' operation. When selecting between these surgical options, women should be advised of all possible consequences [32].

The LACC trial's unanticipated findings, as well as those of other retrospective studies, have sparked a debate over the best surgical technique for patients with early cervical cancer. Furthermore, given the difficulties of presenting an alternative of therapy that has been regarded oncologically inferior, establishing new studies with a less invasive method arm has been problematic. Furthermore, the causes behind minimally invasive surgery's poor results have yet to be discovered [3].

The SUCCOR (surgery in cervical cancer, observational, retrospective) research evaluated minimally invasive versus open abdominal radical hysterectomy in patients with FIGO 2009 Stage IB1 cervical cancer in an observational retrospective analysis. It found that patients who had a minimally invasive radical hysterectomy had a lower disease-free survival rate than those who had an open hysterectomy. Avoiding the use of the uterine manipulator or sealing the vaginal opening above the tumour, on the other hand, might theoretically improve the results of minimally invasive radical hysterectomy. However, prospective studies are needed to corroborate these findings [33].

Recently two RCTs are underway to further unravel outcomes of surgical management in early-stage cervical cancer: one, a Chinese trial with a planned recruitment of 1448 patients will require high level surgical expertise to perform radical hysterectomies; other the RACC trial, enrolling 800 patients will provide insight about robot-assisted radical hysterectomies [33, 34].

Daniel Dargent discovered and described radical vaginal trachelectomy for cervical cancer in 1987 as a fertility-sparing operation for women with cervical cancer [35]. Cibula et al. published the first instance of a complete laparoscopic trachelectomy in 2005, with no known intraoperative or postoperative problems [36].

Results of the multicentric retrospective International Radical Trachelectomy Study published in *AJOG* in 2021 revealed similar oncologic outcome in open and MIS approach for radical trachelectomy. The overall survival rate was 99.2% for open surgery and 99% for MIS [37].

Ovarian transposition is often done laparoscopically in young female patients with early squamous cell carcinoma of the cervix who have scheduled brachytherapy or definitive pelvic radiation to maintain their hormonal or reproductive potential.

With a combined pregnancy rate of 36.2% and a live birth rate of 57.1% [38], fertility results following MIS are comparable to other treatments.

9 Role of Sentinel Lymph Node Mapping in Minimally Invasive Gynaecologic Oncology

In early-staged endometrial cancer, SLN assessment (Fig. 1) is still the gold standard for detecting lymph node metastases. In select patients with cervical cancer, SLN biopsy has been found to be reliable, reducing morbidity without affecting disease-free survival. Large prospective trials have demonstrated the methodology and high sensitivity of SLN biopsy in vulvar cancer. There are no randomised controlled trials evaluating the influence of SLN biopsy on therapy and outcome in ovarian cancer; current SLN evaluation is still experimental [39].

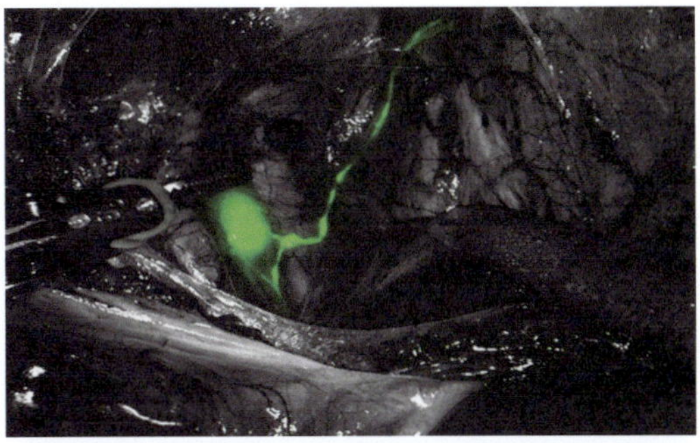

Fig. 1 SLN in endometrial cancer seen using the firefly during robotic surgery. (Picture courtesy Dr. Anupama Rajanbabu)

ICG-based SLN detection rates and bilateral SLN detection rates are comparable to or better than those achieved using blue dye alone or radiocolloid. Many institutions are now using ICG as their preferred imaging dye, particularly those with robotic and laparoscopic platforms equipped with near-infrared mapping equipment. New technological advancements are always being made to improve the surgeon's ability to see lymphatics. Colour-segmented fluorescence (CSF), which is available on the PINPOINT system by Novadaq (Burnaby, British Columbia, Canada) is one approach currently available for clinical application. The current platform supports a picture-in-picture view with four modes running at the same time: high-definition white light, high-precision Spy mode (black and white), PINPOINT mode (green overlay), and CSF mode.

The CSF mode can provide a heat map, which helps the surgeon to detect the more prevalent lymphatics and improve surgical precision by avoiding nonnodal tissue removal. Colour-segmented fluorescence (CSF), which is available on the PINPOINT system by Novadaq

(Burnaby, British Columbia, Canada), is one approach currently available for clinical application. The current platform provides for a picture-in-picture view with four modes running at the same time, including high-definition white light, Spy mode (black and white) with the highest precision, and a picture-in-picture view with four modes running at the same time.

10 Oncological Hazards

10.1 Port Site Recurrences

The topic of tumour development and abdominal wall metastases following CO_2 laparoscopic surgery has been the subject of several (old) research studies, with mixed outcomes. Tumour development is always faster after a laparotomy than it is after a laparoscopy. When a high number of tumour cells are present, pneumoperitoneum, not carbon dioxide, may generate seeding conditions.

Aerosolisation of live tumour cells and efflux with gas via trocar sites, as well as decrease of inflammatory response utilising minimally invasive vs open laparotomy incisions, are among the different research suggested to explain the genesis of port site metastases. Low pressure, avoidance of gas exsufflation via trocar apertures, avoiding tumour tearing, use of bags to recover operational specimens, and meticulous closing of trocar openings can all help to minimise abdominal wall metastases [40, 41].

10.2 Tumour Rupture

Another concern that has kept many gynaecologic oncologists from using laparoscopy for EOC is the increased risk of capsular rupture. Because big tumours frequently require drainage before removal, either to allow specimen retrieval or to gain appropriate working space, minimal access surgery is more likely to result in capsular rupture than laparotomy. This has been elucidated in retrospective reviews by Vergotte et al. and Gammez et al. that have emphasised on poorer outcomes with tumour rupture in MIS [42, 43].

10.3 Morcellation

There is no preoperative procedure that can definitively identify sarcomas from uterine myomas in patients who are about to be operated on. When compared to endometrial cancers, uterine sarcomas have a worse prognosis, especially in the early stages. In comparison to non-morcellation, sarcoma morcellation can cause disease progression and poor survival rates. Although morcellation with tissue containment is thought to guard against undesirable effects, there is insufficient evidence to support this claim. To develop conclusive facts, more research is required [44].

11 Conclusions

Minimally invasive procedures have been created in an effort to reduce surgical morbidity. They have been proved to be practical and safe alternatives to open surgery, with shorter LOS, less blood loss, and equivalent or reduced postoperative complications.

MIS has allowed gynaecologic surgeons to do far more intricate procedures on a diverse set of patients thanks to the technical advancements given by robotic surgery.

Prior laparoscopic expertise is advantageous, at least in the early stages of robotics adaptation; nevertheless, the robotic platform translates well from laparotomy since surgeons may robotically duplicate the technique based on their previous laparotomy experience.

Subspecialty training, surgical expertise and judgement, and understanding of illness and anatomy are not replaced by technological developments. It is also a foregone conclusion that technology will continue to evolve and develop, and, ideally, become less expensive.

LESS and OASIS are two examples of additional methods. LESS entails a single incision, usually in the umbilicus, through which numerous ports or a single port that may handle multiple ports and instruments are implanted. OASIS, or orifice-assisted small-incision surgery, is a novel method used in LESS to alleviate tool clutter.

References

1. Querleu D, Leblanc E, Castelain B. Pelvic lymphadenectomy under celioscopic guidance. J Gynecol Obstet Biol Reprod. 1990;19:576–8.
2. Nezhat CR, Burrell MO, Nezhat FR, et al. Laparoscopic radical hysterectomy with paraaortic and pelvic node dissection. Am J Obstet Gynecol. 1992;166:864–5.
3. Ramirez PT, Frumovitz M, Pareja R, Lopez A, Vieira M, Ribeiro R, et al. Minimally invasive versus abdominal radical hysterectomy for cervical cancer. NEJM. 2018;379(20):1895–904.
4. Rauh R, Hemmerling TM, Rist M, Jacobi KE. Influence of pneumoperitoneum and patient positioning on respiratory system compliance. J Clin Anesth. 2001;13:361–5.
5. Bouchard-Fortier G, Geerts W, Covens A, Vicus D, Kupets R, Gien LT. Is venous thromboprophylaxis necessary in patients undergoing minimally invasive surgery for a gynecologic malignancy? Gynecol Oncol. 2014;134:228–32.
6. Barnett JC, Hurd WW, Rogers RM, Williams NL, Shapiro SA. Laparoscopic positioning and nerve injuries. J Minim Invasive Gynecol. 2007;14:664–72.
7. Palmer R. Safety in laparoscopy. J Reprod Med. 1974;13:1–5.
8. Molloy D, Kalloo PD, Cooper M, Nguyen TV. Laparoscopic entry: a literature review and analysis of techniques and complications of primary port entry. Aust NZJ Obstet Gynaecol. 2002;42:246–54.
9. Shirk GJ, Johns A, Redwine DB. Complications of laparoscopic surgery: how to avoid them and how to repair them. J Minim Invasive Gynecol. 2006;13:352–9.
10. Chapron C, Cravello L, Chopin N, Kreiker G, Blanc B, Dubuisson JB. Complications during set-up procedures for laparoscopy in gynecology: open laparoscopy does not reduce the risk of major complications. Acta Obstet Gynecol Scand. 2003;82:1125–9.
11. Tonouchi H, Ohmori Y, Kobayashi M, Kusunoki M. Trocar site hernia. Arch Surg. 2004;139:1248–56.
12. Wang J, Li X, Wu H, Zhang Y, Wan F. A meta-analysis of robotic surgery in endometrial cancer: comparison with laparoscopy and laparotomy. Dis Markers. 2020;12:2503753.
13. O'Reilly BA. Patents running out: time to take stock of robotic surgery. Int Urogynecol J. 2014;25:711–3.
14. Lim PC, Kang E, Park DH. A comparative detail analysis of the learning curve and surgical outcome for robotic hysterectomy with lymphadenectomy versus laparoscopic hysterectomy with lymphadenectomy in treatment of endometrial cancer: a case-matched controlled study of the first one hundred twenty two patients. Gynecol Oncol. 2011;120:413–8.
15. Walker JL, Piedmonte MR, Spirtos NM, et al. Recurrence and survival after random assignment to laparoscopy versus laparotomy for comprehensive surgical staging of uterine cancer: gynecologic oncology group LAP2 study. J Clin Oncol. 2012;30:695Y700.
16. Baker J, Janda M, Gebski V, et al. Lower preoperative quality of life increases postoperative risk of adverse events in women with endometrial cancer: results from the LACE trial. Gynecol Oncol. 2015;137:102–5.
17. Kohler C, Tozzi R, Klemm P, Schneider A. Laparoscopic paraaortic left-sided transperitoneal infrarenal lymphadenectomy in patients with gynaecological malignancies: techniques and results. Gynecol Oncol. 2003;91:139–48.
18. Scribner DR, Walker JL, Johnson GA, McMeekin SD, Gold MA, Mannel RS, et al. Laparoscopic pelvic and paraaortic lymph node dissection: analysis of first 100 cases. Gynecol Oncol. 2001;82(3):498–503.
19. Lu D, Liu Z, Shi G, Liu D, Zhou X. Robotic assisted surgery for gynaecological cancer. Cochrane Database Syst Rev. 2012;1:Cd008640.
20. Siegel RL, Miller KD, Jemal A. Cancer statistics, 2018. CA Cancer J Clin. 2018;68(1):7–30.
21. Taussig FJ. Cancer of the vulva. Am J Obstet Gynecol. 1940;40(5):764–79.
22. Lu Y, Yao D, Pan Z, et al. Laparoscopic inguinal lymphadenectomy: a new minimally invasive technique to treat vulva carcinoma. Int J Clin Exp Med. 2016;9:4035–40.
23. Jain V, Sekhon R, Giri S, et al. Robotic-assisted video endoscopic inguinal lymphadenectomy in carcinoma vulva: our experiences and intermediate results. Int J Gynecol Cancer. 2017;27(1):159–65.
24. Vergote I, Marquette S, Amant F, et al. Port-site metastases after open laparoscopy: a study in 173 patients with advanced ovarian carcinoma. Int J Gynecol Cancer. 2005;15:776–9.
25. Fagotti A, Vizzielli G, De Iaco P, Surico D, Buda A, Mandato VD, Petruzzelli F, Ghezzi F, Garzarelli S, Mereu L, et al. A multicentric trial (Olympia–MITO 13) on the accuracy of laparoscopic to assess peritoneal spread in ovarian cancer. Am J Obstet Gynecol. 2013;209(462):e1–462.e11.
26. Nezhat FR, Ezzati M, Chuang L, et al. Laparoscopic management of early ovarian and fallopian tube cancers: surgical and survival outcome. Am J Obstet Gynecol. 2009;200:83–5.
27. Davidson BA, Broadwater G, Crim A, Boccacio R, Bixel K, Backes F, et al. Surgical complexity score and role of laparoscopy in women with advanced ovarian cancer treated with neoadjuvant chemotherapy. Gynecol Oncol. 2019;152(3):554–9.
28. Fagotti A, Gueli Alletti S, Corrado G, Cola E, Vizza E, Vieira M, et al. The international Mission study: minimally invasive surgery in ovarian neoplasms after neoadjuvant chemotherapy. Int J Gynecol Cancer. 2019;29(1):5–9.
29. Melamed A, Nitecki R, Boruta DM, del Carmen MG, et al. Laparoscopy compared with laparotomy for debulking ovarian cancer after neoadjuvant chemotherapy. Obstet Gynecol. 2017;129(5):861–9. [PubMed: 28383367]

30. Nitecki R, Rauh-Hain JA, Melamed A, Scambia G, Pareja R, Coleman RL, Ramirez PT, Fagotti A. Laparoscopic cytoreduction after Neoadjuvant ChEmotherapy (LANCE). Int J Gynecol Cancer. 2020;30(9):1450–4. https://doi.org/10.1136/ijgc-2020-001584.
31. Recommendations, 1 April 2020. Authors: esmo guidelines Committee. https://www.esmo.org/guidelines/gynaecological-cancers/cervical-cancer/eupdate-cervical-cancer-treatment-recommendations. Accessed 3 Jul 2020.
32. Figo Gynecologic Oncology Committee. Figo statement on minimally invasive surgery in cervical cancer. Int J Gynaecol Obstet. 2020;149(3):264.
33. Chiva L, Zanagnolo V, Querleu D, On Behalf of the Succor Study Group, et al. Succor study: an International European Cohort Observational Study comparing minimally invasive surgery versus open abdominal radical hysterectomy in patients with stage ib1 cervical cancer. Int J Gynecol Cancer. 2020;30:1269–77.
34. Chao X, Li L, Wu M, et al. Efficacy of different surgical approaches in the clinical and survival outcomes of patients with early-stage cervical cancer: protocol of a phase III multicentre randomised controlled trial in China. BMJ Open. 2019;9(7):e029055. https://doi.org/10.1136/bmjopen-2019-029055.
35. Falconer H, Palsdottir K, Stalberg K, et al. Robot assisted approach to cervical cancer (RACC): an international multi-center, open label randomized controlled trial. Int J Gynecol Cancer. 2019;29(6):1072–6. https://doi.org/10.1136/ijgc-2019-000558.
36. D'Argent D, Brun JL, Roy M, Remi I. Pregnancies following radical trachelectomy for invasive surgical cancer. Gynecol Oncol. 1994;52:105.
37. Cibula D, Ungár L, Pálfalvi L, Binó B, Kuzel D. Laparoscopic abdominal radical trachelectomy. Gynecol Oncol. 2005;97(2):707–9.
38. Salvo G, Ramirez PT, Leitao M, Cibula D, Fotopoulou C, Kucukmetin A, et al. International radical trachelectomy assessment: IRTA study. Int J Gynecol Cancer. 2019;29(3):635–8.
39. Kuznicki ML, Chambers LM, Morton M, Son J, Horowitz M, Creantate KK, et al. Fertility-sparing surgery for early-stage cervical cancer: a systematic review of the literature. J Minim Invasive Gynecol. 2021;28(3):513–26.
40. Fotopoulou C, Ind T, Baldwin P, et al. Sentinel lymph node consensus document of the British Gynaecological cancer society for endometrial, vulvar, and cervical cancers. Int J Gynecol Cancer. 2019;29:1348–50.
41. Wang PH, Yen MS, Yuan CC, et al. Port site metastases after LAVH for endometrial cancer: possible mechanisms and prevention. Gynaecol Oncol. 1997;66:151.
42. Vergote I, De Brabanter J, Fyles A, Bertelsen K, Einhorn N, Sevelda P, Gore ME, Kaern J, Verrelst H, Sjovall K, Timmerman D, Vandewalle J, Van Gramberen M, Trope CG. Prognostic importance of degree of differentiation and cyst rupture in stage I invasive epithelial ovarian carcinoma. Lancet. 2001;357:176–82.
43. Bakkum-Gamez JN, Richardson DL, Seamon LG, Aletti GD, Powless CA, Keeney GL, O'Malley DM, Cliby WA. Influence of intraoperative capsule rupture on outcomes in stage I epithelial ovarian cancer. Obstet Gynecol. 2009;113:11–7.
44. Taşkın S, Varlı B, Yalçın İ, Ortaç F, Taşkıran Ç, Güngör M. Morcellation in gynecology: short review and suggestions from Turkish society of minimally invasive gynecologic oncology. J Turk Ger Gynecol Assoc. 2021;22(1):53–7.

Hormone Replacement Therapy after Gynaecological Cancer

Eshwarya Jessy Kaur, Upasana Baruah, Amita Maheshwari, and Amal Chandra Kataki

1 Introduction

Female hormones and their optimal level play a pivotal role in a woman's ability to smoothly carry out her daily activities. There is significant data in the literature that hormones affect the biochemical and physiological functions and have a more profound impact on her psychosocial interactions and existence, increased risk of overall mortality, cardiovascular diseases, neurological diseases, psychiatric diseases, osteoporosis, and other sequelae [1].

The treatment of gynaecological cancers has conventionally been associated with premature loss of ovarian function and childbearing abilities. HRT needs consideration about the potential for inducing tumours in patients without any oncologic history or in causing a recurrence or progression in previously diagnosed cases. Cancer characteristics are critical determining factors in decision making. The affected organ, grade and stage of tumour, molecular characteristics, therapy received, and disease-free survival are equally important apart from tumour hormone receptor status. Young patients who have premature menopause after treatment for a gynaecological malignancy usually suffer from severe menopausal symptoms because of sudden drop in oestrogen and progesterone levels. Hormone replacement therapy (HRT) has proven to alleviate these symptoms and improve quality of life effectively. However, often the clinicians may hesitate to use it, fearing a disease resurgence. Present data is encouraging to health providers, in that HRT can be safely used for most gynaecological cancer survivors, after adequately informing the patients as large randomised controlled trials are still awaited [2].

Evidence-based application for hormonal therapy in mitigating the adverse effects of sudden and premature fall in ovarian function has resulted in significant increase in quality of life (QOL) indicators of cancer patients. However, data is lacking on the proportion of gynaecological cancer patients receiving hormonal replacement, and therefore there lies a significant gap in the unmet needs and present prescription rates of hormones in this specific subset of patients [3].

The importance of providing appropriate HRT has been addressed in both SGO and NCCN guidelines [4, 5]. In fact, assessing for hormone-related symptoms is an important component of survivor assessment. HRT has not proven to have detrimental effect on survival in patients with high-grade serous ovarian cancer, cervical cancer, vulval tumours, and early-stage endometrial can-

E. J. Kaur (✉) · U. Baruah · A. C. Kataki
Department of Gynaecologic Oncology, Dr. Bhubaneswar Borooah Cancer Institute (A Unit of Tata Memorial Centre, Mumbai), Guwahati, Assam, India

A. Maheshwari
Department of Gynaecological Oncology, Tata Memorial Centre, Parel, Mumbai, Maharashtra, India
e-mail: maheshwaria@tmc.gov.in

A. C. Kataki, D. Barmon (eds.), *Fundamentals in Gynaecologic Malignancy*,
https://doi.org/10.1007/978-981-19-5860-1_26

cer. However, it is contraindicated in low-grade endometrial stromal sarcomas and preferably avoided in granulosa cell ovarian tumours [4–6]. The Women's Health Initiative (WHI) study was a landmark trial that demonstrated the effects of unopposed oestrogen therapy in increasing the risk of endometrial cancer significantly and established that such a treatment is only appropriate in women who have had a previous hysterectomy [7]. In addition, negative impact was also seen with the combination of oestrogen with progesterone in cardiovascular system and breast as was evident by increased incidence of stroke, pulmonary embolism, and breast cancer in this study [8].

WHI study results led to a significant change in the clinicians' overall approach of HRT, and the prescription rates dwindled in cancer survivors. A German study looked at the preference of physicians treating endometrial cancers showed that the vast majority (88%) preferred to use other non-hormonal regimens, and 75% were convinced that in high-grade disease, HRT is absolutely contraindicated [9].

The consequences of gynaecological cancers and their treatment on sexual quality of life of patients are often neglected. Nearly 65% of gynaecological cancer survivors develop sexual dysfunction and decreased libido is the most frequently reported symptom (70%) followed by genitopelvic pain (60%) and orgasmic disorder (20%) [10]. Hot flashes, dryness of vagina, mood changes following induced menopause, fatigue, weight loss, insomnia, and alopecia associated with chemotherapy are the multifactorial causes of decreased sexual quality of life. Pelvic radiotherapy causes more deleterious effects on the vagina with pronounced vaginal stenosis, shortening, and atrophy [11]. This issue needs more intensive research in the future [12].

2 HRT in Ovarian Cancer

Ovarian cancers comprise a heterogeneous group of tumours. Although 90% tumours are of epithelial origin, the biological behaviour and hormone sensitivities of other types also need to be ascertained when prescribing HRT to these patients. Combined oral contraceptives have a definite role in the prevention of epithelial ovarian tumours, and no convincing evidence has implicated oestrogen as a contributing factor towards epithelial ovarian cancer (EOC) [13]. Also, there is no data which could exhibit any adverse outcomes in ovarian cancer patients who have been taking HRT [14–17]. An observational study by Chantal Mascarenhas comprising women diagnosed with invasive EOC ($n = 649$) or borderline ovarian tumours ($n = 150$) demonstrated no significant difference in 5-year survival in the hormone versus non-HRT users, especially in the EOC group and in fact a survival advantage in the borderline tumours subcategory [16]. It is, however, noted that low-grade and borderline serous ovarian tumours exhibit a diffuse positivity for oestrogen, progesterone, and androgen receptors [18]. French national network's 2019 guidelines advise caution while using HRT in borderline serous ovarian tumours with high-risk histological features, e.g. micropapillary pattern, stromal microinvasion, or peritoneal implants as these patients are at risk of potentially hormone-sensitive recurrence [19].

A Cochrane review by Saeaib et al. in 2020 concluded that hormone replacement therapy might be beneficial in improving the overall survival in women who have undergone surgical treatment for EOC. However, it was stated that the evidence in this regard is of low quality, and well-designed RCTs are necessary before HRT use is refuted or encouraged in this population [20]. Here it is noteworthy to mention the findings of Adjuvant Hormonal Therapy trial (AHT) by Rosalind A. Eeles et al. which was designed to study the effect of adjuvant hormonal therapy in epithelial ovarian cancer [21]. The patients were randomly assigned to AHT ($n = 75$) versus follow-up only. Both the groups had similar baseline characteristics with median age of patients being 58 years and predominant histology being serous followed by mucinous, endometroid, and clear cell variety. Though the study failed to recruit adequate number of patients as determined in the initial protocol ($n = 570$) thus decreasing the power of the study, the long-term follow-up of these patients after 19.1 years revealed that AHT can be safely taken by patients with epithelial ovarian cancer, with benefits of improved quality of life and possible improved overall survival.

BRCA mutation carriers who undergo prophylactic risk-reducing salpingo-oophorectomy enter premature menopause, and it is reasonable to give HRT to these patients, at least up to the age of natural menopause [22]. However, there are concerns about increased risk of breast cancer in BRCA mutation carriers with the use of HRT [23]. A 10-year follow-up of 872 women who were BRCA1 mutation carriers reflected that the overall incidence of breast cancer amongst combined oestrogen plus progesterone users was 22%, while it was 12% in oestrogen-alone HRT users [24].

The evidence regarding use of HRT in rare ovarian tumours is deficient due to limited numbers and lack of large population-based trials. Following treatment of germ cell tumours, HRT has not been demonstrated to carry any additional risk of recurrence and is thus recommended [17]. Endometrioid ovarian cancer is oestrogen-sensitive and residual disease after treatment could be stimulated by HRT. Considering therapeutic potential of anti-oestrogenic therapies in advanced endometrioid ovarian cancers, HRT can only be used with discretion in an early-stage completely resected subset of patients [25]. However as per SGO guidelines HRT is not recommended in patients with endometrioid as well as low-grade serous histology [5].

In granulosa cell tumour of ovary, the general advice is to avoid HRT due to oestrogen-dependent nature of this tumour. Caution is therefore encouraged when prescribing both systemic and topical hormones in women with low-grade serous and granulosa cell tumours because of their hormone dependence [26].

3 HRT in Endometrial Cancer

Although endometrial cancer is generally diagnosed in postmenopausal women, almost 25% of women are premenopausal, and 4% develop under 40 years of age [27]. Hot flashes and other menopausal symptoms are commonly reported by premenopausal women treated for endometrial cancer, and these symptoms may be more severe, being surgically induced. More than 90% of women have type-1 endometrial cancers, which are oestrogen-dependent; thus, it is reasonable that hormone therapy after type 1 cancer may be best withheld [28]. However, no data has demonstrated the use of hormone therapy, oestrogen alone or in combination with progestational agent with an increased rate of recurrence. There is no decrease in cancer-specific survival in both lower grades and higher grades, non-oestrogen-dependent, endometrial cancers, and carcinosarcomas [29].

There are limited studies that can guide the use of HRT in uterine sarcomas. Uterine sarcomas are rare cancers and include endometrial stromal sarcomas, leiomyosarcomas, carcinosarcomas, and adenosarcomas. Some endometrial tumours like endometrial stroma sarcomas are well known to express oestrogen and progesterone receptors significantly, and in this specific subgroup HRT is not recommended, irrespective of the degree of differentiation [29, 30]. Leiomyosarcomas also very often overexpress oestrogen and progesterone receptors [31]. However, in a study published by Kapp and colleagues, removal of the ovaries during hysterectomy did not result in improvement in 5-year overall survival [32, 33]. Due to limited data on the safety of HRT, many clinicians consider it not to be safe in these patients [34]. In other uterine sarcomas like carcinosarcomas and adenosarcomas, HRT can be used [33].

The National Comprehensive Cancer Network Panel advocates oestrogen replacement for low-risk patients in terms of tumour recurrence; however initiation of any such therapy should be preceded by comprehensive discussion with the patient, explaining the risk benefit profile. A 6–12 months time should preferably elapse before initiating HRT after completion of adjuvant therapy [35].

4 HRT in Cervical Cancers

Squamous cell carcinomas contribute about 80% of all cervical cancer cases, and the hormone dependency has not been observed, so it seems logical that such patients may be prescribed HRT comfortably.

The rates of ovarian metastasis in patients with squamous cell carcinoma are lower (up to 1.3%) in comparison to adenocarcinoma (up to 6.3%), so the ovarian preservation with or without transposition is feasible in the former group [36]. However, it may also be considered in early-stage adenocarcinomas of cervix [37, 38]. Hormone therapy per se has been associated with a decreased incidence of squamous cell carcinoma and a slight increase in adenocarcinoma [39–41]. Use of HRT has not been shown to adversely affect oncological outcomes for SCC patients irrespective of hysterectomy was undertaken or not [42]. Although there is a slight increase in adenocarcinoma cervix in HRT users, whether HRT use in established cases of cervical adenocarcinoma causes an increase in recurrence rate is yet not addressed. Due to the paucity of data on recurrence and disease-free survival in HRT users, the patients need to be adequately informed and care given on individualised basis. As per European Menopause and Andropause Society (EMAS) and International Gynaecologic Cancer Society (IGCS) guideline, the choice of regimen (unopposed or opposed oestrogen) depends on the hysterectomy status of the patient, as with unopposed oestrogen, there is a risk of stimulation of residual endometrium [26].

5 HRT in Vulval Cancer

Vulvar cancer is more frequent in postmenopausal women; however, the incidence is increasing in women under 50 years over the past three decades, attributed to the increasing incidence of human papillomavirus infection due to changing sexual behaviour and the superadded effects of cigarette smoking [43, 44]. In situ and invasive vulvar cancer are not hormone-dependent tumours. Women with vulvar cancers who have undergone local or extended field radiotherapy may need local oestrogen or systemic HRT, once the treatment has been initiated in the upfront or adjuvant setting. No study has documented an increase in invasive vulval malignancies associated with hormone use, and thus, both systemic and topical hormonal therapy can be used [45, 46].

6 HRT in Vaginal Cancer

Vaginal carcinoma are rare cancers of the genital tract [47]. Like carcinoma cervix SCC histology comprise the majority and therefore HRT can be prescribed when required. Data on uncommon histology like adenocarcinoma is scarce. Therefore, any recommendation for such patients should be made after explaining about the unknown risks involved.

7 HRT in Breast Cancer

Menopause in breast cancer survivors may result from various factors like chemotherapy or radiotherapy to the pelvis for ovarian ablation, endocrine therapy or prophylactic oophorectomy to induce surgical menopause before endocrine therapy. Majority of women with breast cancer express oestrogen and progesterone receptors and therefore the tumour cells have the potential to be stimulated by HRT. A small subset of patients are receptor negative and comprise the triple negative breast cancer (TNBC) group and are considered hormone insensitive [48]. A landmark trial on HRT in postmenopausal women had shown an increased risk of recurrence in women with breast cancer. The HABITS trial (Hormone Replacement Therapy After Breast Cancer—Is it Safe?) was started in May 1997 to evaluate safety of 2-year HRT for menopausal symptoms in women with a previously treated breast cancer. Four hundred and thirty-four women were recruited in the trial. The primary endpoint was any new breast cancer event. The trial was prematurely terminated shortly after 2 years in 2003 as a significant and alarming increased breast cancer risk of recurrence was observed in HRT group (26 recurrences in the HRT group vs. 7 in the non-HRT group). Although more women in the HT arm were receptor positive (62.3% vs. 54.5%), the subset analysis did not reveal any effect of hormone status on effect modification [49]. The Stockholm Trial, which was another trial similar to the HABITS trial, was also prematurely terminated after the results of the HABITS trial. The HABITS and the Stockholm trials have indicated a relative risk (RR) of recurrence between 2.0 and 3.6 for breast cancer recurrence after different HRT regimens [50, 51]. Apart from oestrogen and progesterone oral regimens, tibolone, a synthetic steroid, is routinely used for HRT. The Long-Term Intervention on Fractures with Tibolone (LIFT) study studied the role of Tibolone and found that in addition to decreasing the fracture risk in osteoporotic postmenopausal population, it significantly reduced the risk of breast cancer (odds ratio 0.32) [52]. The Livial Intervention Following Breast Cancer: Efficacy, Recurrence and Tolerability Endpoints Trial (LIBERATE) was undertaken to see effects of tibolone in breast cancer survivor subgroup. Although there was a significant improvement in bone mineral density (BMD) and menopausal symptoms such as hot flashes, the trial was prematurely terminated due of the increasing breast cancer recurrence risk observed (15.2% with tibolone versus 10.7% with placebo) [53–55]. Hence LIFT and Liberate study are contradictory in terms of breast cancer incidence in tibolone users.

Being hormone receptor negative TNBC patients may be considered to benefit from HRT. But there are many pitfalls which need to be considered before one can issue a generalised statement. The cut off to consider hormone negative varies from 1% to 10% as per different guidelines [56]. Secondly there are instances of ER conversion later in these patients and therefore HRT may prove to be detrimental in such instances [57]. Therefore, presently various societies have advised that no hormone replacement therapy should be given to patients with personal history of breast cancer irrespective of hormone receptor status [58]. To alleviate postmenopausal symptoms like hot flashes, non-hormonal methods like lifestyle changes, behavioural modification, and use of non-hormonal drugs like gabapentin, venlafaxine, or fluoxetine are preferred [59].

A distinct entity is the BRCA positive women following prophylactic bilateral salpingo-oophorectomy. In a review by Finch and colleagues it was recommended that in both BRCA1 and BRCA2 mutant patients without breast cancer history, with breasts not removed, HRT may be advised till the age of natural menopause. Similarly, with prophylactic mastectomy done, but no history of breast cancer, HRT may be offered to the age of natural menopause. However, if the patient has already been diagnosed with breast cancer, HRT is contraindicated [60].

8 Hormonal Versus Non-Hormonal Therapy

Systemic menopausal hormone therapy can be delivered either orally or transdermally. In a woman who has undergone hysterectomy, oestrogen alone is given whereas progestogens or the selective oestrogen receptor modulator are prescribed alongside in women with an intact uterus to subvert the stimulatory effects on endometrium [61]. Presently Bazedoxefene (BZE) is the only SERM to be evaluated for such a situation as shown by the SMART trials which showed that CE (conjugated oestrogen) 0.45 mg/BZA 20 mg and CE 0.625 mg/BZA 20 mg provide endometrial protection without breast side effects such as pain or density, episodes of abnormal bleeding, or ovarian stimulation and cysts in women with intact uterus when studied up to 2 years [62, 63]. With early or premature menopause, systemic HRT is recommended until the average age of natural menopause after ruling out all contraindications [26]. Low doses of HRT or non-oestrogen-based therapies should be considered for older women [64]. Low-dose vaginal oestrogen therapy may help in managing moderate or severe genitourinary symptoms. The preparations used may be regimens with ≤50 μg oestradiol or ≤0.3 mg conjugated oestrogens or ≤0.5 g cream. In managing genitourinary syndromes, local oestrogen therapy is often seen to be more effective than systemic therapy [26, 65, 66]. In addition, intravaginal Dehydroepiandrosterone has been approved by the Food and Drug Administration (FDA) for the management of dyspareunia. Its mechanism of action lies in the aromatisation of androstenedione and testosterone to estrone and oestradiol [67, 68]. Another selective oestrogen receptor modulator Ospemifene has an agonist effect in the vagina on oestrogen receptors and is approved by the FDA for managing moderate to severe dyspareunia [69]. However, Ospemifene is associated with increased frequency of hot flushes and a potential increase in the thromboembolism risk is of concern. Its safety in patients with breast cancer has not been evaluated, although early research indicates an anti-oestrogenic to a neutral role in breast tissues [70]. With the currently available low-dose vaginal oestrogen preparations containing 10 μg of oestradiol, the plasma levels stay in the range of ≤20 pg/mL. Intermediate doses (i.e. 25 μg oestradiol or 0.3 mg conjugated equine oestrogen) result in plasma levels reaching up to 20 pg/mL. The higher doses (50–2000 μg oestradiol or 0.625–2.5 mg conjugated equine oestrogen) result in significantly higher plasma levels [65, 71]. In women who are taking aromatase inhibitors, which are inherently anti-oestrogenic, it does not seem prudent to use systemic oestrogen-based therapies. Here, non-hormonal options should be used as the initial therapy [72, 73].

Non-hormonal therapies are not commonly used and hence minimally studied for menopausal symptoms in cancer survivors. Non-hormonal options can range from behavioural cognitive therapy and hypnosis, as well as medical interventions like clonidine, gabapentin, selective serotonin reuptake inhibitors, and serotonin noradrenaline reuptake inhibitors. Lubricants can be used to help with dyspareunia [74]. Cognitive behavioural therapy may not decrease the frequency of vasomotor symptoms, but it certainly helps in reducing the overall impact of menopause. Clinical hypnosis has been noted to decrease measurable hot flush scores as well as patient's perception of symptoms and improvement of overall mood and sleep. This has been exhibited in women with and without history of breast cancer via randomised controlled trials [75, 76]. A systematic review published in 2013 reported that acupuncture may have a placebo effect on vasomotor symptoms but had more effect than no treatment [77]. Exercise and yoga have been known to improve sleep quality. Although exercise does help in mood elevation, there is no evidence to support that yoga or exercise helps in alleviating vasomotor symptoms [78, 79]. There is some evidence in literature to suggest that the use of supplementary phytoestrogens and isoflavonoids may help with vasomotor and genitourinary symptoms [80]. It should be noted that the mechanism of isoflavonoids is via oestrogen receptors, hence best avoided in ER positive breast cancer.

Pharmacological options for vasomotor symptoms include selective serotonin reuptake inhibitors and serotonin-norepinephrine reuptake inhibitors, clonidine, and gabapentin [81]. However, consideration should be given to any inadvertent drug interaction with other adjuvant anticancer therapies. Paroxetine salt 7.5 mg/day is the only FDA-approved drug for hot flashes [82]. The primary options for the prevention and management of osteoporosis are bisphosphonates, denosumab, and parathyroid hormone. Calcium and various metabolically active forms of vitamin D may be used as well [64]. Herbal supplements and botanicals are not recommended as there is a paucity of data regarding safety and efficacy [83]. Also, there is a chance that undisclosed compounds in these products may act on oestrogen receptors or interact with anticancer therapies. A summary of the various evidences of use is represented in Table 1.

Table 1 Summary of the various evidences available

Primary tumour	Histological classification	Recommendation
Breast cancer	Invasive breast cancer	Contraindicated
	DCIS	No data
Endometrial cancer	Type I	Contraindicated
	Type II	Limited data
Uterine sarcoma	Leiomyosarcoma	Limited data
	Endometrial stromal sarcoma	Primarily contraindicated
	Carcinosarcoma, adenosarcoma	Can be considered (+)
Ovarian cancer	High-grade serous	Recommended (+)
	Endometroid	Not recommended (may consider in early stages completely resected ds)
	Low-grade serous	Not recommended
	Granulosa cell tumours	Primarily contraindicated
	Germ cell tumours	Recommended (+)
Cervical cancer	Squamous cell carcinoma	Recommended (+++)
	Adenocarcinoma	May consider in early stages completely resected ds (+/−)
Vaginal cancer	Squamous epithelial cancer	Recommended (+++)
	Adenocarcinoma	Limited data
Vulval cancer	Squamous cell cancer	Recommended (+++)

9 Conclusion

With the advancement in oncological treatments and overall survival, more women are now able to reach the age of natural menopause. Some women experience the sudden cessation of gonadal function, leading to premature ovarian failure as a consequence of treatment. The distressing symptoms with natural or premature ovarian failure are not given adequate importance by both the physician and the patient. This is compounded by the fear of recurrence with the use of HRT. Although as per guideline any form of hormone replacement is contraindicated in women with a personal history of breast cancer, many patients with ovarian, cervico-vaginal, and early endometrial cancer can still benefit from it. The reduced quality of life because of menopausal symptoms should not be ignored. However, the final decision on initiation of HRT should always be individualised and made together with the patient after adequate disclosures and information. Also, options for non-hormonal therapy with their risks and benefits should be discussed with the patient, and a tailor-made regimen, either hormonal or non-hormonal, should be designed.

References

1. Shuster LT, Rhodes DJ, Gostout BS, Grossardt BR, Rocca WA. Premature menopause or early menopause: long-term health consequences. Maturitas. 2010;65:161–6.
2. Biliatis I, Thomakos N, Rodolakis A, Akrivos N, Zacharakis D, Antsaklis A. Safety of hormone replacement therapy in gynaecological cancer survivors. J Obstet Gynaecol. 2012;32:321–5.
3. Molassiotis A, Chan CWH, Yam BMC, Chan SJ. Quality of life in Chinese women with gynaecological cancers. Support Care Cancer. 2000;8(5):414–22.
4. Guidelines N. Survivorship. Natl Compr Cancer Netw [Internet]. 2021. https://www.nccn.org/professionals/physician_gls/pdf/survivorship.pdf.
5. Sinno AK, Pinkerton J, Febbraro T, Jones N, Khanna N, Temkin S, et al. Hormone therapy (HT) in women with gynecologic cancers and in women at high risk for developing a gynecologic cancer: a Society of Gynecologic Oncology (SGO) clinical practice statement: this practice statement has been endorsed by the north American Meno. Gynecol Oncol. 2020;157(2):303–6.
6. Hinds L, Price J. Menopause, hormone replacement and gynaecological cancers. Menopause Int. 2010;16:89–93.
7. Hulley SB, Grady D. The WHI estrogen-alone trial—do things look any better? JAMA. 2004;291:1769–71.
8. Manson JAE, Chlebowski RT, Stefanick ML, Aragaki AK, Rossouw JE, Prentice RL, et al. Menopausal hormone therapy and health outcomes during the intervention and extended poststopping phases of the women's health initiative randomized trials. JAMA. 2013;310(13):1353–68.
9. Jaursch-Hancke C. Online-Datenbank mit Autoren- und Stichwortsuche Androgenmangel bei Frauen: Wann klinisch relevant? Neuroimaging-Verfahren in der Adipositasforschung Androgenmangel bei

Frauen: Wann klinisch relevant? Austrian. J Clin Endocrinol Metab. 2011;4(3):12–6. www.kup.at/klinendokrinologie.
10. Lin H, Fu HC, Wu CH, Tsai YJ, Chou YJ, Shih CM, et al. Evaluation of sexual dysfunction in gynecologic cancer survivors using DSM-5 diagnostic criteria. BMC Womens Health. 2022;22(1):1–7.
11. Vistad I, Cvancarova M, Fosså SD, Kristensen GB. Postradiotherapy morbidity in long-term survivors after locally advanced cervical cancer: how well do physicians' assessments agree with those of their patients? Int J Radiat Oncol. 2008;71(5):1335–42.
12. Kapoor E, Benrubi D, Faubion SS. Menopausal hormone therapy in gynecologic cancer survivors: a review of the evidence and practice recommendations. Clin Obstet Gynecol. 2018;61:488–95.
13. Persson I, Yuen J, Bergkvist L, Schairer C. Cancer incidence and mortality in women receiving estrogen and estrogen-progestin replacement therapy-long-term follow-up of a Swedish cohort. Int J Cancer. 1996;67:327–32.
14. Eeles RA, Tan S, Wiltshaw E, Fryatt I, A'Hern RP, Shepherd JH, et al. Hormone replacement therapy and survival after surgery for ovarian cancer. Br Med J. 1991;302(6771):259–62.
15. Guidozzi F, Daponte A. Estrogen replacement therapy for ovarian carcinoma survivors: a randomized controlled trial. Cancer. 1999;86(6):1013–8.
16. Mascarenhas C, Lambe M, Bellocco R, Bergfeldt K, Riman T, Persson I, et al. Use of hormone replacement therapy before and after ovarian cancer diagnosis, and ovarian cancer survival. Int J Cancer. 2006;119(12):2907–15.
17. Deli T, Orosz M, Jakab A. Hormone replacement therapy in cancer survivors—review of the literature. Pathol Oncol Res. 2020;26:63–78.
18. Buttarelli M, Mascilini F, Zannoni GF, Ciucci A, Martinelli E, Filippetti F, et al. Hormone receptor expression profile of low-grade serous ovarian cancers. Gynecol Oncol. 2017;145(2):352–60.
19. Rousset-Jablonski C, Selle F, Adda-Herzog E, Planchamp F, Selleret L, Pomel C, et al. Fertility preservation, contraception and menopause hormone therapy in women treated for rare ovarian tumours: guidelines from the French national network dedicated to rare gynaecological cancers. Eur J Cancer. 2019;116:35–44.
20. Saeaib N, Peeyananjarassri K, Liabsuetrakul T, Buhachat R, Myriokefalitaki E. Hormone replacement therapy after surgery for epithelial ovarian cancer. Cochrane Database Syst Rev. 2020;1:CD012559.
21. Eeles RA, Morden JP, Gore M, Mansi J, Glees J, Wenczl M, et al. Adjuvant hormone therapy may improve survival in epithelial ovarian cancer: results of the AHT randomized trial. J Clin Oncol. 2015;33(35):4138–44.
22. Sullivan SD, Sarrel PM, Nelson LM. Hormone replacement therapy in young women with primary ovarian insufficiency and early menopause. Fertil Steril. 2016;106(7):1588–99.
23. Gordhandas S, Norquist BM, Pennington KP, Yung RL, Laya MB, Swisher EM. Hormone replacement therapy after risk reducing salpingo-oophorectomy in patients with BRCA1 or BRCA2 mutations; a systematic review of risks and benefits. Gynecol Oncol. 2019;153:192–200.
24. Kotsopoulos J, Gronwald J, Karlan BY, Huzarski T, Tung N, Moller P, et al. Hormone replacement therapy after oophorectomy and breast cancer risk among BRCA1 mutation carriers. JAMA Oncol. 2018;4(8):1059–65.
25. Langdon SP, Herrington CS, Hollis RL, Gourley C. Estrogen signaling and its potential as a target for therapy in ovarian cancer. Cancers (Basel). 2020;12(6):1–17.
26. Rees M, Angioli R, Coleman RL, Glasspool RM, Plotti F, Simoncini T, et al. European menopause and Andropause society (EMAS) and international gynecologic cancer society (IGCS) position statement on managing the menopause after gynecological cancer: focus on menopausal symptoms and osteoporosis. Int J Gynecol Cancer. 2020;30(4):428–33.
27. Londero AP, Parisi N, Tassi A, Bertozzi S, Cagnacci A. Hormone replacement therapy in endometrial cancer survivors: a meta-analysis. J Clin Med. 2021;10(14):128.
28. Lobo F, Thomas E. Type II endometrial cancers: a case series. J Midlife Health. 2016;7(2):69–72.
29. del Carmen MG, Rice LW. Management of menopausal symptoms in women with gynecologic cancers. Gynecol Oncol. 2017;146(2):427–35.
30. Deli T, Orosz M, Jakab A. Hormone replacement therapy in cancer survivors—review of the literature. Pathol Oncol Res. 2020;26(1):63–78.
31. Zang Y, Dong M, Zhang K, Gao C, Guo F, Wang Y, et al. Hormonal therapy in uterine sarcomas. Cancer Med. 2019;8(4):1339.
32. Kapp DS, Shin JY, Chan JK. Prognostic factors and survival in 1396 patients with uterine leiomyosarcomas: emphasis on impact of lymphadenectomy and oophorectomy. Cancer. 2008;112(4):820–30.
33. Guidozzi F. Estrogen therapy in gynecological cancer survivors. Climacteric. 2013;16(6):611–7.
34. del Carmen MG, Rice LW. Management of menopausal symptoms in women with gynecologic cancers. Gynecol Oncol. 2017;146:427–35.
35. Nicole McMillian N, Angela Motter M, Frederick P, Gaffney DK, George S, Giuntoli RI, et al. NCCN Guidelines Version 1.2022 Uterine Neoplasms Continue NCCN Guidelines. 2021. https://www.nccn.org/home/member-. Accessed 6 Nov 2021.
36. Nakanishi T, Wakai K, Ishikawa H, Nawa A, Suzuki Y, Nakamura S, et al. A comparison of ovarian metastasis between squamous cell carcinoma and adenocarcinoma of the uterine cervix. Gynecol Oncol. 2001;82(3):504–9.
37. Jiao XB, Hu J, Zhu LR. The safety of ovarian preservation in early-stage adenocarcinoma compared with squamous cell carcinoma of uterine cervix. Int J Gynecol Cancer. 2016;26(8):1510–4.

38. Bodner K, Laubichler P, Kimberger O, Czerwenka K, Zeillinger R, Bodner-Adler B. Oestrogen and progesterone receptor expression in patients with adenocarcinoma of the uterine cervix and correlation with various clinicopathological parameters. Anticancer Res. 2010;30(4):1341–5.
39. Asthana S, Busa V, Labani S. Oral contraceptives use and risk of cervical cancer—a systematic review & meta-analysis. Eur J Obstet Gynecol Reprod Biol. 2020;247:163–75.
40. Cervical Cancer and Hormonal Contraceptives. Collaborative reanalysis of individual data for 16 573 women with cervical cancer and 35 509 women without cervical cancer from 24 epidemiological studies. Lancet. 2007;370(9599):1609–21. http://www.thelancet.com/article/S0140673607616845/fulltext.
41. Lacey JV, Brinton LA, Barnes WA, Gravitt PE, Greenberg MD, Hadjimichael OC, et al. Use of hormone replacement therapy and adenocarcinomas and squamous cell carcinomas of the uterine cervix. Gynecol Oncol. 2000;77(1):149–54.
42. Vargiu V, Amar ID, Rosati A, Dinoi G, Turco LC, Capozzi VA, et al. Hormone replacement therapy and cervical cancer: a systematic review of the literature. Climacteric. 2021;24(2):120–7.
43. Robinson Z, Edey K, Murdoch J. Invasive vulval cancer. Obstet Gynaecol Reprod Med. 2011;21(5):129–36.
44. Gajjar K, Shafi M. Invasive vulval cancer. Obstet Gynaecol Reprod Med. 2014;24(6):177–85.
45. Singh P, Oehler MK. Hormone replacement after gynaecological cancer. Maturitas. 2010;65(3):190–7.
46. Kuhle CL, Kapoor E, Sood R, Thielen JM, Jatoi A, Faubion SS. Menopausal hormone therapy in cancer survivors: a narrative review of the literature. Maturitas. 2016;92:86–96.
47. Hinds L, Price J. Menopause, hormone replacement and gynaecological cancers. Menopause Int. 2010;16(2):89–93.
48. Boyle P. Triple-negative breast cancer: epidemiological considerations and recommendations. Ann Oncol. 2012;23(Suppl. 6):7–12.
49. Holmberg L, Anderson H. HABITS (hormonal replacement therapy after breast cancer—is it safe?), a randomised comparison: trial stopped. Lancet. 2004;363(9407):453–5.
50. Lupo M, Dains JE, Madsen LT. Hormone replacement therapy: an increased risk of recurrence and mortality for breast cancer patients? J Adv Pract Oncol. 2015;6(4):322.
51. Brewster AM, Do KA, Thompson PA, Hahn KM, Sahin AA, Cao Y, et al. Relationship between epidemiologic risk factors and breast cancer recurrence. J Clin Oncol. 2007;25(28):4438–44.
52. Cummings SR, Ettinger B, Delmas PD, Kenemans P, Stathopoulos V, Verweij P, et al. The effects of Tibolone in older postmenopausal women. N Engl J Med. 2008;359(7):697–708.
53. Kenemans P, Bundred NJ, Foidart JM, Kubista E, von Schoultz B, Sismondi P, et al. Safety and efficacy of tibolone in breast-cancer patients with vasomotor symptoms: a double-blind, randomised, non-inferiority trial. Lancet Oncol. 2009;10(2):135–46.
54. Bundred NJ, Kenemans P, Yip CH, Beckmann MW, Foidart JM, Sismondi P, et al. Tibolone increases bone mineral density but also relapse in breast cancer survivors: liberate trial bone substudy. Breast Cancer Res. 2012;14(1):1–11.
55. Sismondi P, Kimmig R, Kubista E, Biglia N, Egberts J, Mulder R, et al. Effects of tibolone on climacteric symptoms and quality of life in breast cancer patients - data from LIBERATE trial. Maturitas. 2011;70(4):365–72.
56. van Barele M, Heemskerk-Gerritsen BAM, Louwers YV, Vastbinder MB, Martens JWM, Hooning MJ, et al. Estrogens and progestogens in triple negative breast cancer: do they harm? Cancers (Basel). 2021;13(11):1–17.
57. Schrijver WAME, Suijkerbuijk KPM, Van Gils CH, Van Der Wall E, Moelans CB, Van Diest PJ. Receptor conversion in distant breast cancer metastases: a systematic review and meta-analysis. J Natl Cancer Inst. 2018;110(6):568–80.
58. Baber RJ, Panay N, Fenton A. 2016 IMS recommendations on womens midlife health and menopause hormone therapy. Climacteric. 2016;19(2):109–50.
59. Murthy V, Chamberlain RS. Menopausal symptoms in young survivors of breast cancer: a growing problem without an ideal solution. Cancer Control. 2012;19(4):317–29.
60. Finch A, Evans G, Narod SA. BRCA carriers, prophylactic salpingo-oophorectomy and menopause: clinical management considerations and recommendations. Womens Health. 2012;8:543–55.
61. Overview | Menopause: diagnosis and management | Guidance | NICE. https://www.nice.org.uk/guidance/NG23. Accessed 4 Apr 2022.
62. Pickar JH, Yeh IT, Bachmann G, Speroff L. Endometrial effects of a tissue selective estrogen complex containing bazedoxifene/conjugated estrogens as a menopausal therapy. Fertil Steril. 2009;92(3):1018–24.
63. Mirkin S, Pinkerton JV, Kagan R, Thompson JR, Pan K, Pickar JH, et al. Gynecologic safety of conjugated estrogens plus Bazedoxifene: pooled analysis of five phase 3 trials. J Womens Health. 2016;25(5):431–42. https://www.liebertpub.com/doi/abs/10.1089/jwh.2015.5351.
64. Armeni E, Lambrinoudaki I, Ceausu I, Depypere H, Mueck A, Pérez-López FR, et al. Maintaining postreproductive health: a care pathway from the European menopause and Andropause society (EMAS). Maturitas. 2016;89:63–72.
65. Biehl C, Plotsker O, Mirkin S. A systematic review of the efficacy and safety of vaginal estrogen products for the treatment of genitourinary syndrome of menopause. Menopause. 2019;26(4):431–53.
66. Palacios S, Castelo-Branco C, Currie H, Mijatovic V, Nappi RE, Simon J, et al. Update on management of genitourinary syndrome of menopause: a practical guide. Maturitas. 2015;82(3):308–13.

67. Labrie F, Archer DF, Koltun W, Vachon A, Young D, Frenette L, et al. Efficacy of intravaginal dehydroepiandrosterone (DHEA) on moderate to severe dyspareunia and vaginal dryness, symptoms of vulvovaginal atrophy, and of the genitourinary syndrome of menopause. Menopause. 2018;25(11):1339–53.
68. Holton M, Thorne C, Goldstein AT. An overview of dehydroepiandrosterone (EM-760) as a treatment option for genitourinary syndrome of menopause. Expert Opin Pharmacother. 2020;21(4):409–15.
69. Portman DJ, Bachmann GA, Simon JA. Ospemifene, a novel selective estrogen receptor modulator for treating dyspareunia associated with postmenopausal vulvar and vaginal atrophy. Menopause. 2013;20(6):623–30.
70. Pinkerton JV, Kagan R. Ospemifene for the treatment of postmenopausal vulvar and vaginal atrophy: recommendations for clinical use. Expert Opin Pharmacother. 2015;16(17):2703–14.
71. Handa VL, Bachus KE, Johnston WW, Robboy SJ, Hammond CB. Vaginal administration of low-dose conjugated estrogens: systemic absorption and effects on the endometrium. Obstet Gynecol. 1994;84(2):215–8.
72. Stuenkel CA, Davis SR, Gompel A, Lumsden MA, Murad MH, Pinkerton JAV, et al. Treatment of symptoms of the menopause: an endocrine society clinical practice guideline. J Clin Endocrinol Metab. 2015;100(11):3975–4011.
73. Runowicz CD, Leach CR, Henry NL, Henry KS, Mackey HT, Cowens-Alvarado RL, et al. American Cancer Society/American Society of Clinical Oncology breast cancer survivorship care guideline. CA Cancer J Clin. 2016;66(1):43–73.
74. Szabo RA, Marino JL, Hickey M. Managing menopausal symptoms after cancer. Climacteric. 2019;22:572–8.
75. Elkins G, Marcus J, Stearns V, Perfect M, Rajab MH, Ruud C, et al. Randomized trial of a hypnosis intervention for treatment of hot flashes among breast cancer survivors. J Clin Oncol. 2008;26(31):5022.
76. Elkins GR, Fisher WI, Johnson AK, Carpenter JS, Keith TZ. Clinical hypnosis in the treatment of postmenopausal hot flashes: a randomized controlled trial. Menopause. 2013;20(3):291–8.
77. Dodin S, Blanchet C, Marc I, Ernst E, Wu T, Vaillancourt C, et al. Acupuncture for menopausal hot flushes. Cochrane Database Syst Rev. 2013;2013(7):151.
78. Newton KM, Reed SD, Guthrie KA, Sherman KJ, Booth-Laforce C, Caan B, et al. Efficacy of yoga for vasomotor symptoms: a randomized controlled trial. Menopause. 2014;21(4):339–46.
79. Sternfeld B, Guthrie KA, Ensrud KE, Lacroix AZ, Larson JC, Dunn AL, et al. Efficacy of exercise for menopausal symptoms: a randomized controlled trial. Menopause. 2014;21(4):330–8.
80. Franco OH, Chowdhury R, Troup J, Voortman T, Kunutsor S, Kavousi M, et al. Use of plant-based therapies and menopausal symptoms: a systematic review and meta-analysis. JAMA. 2016;315:2554–63.
81. Li T, Zhang Y, Cheng Q, Hou M, Zheng X, Zheng Q, et al. Quantitative study on the efficacy of acupuncture in the treatment of menopausal hot flashes and its comparison with nonhormonal drugs. Menopause. 2021;28(5):564–72.
82. Stubbs C, Mattingly L, Crawford SA, Wickersham EA, Brockhaus JL, McCarthy LH. Do SSRIs and SNRIs reduce the frequency and/or severity of hot flashes in menopausal women. J Okla State Med Assoc. 2017;110(5):272.
83. Anagnostis P, Bitzer J, Cano A, Ceausu I, Chedraui P, Durmusoglu F, et al. Menopause symptom management in women with dyslipidemias: an EMAS clinical guide. Maturitas. 2020;135:82–8.

The Perioperative and Critical Care Aspects in Gynaecology-Oncology

Anupam Das, Kailash Sharma,
and Amal Chandra Kataki

Cancer is one of the leading causes of morbidity and mortality the world over. Gynaecological malignancies are among the commonest malignancies an anaesthesiologist has to encounter both in the diagnostic and therapeutic stage. Thorough knowledge of the pathophysiology of cancer and the systemic effects of primary cancer, metastasis and its treatment (chemotherapy and radiotherapy) is of utmost importance for a comprehensive perioperative and critical care management of these patients. Chemotherapy may affect various organ systems of the body, and radiotherapy to the pelvic region may lead to fibrosis and adhesions, surgical difficulty and increased blood loss. The key is proper planning and good coordination amongst the perioperative team members (Anaesthesiologists, Intensivists, Surgeons, Dieticians and Physiotherapists).

This chapter attempts to provide insights into all these aspects of gynaecological malignancies.

A. Das (✉)
Department of Anaesthesiology, Dr. Bhubaneswar Borooah Cancer Institute (A Unit of Tata Memorial Centre Mumbai), Guwahati, Assam, India

K. Sharma
Tata Memorial Centre, Mumbai, Maharashtra, India

A. C. Kataki
Department of Gynaecologic Oncology, Dr. Bhubaneswar Borooah Cancer Institute (A Unit of Tata Memorial Centre, Mumbai), Guwahati, Assam, India

A cancer patient is subjected to surgery either as a primary treatment for the disease (primary debulking surgery) or as a follow-up to other modalities of cancer treatment (interval debulking surgery) like chemotherapy or radiotherapy or for palliative purposes to relieve distressing symptoms.

Depending on the primary disease, stage of presentation, various patient-related factors and the primary goal and the urgency of the contemplated surgery, the patient needs to be optimised prior to the surgery to whatever extent possible for an uneventful perioperative period.

1 Common Concerns and Challenges

1. *Psychological stress and associated poor nutritional status*: Almost all cancer patients suffer some degree of emotional stress at some stage of the disease. Psychological stress is one of the commonest causes of poor feeding and malnutrition. Depression, anxiety and malnutrition have all been linked to an impaired immune system [1–3].
2. *Difficult vascular access*: Thrombosed peripheral veins as a result of preoperative chemotherapy, long-term intravenous fluid administration or repeated blood sampling are often encountered. Even central venous

A. C. Kataki, D. Barmon (eds.), *Fundamentals in Gynaecologic Malignancy*,
https://doi.org/10.1007/978-981-19-5860-1_27

cannulation is a concern as these patients may have an underlying coagulopathy.

3. *Effects of chemotherapy and radiotherapy*: Many gynaecological cancer patients are subjected to chemotherapy and radiotherapy before surgery. These modalities of treatment can have long-term effects on various organ systems of the body. Most relevant amongst these are the effects of these agents on the cardiovascular and respiratory systems.

   The cardiovascular system: Various chemotherapeutic agents affect the cardiovascular system. Most significant amongst them are the anthracycline group of drugs. However, other agents like cyclophosphamide, busulphan, cisplatin and 5 fluorouracil are all implicated in causing cardiac toxicity. The anthracycline group consists of doxorubicin (Adriamycin), daunorubicin and epirubicin. Acute cardiotoxicity following anthracyclines generally manifests as transient alterations in blood pressure, heart rate and ECG changes (non-specific ST and T wave changes, prolonged QT interval, decreased QRS voltage). They are self-resolving within a week. Arrhythmias including supraventricular, junctional and ventricular tachycardia are seen in 0.5–3% of patients [4]. These changes resolve within 1–2 months of cessation of therapy without any long-term consequence. Chronic cardiotoxicity following anthracycline therapy is generally more significant clinically. It progresses from subclinical to overt clinically manifested congestive cardiac failure over the years. The risk of left ventricular failure increases with an increase in the period of exposure. Mediastinal irradiation and co-existing cardiac disease increase the risk. Alkylating agents like cyclophosphamide cause an acute form of cardiotoxicity within 10 days of its administration [5–7]. It can cause congestive cardiac failure and cardiac tamponade within a week of administration [5, 6, 8]. However, this cardiotoxicity resolves within 6 days without any long-term sequel. 5-fluorouracil, a synthetic pyrimidine antimetabolite, can induce coronary spasm and lead to myocardial ischaemia. This is especially relevant in patients of ischaemic heart disease. The Taxanes (paclitaxel/docetaxel) are antimicrotubule agents, leading to many types of cardiac arrhythmias, with sinus bradycardia being the most common [9]. However, normal sinus rhythm is restored after discontinuation of therapy and do not lead to any long-term squeal. In combination with doxorubicin, Paclitaxel increases the toxicity of doxorubicin by decreasing the clearance of doxorubicin by 30%. Radiotherapy-induced cardiotoxicity is generally not seen in gynaecological oncology cases as most commonly radiotherapy exposure is limited to pelvic areas (as in carcinoma cervix or vulva). However, an anaesthesiologist must be aware of the radiotherapy-induced cardiotoxicity if the patient has a history of mediastinal irradiation in the past for some other primary cancer. These patients are at an increased risk of valvular heart disease, coronary artery disease, congestive cardiac failure, cardiomyopathy, pericardial disease and sudden death. The risk is more when the patients receive radiotherapy at a young age [10–13].

   The pulmonary system: Cancer patients generally have a diminished respiratory reserve. This may be due to advanced age, inability to cough out secretions because of decreased respiratory muscle strength from poor nutrition. This leads to atelectasis of the dependent alveoli. Prolonged immobilisation in bed further contributes to atelectasis. Chemotherapy with drugs like Bleomycin and Mitomycin is implicated in causing pulmonary toxicity. Interstitial pneumonitis progressing to chronic fibrosis is the most common pattern of bleomycin and mitomycin lung toxicity. The risk increases with advanced age, high inspired oxygen concentration, pre-existing lung disease like COPD, etc. Cyclophosphamide and Methotrexate can cause pneumonitis with fibrosis. The most common symptom is cough and fever. If severe, there may be dyspnoea on exertion or even at rest. Ronchi and rales may be heard on auscultation in the basal regions of the lungs. A chest X-ray may reveal bilateral infiltrates along with fibrosis. Spirometry may show a restrictive type of lung disease with decreased lung volumes. Occasionally, pulmonary toxicity may manifest as non-cardiogenic pulmonary oedema or hypersensitivity pneumonitis [14].

The genitourinary system: Dehydration and prolonged NSAIDs for pain relief can lead to intrinsic renal failure. Obstruction to the flow of urine by a large pelvic mass can cause post-renal failure. Cisplatinum may cause coagulation necrosis of the proximal and distal renal tubular epithelial cells and the collecting ducts leading to a reduction in the renal blood flow and glomerular filtration rate (GFR). Methotrexate causes acute nephrotoxicity as a result of intratubular precipitation. Concomitant administration with other nephrotoxic drugs like aminoglycosides increases nephrotoxicity.

Hepatic system: Hepatocellular dysfunction because of systemic metastasis or the adverse effects of therapy manifests as diminished synthetic function of the liver with low serum proteins and coagulation abnormalities. Hypoalbuminaemia can predispose to ascites and its consequences.

Haematological complications: Bone marrow suppression because of myelosuppressive chemotherapy is common. Production of blood cells and coagulation factors is impaired, leading to impaired immunity (from neutropenia) or coagulopathy. Anaemia is common. Serum erythropoietin levels are low because of either direct suppression of erythropoietin-producing cells by malignancy or chemotherapy/radiotherapy. Thrombocytopenia may be due to chemotherapy/radiotherapy or splenic sequestration by the primary neoplastic process [15, 16].

Implications: A thorough knowledge of all the above-mentioned changes in various organ systems of the body is crucial in planning proper perioperative management of any patient. A meticulous history and good clinical examination may reveal a compromised organ system which can then be optimised prior to surgery. At the same time, a sound knowledge of the transient effects of various chemotherapeutic agents on the organ systems will avoid unnecessary and unwanted investigations and evaluations.

2 Perioperative Variables and Long-Term Cancer Outcome

In recent times, the perioperative period has gained tremendous importance in terms of cancer recurrence. This period represents a vulnerable phase for any residual disease to spread and cancer re-expression.

Surgical stress induces an inflammatory response, immune suppression, sympathetic nervous system stimulation and neuroendocrine response. All these can favour cancer metastasis and recurrence.

The inflammatory response is mediated by the release of inflammatory cytokines, which helps in wound healing. While promoting antitumour cytotoxicity, it can paradoxically contribute to the tumour growth by angiogenesis to promote wound healing.

Post-surgery, the immune system is depressed, as evident by suppression of NK cell activity, attenuation of inflammatory cytokines, production of anti-inflammatory cytokines and suppression of lymphocyte proliferation along with a downregulation of cell-mediated immunity.

Surgery activates the sympathetic nervous system. This stimulates the hypothalamic-pituitary-adrenal axis and releases catecholamines and glucocorticoids, which has immunomodulating effects [17].

There is a relationship between the sympathetic nervous system and the immune system. There is sympathetic innervation of the lymphoid organs, and they express adrenergic receptors on their cell membranes. Catecholamines also have a direct local modulatory effect on steroid secretions. Catecholamines can exert their immune-suppressive effects by suppressing cellular immunity by decreasing the production of proinflammatory cytokines in addition to suppressing the NK cell, macrophages and cytotoxic T lymphocyte activities.

Multiple perioperative variables like the anaesthesia technique, adequate control of perioperative pain, type of analgesics, blood transfusion, temperature control, and use of β-blockers which influence the inflammatory, immune system, sympathetic nervous system and neuroendocrine system are proposed to influence cancer metastasis and recurrence in recent times. Regional anaesthesia is proposed to reduce cancer recurrence rates by attenuating the sympathetic nervous system response to surgery. Inadequate control of pain theoretically can stimulate the sympathetic nervous system and the neurohumoral response, leading to increased circulating catecholamines and cortisol levels in the perioperative period. Both these can result in immune suppression. Opioids promote cancer recurrence by suppressing the hypothalamic-pituitary-adrenal axis and suppressing stress response, thereby decreasing cortisol levels. Few retrospective studies are done on the association between perioperative blood transfusion and cancer recurrence, and most of these studies are done in the colon and hepatocellular carcinomas [18–20]. Downregulation of the antigen-presenting cells and decreasing number of lymphocytes are few immune-modulating effects of blood transfusion, which are proposed to be the mechanism behind this hypothesis. Intraoperative hypothermia has been linked to immune suppression, which hinders wound healing. This hypothermia-induced immune depression is the reason behind the hypothesis of an association of intraoperative hypothermia and cancer recurrence.

3 Perioperative Fluid Management

Judicious perioperative fluid management is an essential component of cancer surgery. Maintaining an optimum balance of body fluids is crucial for an optimum outcome. ERAS (enhanced recovery after major surgery) protocols aim to maintain euvolemia in preoperative and throughout the surgery [21].

Fluid imbalance is commonly encountered in onco-surgery because of prolonged preoperative fasting, excessive bowel preparation, or an ongoing pathology like bowel obstruction. Blood loss and inadequate fluid replacement further contribute to fluid depletion. In addition, long duration surgery with bowel exposure for prolonged periods, extensive tissue dissection and anaesthesia-related vasodilatation adds to fluid imbalance in the intraoperative period.

ERAS protocol advocates decreasing the preoperative fasting period, limiting bowel preparation to a minimum and carbohydrate loading 2 h before surgery [21].

During the intraoperative period, goal-directed fluid therapy is aimed at striking a balance between intravascular and extravascular compartments. Goal-directed fluid therapy (GDFT) is defined as "the concept of using indices of continuous blood flow and tissue oxygen saturation to optimise end-organ function". ERAS protocol advises balanced electrolyte solution at 1–3 mL/kg/h [21]. GDFT decreases the length of ICU stay, hospital stay and significant complications leading to an improved outcome.

Optimal fluid therapy improves perioperative outcomes and recovery and plays a crucial role in enhanced recovery pathways (ERPs). Improved perioperative fluid management leads to several benefits, including improved pulmonary function, tissue oxygenation, gastrointestinal motility and wound healing.

The three principles of management of fluid balance include:

1. Correct any abnormalities
2. Provide the daily requirements
3. Replace any abnormal and ongoing losses

It is recommended that patients receive 25–35 mL/kg of water per day in the recovery period.

In ERAS guidelines, early oral intake is encouraged postoperatively in all patients whenever possible. This enables IV fluid administration to be discontinued, sometimes even before the patient leaves the post-anaesthesia care unit. This early transition to oral hydration leads to early healing and recovery from surgery and early discharge.

Maintenance fluid therapy should be achieved with an isotonic, balanced crystalloid solution at a rate of 1–3 mL/kg/h.

Excessive fluid administration in the perioperative period must be avoided as it can lead to many detrimental effects. Increased interstitial fluid accumulation can lead to organ dysfunction like pulmonary oedema leading to poor tissue oxygenation, gut oedema leading to bacterial translocation, postoperative ileus, impaired GI function and intolerance for enteral nutrition, delayed wound healing and an increase in acute kidney injury. We should avoid treating perioperative oliguria with excessive IV fluids.

3.1 Recommendations for Perioperative Fluid Therapy in Major Surgery

1. Minimise preoperative fasting times. Encourage unrestricted intake of clear fluids until 2 h before elective surgery [19, 20, 22, 23].
2. A passive leg raising test is useful for predicting fluid responsiveness in haemodynamically unstable adults throughout the perioperative period.
3. Aim for a moderately liberal IV fluid regimen with an overall positive fluid balance of 1–2 L at the end of surgery. For major abdominal surgery, an average crystalloid fluid infusion rate of 10–12 mL/kg/h during surgery and 1.5 mL/kg/h in the first 24 h postoperative period should be used.
4. Ensure that intravascular volume status is optimised before adding vasopressor therapy.
5. Use advanced haemodynamic monitors to measure fluid responsiveness in higher-risk patients.
6. A goal-directed haemodynamic strategy may perform better if a patient's IV fluid status is first optimised, and if needed, introduce a vasopressor or inotrope.
7. Aim for an early transition from IV to oral fluid therapy after surgery.

Goal-directed haemodynamic therapy (GDHT) comprises rational use of fluids, inotropes, vasopressors and red blood cell (RBC) transfusion according to haemodynamic targets to improve oxygen delivery. It can provide outcome benefits in high-risk patients. It has been shown to decrease morbidity and mortality, and it is recommended in enhanced recovery protocols. Although GDHT has not been shown to decrease the overall rate of complications and death in high-risk cancer patients undergoing major abdominal surgeries, it has been associated with a reduced length of hospital stay.

For major surgeries with significant fluid shifts, invasive arterial lines or cardiac output monitors guide fluid therapy. Pulse pressure variation (PPV), stroke volume variation (SVV), systolic blood pressure variation (SVP) and change in inferior vena cava diameter are used as parameters for fluid responsiveness [24].

3.2 Blood Product Replacement

An appropriate assessment of blood loss guides us for adequate blood products replacement. We can use point of care tests to avoid unnecessary transfusion and provide blood and blood products at the earliest. Preoperative correction of anaemia is of utmost importance. It is crucial to follow massive blood transfusion guidelines, use fluid warming devices, point of care testing and maintain electrolyte balance by serial ABG monitoring. Intraoperative use of TEG (thromboelastography) can give additional information on the management of blood and blood products [25]. Coagulation factor replacement can be considered in the presence of bleeding associated with warfarin therapy or vitamin K deficiency, as a part of massive blood transfusion protocol or in the presence of disseminated intravascular coagulation (DIC).

4 Concerns for Gynaecological Cancer Surgery

In addition to the general concerns discussed earlier in the chapter, gynaecological cancers present surgical difficulties because of inaccessible surgical site deep in the pelvic cavity, involvement of other abdominal and pelvic organs and the infiltration of abdominal and pelvic neurovascular bundle involvement. Past history of surgery or radiotherapy further complicates the surgical site by causing adhesions and fibrosis. These patients are prone to deep vein thrombosis (DVT) due to the primary disease, prolonged compression of pelvic vessels by tumour, prolonged surgery, prolonged immobilisation or chemotherapy and erythropoietin-stimulating agent therapy. These patients generally need DVT prophylaxis with low molecular weight heparin. Mechanical thromboprophylaxis devices and early mobilisation also help in preventing DVT. Major fluid shifts are common, especially with hypoalbuminaemia and associated ascites. Careful GDFT starting from the preoperative period is essential for a favourable outcome. Maintaining core body temperature by use of fluid warmers and warming blankets are crucial. Gynaecological cancer surgery involves large abdominal incisions. Adequate pain relief is of utmost importance to decrease the stress response to surgery, facilitate early mobilisation, and prevent atelectasis to the dependent portion of the lungs by making the patient comfortable and encouraging postoperative spirometry and deep breathing exercises. Multimodal analgesia is considered. Epidural catheter insertion, patient-controlled epidural analgesia, patient-controlled intravenous analgesia, TAP block, transversus abdominis plane blocks, etc. are to be considered. Whenever possible, minimally invasive surgical techniques are preferred.

4.1 Anaesthetic Considerations for Carcinoma Vulva and Cervix

Carcinoma vulva and cervix are primarily squamous cell carcinomas. Lymph node involvement is common for cancer vulva. Cancer cervix may spread locally to adjacent structures like vaginal mucosa, paracervical lymph nodes, urinary bladder and rectum. Through bloodstream, it can spread to distant organs like lungs, liver and bones. Vulvectomy with lymph node dissection is the surgery commonly performed for carcinoma vulva. For cancer cervix majority of patients requires radical hysterectomy. In a few cases, patients are subjected to preoperative neoadjuvant chemotherapy and radiotherapy with its resultant complications. Video endoscopic inguinal lymphadenectomy (VEIL) is performed in some centres for carcinoma vulva. These patients are prone to lymphoedema and venous thromboembolism in the postoperative period, requiring DVT prophylaxis, elastic stockings, limb physiotherapy and early mobilisation. Good preoperative optimisation of all the systems and correction of anaemia are vital for a successful outcome. Surgery can be done under regional anaesthesia (subarachnoid block/epidural anaesthesia) or general anaesthesia. Radical hysterectomies are generally done under general anaesthesia supplemented by epidural analgesia. Careful spine assessment should be done in PAC clinic while planning anaesthesia. Maintenance of fluid balance, avoiding dyselectrolytaemia, adequate pain relief, good antibiotic prophylaxis and temperature regulation are vital in the perioperative period.

4.2 Anaesthetic Considerations for Endometrial Cancers

Endometrial cancers are commonly adenocarcinomas. They can be posted for staging laparotomies or definitive resections (total abdominal hysterectomies with bilateral salpingo-oophorectomy and pelvic lymph node dissection). Advanced disease may be posted for palliative procedures. Anaesthetic preparations and considerations are similar to cervical cancer with careful preoperative organ systems optimisation, correction of nutrition, anaemia and dyselectrolytaemia. Maintenance of fluid balance, core body temperature, adequate blood products arrangements in the preoperative period and DVT prophylaxis in the postoperative period is vital.

4.3 Anaesthetic Considerations for Ovarian Cancers

Amongst all gynaecological cancers, ovarian cancer has the poorest prognosis. This is mainly due to late presentation and peritoneal carcinomatosis. Primary cell types of ovarian cancer origin are germ cell tumours, surface epithelium, stromal tumours and primary peritoneal carcinomatosis. These patients may be posted for staging laparotomies or total abdominal hysterectomies with bilateral salpingo-oophorectomy, lymphadenectomy, omentectomy, peritonectomy and search for metastatic deposits (random biopsies) and tumour debulking. More extensive disease with spread to other abdominal and pelvic organs may necessitate a greater extent of resection (cytoreductive surgery). Some patients are posted for interval debulking surgery (surgery planned after a course of induction chemotherapy). Radiotherapy is generally reserved for metastasis.

As is evident from above, these patients pose a significant challenge to the anaesthesiologist. A thorough preoperative history, clinical examination and optimisation are vital for a favourable outcome in the postoperative period. The effect of preoperative chemotherapeutic agents on various organ systems needs to be considered. A thorough cardiac evaluation, including echocardiography and assessment of the left ventricular function, is mandatory. Nutritional status must be improved before surgery to whatever extent possible. The patient must be referred to a physiotherapist, and lung expansion exercises must be started preoperatively. Patients on preoperative diuretics because of impending congestive cardiac failure or ascites are at risk of developing dyselectrolytaemia, which must be corrected preoperatively. Blood loss estimation is difficult in the presence of ascites because of mixed fluids. Large volume fluid shifts may necessitate invasive blood pressure monitoring, central venous catheterisation and adequate blood products arrangement in the preoperative period. Meticulous attention to infection prophylaxis, temperature control avoiding hypothermia, good perioperative analgesia, repeated electrolyte and arterial blood gas analysis and necessary correction, DVT prophylaxis in the postoperative period, early mobilisation, active postoperative physiotherapy and incentive spirometry are crucial. The patient may be electively mechanically ventilated in the postoperative period until stabilisation of all haemodynamic, arterial blood gas parameters and correction of all dyselectrolytaemias. After recovery from anaesthesia, patient-controlled epidural analgesia may be continued. HIPEC (hyperthermic intraperitoneal chemotherapy) involves instilling a high dose heated chemotherapeutic solution into the peritoneal cavity after completion of cytoreductive surgery. This can lead to altered thermoregulation, coagulation abnormalities and haemodynamic abnormalities. There may be protein loss, increased intra-abdominal pressure, increased airway pressure, reduced functional residual volume and increased basal metabolic rate. The carbon dioxide level in blood increases with resultant peripheral vasodilatation and fall in systemic vascular resistance. It is recommended to maintain core body temperature between 35 and 36 °C before starting HIPEC and maintain core body temperature below 38 °C during the procedure.

5 Recent Advances

With advancements in surgical techniques and medical infrastructure, minimally invasive and robotic surgeries are gaining widespread popularity for their apparent advantages over open laparotomies in reducing morbidity and mortality. Common gynaecological robotic surgeries are radial hysterectomy, robotic-assisted vaginal hysterectomy, pelvic and inguinal lymphadenectomy.

5.1 Anaesthetic Considerations for Robotic Surgery

The primary anaesthetic concern in robotic surgery is equipment positioning and avoiding accidental injuries to the patient by the robotic arms and dislodgement of monitor cables, catheters and IV lines by robotic arms. All these need to be secured before the robot is docked, and similar precautions need to be practised when the robot is de-docked. The surgery involves extremes of patient table positioning; as such, the patient needs to be properly secured to the surgical table and all pressure points need to be properly padded. Other concerns are the physiological changes of the steep Trendelenburg position. This can have an effect on the cardiovascular system, pulmonary system, etc. Robotic abdominal surgeries involve peritoneal insufflation with gases. Pneumoperitoneum increases intra-abdominal pressure increasing systemic vascular resistance and mean blood pressure and reducing mesenteric, renal and hepatic blood flow. Pneumoperitoneum also decreases the functional residual capacity. This can lead to atelectasis, increased shunt and a fall in oxygen saturation. In a nutshell, proper patient positioning, avoiding inadvertent injuries from robotic arms, dealing with the physiological changes associated with surgical table positioning and pneumoperitoneum are the keys for robotic surgery anaesthesia management.

6 Conclusion

Gynaecological cancers are on the rise, and more and more patients are subjected to surgery for curative or palliative purposes. These patients need special considerations because of advanced age, late presentation with systemic metastasis, preoperative chemotherapy and radiotherapy effects on other organ systems, poor nutritional status, risk of DVT and difficult surgical access. Minimally invasive surgical techniques and robotic surgeries are coming up, bringing in their challenges and advantages. Good preoperative planning and good teamwork can be a game changer.

References

1. van't Spijker A, Trijsburg RW, Duivenvoorden HJ. Psychological sequelae of cancer diagnosis: a metanalytical review of 58 studies after 1980. Psychosom Med. 1997;59(280):280.
2. Kiecolt-Glaser JK, McGuire L, Robles T, Glaser R. Psychoneuroimmunology: psychological influences on immune function and health. J Consult Clin Psychol. 2002;70:537–47.
3. Nixon DW, Heymsfield SB, Cohen AE, et al. Protein calorie undernutrition in hospitalised cancer patients. Am J Med. 1980;68:683.
4. Frishman WH, Sung HM, Yee HC, et al. Cardiovascular toxicity with cancer chemotherapy. Curr Probl Cancer. 1997;21:301–60.
5. Goldberg MA, Antin JH, Guinan EC, Rappeport JM. Cyclophosphamide cardiotoxicity: an analysis of dosing as a risk factor. Blood. 1986;68:1114–8.
6. Dow E, Schulman H, Agura E. Cyclophosphamide cardiac injury mimicking acute myocardial infarction. Bone Marrow Transplant. 1993;12:169–72.
7. Gardner SF, Lazarus HM, Bednarczyk EM, et al. High-dose cyclophosphamide-induced myocardial damage during BMT: assessment by positron emission tomography. Bone Marrow Transplant. 1993;12:139–44.
8. Gottdiener JS, Appelbaum FR, Ferrang VJ, Deisseroth A, Zeigler J. Cardiotoxicity associated with high dose cyclophosphamide therapy. Arch Intern Med. 1981;141:758–63.
9. Rowinsky EK, McGuire WP, Guarnieri T, et al. Cardiac disturbances during the administration of taxol. J Clin Oncol. 1991;9:1704–12.
10. Aleman BMP, van den Belt-Dusebout AW, Klokman WJ, Van't Veer MB, Bartelink H, van Leeuwen FE. Long-term cause-specific mortality of patients treated for Hodgkin's disease. J Clin Oncol. 2003;21(18):3431–9.
11. Hoppe RT. Hodgkin's disease: complications of therapy and excess mortality. Ann Oncol. 1997;8(1):S115–8.
12. Ng AK, Bernardo MP, Weller E, et al. Long-term survival and competing causes of death in patients with early-stage Hodgkin's disease treated at age 50 or younger. J Clin Oncol. 2002;20(8):2101–8.
13. Swerdlow AJ, Higgins CD, Smith P, et al. Myocardial infarction mortality risk after treatment for Hodgkin disease: a collaborative British cohort study. J Natl Cancer Inst. 2007;99(3):206–14.
14. Rosenow EC III, Myers JL, Swensen SJ, et al. Drug-induced pulmonary disease: an update. Chest. 1992;102:239–50.
15. Gehdoo RP. Anticancer chemotherapy and it's anaesthetic implications (current concepts). Indian J Anaesth. 2009;53(1):18–29.
16. Heyman MR. Cancer and therapy-related hematologic abnormalities. In: Lefor AT, editor. Surgical problems affecting the patient with cancer. Philadelphia: Lippincott Raven; 1996. p. 373–92.
17. Nelson CJ, Lysle DT. Severity, time, and beta-adrenergic receptor involvement in surgery-induced immune alterations. J Surg Res. 1998;80:115–22.
18. Amato A, Pescatori M. Perioperative blood transfusions for the recurrence of colorectal cancer. Cochrane Database Syst Rev. 2006;1:CD005033.
19. Acheson AG, Brookes MJ, Spahn DR. Effects of allogeneic red blood cell transfusions on clinical

outcomes in patients undergoing colorectal cancer surgery: a systematic review and meta-analysis. Ann Surg. 2012;256:235–44.
20. Kuroda S, Tashiro H, Kobayashi T, et al. No impact of perioperative blood transfusion on recurrence of hepatocellular carcinoma after hepatectomy. World J Surg. 2012;36:651–8.
21. Miller TE, Roche AM, Mythen M. Fluid management and goal-directed therapy as an adjunct to Enhanced Recovery After Surgery (ERAS). Can J Anaesth. 2015;62(2):158–68.
22. Ljungqvist O, Søreide E. Preoperative fasting. Br J Surg. 2003;90(4):400–6.
23. Sarin A, Chen LL, Wick EC. Enhanced recovery after surgery—preoperative fasting and glucose loading—a review. J Surg Oncol. 2017;116(5):578–82.
24. Marik PE, Cavallazzi R, Vasu T, Hirani A. Dynamic changes in arterial waveform derived variables and fluid responsiveness in mechanically ventilated patients: a systematic review of the literature. Crit Care Med. 2009;37(9):2642–7.
25. De Pietri L, Montalti R, Begliomini B, et al. Thromboelastographic changes in liver and pancreatic cancer surgery: hypercoagulability, hypocoagulability or normocoagulability? Eur J Anaesthesiol. 2010;27(7):608–16.

Palliative Care in Advanced Gynaecological Malignancy

Kabindra Bhagabati, Sukhdev Nayak, Amal Chandra Kataki, and Debabrata Barmon

Palliative care is the active total care of patients as well as family members to enhance the quality of life with the help of proper symptom control and psychosocial and spiritual supports. It incorporates efforts to relieve sufferings from the time of diagnosis. Palliative care supports the goals of care as well as bereavements after demise [1].

The patient diagnosed with gynaecological malignancy faces myriads of problems encompassing physical as well as psycho-social and spiritual. Early incorporation of palliative care principles is crucial for total care of patients [2]. The four specific aims to care for patients—gather information, transmit information, building relationship, and support patient—as well as the family members help to achieve goals of treatment in gynaecologic cancer patients [2]. With the increased number of cases diagnosed early due to increased awareness and screening camps as well as the advent of newer medicines for chemotherapy, the survival of women with cancer has increased manifold, so also the chances of remission along with lesser physical and mental trauma. Whether medical improvement is possible or not, amelioration of patient's subjective symptoms should be cared for.

A collaborative effort of gynaecologic oncology, palliative care, and other specialties will address the physical, psycho-social, and spiritual needs of the patient. This support should begin at the time of diagnosis transmitted through various treatment procedures culminating in death and bereavement process [1].

1 Communication with Patients

Proper and effective communication with the patient and family members is of utmost importance in advanced gynaecological malignancy. To accept the disease status and prognosis by the patient and relatives, the doctor must have a good communication skill along with a good long-standing relationship with the patient [3]. The relationship can be built over a period of time since the diagnosis of the disease with mutual respect between patient and caregiver with caring team, listening and responding to patient's queries, agreeing on priorities of patient, discussing treatment options, accepting treatment refusals, etc. [4]

K. Bhagabati (✉)
Department of Palliative Medicine, Dr. B. Borooah Cancer Institute (A Unit of Tata Memorial Centre, Mumbai), Guwahati, Assam, India

S. Nayak
Department of Anaesthesiology, AIIMS Bhubaneswar, Oddisha, India

A. C. Kataki · D. Barmon
Department of Gynaecologic Oncology, Dr. Bhubaneswar Borooah Cancer Institute (A Unit of Tata Memorial Centre, Mumbai), Guwahati, Assam, India
e-mail: dydiracademic@bbci.tmc.gov.in

A. C. Kataki, D. Barmon (eds.), *Fundamentals in Gynaecologic Malignancy*,
https://doi.org/10.1007/978-981-19-5860-1_28

Strengths in the Indian health care delivery system need to be built upon, while attention should be paid to developing effective psychosocial interventions, with a robust financial protection plan for patients and their involvement in decision making. Counseling of patients should be made part of a routine protocol. The main themes of communication interview with the patients and the family should cover the six main areas, e.g., Best and worst experiences during the treatment process; Financial and emotional stress; Care giving and social support; Satisfaction with the medical staff; Preferences for a female gynecologist and/or female gynaecology ward; and Prompt and free treatment [5].

The survivals for women with advanced ovarian cancer and others have increased over the years, and it is also common that patients experience recurrences in their course of disease [6].

Supportive communication skills can help reduce anxiety, facilitate coping, and enhance hope in patients and family members.

2 Breaking Bad News

Like other oncology patients, gynaecological cancer patients also need to be communicated the bad news on several occasions, such as disclosing the diagnosis, discussing unexpected findings in surgery, not responding to treatments, cancer progression, etc. If the bad news is communicated poorly, it can lead to stress and anxiety [7]. This has to be learned by meticulous training. A structured training in palliative care improves the medical trainees comfort level in breaking bad news and in communication skill [8]. The "SPIKES method" by Baile et al. from MD Anderson Cancer Centre is a six-step protocol for breaking bad news (Table 1) [9].

It is also important to know certainty of the bad news delivered. A discussion about prognosis and goals of treatment with the patient and relatives will provide a good symptom relief of advanced gynaecologic malignancy [1].

Table 1 SPIKES—a six-step protocol for breaking bad news (Baile et al. The Oncologist 2000, **5**:302–311)

Step I SPIKES	Setting up the interview	– Privacy – Sit down – Make connection with the patient – Interruptions should be avoided
Step II SPIKES	Patient's perception	– What the patient knows – Whether the patient wants to know the diagnosis or status
Step III SPIKES	Invitation	– How the patient wants to have the information about disease
Step IV SPIKES	Knowledge	– Give a warning shot – Wait for reactions – Acknowledge feelings – Avoid giving too much news at a time – Give information in small chunks & reassess patient's understanding
Step V SPIKES	Emotion & empathetic response	– Acknowledge emotions – Know the reasons of emotion – Make empathetic statements
Step VI SPIKES	Strategy & summary	– Know patient's goals/fears – Plan to achieve goals

3 Management of Symptoms

Advanced gynaecologic malignancies lead to several distressing common symptoms in females. Symptomatic management is one of the major arms of palliative care. Scientific principles of symptom management consist of Evaluation, Explanation, Management, Monitoring, and Attention to detail [10].**Evaluation**: To know the cause and pathology of the symptom. It also includes what has been tried and the impact of symptoms on patient's life.

Explanation: To explain to patients and family members about the symptoms in their own language. Also, it is important to answer their questions about symptoms and discuss the treatment options.

Management: To treat the cause if it is treatable. Otherwise, proper medications at adequate dosage to relieve the symptoms should be given. Use of non-drug measures like relaxation therapy also help. Help from other specialties can also be sought for proper management.

Monitoring: The effects of medications should always be reviewed at regular intervals.

Attention to detail: Detailed attention to each and every aspect is necessary for adequate relief from symptoms. An inquisitive mind is necessary for attention to detail [10].

3.1 Dyspnea

Dyspnea is unpleasant awareness of difficulty in breathing. It is a common symptom in advanced cancer patients. It is a subjective symptom and can vary in intensity. If the patient is breathless at rest, the patient is likely to be anxious as well. Dyspnea can be caused by several factors (Table 2) [11].

Table 2 Causes of dyspnea

Caused by cancer	• Pleural effusion • Obstruction of main bronchus • Replacement of lung by cancer • Lymphangitis carcinomatosis • Mediastinal obstruction • Pericardial effusion • Massive ascites • Cachexia–anorexia syndromes
Caused by treatment	• Pneumonectomy • Radiation-induced fibrosis • Chemotherapy – Bleomycin – Doxorubicin
Related to cancer and/or debility	• Anemia • Atelectasis • Pulmonary embolism • Pneumonia • Empyema • Weakness
Concurrent causes	• COPD • Asthma • Heart failure • Acidosis

The management of dyspnea include correct the correctable causes [11]. Opioids like morphine is used to relieve dyspnea. It is started in a low dose like 2.5 mg Q4H and carefully titrated up as side effects like drowsiness may develop. Benzodiazepines like lorazepam 0.5–1 mg PO is useful for patient with anxiety [12]. Bronchodilators may help in COPD, and in patient with smoking history. Diuretics and glucocorticoids may help is heart failure, lymphangitis carcinomatosis, or radiation/chemotherapy-induced pneumonitis [1].

Some supportive measures may be helpful in dyspnea. Relaxation techniques like music, guided imagery, and slow regular deep breathing help to reduce dyspnea. Blowing a gush of air into the face with the help of a fan helps to reduce feelings of dyspnea [1, 11].

3.2 Hemorrhage

Hemorrhage in terminal phases becomes difficult to manage. The blood loss is usually rapid and if not managed on an emergency basis death is inevitable [1].

Hemorrhage can be caused by (i) tumour invasion of blood vessels, (ii) related to causes of treatment—thrombocytopenia and coagulopathy, and (iii) combination of the two. Common sites are usually internal like gastrointestinal, genitourinary, and respiratory tract [1].

Mild bleeding can be controlled by Tranexamic Acid and Ethamsylate. Any hematological deficiency should be corrected. Decision about volume replacement with blood should be on an individual basis. For vaginal bleeding, packing may be necessary to control bleeding. Radiotherapy in high dosage may be successful to control bleeding in vaginal, vulvar, cervical, or uterine cancer.

Hematuria is caused by tumour invasion in vasculature of the genitourinary tract. Hemorrhagic cystitis due to urotoxins from chemotherapy and radiation is another cause of hematuria. Bladder irrigation is first to be tried for the treatment of hematuria. If not controlled then cystoscopy evaluation should be done and coagulation may be necessary [13]. If all fail, then infusion of 1% alum is recommended. If that also doesn't work, administration of PGE2 and silver nitrate is the next step. Formalin can be the last resort to be administered [14].

Identification of patients at risk for bleeding is important. Patient and family members should be empowered to do the following at the earliest [1].

- Use dark towels.
- Apply pressure with pad over the area, if possible.
- Consider narcotics.
- Provide psychological support.
- Ensure presence of a trained personal.
- Bring the patient to hospital, if possible.

3.3 Nausea and Vomiting

Sixty percent of advanced malignancy patients experience nausea and vomiting. Nausea occurs by stimulation of receptors present in the GI tract, chemoreceptor trigger zone, vestibular apparatus, cerebral cortex, etc. [1] The causes include malignant bowel obstruction, cerebral metastasis, drugs like opioids, uremia, electrolyte imbalance, hypercalcemia, etc.

Management include correct the correctable causes—drugs, infection, cough, hypercalcemia, constipation, severe pain, etc. First the anti-emetic for most likely cause should be prescribed on a regular basis. At first, IM or SC route can be used instead of enteral route. Metoclopramide 30–100 mg/24 h SC for gastritis, gastric stasis, and functional bowel obstruction can be used.

For drugs and biochemical causes, Haloperidol 1.5–3 mg PO stat and HS or 2.5–10 mg/24 h SC is the drug of choice. Hyoscine butylbromide 80–160 mg/24 h SC is used for bowel colic or to reduce gastrointestinal secretion. For organic bowel obstruction, raised intracranial pressure, motion sickness, etc., Cyclizine 100–150 mg/24 h can be used [15].

The patient should be reviewed after 24 h. If there is no relief then review the causes; if cause is wrong, alternative first-line anti-emetic should be used in optional dosage. If the cause is right, use first-line in optimal dosage and add second-line anti-emetic [15]. For prokinetic effect, Cisapride 20 mg BD can be used. Broad-spectrum antiemetics Levomepromazine 12.5–25 mg PO HS is the option if first-line anti-emetic does not work. Corticosteroids like Dexamethasone 8–16 mg OD can work as adjuvant anti-emetic. $5HT_3$ receptor antagonist Tropisetron 5 mg PO/SC OD can be used in massive release of 5HT (serotonin) in chemotherapy, abdominal radiation, bowel obstruction, renal failure, etc. [15].

3.4 Anorexia

Anorexia is one of the common symptoms in advanced cancer and is very distressing for family members. Patients having anorexia usually have poor prognosis, lower response rate to treatments, and decreased performance status [16]. In advanced gynaecologic malignances, bowel obstruction is very common and lead to anorexia.

Reversible causes of anorexia, e.g., pain, constipation, hypercalcemia, mucositis, etc., should be treated promptly. Medications can be used in various causes: [1] Prokinetic agents like metoclopramide is helpful for nausea and early satiety; [2] Corticosteroids in low dosage and progesterone agents may be helpful to increase the appetite [17]. It is important to educate the family members about to keep away from force feeding which may cause more suffering to patients. The metabolic derangements due to anorexia and cachexia in terminal phase cannot be reversed by enteral and parenteral nutrition [18]. It is important to listen to and acknowledge the familial worries about not eating and emphasis on balanced diet in terminal stage. Feeding by loved family member with food in a smaller plate is usually encouraging. Providing food of choice when the patient feels like hungry can help [15].

3.5 Malignant Ascites

Ovarian cancer is the most common cause of malignant ascites [1]. The pathophysiology includes lymphatic drainage obstruction, obstruction of hepatic venous system due to tumour invading liver parenchyma. Ascites leads to physical symptoms like distension of abdomen, early satiety, pain, loss of appetite, and dyspnea. Paracentesis is the choice for relief of symptoms [1]. In the terminal phase, it is advisable to do paracentesis when patient has dyspnea. Diuretic therapy is effective for portal hypertension from liver metastasis.

Agents that target vascular endothelial growth factors suppress formation of ascites [19]. Intraperitoneal hypothermic chemotherapy and immunologic therapies are two novel methods is ascites.

3.6 Malignant Bowel Obstruction

Malignant bowel obstruction is very common in gynaecological malignancies, especially in relapsed ovarian cancer. Thirty-five percent relapsed ovarian cancer can lead to intestinal obstruction [1]. Obstruction may be partial or complete and transient or persistent. Patients may commonly have multiple sites of obstruction involving both small and large bowels.

The clinical features of malignant bowel obstruction are abdominal pain, vomiting, intestinal colic, abdominal distension, and constipation. Bowel sounds may vary from absent to hyperperistaltic (Borborygmi) [15].

On diagnosis, conservative treatment should start immediately with intravenous fluid, nasogastric tube aspiration, electrolyte imbalance correction with adequate pain and vomiting control. If it fails, then we may consider surgery, chemotherapy, or medical management [1]. The decision should be individualized for patients and will depend on many factors like extent of disease, overall life expectancy, patient preferences, etc. In malignant bowel obstruction, chemotherapy has no role to play [20, 21].

Surgical intervention is contraindicated in intra-abdominal carcinomatosis and massive ascites; previous operative findings nullify a successful procedure [15]. Surgery can be considered if the cause is easily reversible like, e.g., postoperative adhesions or single neoplastic obstruction; patient's general condition is good and willing to go for surgery [15].

Apart from the conservative measurement, management of intestinal obstruction focuses on relief of nausea and vomiting. If the patient has no or mild colic and passing flatus, a prokinetic drug like Metoclopramide 10 mg Q8H is the choice. Patients with severe colic or not passing flatus, antispasmodic and antisecretory drugs are the choice. Bulk forming, stimulant, and osmotic laxatives should also be stopped [15]. For constant cancer pain, morphine should be continued regularly. If the patient is receiving parenteral medications, opioids can also be administered subcutaneously.

If constipation is a probable cause, then phosphate enema should be given along with a fecal softener, i.e., Docusate Sodium Table 100–200 mg BD. If small bowel is only affected, a colonic stimulant laxative will be useful.

A corticosteroid helps in reducing local edema and improves bowel lumen patency. It also reduces pressure on intestinal nerves and thereby reducing functional obstruction [22].

A persistent complete obstruction may need two classes of drugs—somatostatin analogs, e.g., octreotide. It is an intestinal antisecretory agent but has no antimuscarinic effects; and $5HT_3$ receptor antagonists like Granisetron, Ondansetron, and Tropisetron. 5HT (serotonin) is released from the enterochromaffin cells in bowel wall on raised intraluminal pressure.

3.7 Constipation

Constipation is very common among gynaecologic cancer patients in palliative care [1]. It may be caused by the disease itself or by the side effects of treatments (e.g., drugs like opioids, serotonin antagonists, $5HT_3$ antagonists, etc.). Stimulant laxatives and stool softeners are the choice of medications used for constipation [15]. Senna, Bisacodyl, and Docusate sodium are mostly used for constipation. Osmotic laxatives like Magnesium Hydroxide, Lactulose, PEG, etc. are also useful in constipation.

If the stool is hard and impacted, firstly lubricants (Glycerin suppositories) and enemas (mineral oil, etc.) can be tried. If not relieved, manual evacuation of stool can be done.

The important thing to keep in mind is to rule out bowel obstruction and fecal impaction before initiating treatment for constipation. A bowel regimen consisting of stimulant and fecal softener laxatives should always be prescribed with opioids.

4 Management of Pain

Pain is a common symptom in gynaecologic oncology patients. Evidence-based guidelines for cancer pain management also applies gynaecologic cancers. There are several factors affecting pain threshold [23]. In fatigue, insomnia, discomfort, fear, anxiety, depression, sadness, mental isolation, social isolation etc., pain threshold is lowered and pain is felt easily whereas in relief of symptoms, sleep, relaxation, elevation of mood, companionship, etc., threshold is increased. Pain is often multidimensional—physical, psychological, social, and spiritual. Treating the pain of cancer patients should include care in all four dimensions with a multiprofessional team to get proper relief from pain.

4.1 Evaluation of Pain

Evaluation of pain should involve [23].

- Description of pain.
- Cause of the pain.
- Underlying mechanism.
- Contribution of nonphysical factors.

4.2 Description of Pain

The description of pain needs to be promoted by questions about PQRST characteristics [23] (Table 3). There are several scales used to determine the intensity of pain (Fig. 1).

Table 3 PQRST characteristics for description of pain

P	Palliative factors Provocative factors	What makes it better? What makes it worse?
Q	Quality	What is it like? Is it stabbing, pinching, gnawing, colicky, tingling, burning type?
R	Radiation	Is there any radiation of pain?
S	Severity	How it affects your life?
T	Temporal factors	Is it continuous or intermittent? Is there any diurnal variation?

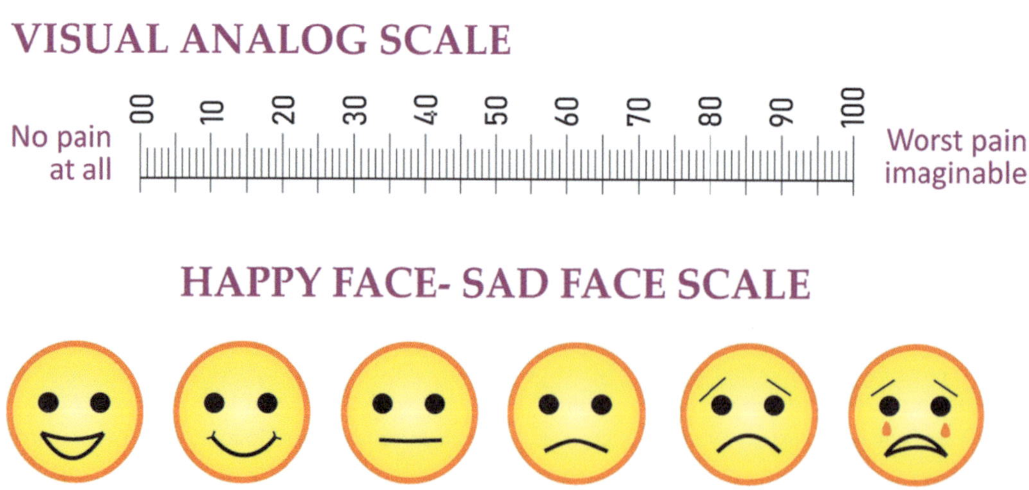

Fig. 1 Pain scales

4.3 Causes of Pain

Pain in cancer can be caused by [24]

- Cancer itself (85% of patients), e.g., soft tissue, visceral, bone, neuropathic.
- Anticancer or other treatment (17%), e.g., chemotherapy-induced mucositis, radiation-induced proctitis.
- Cancer-related debility (9%), e.g., constipation, muscle spasm.
- A concurrent disorder (9%), e.g., spondylosis, osteoarthritis.

4.4 Mechanisms of Pain

It is important to distinguish between functional and pathological pain. Functional pains are caused by everyone's day-to-day activities. Pathological pains can be of two types [23]:

- Nociceptive.
- Neuropathic.

Nociceptive pain is associated with tissue injury. Tissue damage may trigger neuronal activities in nociceptors, which transmit the impulses through dorsal horn of the spinal cord [23].

Neuropathic pain is associated with nerve compression or injury. Causes of neuropathic pain can be due to compression/infiltration of nerve fibers by a tumour in the spinal cord, plexopathy, etc. Anticancer treatment like post-surgical incisional pain, phantom limb pain, chemo- and radiation-induced neuropathy, and concurrent disorders like diabetic neuropathy etc. also can be causes of neuropathic pain.

It is important to distinguish nociceptive pain from neuropathic pain. Nociceptive pain is usually sharp, located in our site, whereas neuropathic pain is described as burning, tingling, shooting type, and have neuro-dermatomal distribution [23].

4.5 Nonphysical Factors

Pain intensity is influenced by nonphysical factors. Help of a psychologist and medical social worker is necessary to evaluate psychosocial factors and to facilitate anxiety, depression, and fears of the patient will lead to success in cancer pain management [23].

4.6 Analgesics

Use of the World Health Organization analgesic ladder helps to control even intractable pain (Fig. 2). Uses of analgesics are governed by the principle—By the mouth, by the clock, and by the ladder. The right dose of a drug for one person may not be suitable for another. There are three classes of analgesics used in cancer pain [23]:

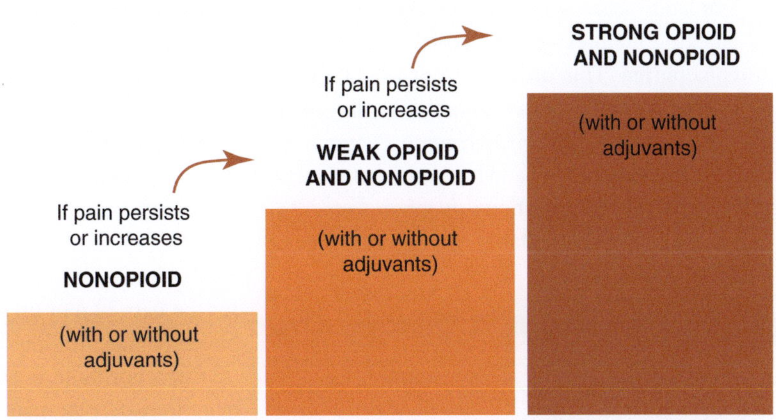

Fig. 2 WHO analgesic ladder

- Nonopioid—NSAIDs, Antipyretics.
- Opioids.
- Adjuvants.

4.7 Nonopioids

NSAIDs are used for pain associated with inflammation [25]. Prostaglandins are produced at the site of inflammation by arachidonic acid pathway which is facilitated by cyclo-oxygenase (COX) [26]. NSAIDs inhibit COX to reduce inflammation and thereby pain.

Paracetamol (Acetaminophen) is an antipyretic analgesic and inhibits cyclo-oxygenase (COX) in the brain [26]. It has peripheral analgesic action but do not have anti-inflammatory property [27].

4.8 Opioids

Weak opioid analgesics available for use are:

Codeine
Dextropropoxyphene
Dihydrocodeine
Pentazocine
Tramadol

Codeine is a prodrug of morphine and is 1/10 as potent as morphine [28]. Dextropropoxyphene is available in combinations only. A study shows that the efficacy of the medicine is not increased with combination.

Tramadol acts via opioid receptors and partly by blocking the presynaptic reuptake of 5HT and norepinephrine. This dual action of tramadol has synergetic action and adverse effects with tramadol are also less [29]. Pentazocine is not used because it is short acting and has psychotomimetic side effects like hallucinations, dysphoria, etc. [23]

Strong opioids available for severe cancer pain are:

Morphine	Methadone
Diamorphine	Fentanyl
Hydromorphone	Buprenorphine
Oxycodone	

Uses of strong opioids are regulated by stringent laws in various countries due to fear of misuse. All the strong opioids are not available in some countries.

Oral morphine is the strong opioid commonly used for relief of severe type cancer pain. Morphine is metabolized to morphine-3-glucuronide (M3G) and morphine-6-glucuronide (M6G). M6G is active and is responsible for pain relief. All are excreted through urine. So, longer duration of action and chances of sedation or respiratory depression seen in renal compromised patients as metabolites are accumulated in the blood [23]. Usually morphine does not cause respiratory depression in patients because pain itself acts as a physiological antagonist to the central depressing effect of morphine [28]. Psychological dependence (addiction) with oral morphine does not occur if the dose of oral morphine is correct for pain relief only [23].

The duration of action of morphine is 3–6 h. So, it is given every 4 h. It is available as immediate release tablets, sustained release tablets, and aqueous solution as injections. The patient should be reviewed after 48 h (24 h in case of elderly). If pain relief is not at least 90%, we can increase the dose by 50% [23]. A double dose at bedtime helps the patient to go through the night without waking up.

Fentanyl is available as transdermal patch and injection. It is a potent μ-receptor agonist. It is used as an alternative strong opioid to oral morphine where:

- Morphine-induced constipation is very severe.
- Intractable vomiting with morphine.
- Difficulty in swallowing food.
- Oral medicine compliance is poor.

Fentanyl has to be applied to a dry, unshaven, non-inflamed, harmless skin for 72 h. It is less constipating and less nauseating than morphine. Plasma concentration is achieved after 36 to 48 h. Rescue dose of oral morphine may be required for the first 24 h or up to 72 h until steady state of plasma concentration of fentanyl is achieved.

Buprenorphine is available as sublingual tablets, transdermal patch, and injection. It is a

Table 4 Side effects of opioids

Side effects	Incidence	Management
Constipation	>90%	Stimulant laxative e.g., bisacodyl 20 mg HS Increase up to 20 mg TDS Stool softener-liquid Paraffin 10 mL TDS
Nausea and vomiting	33%	Haloperidol 1–3 mg HS or Metoclopramide 10 mg TDS Prophylactic antiemetics can be given for first 3 days
Sleepiness	33%	Self-limiting in a week Reduce dose and review
Dry mouth		Mouth care, frequent sips of water, ice cubes
Urinary hesitancy		Tamsulosin 0.4 mg HS
Itching		Keep skin moist, antihistaminic

potent μ-receptor agonist, δ-receptor agonist, and κ-receptor antagonist [23]. Sublingual tablets are 60 times more potent than morphine and are given 8 h. Buprenorphine patch acts for 7 days. It is excreted in stool in unchanged form. Absence of excretion through kidneys makes it a safer drug to use in renal dysfunction [28].

Though opioid-related side effects are common, these can be managed easily. On the other hand, uses of opioid should not be restricted to fear of side effects. The common side effects of opioids and their management are given in Table 4.

5 Bone Metastasis

Though bony metastasis is seen in 1% patients with gynaecological cancer [30], it causes significant symptoms like pain, hypercalcemia, spinal cord compression, pathological fractures, etc. Treatment should be aimed at maintaining a good quality of life and functional independence of patient. Chemotherapy can be considered to control the disease as this will help to control the bony symptoms [31].

Radiation therapy is the treatment of choice for painful bony metastasis and is highly effective with localized symptoms [32]. External beam radiotherapy is given in high-dose single fraction or low-dose multiple fractions depending on extension of disease. Paracetamol is the drug of choice for bony pain. Low-dose opioids may also be needed for proper pain control.

Bisphosphonates help to reduce pain and bone resorption [33]. Zoledronic acid is used as 4 mg in 50 mL of N/S given IV over 15–30 min. Pamidronic acid is used as 60–90 mg in 1000 mL of 0.9% NS over at least 2 h.

Denosumab is a human monoclonal antibody that also protects bone degradation [34]. Metastatic disease to vertebrae may lead to spinal cord compression. Immediate surgical intervention is required to prevent progressive neurological deterioration followed by radiotherapy [35]. It helps to maintain the ability to walk. If neurological damage has started before operation, then our aim would be to prevent further damage with high-dose steroid and radiotherapy [36].

6 Hypercalcemia

Hypercalcemia is an emergency state and is seen in up to 30% of advanced cancer patients [37]. Hypercalcemia may be asymptomatic; when symptomatic, commonly gastrointestinal symptoms like nausea, vomiting, anorexia, constipation, etc. are seen. Polyuria is seen due to impairment of nephron to concentrate urine. As a result, dehydration and neurological symptoms are developed. It starts with irritability and depression and progresses to muscle weakness, delirium, and coma.

Treatment of hypercalcemia should begin promptly with intravascular volume expansion with normal saline. Bisphosphonates can be added for symptomatic patients. For severe hypercalcemia, calcitonin (2–8 IU/kg IM 12 hourly) should be added with bisphosphonates [1].

7 Brain Metastasis

Brain metastasis incidence in gynaecologic malignancies is very low. Brain metastasis should be suspected if the patient presents symptoms like headache, seizures, nausea and vomiting, hemiparesis, disturbances in gait, etc. [38] After proper diagnosis, first-line therapy includes steroids. This helps to reduce the perilesional edema and provides symptom relief. For mild to moderate symptoms, dexamethasone 4–8 mg/day orally is the starting dose which can be increased up to 16 mg/day. For patients with severe symptoms (e.g., intractable vomiting), injectable dexamethasone can be started as 8 mg Q8H or 16 mg/day (single dose) and increased up to 100 mg/day [39]. If radiation is planned, to counteract cerebral edema which can be a side effect of radiation and may worsen in situation, steroids should be started 48 h prior to starting radiation and continued through the course and then taper off after completion of radiation therapy [40]. If seizures are present, antiepileptic drugs like Phenytoin sodium 100 mg TDS should be initiated [41].

Involvement of radiation oncology and neurosurgery is important for providing good symptomatic relief in brain metastasis. If the brain lesions are 1–3 in numbers with poor control of systemic disease, best supportive care or whole brain radiotherapy is recommended [42]. In Patients with stable systemic disease, neurosurgery opinion is taken, whether resectable. With 4 or more metastatic lesion whole brain radiotherapy or stereotactic radio-surgery is recommended [42].

8 As Death Approaches

Increasing weakness day by day may indicate that death is imminent. Companionship and support at this time is of utmost importance. Most patients would prefer to stay and die at home [43]. But one-third of terminally ill cancer patients will spend their last days in a hospital [44]. Quality of life of these patients is worse than those staying at home [45]. With good support from relatives, high quality of care is possible at home. Empowering the caregivers/relatives to care for their patient and an attentive home care team from the hospital responding quickly to new problems are keys to good quality of life of the patient at this hour. Nonsupportive drugs, laboratory tests, and imaging should be stopped. Necessary drugs like opioids, antiemetics, anxiolytics, etc. should be continued as per situation and can be converted to SC or IM or IV route if needed.

Accumulation of bronchial secretions in the airways leading to death rattle is a common symptom in dying patients. Treatment is initiated only if it causes distress to the family members present at the bedside. Repositioning of patient's head helps reduce the airway noise. Glycopyrrolate injection (0.1–0.2 mg IV/SC every 4 h) is usually helpful [46].

Planning for the last days is important, and it requires understanding by the patient and family members of what might happen. Common problems must be discussed beforehand and explained in their languages about the reason and what should be done. Relatives should also be prepared psychologically to cope at that situation. Family members usually want the physical presence of somebody at home who knows the disease or someone whom they can talk to at any time.

References

1. Landrum LM, Blank S, Chen L, Duska L, Bae-Jump V, Lee PS, et al. Comprehensive care in Gynaecologic oncology: the importance of palliative care. Gynecol Oncol. 2015;137:193–202.
2. Smith TJ, Temin S, Alesi ER, Abermethy AP, Balboni TA, Basch EM, et al. American Society of Clinical

Oncology provisional clinical opinion: the integration of palliative care into standard oncology care. J Clin Oncol. 2012;30(8):880–7.
3. Buckman R, Baile WF. Communication Skills. In: Berek JS, Hacker NF, editors. Berek & Hacker's Gynecologic Oncology. 5th ed. Philadelphia: Lippincott Williams & Wilkins, Wolters Kluwer; 2010. p. 820–32.
4. Twycross R. Introducing palliative care. 3rd ed. Oxford: Radcliff Medical Press; 1999. p. 21–36.
5. Pati S, Chauhan AS, Mahapatra S, Nayak S, Nayak S, Weller D. Treatment experiences of women with reproductive cancers in Odisha, India: a qualitative exploration of enablers and barriers. Asian Pac J Cancer Prev. 2017;18(4):1019–24.
6. Armstrong DK. Relapsed ovarian cancer: challenges and management strategies for a chronic disease. Oncologist. 2002;7(Suppl. 5):20–8.
7. Epstein R, Street RL Jr. Patient Centred communication in cancer care : promoting healing and reducing suffering. Bethesda, MD: National Cancer Institute, NIH Publications; 2007.
8. Barth J, Lannen P. Efficacy of communication skills training courses in oncology: a systematic review and meta-analysis. Ann Oncol. 2011;22(5):1030–40.
9. Baile WF, Buckman R, Lenzi R, Glober G, Beale EA, Kudelka AP. SPIKES—a six step protocol for delivering bad news: application to the patient with cancer. Oncologist. 2000;5(4):302–11.
10. Twycross R. Introducing palliative care. 3rd ed. Oxford: Radcliff Medical Press; 1999. p. 61–5.
11. Twycross R. Introducing palliative care. 3rd ed. Oxford: Radcliff Medical Press; 1999. p. 120–6.
12. NCCN Practice Guidelines in Oncology: Palliative care version 2.2014:2014.
13. Bagley D. In: Smith A, editor. Treatment of hematuria. Philadelphia: WB Saunders; 1999.
14. Donahue IA, Frank IN. Intravesical formalin for hemorrhagic cystitis: analysis of therapy. J Urol. 1989;141(4):809–12.
15. Twycross R. Introducing palliative care. 3rd ed. Oxford: Radcliff Medical Press; 1999. p. 113–20.
16. DeWys WD, Begg C, Lavin PT, Band PR, Bennet JM, Bertino JR, et al. Prognostic affect of weight loss prior to chemotherapy in cancer patients. Eastern co-operative Oncology Group. Am J Med. 1980;69(4):491–7.
17. Miller S, Mc Nutt L, McCann MA, McCorry N. Use of corticosteroids for anorexia in palliative medicine: a systematic review. J Palliat Med. 2014;17(4):482–5.
18. Mercadante S. Parenteral versus enteral nutrition in cancer patients: indications and practice. Support Care Cancer. 1998;6(2):85–93.
19. Yukita A, Asano M, Okamoto T, Mizutani S, Suzuki H. Suppression of ascites formation and re-accumulation associated with human ovarian cancer by an anti-VPF monoclonal antibody in vivo. Anticancer Res. 2000;20(1A):155–60.
20. Kolomainen DF, Barton DP. Surgical management of bowel obstruction in gynecological malignancies. Curr Opin Support Palliat Care. 2011;5(1):55–9.
21. Diver E, O'Connor O, Garett L, Bornta D, Goodman A, Del CM, et al. Modest benefit of total parenteral nutrition and chemotherapy after venting gastrostomy tube placement. Gynecol Oncol. 2013;129(2):322–5.
22. Harris AL, Cantwell BMJ. Mechanisms and treatment of cytotoxic induced nausea and vomiting. In: Devis CJ, Lake-Bakaar GV, Grahame-Smith DG, editors. Nausea and vomiting : mechanisms and treatment. Berlin: Springer-Verlag; 1986. p. 78–93.
23. Twycross R. Introducing palliative care. 3rd ed. Oxford: Radcliff Medical Press; 1999. p. 65–99.
24. Grond S, et al. Assessment of cancer pain: a prospective evaluation in 2266 cancer patients referred to a pain service. Pain. 1996;64:107–14.
25. Yaksh TL, et al. Mechanism of action of non-steroidal anti-inflammatory drugs. Cancer Investig. 1998;16:509–27.
26. Flower RJ, Vane JR. Inhibition of prostaglandin syntheses in brain explains the antipyretic activity of paracetamol. Nature. 1972;240:410–1.
27. Moore UJ, et al. The efficacy of locally applied aspirin and acetaminophen in postoperative pain after third molar surgery. Clin Pharmacol Ther. 1992;52:292–6.
28. Fallon M, Cherny NI, Hanks G. Opioid analgesic therapy. In: Hanks G, Cherny NI, Christakis NA, Fallon M, Kassa S, Portenoy RK, editors. Oxford textbook of palliative medicine. 4th ed. Oxford: Oxford University Press; 2010. p. 661–98.
29. Vickers MD, et al. Tramadol: pain relief by an opioid without depression of respiration. Anaesthesia. 1992;47:291–6.
30. Thanapprapasr D, Nartthanarung A, Likittanasombert P, Na Ayudhya NI, Charakom C, Udomsubpayakul U, et al. Bone metastasis in cervical cancer patients over a 10 year period. Int J Gynecol Cancer. 2010;20(3):373–8.
31. Uccella S, Morris JM, Bakkum Gomez JN, Keeney GL, Podratz KC, Mariani A. Bone metastasis in endometrial cancer: report on 19 patients and review of the medical literature. Gynecol Oncol. 2013;130(3):474–82.
32. Chow E, Harris K, Fan G, Tsao M, Sze WH. Palliative radiotherapy trials for bone metastasis: a systematic review. J Clin Oncol. 2007;25(11):1423–36.
33. Kohno N, Aogi K, Minami H, Nakamura S, Asaga T, Lino Y, et al. Zoledronic acid significantly reduces skeletal complications compared with placebo in Japanese women with bone metastases from breast cancer: a randomized placebo controlled trial. J Clin Oncol. 2005;23(15):3314–21.
34. Stopeck AT, Lipton A, Body JJ, Stegger GG, Toukin K, de Boer RH, et al. Denosumab compared with Zoledronic acid for the treatment of bone metastasis in patients with advanced breast cancer: a randomized double-blind study. J Clin Oncol. 2010;28(35):5132–9.
35. Patchell RA, Tibbs PA, Regine WF, Payne R, Saris S, Kryscio RJ, et al. Direct de-compressive surgical resection in the treatment of spinal cord compression caused by metastatic cancer: a randomized trial. Lancet. 2005;366(9486):643–8.

36. Chi JH, Gokaslan ZL. Vertebroplasty and kyphoplasty for spinal metastases. Curr Opin Support Palliat Care. 2008;2(1):9–13.
37. Grill V, Matin TJ. Hypercalcemia of malignancy. Rev Endocr Metab Disord. 2000;1(4):253–63.
38. Ratner ES, Toy E, Q' Malley DM, McAlpine J, Rutherford TJ, Azodi M, et al. Brain metastases in epithelial ovarian and primary peritoneal carcinoma. Int J Gynecol Cancer. 2009;19(5):856–9.
39. Vick NA, Wilson CB. Total care of the patient with a brain tumour with consideration of some ethical issues. Neurol Clin. 1985;3(4):705–10.
40. Ryken TC, McDermott M, Robinson PD, Ammirati M, Andrews DW. Asher Al et al. the role of steroids in the malignant of brain metastasis: a systematic review and evidence based clinical practice guideline. J Neurooncol. 2010;96(1):103–14.
41. Mikkelsen T, Paledogos NA, Robinson PD, Ammirati M, Andrews DW, Al A, et al. The role of prophylactic anticonvulsants in the management of brain metastases: a systematic review and evidence based clinical practice guideline. J Neurooncol. 2010;96(1):97–102.
42. NCCN Practice Guidelines in Oncology: Central Nervous System Cancers version 2. 2014: 2014.
43. Bruera E, Russel N, Sweeney C, Fisch M, Palmer JL. Place of death and its predictors for local patients registered at a comprehensive cancer center. J Clin Oncol. 2002;20(8):2127–33.
44. Goodman DC, Morden NE, Chang CH, Fisher ES, Wennberg JE. In: Bronner KK, editor. Trends in cancer care near the end of life: a dartmouth atlas of health care brief. Lebanon, NH: The Dartmouth Institute for Health Policy and Clinical Practices; 2013.
45. Wright AA, Keating NL, Balboni TA, Matulonis UA, Block SD, Prigerson HG. Place of Death: correlations with Quality of Life of Patients with Cancer and Predictors of bereaved caregivers' mental health. J Clin Oncol. 2010;28(29):4457–64.
46. Bennet M, Lucas V, Brennan M, Hughes A, O'Donnel V, Wee B. Using anti-muscarinic drugs in the management of death rattle: evidence-based guidelines for palliative care. Palliat Med. 2002;16(5):369–74.

Gynaecological Cancers and Nursing

Minoti Baruah, Anil K. Mathew, Amal Chandra Kataki, and Debabrata Barmon

Nursing roles have been evolving to meet the demands of the ever-changing landscape of cancer care and improved survival. The treatment for gynaecological cancer varies depending on the type and stage of cancer. The treatment for gynaecological cancer may be a single approach or a multi-modality treatment with the options ranging from surgery, radiotherapy, chemotherapy, hormonal and targeted therapies [1].

Cancer care has eleven areas identified by the Oncology Nursing Society (ONS) and the American Nurses Association (ANS) [2] which need focused attention. These are Prevention and Early Detection, Information, Coping, Comfort, Nutrition, Protection, Mobility, Elimination, Sexuality, Ventilation, and Circulation.

ONS and ANA in 2004 added establishing research priorities, focusing nursing research on problems experienced in the real world of nursing practice and evidence-based practice into their scope and standards [2]. In the systemic review conducted by Cook et al., it was seen that the specialist nurse offers tailored, accessible, and expert care to women with gynaecological cancer. Specialist nurses could afford more time to spend with patients hence enable greater exploration and identification of patient needs and the provision of personalized care [3].

The scope of oncology nursing practice thus encompasses clinical practice, education, consultation, research, and administration. Nurses involved in cancer care have the responsibility to develop and demonstrate knowledge and skills that display competence in the field.

To render effective nursing care, the patient's actual and potential problems have to be assessed. The assessment is either:

(a) **Subjective**—wherein the clients' awareness of diagnosis, modality of treatment, and prognosis has been understood or misinterpreted is assessed.

Coping skills of the patient are assessed and need for verbalization or further counseling is identified. Emotional reactions to diagnostic tests and prognosis are assessed, as is the ability to cope with many assaults to body image throughout the course of disease and treatment.

M. Baruah (✉)
Department of Anaesthesiology, Dr. B. Borooah Cancer Institute (A Unit of Tata Memorial Centre, Mumbai), Guwahati, Assam, India
e-mail: med.sup.bbci@gamail.com

A. K. Mathew
Dr. B. Borooah Cancer Institute, Guwahati, Assam, India

A. C. Kataki · D. Barmon
Department of Gynaecologic Oncology, Dr. Bhubaneswar Borooah Cancer Institute (A Unit of Tata Memorial Centre, Mumbai), Guwahati, Assam, India
e-mail: dydiracademic@bbci.tmc.gov.in

A. C. Kataki, D. Barmon (eds.), *Fundamentals in Gynaecologic Malignancy*,
https://doi.org/10.1007/978-981-19-5860-1_29

(b) Objective
  (i) Assess for factors that can promote infection.
  (ii) Monitor factors that may contribute to bleeding.
  (iii) Assess nutritional status.
  (iv) Pain assessment.
  (v) Rehabilitation.

1 Pre- and Postoperative Care of a Patient Undergoing Surgery for Gynaecologic Cancers

Cancer patients undergoing surgery often present with unusual and challenging problems. Chronic illness and risk factors such as malnutrition, anemia, and substance abuse increase the risks associated with surgical interventions. Detailed counseling and preoperative education should be undertaken so that patients are psychologically prepared and have clear expectations and goals for their recovery.

Enhanced and early recovery after surgery, needs patient to be mobilized early and encouraged to walk in the ward. Prolonged postoperative stay in bed is associated with atelectasis and deep vein thrombosis. Prolonged bed rest after abdominal surgery is associated with a threefold increase in pulmonary complications. A multimodal postoperative pain regime is utilized for adequate pain relief.

Patients may be allowed liquids on the evening of surgery and low-residue diet early, if tolerated, as a part of ERAS. Delayed resumption of diet leads to increased morbidity and prolonged postoperative ileus, leading to increased morbidity and prolonged postoperative ileus, leading to an increased length of stay.

2 Management of Patients with Stoma

Preoperative counseling where the patient's attitude towards the surgery and feeling about having a stoma is assessed and discussed with patients and caregivers. Need for thorough bowel preparation and dietary restrictions is explained to the patient. The procedure is explained so that the patient is fully conversant with what to expect after surgery.

Immediate postoperative care includes pouching the stoma with a clear and drainable pouch and assessing for bleeding and necrosis. Temperature of the stoma should be warm, color reddish pink and shiny while protrusion from abdominal wall should be 1-3 cm. Peristomal skin should be normal and healthy. To see for functioning of the stoma, colostomy will function within 4–5 days when peristalsis starts while ileostomy functions within 24–48 h. Intensive counseling is to be done to improve psychological and emotional health and to achieve independence in stoma care and resumption of normal activities.

Late postoperative care, prior to discharge from hospital, is where the patient should be able to carry out appliance change correctly without aid. The patient or caregiver should be able to prepare an appliance correctly, empty drainable appliances, and correctly use the clip. Irrigation of end colostomy should be taught as should be skin care and appliance hygiene. Normal low residual food should be advised and encouragement provided to lead a healthy life.

Most cancer patients undergo treatment with some form of chemotherapy and have central venous catheters implanted for ease of intravenous access and to avoid multiple punctures to administer the chemotherapeutic agents. These central venous catheters are in place for prolonged periods and need proper care and maintenance to maintain patency and to keep the site free from infection. Table 1 depicts standard care and maintenance of central venous catheter devices.

Nursing considerations in gynaecological cancers can be tumour specific and site specific. Common manifestations of symptoms and their associated sites are grouped together for an overview, while the associated nursing actions and interventions are in Table 2.

Table 1 Care and maintenance of central venous catheter devices

	Tunneled	Non-tunneled	Port
Site care	Transparent dressing weekly Gauze dressing every 48 h	Transparent dressing weekly Gauze dressing every 48 h	No need First 10 postoperative days clean and keep dry
Flushing	**Open end**—Heparin solution, 5 mL (10 i.u/mL) twice weekly **Close end**—Normal saline volume 10 mL once a week	**Open end**—Heparin solution 5 mL (10 i.u/mL) twice a week **Closed end**—Normal saline volume 10 mL once a week	**Open end**—Heparin solution volume 10 mL (100 i.u/mL) once a month **Closed end**—Heparin solution volume 10 mL (100 i.u/mL) once in three months

Table 2 Actions and interventions (nursing)

Identification	Dysfunction	Action/intervention
Removal of organ/tissue Uterus Ovaries Cervix Shortened vagina Bowel Bladder Lymph nodes	Physical Structural Functional changes Psychological changes: Loss of fertility Loss of self-identity Loss of feminity	Infertility support Dilator support Psychosexual counselling Pain therapy Psychosocial support
Removal of organs Clitoris Labia majora Labia minora **Alteration of structure** Clitoris Anal sphincter Urethra Introitus	Impacts sexual health Body image Fibrosis of orifices Interruption/damage to muscle control Urine dysfunction Fecal incontinence	Continence advisor Use of funnel to avoid spraying of urine Enhance positive body image
Assessment of wound	Infection Poor healing Disease—fungation Hygiene Excoriation Contamination by urine or feces	Early intervention Measures to eliminate odor Address hygiene issues
Lymphedema	Altered body image Social implications viz. clothes/shoes/equipment/financial Physical pain Infection Mobility issues	Encourage mobility Body positivity Skin care Compression hosiery
Pruritus	Cause Biochemical Drug related Environmental Clothing	Keep the area cool Rub rather than scratch Dry skin emollients Menthol Calamine Cotton bedding and clothing
Fibrosis of vagina	Pain/discomfort Sexual health	Topical lubricants Psychosexual support
Urinary disturbances **Bowel problems** **Stoma formation**	Continence Body image Skin care Underwear Pads	Medication—Codeine, Imodium Maintain comfort Skin care

3 Tumour-Specific Considerations (Nursing) [4]

Site-wise most common problems include:

3.1 Cervical Cancer

Pain.
Vaginal bleeding and discharge.
Fistula/stoma formation.
Difficulty in passing urine/feces.
Renal failure.
Lymphedema.
Hypercalcemia.
Deep venous thrombosis.

Advanced disease—palliative care.

Palliative care aims to improve the quality of life. As the disease advances, it needs to be holistically managed considering the woman as a whole individual entity within the frame of physical, psychological, and social well-being.

3.2 Vulva

Fungation of wound.
Neuropathic pain.
Bleeding or discharge.
Deep vein thrombosis.
Renal failure.
Skin problems.
Positioning.
Mobility.
Sexual health.

3.3 Endometrium and Ovary

Pain.
Ascites.
Breathlessness.
Neuropathic pain.
Bleeding or discharge.
Renal failure.
Difficulty in passing urine/feces.
Lymphedema.
Deep vein thrombosis.
Hypercalcemia.

Over time women suffering from gynaecologic cancers under multiple procedures and treatment protocols have a negative effect on the quality of life with respect to sexual and reproductive ability as well as body image [5, 6]. Patients can experience numerous symptoms during diagnosis and treatment [7–10]. Symptoms-related discomforts adversely affect the patients and their families resulting in poor treatment adherence [10].

The Society for Gynaecologic Oncology (SGO) has laid stress that women with terminal or relapsed gynaecological cancers should receive basic palliative care without delay and should get special palliative care when appropriate. [11, 12] Nurses are in constant touch with patients and their families, thus most suited to assess needs and deliver care to such patients [13, 14].

A significant number (83%) of admitted patients with gynaecologic cancers require supportive nursing care in contrast with 40% of outpatients with akin disease [15]. These two groups of cancer patients may necessitate different supportive care to meet their physical, psychological, social, spiritual, sexual, and practical information needs [16].

Palliative care can be used as a treatment for patients with advanced cancer diagnosis; early palliative care can improve quality of life and prolong survival [17]. Palliative care focuses on improving quality of life of patients and families in the face of life-threatening problems, through prevention, recovery by identifying early treatment of physical, psychosocial, and spiritual needs [18].

Nurses by the very nature of their jobs develop a uniquely empathetic relationship with their patients afflicted by cancer, where the nurse can access and assess the needs of the patient. The key to all nursing and supportive care is through assessment.

- It identifies people who need help/support with physical, psychological, spiritual, social, and sexual effects.
- It provides the opportunity for the person to think through their needs and together with the nurse make a plan about how to best meet this need.
- It promotes and helps with self-management.
- It helps health teams target support and care effectively and efficiently by making appropriate informed decisions.

Despite the availability of the Papanicolaou's smear for over 60 years and the cervix being an accessible part of the anatomy a significant percentage of women remain unscreened. The nursing professional can play a pivotal role in increasing the number of women who participate in cervical cancer screening programs. Nursing professionals have made immense contributions to the development of behavioral interventions that influence PAP testing [19] or alternative proven method of screening.

4 Special Roles of the Oncology Clinical Nurse Specialist

With respect to oncology nursing there is a considerable overlap of responsibilities. But there are aspects in the context of gynaecological nursing, and in particular vulvar cancer which the specialized nursing personal needs to address and emphasize.

(A) As a communicator:

For a patient who has just been diagnosed with gynaecological cancer the emotional and psychological turmoil is very detrimental. It affects the patient's personal as well as social life equally. The sense of disfigurement is arguably greater for vulval cancer than other gynaecological cancers. Now this is a juncture where the patient compliance is necessary to progress with the best possible treatment. Naturally, the patient would look up for help and the Clinical Nurse Specialist (CNS) can be a great source of support and strength for her as well as her relatives. When a medically specialized nurse is alongside the patient across the length of the treatment, she would be able to answer most of her queries and attend to her nursing needs [20].

(B) The role of specialized oncology nurse in sexuality and other quality-of-life issues:

All sexually active patients as well as their partners should receive specific information with the emphasis on the effects of surgery or adjunct treatment on their relationship. Addressing sexuality issues requires training, speaking skills, and confidence. The person delivering the counseling should be comfortable as well as in a position to talk comprehensively about the subject. This is a very important role which a specialized clinical nurse can execute through a proactive and holistic approach. [21]

Maughan et al. conducted a randomized control trial involving 36 women and data collected using the quality-of-life measure (the EORTC QLQ-30) and the Lasry Sexual functioning scale. The group which received specialist psychosexual counseling showed better results as well as treatment compliance. [22]

(C) Informational needs:

A nursing personnel trained in gynaecological cancer has a holistic knowledge of the disease, its treatment modalities, respective complications as well as its management. The patient interaction with nursing specialist will begin right from the diagnosis progressing through her counseling, treatment, and follow-up period at the center. This cumulative experience will eventually affect the quality of life (QoL) of the patient.

When a treatment decision is taken a clear rationale behind the treatment option is chosen and the potential outcome of the same has to be explained to the patient. Ideally, the patient should have an understanding to her level of satisfaction. [23]

It is usually seen that the preoperative ward rounds are done by the consultant and residents. If the oncology nursing specialist accompanies the team during the discussion this can be a good practice and a great platform for patient-centered discussion.

5 Conclusion

The optimum care of gynaecologic cancer patients not only depends on the correct diagnosis and appropriate treatment but also seeing to the concern that the patient is involved in the decision-making process. Without the involvement of a trained oncology nursing professional, many women would not truly understand their illness and treatment rationale. This in turn will adversely affect the prognosis as well as their response to life crisis. The nursing focus on healthcare for women with gynaecologic cancers includes both rational and human approach. The primary need of the patients to achieve cure and be given emotional support necessitates nursing care which is available, competent and coordinated.

References

1. BGCS. BGCS: Guidelines. British Gynaecologic Cancer Society. Available from: http://www.esmo.org/Guidelines/GynaecologicalCancers. Accessed 10 May 2018.
2. Lubejko B, Wilson B. Scope and standards of oncology nursing practice. Oncology Nursing Society guidelines 2019.
3. Cook O, McIntyre M, Recoche K, Lee S. Experiences of gynecological cancer patients receiving care from specialist nurses: a qualitative systematic review. JBI Database System Rev Implement Rep. 2017;15(8):2087–112. https://doi.org/10.11124/JBISRIR-2016-003126.
4. https://www.nwcscnsenate.nhs.uk/files/gynae
5. Nazik E, Ozdemir F, Soydan S. Social support and quality of life in Turkish patients with gynaecologic cancer. Asian Pac J Cancer Prev. 2014;15:3081–6.
6. Terzioglu F, Sahan UF. Palliative care in gynaecologic cancers. J Palliat Care Med. 2016;6:1–3.
7. Pathy S, Raheja SG, Rakhi S. Palliative care in advanced gynaecologic cancers: Institute of Palliative Medicine experience. Indian J Palliat Care. 2008;14:86–9.
8. Mishra K. Gynaecological malignancies from palliative care perspective. Indian J Palliat Care. 2011;17:45–51.
9. Rezk Y, Timmins PF, Smith HS. Palliative care in gynaecologic oncology. Am J Hosp Palliat Care. 2011;28:356–74.
10. Smith TJ, Temin S, Alesi ER, Abernethy AP, Balboni TA. American Society of Clinical Oncology, provisional clinical opinion: the integration of palliative care into standard oncology care. J Clin Oncol. 2012;30:880–7.
11. https://www.sgo.org/choosingwisely
12. https://www.who.int/cancer/media/FINAL-palliativecare module.pdf
13. Prem V, Karvannan H, Kumar SP, Karthikbabu S, Syed N, et al. Study of nurses knowledge about palliative care: a quantitative cross-sectional survey. Indian J Palliat Care. 2012;18:122–7.
14. Mawardika T, et al. BMC Nurs. 2019;18(Suppl. 1):28.
15. Bonnachi A, et al. Use of needs evaluation questionnaire with cancer outpatients. Support Care Cancer. 2016;24(8):3507–15.
16. Temel JS, et al. Early palliative care for patients with metastatic non-small-cell lung cancer. New Eng JMed. 2010;363:733–42.
17. https://www.who.int/cancer/palliative/def/en
18. Hilton LW, et al. The role of nursing in cervical cancer prevention and treatment. Presented at Second International Conference on Cervical Cancer, Houston, Texas 2002 11–14.
19. Ekwall E, et al. Important aspects of healthcare for women with gynaecologic cancer. Oncol Nurs Forum. 2003;30(2):313–9.
20. McCreadie M. The role of the clinical nurse specialist. Nurs Stand. 2001;16:33–5.
21. Corney R, Everett H, Howells A, Crowther M. The care of patients undergoing surgery for gynaecological cancer: the need for information, emotional support and counselling. J Adv Nurs. 1992;17:667–71.
22. Maughan K, Clarke C. The effect of a clinical nurse specialist in gynaecological oncology on quality of life and sexuality. J Clin Nurs. 2001;10(2):221–9.

NHS Centre for Reviews and Dissemination. University of York, informing, communicating and sharing decisions with people who have cancer. Effective Health Care Bull. 2000;6:1–8.

Prevention and Screening in Gynaecological Cancer

Abhishek Shankar, Amal Chandra Kataki, Deepak Saini, and Pritanjali Singh

1 Introduction

Women comprise nearly half of the overall population, and cancer is one of the leading causes among women in both developed and developing countries. According to the International Agency for Research on Cancer (IARC), 20% of the population develop cancer at some stage of their lives and mortality among women remains 1 out of 11 in comparison to one out of eight in men [1]. Around half of new cases and nearly 60% of deaths in women were contributed by cancer in low- and middle-income countries (LMICs) [2]. Every fourth cancer diagnosed in women is breast cancer followed by colorectum, lung, and cervix uteri. Gynaecological cancers, i.e., breast, cervix, ovary, uterus or endometrium, vagina, and vulva, account for nearly one fourth of incidence and deaths of overall cancer cases in LMICs [3]. Breast cancer incidence has surpassed lung cancer due to increasing number of new cases in LMICs and particularly in Asian region. Almost two in every five cases of breast cancer and uterine cancer and every second case of cervical, ovarian, and vaginal cancer are reported in terms of incidence, mortality, and prevalence [1, 3].

High incidence and prevalence of gynaecological cancers remain a challenging issue despite availability of preventive methods such as improved disease awareness and health seeking behavior, effective screening, chemoprevention, and vaccination [4]. LMICs report higher cases of gynaecological cancer in comparison to High Income Countries (HICs) [2, 3]. Advanced stage at presentation of gynaecological cancers is common in LMICs where effective preventive strategies and screening of gynaecological cancers can play an important role in reducing the burden and early detection and treatment [4].

A. Shankar (✉) · P. Singh
Department of Radiation Oncology, All India Institute of Medical Sciences, Patna, Bihar, India

A. C. Kataki
Department of Gynaecologic Oncology, Dr. Bhubaneswar Borooah Cancer Institute (A Unit of Tata Memorial Centre, Mumbai), Guwahati, Assam, India

D. Saini
Department of Materia Medica, State Lal Bahadur Shastri Homoeopathic Medical College & Hospital, Prayagraj, India

2 Primary Prevention in Gynaecological Cancers

2.1 Health Promotion

Healthy activities play an important role in reducing cancer risks. Risk factors such as obesity, smoking, tobacco and alcohol consumption, and low dietary fiber intake increase the chances of developing gynaecological cancer. Health

A. C. Kataki, D. Barmon (eds.), *Fundamentals in Gynaecologic Malignancy*,
https://doi.org/10.1007/978-981-19-5860-1_30

promotion is the cost-effective intervention to address the risk factors through various awareness campaigns using all the health communication channels [4, 5]. Physical activity reduces the development of breast cancer and endometrial cancer while smoking is emerging as a major risk factor for gynaecological cancers. Just 1 h/day for 5 days in a week of exercise is enough for risk reduction of breast cancer [4, 6, 7]. A study conducted in Canada demonstrated the role of obesity in increasing the risk of breast and ovarian cancers by twofold [8]. Also, sanitization and personal hygiene reduce the infectious causes of cervical cancer, which is caused primarily by Human Papilloma Virus (HPV) [4].

2.2 Cancer Education

Awareness and education regarding knowledge and information about signs and symptoms of gynaecological cancers may help in reducing the morbidity and mortality by ensuring early detection through screening. Breast lump is the most common presentation in case of breast cancer, whereas abnormal bleeding or discharge per vagina and back pain with fatigue are common presentations for cervical, endometrial, and ovarian cancers [9–11]. Many signs and symptoms of various gynaecological cancers are similar in presentation except breast [12–16].

There is an increase in general awareness about signs and symptoms of gynaecological cancers in LMICs but there is a rural and urban divide [17, 18]. Table 1 contains information about common signs and symptoms of various gynaecological cancers.

3 Prevention and Screening in Gynaecological Cancers

3.1 Breast Cancer

Every fourth cancer diagnosed in women is breast cancer. Every one tenth new cases of cancer is breast cancer and nearly every 1 in 20 deaths is due to breast cancer. Currently LMICs are contributing nearly two thirds of overall breast cancer burden with Asia region on the top [3].

There are few methods for early detection of breast cancer including Breast Self-Examination,

Table 1 Common signs and symptoms of gynaecological cancers

Cancer type	Signs and symptom
Breast	• Breast lump
	• Lump in axilla
	• Thickening or changes of breast skin, shape, or size
	• Nipple retraction or discharge
	• Pain or redness in region of breast
Cervical	• Bleeding—between periods, after menopause, after intercourse
	• Offensive vaginal discharges
	• Lower back or abdominal pain
Ovarian	• Bleeding after menopause
	• Abnormal vaginal discharges
	• Continuous pelvic or abdominal pain
	• Change in stool or micturition habit
Endometrial	• Abnormal vaginal bleeding or discharges
	• Pelvic pain
Vaginal	• Abnormal vaginal bleeding or discharges
	• Change in stool or micturition habit
	• Lower back or abdominal pain
Vulval	• Skin or color change at vulvar region
	• Pain during micturition or intercourse
	• Itching, lump or ulcer at vulvar region

Clinical breast examination, and Mammography. Mammography is widely practiced and recommended for breast cancer screening [4]. Various organizations recommend mammography as age-specific screening for breast cancer and are listed in Table 2.

Chemoprevention of breast cancer is an active area of research where many therapeutic agents have been tested so far. Currently, Tamoxifen and Raloxifene are being recommended by US health authorities for chemoprevention of breast cancer. In high-risk and asymptomatic groups, use of Tamoxifen decreases the risk of developing breast cancer by half [4].

3.2 Cervical Cancer

Cervical cancer is the second most common gynaecological cancer in LMICs. Though preventable, nearly 83% of total diagnosed cervical cancer cases and 85% cervical cancer deaths are reported from LMICs [19]. Human Papilloma Virus (HPV) is the causative agent of every nine in ten cases of cervical cancer; HPV 16 and HPV 18 strain accounts for nearly 3/4th of the total cervical cancer cases. HICs have successfully managed to reduce cervical cancer burden through HPV vaccination and with continuation of screening services [4, 19].

Cervical cytology examination and HPV DNA examination have been found to be associated with reduction in total burden of cervical cancer in high income countries. Screening practices are limited to urban areas and that too is very limited. Visual inspection with acetic acid (VIA) has been found cost-effective in screening cervical cancer in population-based settings, but HPV DNA and cervical cytology examinations are most effective and accurate [20].

Different screening methods for cervical cancer are listed in Table 3.

3.2.1 HPV Vaccination

HPV vaccination is the most effective method for cervical cancer prevention with efficacy of nearly

Table 2 Breast cancer screening recommendations

Organization	Age	Recommendations
US Preventive Services Task Force (USPSTF)	40–50 years	Individual choice of screening
	50–74 years	Every 2 years
	>74 years	No clinical benefit
American Cancer Society (ACS)	30–40 years	Mammography + MRI every year for known case of BRCA gene mutation
	40–44 years	Individual choice and every year
	45–54 years	Every year
	>55 years	Every 2 years
Canadian Task Force	40–49 years	No screening
	50–74 years	Every 2 or 3 years
NPCDCS and operational framework for management of common cancers, MoHFW, Government of India	30–65 years	Clinical Breast Examination (CBE) by health care professional every 5 years (suspected cases are referred for mammography)

Table 3 Cervical cancer screening recommendation [4]

Organization	Age	Recommendation
US Preventive Services Task Force (USPSTF)	21–29 years	Cervical cytology examination every 3 years
American Cancer Society (ACS)	30–65 years	Cervical cytology examination every 3 years and HPV DNA test every 5 years
American Society for Colposcopy and Cervical Pathology		Pap test + HPV DNA test every 5 years
American Society for Clinical Pathology	<21 years	No screening
NPCDCS and operational framework for management of common cancers, MoHFW, Government of India	30–65 years	Visual inspection with acetic acid (VIA) every 5 years

Table 4 HPV vaccines (adapted from Shankar et al. [4])

Vaccine name	HPV coverage	Age group	Recommended regimen and route
Cervarix (bivalent)	HPV type 16 and 18	9–25 years	0, 1, and 6 months; IM
Gardasil (quadrivalent)	HPV type 6, 11, 16, and 18	9–26 years	0, 2, and 6 months; IM
Gardasil (nonavalent)	HPV type 6, 11, 16, 18, 31, 33, 45, 52, and 58	9–26 years	0, 2, and 6 months; IM

HPV human papilloma virus, *IM* intramuscular

95–100%. HPV vaccination not only provides protection against cervical cancer but also for other types of cancer caused by HPV. There is a low coverage of HPV vaccination in LMICs in comparison to HICs along with screening for cervical cancer [4, 21].

HPV vaccines are available in bivalent, quadrivalent, and nonavalent combinations, providing up to 90% protection [21]. HPV vaccine is recommended for age group 9–26 years with 3 doses in 6 months (before sexual initiation), though few studies have found that only two doses are sufficient for protection against cervical cancer for age group 9–18 years [4]. Details of various HPV vaccines are summarized in Table 4.

3.3 Ovarian Cancer

Nearly two thirds of women are diagnosed with ovarian cancer at an advanced stage leading to poor survival. Currently there is no recommendation regarding any screening method for ovarian cancer [22]. There are certain risk factors that predispose to the development of ovarian cancer. History of ovarian cancer in close relatives increases the relative risk of developing ovarian cancer up to 10, and there is more risk if diagnosis of ovarian cancer in relatives is before 50 years of age [23].

Various studies have been conducted to find a suitable screening method to detect ovarian cancer early. European Group on Tumour Markers and UK Collaborative Trial of Ovarian Cancer Screening (UKCTOCS) trial used estimation of CA-125 as a screening method, but none of these studies recommended the use of CA-125 in view of no benefit in mortality and cost-effectiveness [22]. Some studies suggested the use of oral contraceptives for carriers of BRCA gene mutation as chemoprevention but not recommended [24].

There are recommendations for ovarian cancer screening for high risk individuals with family history of ovarian cancer, although there are no mortality benefits. Combination of serum CA-125 and transvaginal ultrasound is suggested by American College of Obstetricians and Gynecologists [4, 25].

3.4 Endometrial Cancer

Aging coupled with increased obesity are two important risk factors for increase in incidence of endometrial cancer. Obesity alone contributes as a risk factor in nearly 60% cases of endometrial cancer. Other countable risk factors are nulliparity, history of polycystic ovary syndrome (PCOS), use of tamoxifen, estrogen therapy, systemic inflammation, and genetic predisposition. Genetic predisposition is most common in women with Lynch syndrome that increases the risk by 70% in comparison to general population with relative low risk [26].

Patients should be counseled and educated about the signs, symptoms, and risk factors of endometrial cancer and asked to report to a doctor in case of any unusual symptoms related to vaginal bleeding [4].

3.5 Other Gynaecological Cancer

Vulvar and vaginal cancers account for a small portion of gynaecological cancers. Squamous cell carcinoma (SCC) is the most common histology. Postmenopausal women have a higher risk of vulvar cancer. HPV infection is the common cause along with other risk factors such as habit of smoking, HIV infection, and genetic predisposition. HPV strain 16 has been associated with SCC of vulva [27]. Vaginal cancer, a rare cancer, may develop secondary to cervical, vulvar cancer, or a result of metastasis. There is no independent screening method recommended for screening for vaginal or vulvar cancer while cervical cytology along with HPV test may detect the malignant lesion [28]. HPV vaccination may play an important function to reduce the risk of development of vaginal and vulvar cancers as studies suggest low incidence of vaginal cancer in HPV-vaccinated individuals [27, 28].

4 Screening Modification for Individuals with High-Risk Gynaecological Cancer

Certain gynaecological malignancies have a high chance of occurrence in individuals with certain genetic mutations or having personal or family history of gynaecological cancers. Such individuals are marked as high-risk individuals. Various guidelines recommend modifications in screening guidelines for such individuals [29]. For persons who are having 20% or more lifetime risk of breast cancer, annual mammography is recommended from the age of 30, while the American Society of Breast Surgeons recommend it from the age of 35. The American Cancer Society recommends annual MRI of the breast along with mammograms from 30 years of age [29, 30]. Cervical cancer screening for high-risk HPV is currently not recommended due to potential harms than benefits [31]. *BRCA 1* and *BRCA 2* gene mutations are potential risk factors for breast and ovarian cancer. Though screening is not recommended for ovarian cancer, experts recommend screening for *BRCA* mutation in individuals with strong family history of breast, ovarian, or fallopian tube cancer [32]. Screening recommendations for high-risk gynaecological cancer are mentioned in Table 5.

Table 5 Screening recommendations for high-risk gynaecological cancer [33]

Cancer type	Recommended screening	Frequency	Age group[a]
Breast	Breast Self-Examination	Monthly	18 years and above
	Clinical Breast Examination	Every 6 months	25 years and above
	Mammography	Every year	25–30 years and above
	MRI		
Ovarian	Transvaginal USG	6–12 months	25–35 years and above
	Serum CA-125		

MRI magnetic resonance imaging, *USG* ultrasonography
[a] Screening recommended 5–10 years prior to the diagnosis of gynaecological cancers in high-risk individuals

5 Conclusion

Women constitute nearly half of the world population, and there is a high risk of developing cancer among women in view of many modifiable and nonmodifiable risk factors. There is an increase in incidence of gynaecological cancers with higher cancer-related mortality in women than men. In spite of the technological advancement and better therapeutic options, relative mortality benefit in gynaecological cancers is yet to be achieved in LMICs. This can be achieved through awareness drives focusing on knowing risk factors for women's cancer, encouraging healthy lifestyle, and intensive screening of eligible populations. There is a need to focus more on cancer vaccination in LMICs, also, more research on other gynaecological cancers. Screening of high-risk individuals for gynaecological cancer is important, and people with a strong family history should be encouraged to undergo age-specific cancer screening.

References

1. Union of International Cancer Care. GLOBOCAN 2020: new global cancer data 2020. Geneva: UICC; 2020. https://www.uicc.org/news/globocan-2020-new-global-cancer-data. Accessed 7 Mar 2022.

2. Torre LA, Islami F, Siegel RL, Ward EM, Jemal A. Global cancer in women: burden and trends. Cancer Epidemiol Biomark Prev. 2017;26(4):444–57.
3. International Association for Research on Cancer. Cancer today. Geneva: World Health Organization; n.d.. https://gco.iarc.fr/today/home. Accessed 5 Mar 2022.
4. Shankar A, Saini D, Singh P, Kataki A, Bhagabaty S, Kataki K. Cancer prevention and screening. In: Kataki A, editor. Principles and practice of oncology. 1st ed. Guwahati: Dr. B. Borooah Cancer Institute Academia; 2020. p. 93–107.
5. Gandhi AK, Kumar P, Bhandari M, Devnani B, Rath GK. Burden of preventable cancers in India: time to strike the cancer epidemic. J Egypt Natl Cancer Inst. 2017;29(1):11–8.
6. Dallal CM, Sullivan-Halley J, Ross RK, Wang Y, Deapen D, Horn-Ross PL, et al. Long-term recreational physical activity and risk of invasive and in situ breast cancer: the California teachers study. Arch Intern Med. 2007;167(4):408–15.
7. Voskuil DW, Monninkhof EM, Elias SG, Vlems FA, van Leeuwen FE. Physical activity and endometrial cancer risk, a systematic review of current evidence. Cancer Epidemiol Biomark Prev. 2007;16(4):639–48.
8. Pan SY, Johnson KC, Ugnat AM, Wen SW, Mao Y. Association of obesity and cancer risk in Canada. Am J Epidemiol. 2004;159(3):259–68.
9. Koo MM, von Wagner C, Abel GA, McPhail S, Rubin GP, Lyratzopoulos G. Typical and atypical presenting symptoms of breast cancer and their associations with diagnostic intervals: evidence from a national audit of cancer diagnosis. Cancer Epidemiol. 2017;48:140–6.
10. Eze JN, Emeka-Irem EN, Edegbe FO. A six-year study of the clinical presentation of cervical cancer and the management challenges encountered at a state teaching hospital in Southeast Nigeria. Clin Med Insights Oncol. 2013;7:151.
11. Goff BA, Mandel LS, Melancon CH, Muntz HG. Frequency of symptoms of ovarian cancer in women presenting to primary care clinics. JAMA. 2004;291(22):2705–12.
12. Prevention CfDCa. Breast cancer. Atlanta, GA: CDC; n.d.. https://www.cdc.gov/cancer/breast/basic_info/symptoms.htm. Accessed 7 Mar 2022.
13. Centers for Disease Control and Prevention. Cervical cancer. Atlanta, GA: CDC; n.d.. https://www.cdc.gov/cancer/cervical/basic_info/symptoms.htm. Accessed 7 Mar 2022.
14. Centers for Disease Control and Prevention. Ovarian cancer. Atlanta, GA: CDC; n.d.. https://www.cdc.gov/cancer/ovarian/basic_info/symptoms.htm. Accessed 7 Mar 2022.
15. Centers for Disease Control and Prevention. Uterine cancer. Atlanta, GA: CDC; n.d.. https://www.cdc.gov/cancer/uterine/basic_info/symptoms.htm. Accessed 7 Mar 2022.
16. Centers for Disease Control and Prevention. Vaginal and vulvar cancers. Atlanta, GA: CDC; n.d.. https://www.cdc.gov/cancer/vagvulv/basic_info/symptoms.htm. Accessed 7 Mar 2022.
17. Prusty RK, Begum S, Patil A, Naik DD, Pimple S, Mishra G. Knowledge of symptoms and risk factors of breast cancer among women: a community based study in a low socio-economic area of Mumbai, India. BMC Womens Health. 2020;20(1):106.
18. Mwaka AD, Orach CG, Were EM, Lyratzopoulos G, Wabinga H, Roland M. Awareness of cervical cancer risk factors and symptoms: cross-sectional community survey in post-conflict northern Uganda. Health Expect. 2016;19(4):854–67.
19. Reichheld A, Mukherjee PK, Rahman SM, David KV, Pricilla RA. Prevalence of cervical cancer screening and awareness among women in an urban community in South India—a cross sectional study. Ann Glob Health. 2020;86(1):30.
20. Sankaranarayanan R, Nene BM, Shastri SS, Jayant K, Muwonge R, Budukh AM, et al. HPV screening for cervical cancer in rural India. N Engl J Med. 2009;360(14):1385–94.
21. Brisson M, Kim JJ, Canfell K, Drolet M, Gingras G, Burger EA, et al. Impact of HPV vaccination and cervical screening on cervical cancer elimination: a comparative modelling analysis in 78 low-income and lower-middle-income countries. Lancet. 2020;395(10224):575–90.
22. Chien J, Poole EM. Ovarian cancer prevention, screening, and early detection: report from the 11th Biennial Ovarian Cancer Research Symposium. Int J Gynecol Cancer. 2017;27(9S Suppl 5):S20–S2.
23. Zheng G, Yu H, Kanerva A, Försti A, Sundquist K, Hemminki K. Familial risks of ovarian cancer by age at diagnosis, proband type and histology. PLoS One. 2018;13(10):e0205000.
24. Menon U, Karpinskyj C, Gentry-Maharaj A. Ovarian cancer prevention and screening. Obstet Gynecol. 2018;131(5):909–27.
25. Trinidad CV, Tetlow AL, Bantis LE, Godwin AK. Reducing ovarian cancer mortality through early detection: approaches using circulating biomarkers. Cancer Prev Res. 2020;13(3):241–52.
26. MacKintosh ML, Crosbie EJ. Prevention strategies in endometrial carcinoma. Curr Oncol Rep. 2018;20(12):101.
27. Rogers LJ, Cuello MA. Cancer of the vulva. Int J Gynaecol Obstet. 2018;143(S2):4–13.
28. Adams TS, Cuello MA. Cancer of the vagina. Int J Gynaecol Obstet. 2018;143(S2):14–21.
29. Lee CS, Monticciolo DL, Moy L. Screening guidelines update for average-risk and high-risk women. Am J Roentgenol. 2019;214(2):316–23.
30. American Cancer Society. American Cancer Society recommendations for the early detection of breast cancer. Atlanta, GA: ACS; n.d..

https://www.cancer.org/cancer/breast-cancer/screening-tests-and-early-detection/american-cancer-society-recommendations-for-the-early-detection-of-breast-cancer.html. Accessed 7 Mar 2022.
31. Melnikow J, Henderson JT, Burda BU, Senger CA, Durbin S, Weyrich MS. Screening for cervical cancer with high-risk human papillomavirus testing: updated evidence report and systematic review for the US Preventive Services Task Force. JAMA. 2018;320(7):687–705.
32. National Cancer Institute. BRCA gene mutations: cancer risk and genetic testing. Bethesda, MD: NCI; n.d.. https://www.cancer.gov/about-cancer/causes-prevention/genetics/brca-fact-sheet. Accessed 7 Mar 2022.
33. Daly MB, Pal T, Berry MP, Buys SS, Dickson P, Domchek SM, et al. Genetic/familial high-risk assessment: breast, ovarian, and pancreatic, Version 2.2021, NCCN Clinical Practice Guidelines in Oncology. J Natl Compr Cancer Netw. 2021;19(1):77–102.

Recent Advances in Gynaecological Oncology

Col Bidhan Roy, T. S. Shylasree, Debabrata Barmon, Amal Chandra Kataki, and Ushashree Das

1 Introduction

In 2020, there were 19.3 million new cancer cases and 9.9 million deaths due to cancer worldwide [1]. Total female cancer reported in 2020 was approximately 9.2 million new cases and about 4.4 million deaths, with breast and cervix cancers being the two leading female cancers [1]. Awareness, prevention, equitable distribution of resources, early diagnosis, and affordable treatment are the prime strategies needed to combat cancer. There has been significant progress in the surgical and medical management of gynaecologic malignancies in the past several years, backed by landmark clinical trials. As a result, there is increasing emphasis on tailored, less morbid but equally efficacious treatment and chronic maintenance therapy. This chapter focuses on integrating various evidence-based updates that helped us to understand and better our current practice in gynaecological oncology.

C. B. Roy (✉)
Department of Obstetrics & Gynaecology, Armed Forces Medical College, Pune, India

T. S. Shylasree
Consultant Gynaecological Oncologist, Aberdeen Royal Infirmary Grampian NHS Trust & North Cancer Alliance, Aberdeen, United Kingdom

D. Barmon · A. C. Kataki
Department of Gynaecologic Oncology, Dr. Bhubaneswar Borooah Cancer Institute (A Unit of Tata Memorial Centre, Mumbai), Guwahati, Assam, India
e-mail: dydiracademic@bbci.tmc.gov.in

U. Das
Department of Gynaecologic Oncology, Tata Memorial Hospital, Homi Baba National Institute, Mumbai, India

2 Cervical Cancer

Worldwide, cancer of the cervix is the fourth most common cancer in females and the second most common cancer in India after breast cancer [1, 2]. China and India contribute more than a third of the global cervical cancer burden [3]. Globally, about 604,127 new cases and 341,831 deaths due to cancer cervix were reported in 2020 [1]. India recorded 123,907 new cases and 77,348 deaths due to cervical cancer.

2.1 Prevention and Screening

The World Health Organization's strategic plan of "90/70/90" targets by 2030 includes 90% of girls covered with an HPV vaccination by age 15, 70% of women screened using a high-performance test by age 35 and again by age 45, and 90% of women identified with preinvasive and invasive cervical cancer adequately managed [4]. Elimination of cervical cancer is defined as an incidence of fewer than 4 cases per 100,000 women [5]. Scaled-up vaccination, screening, and pre-cancer treatment are essential elements of management strategy, especially in low-resource countries. The recom-

A. C. Kataki, D. Barmon (eds.), *Fundamentals in Gynaecologic Malignancy*,
https://doi.org/10.1007/978-981-19-5860-1_31

mended starting age for screening is 25 years with a primary HPV test (Cobas or Onclarity HPV test) every 5 years. However, co-testing with pap smear and HPV DNA test remains an essential modality until the wide availability of primary HPV tests [6]. WHO recommends HPV DNA-based study as the preferred cervical cancer primary screening modality compared to visual inspection with acetic acid or cytology [7]. The Federation of Obstetric and Gynaecologic Societies of India (FOGSI) concurs with the recommendation but advises visual inspection with acetic acid in low-resource settings till affordable HPV tests are available [8]. Another FDA-approved new method, namely dual stain testing (p16 and Ki-67) in the liquid-based cytology (LBC) sample, has emerged to predict pre-cancerous lesions in HPV-positive patients more accurately [9].

Previously the protective role of HPV vaccination against preinvasive cancers has been proven in multiple RCTs. The human papillomavirus (HPV) vaccine's protective effect against invasive cervical cancers is documented. A Swedish study reported an incidence of cervical cancer of 47 cases per 100,000 persons among vaccinated women and 94 cases per 100,000 persons among unvaccinated. The protective effect was more significant among women who were vaccinated before the age of 17 [10]. Another study by Jacqueline et al. reported a decline in the rates of both cervical squamous carcinoma and adenocarcinoma since the introduction of HPV vaccination in the U.S. [11] Recently, vaccination armament has been augmented with the introduction of second-generation nonavalent HPV vaccine with an efficacy of around 96% [12]. In the future, HPV vaccination in national immunization schedule and single-dose HPV vaccine would be the best cost-effective way to overcome cancer cervix.

2.2 Human Papillomavirus-Negative Cervical Cancer and Classification of Adenocarcinoma

Approximately 5.5–11% of all cervical cancers are HPV-negative [13]. The truly HPV-negative cervical cancers are almost all cervical adenocarcinomas, most likely caused by mutations of PI3K-AKT [13]. The median age of patients with HPV-associated adenocarcinoma (HPVA) was 42 years, compared to 55 years for patients with non-HPV-associated adenocarcinoma (NHPVA) [14]. The median size of HPVA was 21 mm, compared to 38 mm in NHPVA [14]. They are often diagnosed at an advanced FIGO stage and have a poor prognosis [13]. Based on this, a new classification of endocervical adenocarcinoma was suggested [14]. Those with easily identified apical mitotic figures and apoptotic bodies were considered HPV-associated adenocarcinoma and further subcategorized based on cytoplasmic features. Tumours with no easily identifiable apical mitotic activity and apoptotic bodies were classified as non-HPV-associated adenocarcinoma. A new 3-tier pattern-based system to classify endocervical adenocarcinoma into patterns A, B, and C is suggested [15]. Pattern A tumours are characterized by well-demarcated glands frequently forming clusters or groups with relative lobular architecture and carries good prognosis. Systematic lymphadenectomy can be avoided in this subset of endocervical adenocarcinoma. Pattern B tumours demonstrated localized destructive stromal invasion along with tumour cells within the stroma. Pattern B is associated with intermediate prognosis. Pattern C showed diffusely infiltrative glands along with extensive desmoplastic response and definitely justifies an aggressive surgical staging.

2.3 FIGO 2018 Staging

The new revised FIGO 2018 staging considers technological developments, tumour size, and poor prognosis of nodal metastases in case of cervical cancer [16]. The lateral extent of the disease is not considered anymore in stage 1A. Stage 1B is further subdivided based on tumour size into Stage 1B1 ≥5 mm depth to <2 cm, 1B2 ≥2 cm to <4 cm, and 1B3 as ≥4 cm. A newer stage IIIC is introduced for positive pelvic and paraaortic nodes either on pathology or radiology irrespective of the tumour size, C1 being positive pelvic nodes only and C2 being paraaortic nodes. FIGO no more recommends any specific modality for imaging but allows the choice on imaging to be based on resource settings and patient affordability. In case of nonavailability of the imaging, FIGO 2009 clinical staging can be used to stage the disease. Many unanswered questions remain, such as measurement of tumour size, the definition of parametrial involvement, ovarian metastases, and lower uterine segment extension [17].

2.4 Minimal Access Surgery

The landmark LACC trial, a prospective multicenter RCT, included stage IA1 with LVSI, IA2, or IB1. The patients were randomly assigned to undergo minimally invasive surgery (laparoscopy or robot-assisted surgery) or conventional open surgery [18]. The study was prematurely stopped and showed that MIS was inferior to open surgery with a low DFS at 4.5 years (86.0% in MIS and 96.5% in the open). The 3-year overall survival was 93.8% vs. 99.0%, with HR for death from any cause being 6.00. The trial was criticized for missing information like tumour size, parametrial size, and involvement, which were essential predictors for recurrence. Similar findings were reported in an epidemiological study [19]. The recommended approach for radical hysterectomy is open and abdominal, according to NCCN and European guidelines [20, 21]. Majority of patients (92%) enrolled in the LACC trial had stage IB1 tumours. In an analysis of NCDB of patients with stage IA disease, there was no difference in survival based on the route of hysterectomy with 4-year survival rates of 97.7% for open and 98.6% for MIS hysterectomy [22].

2.5 Nodal Assessment

The presence of lymph node metastases is an important prognostic factor for survival in cervical cancer. Sentinel lymph node (SLN) appears feasible in cervical cancer due to systematic lymphatic drainage of the cervix and ease of administration of the dye. It has been increasingly used in the management of early cervical cancer. In a prospective French study (Senticol), the use of dual dye yielded a detection rate of 97.8% with a sensitivity of 92%, with a negative predictive value of 98.2% [23]. Sentix, a multicenter prospective observational trial, evaluated sentinel lymph node (SLN) biopsy without pelvic lymph node dissection in patients with early-stage cervical cancer. Though the bilateral detection rate was 91%, the frozen section failed to detect 54% of positive lymph nodes (pN1), including 28% of cases with macrometastases and 90% with micrometastases [24]. Senticol II compared the effect of sentinel-lymph-node biopsy (SLNB) to that of SLNB + pelvic lymphadenectomy (PLND) to determine the postoperative lymphatic morbidity in the two groups [25]. Disease-free survival and overall survival at 4 years were similar in patients treated with SLN biopsy and patients who underwent a lymphadenectomy. The European guideline strongly recommends sentinel node biopsy before pelvic lymphadenectomy with a combination of blue dye with radiocolloid or indocyanine green alone [21].

The uterus-11 study evaluated the impact of surgical staging with transperitoneal laparoscopy compared to standard clinical/radiological staging, followed by chemoradiation (CR) in locally advanced cervical cancer [26]. A total of 255 LACC patients (FIGO2009 IIB-IVA) were included. Though 33% of patients were upstaged because of surgical staging, improvements in PFS and OS were not statistically significant. An analysis of NCDB of stage IA2-IB2 cervical cancer patients who underwent radical hysterectomy with pelvic lymph node dissection with or without paraaortic node dissection showed extending paraaortic lymphadenectomy during radical hysterectomy has no survival advantage [27].

ABRAX, a retrospective cohort study, reported similar DFS, OS, and local control rates between patients who underwent planned surgery and patients who abandoned further surgery after intraoperative detection of pelvic node metastases. The result was published as an abstract in ESMO 2020 virtual congress.

2.6 Role of Conservative Surgery

The rationale for a conservative procedure in early cervical cancer is a low rate of parametrial involvement (<1%) with favorable characteristics like tumour size <2 cm, no deep stromal invasion, no LVSI, and negative nodes [28]. The prospective, single-arm, multicenter ConCerv trial included early-stage cervical cancer with squamous and grade 1/2 adenocarcinoma [29]. They were offered cervical conization or simple hysterectomy with pelvic lymph node dissection or sentinel node dissection. With a median follow-up of 36.3 months, the cumulative incidence of recurrence was 3.5%. The LESSER (LESs Surgical radicality for EaRly stage cervical cancer) study was a proof of concept randomized phase 2 noninferiority trial evaluating the safety and efficacy of simple hysterectomy compared to modified radical hysterectomy in patients with stages IA2-IB1 cervical cancer and tumours of ≤2 cm in size [30]. There were no significant differences in adjuvant therapy between groups (30% vs. 20%, $p = 0.48$) or quality-of-life. At 31 months of follow-up, there was no difference in disease-free survival. A population-based study compared less radical surgery like conization, trachelectomy, or hysterectomy with more radical surgery like modified radical or radical hysterectomy [31]. The disease-specific survival was similar in both groups.

2.7 Role of Chemotherapy in Advanced Cervical Cancer

The advantages of NACT include a decrease in tumour burden, increased tumour oxygenation, distant micrometastases are cured, and increased chances of operability in locally advanced cases. Two phase III trials have been conducted. A study done in India evaluated 633 patients with squamous cervical cancer with stage IB2, IIA, and IIB who were randomized between three cycles of NACT (paclitaxel + carboplatin) three weekly followed by radical hysterectomy versus standard CTRT [32]. The 5-year DFS in the neoadjuvant chemotherapy plus surgery group was 69.3% compared with 76.7% in the concomitant chemoradiation group ($p = 0.038$); the corresponding 5-year OS rates were 75.4% and 74.7%, respectively ($p = 0.87$). Preliminary results of EORTC 55994 show no difference in 5-year OS between NACTS and CCRT with increased short-term severe adverse effects in the neoadjuvant group [33]. Similarly, NACT prior to definitive CTRT in locally advanced cervical cancer has been studied in a phase II trial, the CIRCE trial (Chemotherapy Induction followed by chemoRadiation for locally advanced CErvical cancer) [34]. The complete response rate, PFS and OS were significantly lower with NACT followed by CTRT group compared to CTRT only group. The OUTBACK trial randomized women who had locally advanced cervical cancer to either cisplatin-based chemoradiation or cisplatin-based chemoradiation followed by adjuvant chemotherapy with four cycles of carboplatin and paclitaxel [35]. The PFS and OS were similar between the groups. The final results of GOG 240 showed significant improvement in OS with the addition of bevacizumab to systemic chemotherapy in recurrent, persistent, or metastatic cervical cancer [36].

2.8 Immune Checkpoint Inhibitor and PARP Inhibitor in Cervical Cancer

Recently, there have been some significant and fruitful researches that got materialized in advanced or recurrent metastatic cancer cervix. Immunotherapy (ADSX11-001) with or without Cisplatin and Pembrolizumab use in PD-L1 positive patients are some of the remarkable milestones [37, 38]. The phase II KEYNOTE-158 trial showed an antitumour activity of pembrolizumab in previously treated advanced cervical cancer (15% in PD-L1-positive tumour vs. 0% in PD-L1-negative tumour). Hence it was approved for patients with recurrent or metastatic cervical cancer with disease progression after chemotherapy and who express PD-L1 (Combined Positive Score [CPS] ≥1) as determined by an FDA-approved test in June 2018 [39]. EMPOWER-

Cervical1/GOG-3016/ENGOT-cx9 investigated the role of anti-programmed cell death (PD)-1 cemiplimab vs. investigator choice single-agent chemo in recurrent or metastatic cervical cancer that has progressed after first-line platinum-based treatment [40]. At the interim analysis, OS, PFS, and ORR were higher with cemiplimab. Conjugated monoclonal antibodies (Tisotumab vedotin) are the latest in oncologic therapeutics, and a phase II study in persistent, recurrent, and metastatic cervical cancer has been carried out with good median overall survival of 8.3 months [41]. Triapine (ribonucleotide reductase inhibitors) in combination with platinum-based concurrent chemotherapy has been tested in a phase II trial with good outcome [41]. New trials revealed increased progression-free survival and overall survival have been noticed with the use of Veliparib (PARP inhibitor) in combination with topotecan or in combination with Cisplatin and paclitaxel in the setting of advanced or recurrent cancer cervix [42].

2.9 Advances in Radiotherapy

The standard of care for the treatment of locoregionally advanced cervical cancer is external beam radiation therapy (EBRT), including brachytherapy with concurrent chemotherapy. Intensity-modulated radiation therapy (IMRT) has the ability to maintain tumouricidal doses to target volumes while reducing the dose to nearby critical structures. NRG Oncology/RTOG 1203 (TIME-C trial) compared patient-reported acute toxicity and health-related quality of life during treatment with standard pelvic radiation or intensity-modulated radiation therapy (IMRT) in women with cervical and endometrial cancer [43]. IMRT was associated with significantly less GI and urinary toxicity than standard RT. PARCER trial compared late toxicity of image-guided intensity-modulated radiotherapy (IG-IMRT) vs. three-dimensional conformal radiation therapy (3D-CRT) in cervical cancer patients undergoing postoperative radiation [44]. The cumulative incidence of late toxicity of grade ≥2 were 28.1% versus 48.9% in the IG-IMRT and 3D-CRT arms respectively. The pelvic relapse-free survival and disease-free survival in the IG-IMRT versus the 3D-CRT arm were 81.8% versus 84% ($p = 0.55$) and 76.9% versus 81.2% ($p = 0.89$), respectively. Gandhi et al. from India reported an RCT comparing Whole Pelvic Conventional Radiotherapy (WP-CRT) versus Intensity Modulated Radiotherapy (WP-IMRT) in 44 locally advanced cervical cancer [45]. Both early and late GI and bladder toxicities were significantly less in the IMRT group with similar 5 year DFS and OS, compared to WP-CRT. Another single-center RCT reported efficacy and feasibility of pelvic bone marrow sparing intensity-modulated radiotherapy (PBMS-IMRT) [46]. Hematologic toxicity in the PBMS-IMRT group was 50.0%, significantly lower than the 69.5% in the control group where only IMRT was given without marrow constraint. The American Society for Radiation Oncology (ASTRO) recommends intensity-modulated radiation therapy (IMRT) for postoperative EBRT and conditionally recommends definitive EBRT to reduce short-term and long-term toxicity [47]. STARS trial investigated the effect of sequential chemotherapy and radiotherapy (SCRT) compared to concurrent chemoradiation (CCRT) or radiation alone after radical hysterectomy in patients with adverse prognostic factors [48]. SCRT was associated with higher DFS and lower cancer deaths than CCRT and RT alone.

Simultaneous development in brachytherapy was reported in the EMBRACE trial. EMBRACE I showed MR-based image-guided adaptive brachytherapy (MR-IGABT) after external beam radiotherapy (EBRT) with concomitant chemotherapy and individualized dose prescription resulted in improved target dose coverage and decreased isodose surface volumes compared to standard plans used with classical Point A-based brachytherapy [49].

3 Ovarian Carcinoma

Ovarian cancer is considered the most lethal gynaecologic malignancy, with a median 5-year survival of just 47% [50]. In India, new ovarian cancer cases were approximately 45,701, and about 32,077 deaths due to ovarian cancer were reported in 2020 [1]. Altogether, 313,959 new cases of ovarian cancer and 207,252 deaths due to ovarian cancer were reported worldwide in 2020 [1]. Most patients with epithelial ovarian cancer have advanced stage at presentation. Of those diagnosed with advanced-stage disease, more than 70% will have recurrence within the first 5 years [51]. The 5-year survival for ovarian cancer (all stages included) was about 47.62% during the years 2009–2015 [52].

3.1 Screening

The long-term follow-up results of the UK Collaborative Trial of Ovarian Cancer Screening (UKCTOCS) were published in 2021 [53]. In this RCT, after a median follow-up of 16.3 years, the incidence of stage I or II disease was 39.2% higher in the MMS group than in the no screening group. In contrast, the incidence of stage III or IV disease was 10.2% lower; however, it did not translate to a significant reduction in ovarian and tubal cancer deaths in the MMS ($p = 0.58$) or USS ($p = 0.36$) groups compared with the no screening group. NCCN recommends no screening method for the population at average risk and transvaginal ultrasound with CA125 starting at 30–35 years, at physicians' discretion [54, 55].

3.2 Neoadjuvant Chemotherapy + IDS vs. PDS

Neoadjuvant chemotherapy has been proven to be noninferior in various RCTs, but all those trials were criticized for various reasons, and primary debulking surgery followed by chemotherapy remains the standard treatment for high-grade serous carcinoma. Scorpion trial randomized 171 patients with high tumour load assessed by a standardized laparoscopic predictive index to either primary debulking surgery (PDS) followed by adjuvant chemotherapy or neoadjuvant chemotherapy (NACT) followed by interval debulking surgery (IDS) and adjuvant chemotherapy. The rate of complete cytoreduction was higher in the IDS arm (47.6% vs. 77.0%; $p = 0.001$); the major complication rate was higher in the PDS arm (25.9% vs. 7.6%; $p = 0.0001$). The PFS (HR 1.05, $p = 0.73$) and OS (HR 1.12, $p = 0.56$) were similar in both arms [56]. PDS is generally preferred, but NACT followed by IDS is an alternative for older patients, women with a large disease burden, or multiple comorbidities [57]. SCORPION trial was a single-center RCT to establish whether neoadjuvant chemotherapy (NACT) followed by interval debulking surgery (IDS) is superior to primary debulking surgery (PDS) [58]. Only patients with high volume disease were included. The rates of complete cytoreduction were different between the arms (47.6% in PDS vs. 77.0% in IDS arm; $p = 0.001$) with significantly higher postoperative complication rate in the PDS arm, 25.9% vs. 7.6% [56]. Median progression-free survival and overall survival for patients assigned to primary debulking surgery were similar to the NACT-IDS arm (HR 1.05, $p = 0.73$; HR 1.12, $p = 0.56$). A Japanese RCT, JCOG0602, failed to show noninferiority of neoadjuvant chemotherapy compared with primary debulking surgery [59]. The median OS was 49.0 and 44.3 months in the PDS and NACT, and the median progression-free survival was 15.1 and 16.4 months in the PDS and NACT. This trial has been criticized for a low rate of complete cytoreduction and a significant percentage of patients in the PDS arm having IDS after initial incomplete surgery.

3.3 Lymph Node Assessment

The lymphatic spread has been an essential prognostic factor in early and advanced ovarian cancer. LION trial was the first RCT to study the benefit of systematic lymph node dissection in advanced ovarian cancer [60]. A total of 647 patients with stage IIB through operable stage IV disease who had undergone macroscopically complete resection and had normal lymph nodes both before and during surgery were intraoperatively randomized to either undergo or not undergo lymphadenectomy. The median OS and PFS between the groups were similar, with serious postoperative complications observed more frequently in the lymphadenectomy group (repeat laparotomy, 12.4% vs. 6.5%; mortality within 60 days after surgery, 3.1% vs. 0.9%).

3.4 Frontline Chemotherapy

Paclitaxel and carboplatin every 3 weeks is the standard chemotherapy regimen for advanced ovarian cancer patients. JGOG 3016 reported a significant improvement in OS with weekly paclitaxel [61]. This benefit could not be replicated in GOG 262 or ICON 8. In GOG 262, 84% received Bevacizumab, and weekly paclitaxel was not associated with more prolonged progression-free survival than paclitaxel administered every 3 weeks [62]. However, among patients who did not receive bevacizumab, weekly paclitaxel was associated with better progression-free survival. ICON 8 randomized patients between three arms, 3 weekly Paclitaxel and Carboplatin vs. 3 weekly carboplatin and weekly Paclitaxel vs. weekly Paclitaxel and Carboplatin [63]. The PFS was not different between the groups. The suggested cause of the difference in JGOG 3016 and ICON 8 is pharmacogenomics and different categories of patients; 50% of ICON8 patients received chemotherapy in the neoadjuvant setting, whereas only 10% of JGOG patients underwent primary surgery [64].

Historically elderly and clinically frail women with advanced ovarian cancers receive single-agent carboplatin at least for the first one or two cycles, which is escalated to combination chemotherapy every 3 weekly after improvement in performance status. A GINECO/GCIG RCT (EWOC-1) compared the feasibility, efficacy, and safety of single-agent carboplatin every 3 weeks, weekly carboplatin-paclitaxel, or conventional every-3-weeks carboplatin-paclitaxel in vulnerable older patients with ovarian cancer [65]. This trial was terminated early because single-agent carboplatin was associated with significantly worse survival compared with every-3-weeks or weekly carboplatin-paclitaxel regimens.

Long-term follow-up results of GOG 0241 were published in 2019 [66]. This multicenter RCT compared four chemotherapy regimens for advanced or recurrent stage I mucinous ovarian cancer. The trial was stopped early because of slow accrual, but the recruited patients did not show any difference in OS or PFS with paclitaxel-carboplatin, oxaliplatin-capecitabine each with or without Bevacizumab [66].

3.5 Intraperitoneal Chemotherapy

Trials on intraperitoneal (IP) chemotherapy (CT) showed significantly better survival with IP CT compared to intravenous (IV) CT [67]. GOG 252 two intraperitoneal regimens (carboplatin and Cisplatin) were studied [68]. All patients received Bevacizumab concomitantly and maintenance for 22 cycles. The median PFS and OS were similar between IV chemotherapy vs. IP Carboplatin and IP Cisplatin arm in patients who received Bevacizumab [68]. The complications associated with the IP route have precluded it from being accepted worldwide even when not using Bevacizumab. Hyperthermic intraperitoneal chemotherapy (HIPEC) during surgery is an option hypothesized to give benefits of IP route of chemotherapy without catheter-related complications. HIPEC has been proposed in primary, interval, consolidation, and recurrent settings, but the most accepted evidence was the Dutch Trial which assessed the efficacy of HIPEC during interval cytoreductive surgery. Van Driel et al. evaluated 245 patients with advanced ovarian cancer who received neoadjuvant chemotherapy (NACT) and were randomized to HIPEC or no HIPEC [69]. The trial showed an improved PFS of 4 months and median overall survival (OS) benefit of almost 12 months (33.9 months versus 45.7 months). Another trial by Lim et al. with 184 patients in a similar setting showed somewhat dissimilar results [70]. The HIPEC was administered at a lower dose of 75 mg/m^2 for 90 min at 42–43 °C. The study showed no superiority of the HIPEC arm over the other in terms of 2-year PFS (43.2% vs. 43.5%) and 5-years OS (16.0% vs. 20.9%). Due to such conflicting results from these trials, more evidence is necessary before HIPEC is integrated as standard care for the management of ovarian cancer. HIPEC has also been explored in the recurrent setting but mainly in retrospective and small prospective settings. Spillotis et al. randomized 120 patients with recurrent ovarian cancer to secondary cytoreduction with or without HIPEC and showed OS benefit (26.7 months vs. 13.4 months) [71]. The study was criticized for no PFS data collection, no data on complications, and the methodology of the procedure. It showed similar results for both platinum-sensitive and resistant patients, with PCI being an independent prognostic factor with PCI > 15 having a worse outcome.

3.6 Surgery vs. Chemotherapy for Recurrence

Despite a good response to primary treatment, nearly ¾th of patients relapse within 2 years of treatment, and platinum-free interval serves as a guide to planning treatment in such patients. Secondary cytoreductive surgery (SCS) has been shown to be beneficial in recurrent settings with careful patient selection criteria. GOG 213 evaluated 485 patients with a platinum-free interval of 6 months or more and had the investigator-determined resectable disease to undergo secondary surgical cytoreduction and then receive platinum-based chemotherapy or to receive platinum-based chemotherapy alone [72]. Complete gross resection was achieved in 67% of the patients who underwent SCS. Carboplatin + Paclitaxel or Gemcitabine with bevacizumab followed by bevacizumab maintenance till progression or unacceptable toxicity was administered to 84% of the patients. The hazard ratio for death (secondary cytoreduction vs. no surgery) was 1.29 ($p = 0.08$). DESKTOP III randomized recurrent ovarian cancer patients with a platinum-free interval of 6 months with positive AGO score (Eastern Cooperative Oncology Group performance status score of 0, ascites ≤500 mL, and complete resection at initial surgery) were randomized to platinum-based chemotherapy alone vs. cytoreductive surgery followed by the same chemotherapy [73]. A complete resection was achieved in 75.5%. The median overall survival was 53.7 months in the cytoreduction group and 46.0 months in the no-surgery group ($p = 0.02$). Patients with a complete resection had a median overall survival of 61.9 months, and patients with surgery and incomplete resection did worse than the no-surgery arm (median 28.8 months) [73]. A Chinese RCT evaluating the benefit of SCS included 357 patients with recurrent ovarian cancer with PFI of at least 6 months and potentially resectable disease according to the international model (iMODEL) score and PET-CT imaging [74]. iMODEL score is calculated using: FIGO stage at presentation, residual disease after primary surgery, platinum-free interval, performance status, presence of ascites, and level of CA-125 at recurrence. In the no-surgery group, 6% had secondary cytoreduction during second-line therapy, while 37% who had disease progression had surgery at a subsequent recurrence. At the interim analysis, median overall survival was 58.1 months in the surgery group and 53.9 months in the no-surgery group (HR 0.82). Median progression-free survival was 17.4 months in the surgery group and 11.9 months in the no-surgery group (HR 0.58, $p < 0.0001$).

3.7 Angiogenesis Inhibitor

GOG 218 established the addition of Bevacizumab to standard frontline chemotherapy for advanced high-grade epithelial ovarian cancer [75]. A total of 1873 women with incompletely resected stage III to IV disease were randomly assigned to carboplatin and paclitaxel versus chemotherapy plus concurrent bevacizumab versus chemotherapy plus concurrent and maintenance bevacizumab. The survival was similar in patients who received bevacizumab compared with chemotherapy alone. However, the median OS for stage IV bevacizumab-concurrent plus maintenance was 42.8 months vs. 32.6 months for the control arm. ENGOT-OV15/AGO-OVAR 17 (BOOST trial) included stage IIB–IV epithelial ovarian cancer who underwent primary cytoreductive surgery followed by chemotherapy and bevacizumab [76]. Patients were randomized to receive bevacizumab for either 15 or 30 months. The PFS or OS were similar in both arms with increased adverse events with a longer duration of Bevacizumab.

3.8 Maintenance Therapy/ Monotherapy with PARP Inhibitors

Patients with BRCA 1 or BRCA 2 mutated ovarian cancer (BMOC) have improved survival, higher response to platinum, and longer treatment-free intervals compared with non-BRCA-mutated patients. This is because of an impaired ability of tumour cells to repair platinum-induced double-strand breaks, thereby conferring increased chemosensitivity and other DNA-damaging agents such as pegylated liposomal doxorubicin (PLD) [77]. The landmark change in the treatment of ovarian cancer has been the introduction of PARP inhibitors (PARPi). The principal mechanism of action is "synthetic lethality" wherein two genetic lesions which are not lethal singly but when combined in a cell become lethal [78].

Olaparib and Niraparib have been approved by FDA as maintenance therapy after first-line platinum-based chemotherapy [79]. SOLO-I randomized BRCA-mutated advanced, high-grade serous or endometrioid ovarian cancer with a complete or partial clinical response after platinum-based chemotherapy between Olaparib and placebo as maintenance monotherapy for up to 2 years [80]. After a median follow-up of 41 months, the risk of disease progression or death was 70% lower with Olaparib than with placebo [81]. After 5-year follow-up, the median progression-free survival was 56.0 months with Olaparib versus 13.8 months with placebo [80]. The most common grade 3–4 adverse events were anemia and neutropenia. PRIMA-III was another phase III RCT evaluating niraparib as maintenance in the frontline setting [82]. Patients with newly diagnosed advanced ovarian cancer were randomized to receive niraparib or placebo once daily after a response to platinum-based chemotherapy. Among the patients who had HR deficiency (50.9%), the median PFS was significantly longer in the niraparib group than in the placebo group. In the overall population, the corresponding progression-free survival was 13.8 months and 8.2 months ($p < 0.001$). At the 24-month interim analysis, the rate of overall survival was 84% in the niraparib group and 77% in the placebo group. Niraparib is the only PARPi approved for frontline maintenance treatment in advanced ovarian cancer regardless of biomarker status [83]. PAOLA-1 trial included all newly diagnosed, advanced, high-grade ovarian cancer after response to first-line platinum–taxane chemotherapy plus bevacizumab [84]. Patients were eligible regardless of the surgical outcome or BRCA mutation status. The patients were randomized to receive Olaparib or placebo for up to 24 months; all the patients received bevacizumab 15 mg/kg every 3 weeks for up to 15 months. The median PFS was 22.1 months with Olaparib plus bevacizumab and 16.6 months with placebo plus bevacizumab. VELIA/GOG-3005 was another three-arm phase III RCT exploring the addition of veliparib to frontline chemotherapy with carboplatin and paclitaxel and then continuing as maintenance therapy [85]. A reduction in risk to disease progression or death by 32% was noted (PFS 23.5 months vs. 17.3 months). The highest benefit was noted for BRCA-mutated (PFS 34.7 months vs. 22.0 months) and HR-deficient group (PFS 31.9 months vs. 20.5 months).

PARPi can be given as maintenance therapy in platinum-sensitive recurrent ovarian cancer (PSROC) or as monotherapy after multiple lines of chemotherapy. SOLO-II evaluated Olaparib in BRCAm PSROC after at least two lines of chemotherapy and demonstrated a benefit in PFS (19.1 months vs. 5.5 months) [86]. Median overall survival was 51.7 months (95% CI 41.5–59.1) with Olaparib and 38.8 months (31.4–48.6) with placebo (hazard ratio 0.74 [95% CI 0.54–1.00]; $p = 0.054$), unadjusted for the 38% of patients in the placebo group who received subsequent PARP inhibitor therapy [87]. NOVA evaluated niraparib in BRCAm PSROC and demonstrated a benefit in PFS (21.0 months vs. 5.5 months) [88]. Similarly, the non-gBRCAm with HRD+ cohort showed a benefit in PFS (12.9 months vs. 3.8 months), and FDA approved niraparib as maintenance therapy in PROC in March 2017 [89]. On long-term follow-up however no difference in survival was observed. The authors concluded that the analysis is confounded by a high rate of crossover and missing data, thus limiting its interpretation [90]. NORA trial evaluated the effect of individualized dose of Niraparib on PFS in Chinese patients with platinum-sensitive recurrent ovarian cancer [91]. A significant improvement in PFS was seen in the Niraparib group even when receiving an individualized starting dose. ARIEL-III evaluated rucaparib in PSROC after at least two lines of chemotherapy and demonstrated the highest benefit in PFS for BRCAm (16.6 months vs. 5.4 months) and HRD+ (13.6 months vs. 5.4 months) versus ITT (10.8 months vs. 5.4 months) and was approved by FDA in April 2018 as maintenance therapy [92]. SOLO-III compared olaparib with investigators' choice of non-platinum chemotherapy (pegylated liposomal doxorubicin, paclitaxel, gemcitabine, or topotecan) in recurrent ovarian cancer (ROC) patients and demonstrated benefit in terms of objective response rate (ORR), with an odds ratio (OR) 2.53. In the subgroup who had already received two prior lines of treatment, the OR was 3.44 [93]. Rucaparib monotherapy vs. investigator's choice chemotherapy in patients with recurrent high-grade epithelial ovarian, fallopian tube, or primary peritoneal cancer with germline or somatic BRCA mutation has been investigated in ARIEL 4. It was presented in the first scientific Plenary Session of the Society of gynaecologic Oncology (SGO) 2021 Virtual Annual Meeting on Women's Cancer (Abstract ID 11479). The median progression-free survival was also 7.4 months in the experimental arm vs. 5.7 months in the chemotherapy arm (HR = 0.67, $p = 0.002$) with a similar objective response rate.

4 Endometrial Cancer

Uterine corpus cancer is the sixth most diagnosed cancer in women, more common in countries with a high human development index [1]. In 2020, the reported number of new uterine cancers was 417,367, and the number of uterine cancer-related deaths was 97,370 [1]. India reported 16,413 new cases and about 6385 deaths due to uterine malignancies. Heterogenicity in endometrial cancer is an emerging facet, and molecular profiling is enhancing the scope of precision medicine in gynaecologic oncology. In recent times, there have been advances in the understanding of molecular biology, adjuvant treatment for high-risk disease and HER2/neu-positive serous tumours, and immunotherapy.

4.1 Fertility Preserving Option

Young patients with well-differentiated endometrioid endometrial adenocarcinoma with no myometrial invasion are traditionally treated with high-dose oral progesterone [94]. The levonorgestrel-releasing intrauterine contraceptive device (LNG-IUS) in such subset of patients provides a possible role with 67–75% overall response at 6 months of use [95]. It has the advantage of lower side effects with respect to weight gain and venous thromboembolism when compared to oral progestins. Hysteroscopic resection in combination with oral progestin therapy is associated with a shorter treatment duration to achieve CR than treatment with progestin therapy alone [96]. There has been some growing evidence of the use of metformin in endometrial cancer. Decreased insulin sensitivity of the body tissues results in elevated levels of circulating insulin (increased insulin resistance). Subsequently, excessive insulin downregulates sex hormone-binding globulin levels and upregulates estrogen and androgen levels in the blood. Thus, insulin resistance leads to an increased risk for endometrial cancer. Metformin (insulin sensitizer) promotes the utilization of insulin by the body tissues and thus reduces the circulating levels of insulin. Metformin also suppresses endometrial cancer cell growth via cell cycle arrest, concomitant autophagy, and apoptosis by inhibition of the LKB1-AMPK-mTOR, PI3K-Akt, IGF-1-associated pathways [97].

4.2 Sentinel Node (SLN) Evaluation

Sentinel lymph nodes showed a high degree of diagnostic accuracy in detecting metastases and can safely replace complete lymphadenectomy in the staging of early stage well-differentiated endometrial cancer. Thus, the morbidity of lymphadenectomy can be avoided. SLN biopsies offer a compromise between omitting lymph node dissection and increased risk of systematic lymphadenectomy like lymphocyst formation or morbidity due to increased duration of surgery. The Fluorescence Imaging for Robotic Endometrial Sentinel lymph node biopsy (FIRES) trial is a multicenter, prospective cohort study evaluating the role of the sentinel node in clinical stage I endometrial cancer [98]. A sensitivity of 97.2% and a negative predictive value of 99.6% were reported. The accuracy of sentinel lymph node procedure compared with lymphadenectomy in women with intermediate- and high-grade endometrial cancer was assessed by Cusimano et al. (SENTOR trial) [99]. In this cohort study of 156 patients with endometrial cancer, including serous carcinoma, carcinosarcoma, and undifferentiated histology, SLNB had a sensitivity of 96% and a negative predictive value of 99% for the detection of nodal metastasis. A total of 26% of patients with node-positive cancer were identified outside lymphadenectomy boundaries or required immunohistochemistry for diagnosis. A prospective validation study by Solimon et al. included only high-risk histology [100]. Only blue dye was used in 28% and a sensitivity of 95% and False-negative rate of 5% was reported. The SHREC trial assessed the diagnostic accuracy of a pelvic sentinel lymph node algorithm in high-risk endometrial cancer [101]. The specific algorithm proposed by the authors had a sensitivity of 100% and a negative predictive value of 100%. The bilateral mapping rate was 95%. Based on these and other retrospective studies, SGO recommends both sentinel lymph node mapping and an algorithm-based approach to staging as acceptable alternatives to complete nodal staging in all grades and types of endometrial cancer [102].

4.3 Molecular Markers Guiding Therapy

The TCGA project determined four molecularly defined subgroups of endometrial cancer, which yielded excellent prognostic results [103]. It grouped endometrial cancer into four groups, namely group 1 (7%), which is an ultra-mutated group with DNA polymerase mutation and is associated with a good prognosis. Group 2 (28%) is a hyper-mutated group with microsatellite instability and defects in mismatch repair; group 3 (39%) has a low-copy number group that also exhibited microsatellite instability. Lastly, group 4 (26%) is characterized by a low mutation group, chromosomal instability, and high-copy number variations, and they are primarily with TP53 mutations, grade 3 tumours, and serous carcinomas. Group 4 is associated with worst prognosis.

However, the methods required for classification are currently quite expensive and require special handling of the tissue, limiting applicability. The Proactive Molecular Risk Classifier for Endometrial Cancer (ProMisE) classification identifies molecularly distinct subgroups with a prognostic signature similar to that of the TCGA classification scheme [104]. The four groups were MMR-deficient (MMR-D), POLE exonuclease domain mutations (POLE EDMs), p53 abnormal, and p53 wild-type. The GOG 210/NRG group classification parallels TCGA classification. In the post-hoc analysis of the PORTEC-3 trial, patients with p53 abnormal tumours regardless of histology had significantly improved recurrence-free survival with combined chemotherapy and radiotherapy group compared to radiotherapy alone. Patients with POLE ultra-mutated cancers had excellent recurrence-free survival regardless of treatment modality [105]. Molecular classification is encouraged in all endometrial carcinomas, especially high-grade tumours, and prognostic risk groups are stratified based on this in recent ESGO/ESTRO/ESP guidelines [94].

HER2/neu overexpression in all histologic types of endometrial cancers is not similar. In the high-risk group of the PORTEC-3 study population, HER2 positivity was seen in 37.5% serous,

25% endometrioid, and 20.8% clear cell histology [106]. The association was strong between HER2 positivity and the p53 abnormal subgroup. Carboplatin and Paclitaxel with and without Trastuzumab in patients with advanced or recurrent uterine serous carcinoma who overexpress HER2/neu showed improved PFS and OS [107].

GOG 3007 evaluated the efficacy of everolimus and letrozole (EL) in women with recurrent endometrial cancer [108]. A 24% response rate in the everolimus/letrozole arm (PFS 6.4 months and OS 20.0 months) and a 22% response rate in the progestin/tamoxifen arm (PFS 3.8 months and OS 16.6 months) were reported.

4.4 Immunotherapy

PD-1 and PD-L1 are overexpressed in 75% and 25–100% of endometrial cancers, respectively [109]. These tumours show mutational overload with neoantigens and tumour-infiltrating lymphocytes, which make them an ideal candidate for immunotherapy. Keynote-028 evaluated the safety and efficacy of pembrolizumab, an anti-programmed death one monoclonal antibody, in patients with programmed death-ligand 1 (PD-L1)-positive advanced solid tumours. Pembrolizumab demonstrated a durable antitumour activity in a subgroup of patients with heavily pretreated advanced PD-L1-positive endometrial cancer [110]. This led to the FDA's first tissue/site-agnostic approval of Pembrolizumab for patients with microsatellite instability-high (MSI-H) or mismatch repair-deficient (dMMR) solid tumours progressed following prior treatment and has no satisfactory alternative treatment options. KEYNOTE-158 reported an overall response rate of 48% with pembrolizumab in patients with heavily pretreated, advanced microsatellite instability-high (MSI-H) or mismatch repair-deficient (dMMR) endometrial cancer [111, 112]. KEYNOTE-775/Study 309 compared pembrolizumab and multikinase inhibitor, Lenvatinib, with single-agent chemotherapy standard single-agent chemotherapy in patients with advanced, metastatic, or recurrent endometrial cancer progressing after a prior platinum-based regimen [113]. Lenvatinib/pembrolizumab led to a doubling in response rate: 31.9% vs. 14.7% with physician's choice of treatment. There was a significant improvement in overall survival and progression-free survival regardless of MMR status. The FDA approved pembrolizumab with lenvatinib for patients with advanced endometrial carcinoma, which is not MSI-H or dMMR, who have disease progression following prior systemic therapy, and who are not candidates for curative surgery or radiation [114].

4.5 Adjuvant Treatment in High-Risk Endometrial Cancers

Approximately 15–20% of endometrial cancer patients are at increased risk of recurrence or distant metastases and are thus classified as high risk [115]. Multiple studies have characterized the risk of postsurgical recurrence and tried to identify adjunctive therapies to reduce it. PORTEC-3 investigates the benefit of adjuvant chemotherapy during and after radiotherapy versus pelvic radiotherapy alone for women with high-risk endometrial cancer [116]. At a median follow-up of 72.6 months, 5-year overall survival was 81.4% with chemoradiotherapy versus 76.1% with radiotherapy alone (HR 0.70, $p = 0.034$), and 5-year failure-free survival was 76.5% versus 69.1% (HR 0.70, $p = 0.016$) [117]. The benefit was mainly for women with stage III and serous cancers. GOG 249 compared vaginal cuff brachytherapy and chemotherapy (VCB/C) with pelvic radiation therapy (RT) in high-intermediate and high-risk early-stage endometrial carcinoma concerning recurrence-free survival (RFS) [118]. The 5-year RFS and OS were similar in both the groups but pelvic or paraaortic nodal recurrences were more common with VCB/C (9% vs. 4%). GOG 258 compared a similar chemoradiotherapy regimen as in PORTEC-3 with six cycles of chemotherapy alone in stage III and IVA endometrial cancer [119]. The relapse-free survival was similar in both groups. Vaginal, pelvic, and para-aortic nodal recurrence was more common in the chemotherapy arm, and distant recurrences were more common with chemoradiotherapy. The use of chemoradiation maximizes RFS and OS and nodal control in women with stage III disease or serous histology. In the translational study of PORTEC-3, patients with p53abn endometrial cancer had the worst outcome. They showed a significant survival benefit of added adjuvant chemotherapy: Mismatch repair-deficient endometrial cancers had an intermediate prognosis, and RFS was similar in radiotherapy and chemoradiation arms. Hence, adding chemotherapy to radiotherapy did not reduce mismatch repair-deficient endometrial cancer recurrence [120].

5 Vulvar Carcinoma

These are rare malignancies, representing 4% of all gynaecological cancers. Emerging evidence suggests an increase in both vulvar intraepithelial neoplasia and invasive vulvar cancer in young women. This rising trend has been attributed to smoking, Human Papilloma Virus (HPV) infection, and changing sexual behavior [121]. HPV positivity in vulval cancer is a good prognostic factor. Recently, genomic alteration revealed a new category of HPV-negative vulval cancer with NOTCH1 and HRAS mutations and normal p53 expression. This new subtype of vulval cancer is considered to have an intermediate 5-year survival rate [122].

5.1 Updated Staging

FIGO staging of vulvar cancer was updated in 2021 for all morphologic types except melanoma [123]. FIGO 2021 staging allows incorporation of cross-sectional imaging findings into vulvar cancer staging similar to cervical cancer, and documentation regarding the HPV status of the carcinoma of the vulva is strongly recommended. Main changes were made in stage III disease; stage IIIA included an extension to upper two-thirds of the urethra and vagina or extension to bladder mucosa, rectal mucosa, or regional lymph node metastases ≤5 mm, stage IIIB being any regional nodal metastases >5 mm, and IIIC being regional lymph node metastases with extracapsular spread.

5.2 Sentinel Node

Groningen International Study on Sentinel nodes in Vulvar cancer, GROINSS V I, was an observational validation study on vulvar cancer's sentinel node (SLN) procedure [124]. After a median follow-up of 105 months, the isolated groin recurrence rate was 2.5% for sentinel node-negative patients, and disease-specific 10-year survival was 91%. This European guideline recommended the SLN procedure in patients with unifocal cancers of less than 4 cm, without suspicious groin nodes [125]. When an ipsilateral sentinel lymph node is not detected, a complete ipsilateral inguinofemoral lymphadenectomy must be done, and if an ipsilateral sentinel lymph node is positive, a complete bilateral inguinofemoral lymphadenectomy is recommended [126]. The sequel to the GROINSS-V trial, GROINSS-V II, investigates the efficacy of groin radiation without inguinofemoral lymphadenectomy for patients with positive sentinel nodes [127]. Among patients with SN micrometastases (≤2 mm), patients who received groin radiotherapy had a groin recurrence rate at 2 years of 1.6%. In patients with SN macrometastases (>2 mm), the isolated groin recurrence rate at 2 years was 22% after radiotherapy only, and 6.9% in those who underwent inguinofemoral lymphadenectomy followed by radiotherapy ($p = 0.011$) [127]. NCCN version 1.2022 incorporates this into the guideline and recommends only EBRT with or without chemotherapy for single sentinel node-positive with ≤2 mm metastases. Complete inguinofemoral lymphadenectomy is the preferred approach for sentinel node metastases more than 2 mm [128]. GROINSS-V III is investigating whether the efficacy of treatment can be increased by enhancing the dose of radiotherapy and by adding concurrent chemotherapy to inguinofemoral radiotherapy.

5.3 Tumour-Free Surgical Margin

NCCN recommends a gross surgical margin of 1 cm and 8 mm pathologic margin [128]. A smaller margin is acceptable to preserve critical structures like the clitoris, urethra, and anal sphincter. Re-excision or adjuvant radiotherapy is advised only for margin positive for invasive cancer [128], whereas FIGO 2021 report on vulvar cancer states, cases with close, i.e., less than 5 mm surgical margin, may benefit from adjuvant radiotherapy if re-excision of the margins is not possible without severe morbidity [126].

5.4 Systemic Therapy

New therapies for recurrent, progressive, and metastatic disease include testing for mismatch repair/microsatellite instability, PD-1 and NTRK gene fusion, and use of Larotrectinib or Entrectinib for NTRK gene fusion-positive tumours [128].

6 Gestational Trophoblastic Neoplasia

Hemida et al. reported an RCT, where patients with low-risk gestational trophoblastic neoplasia were randomized to a second curettage or no curettage group before methotrexate treatment, and its effect on the number of chemotherapy courses and the relapse rate was studied [129]. The mean number of chemotherapy courses required to reach hCG normalization was 4.4 in the control group vs. 3.8 in the intervention group ($p = 0.14$). Immunotherapy has made its way into the armamentarium against chemotherapy-resistant gestational trophoblastic neoplasia (GTN) since PD-L1 is constitutively expressed in all subtypes of GTN. TROPHIMMUN is a phase II trial that assessed avelumab in women with chemotherapy-resistant GTN [130]. In patients with single-agent chemotherapy-resistant GTN, 53.3% had hCG normalization after a median of 9 avelumab cycles with a favorable safety profile. CAP 01 trial evaluated the activity and safety of camrelizumab (PD-1 inhibitor) plus apatinib (VEGF receptor inhibitor) in patients with high-risk chemorefractory or relapsed gestational trophoblastic neoplasia [131]. This is a single-center phase II study including 20 patients. The objective response rate was 55%; ten (50%) patients had a complete response.

7 Uterine Mesenchymal Tumours

ESMO-EURACAN-GENTURIS Clinical Practice Guideline for soft tissue and visceral sarcoma has outlined some definitive recommendations for managing uterine sarcoma [132]. Adjuvant radiotherapy does not improve RFS or OS. Still, it can be an option in selected cases, considering risk factors, including local relapse, cervical involvement, parametrial involvement, serosal involvement, and UES histology. Adjuvant chemotherapy in the uterus-confined leiomyosarcoma is not the standard. Adjuvant hormonal therapy (HT) is not the standard treatment for endometrial stromal sarcoma, though there is retrospective evidence of decreased relapse [133]. GOG 277 is a phase III trial to determine whether adjuvant chemotherapy with gemcitabine-docetaxel followed by doxorubicin improves survival compared to observation in women with resected, uterus-confined, high-grade LMS [134]. Despite international collaboration, the study was closed for accrual futility. The observed OS and RFS data do not suggest superior outcomes for patients treated with additional doxorubicin after gemcitabine and docetaxel.

8 Conclusion

Genetic and molecular alterations in oncology are now being integrated and translated into clinical practice with significant benefits. Precision surgery is individual tumour biology coupled with image-guided surgery, and new developments are giving encouraging results [135]. Emerging and meaningful contemporary research is being carried out worldwide to evolve the best practice available in the treatment of cancer patients. The social media platform is a helpful tool wherein any latest development can be shared for the benefit of humankind. In the future, the advancement and integration of preventive oncology into primary health care facilities would be an important milestone to combat the increasing trend of cancers worldwide.

References

1. Sung H, Ferlay J, Siegel RL, et al. Global cancer statistics 2020: GLOBOCAN estimates of incidence and mortality worldwide for 36 cancers in 185 countries. CA Cancer J Clin. 2021;71(3):209–49.
2. Mathur P, Sathishkumar K, Chaturvedi M, et al. Cancer statistics, 2020: report from National Cancer Registry Programme, India. JCO Glob Oncol. 2020;6:1063–75.
3. Arbyn M, Weiderpass E, Bruni L, et al. Estimates of incidence and mortality of cervical cancer in 2018: a worldwide analysis. Lancet Glob Health. 2020;8(2):e191–203.
4. Simelela PN. WHO global strategy to eliminate cervical cancer as a public health problem: an opportunity to make it a disease of the past. Int J Gynecol Obstet. 2021;152(1):1–3.
5. WHO. Global strategy to accelerate the elimination of cervical cancer as a public health problem. Geneva: WHO; 2020. https://www.who.int/publications/i/item/9789240014107. Accessed 5 Dec 2021.
6. Perkins RB, Guido RL, Saraiya M, et al. Summary of current guidelines for cervical cancer screening and management of abnormal test results: 2016-2020. J Women's Health (Larchmt). 2021;30(1):5–13.
7. WHO Guidelines Approved by the Guidelines Review Committee. WHO guideline for screening and treatment of cervical pre-cancer lesions for cervical cancer prevention. 2nd ed. Geneva: World Health Organization; 2021.
8. Bhatla N, Singhal S, Saraiya U, et al. Screening and management of preinvasive lesions of the cervix: good clinical practice recommendations from the Federation of Obstetrics and Gynaecologic Societies of India (FOGSI). J Obstet Gynaecol Res. 2020;46(2):201–14.
9. Prigenzi KCK, Heinke T, Salim RC, Focchi GRA. Dual p16 and Ki-67 Expression in liquid-based cervical cytological samples compared to pap cytology findings, biopsies, and HPV testing in cervical cancer screening: a diagnostic accuracy study. Acta Cytol. 2018;62(2):104–14.
10. Lei J, Ploner A, Elfström KM, et al. HPV Vaccination and the risk of invasive cervical cancer. N Engl J Med. 2020;383(14):1340–8.
11. Mix JM, Van Dyne EA, Saraiya M, Hallowell BD, Thomas CC. Assessing impact of HPV vaccination on cervical cancer incidence among women aged 15-29 years in the United States, 1999-2017: an ecologic study. Cancer Epidemiol Biomark Prev. 2021;30(1):30–7.
12. Huh WK, Joura EA, Giuliano AR, et al. Final efficacy, immunogenicity, and safety analyses of a nine-valent human papillomavirus vaccine in women aged 16-26 years: a randomised, double-blind trial. Lancet. 2017;390(10108):2143–59.
13. Xing B, Guo J, Sheng Y, Wu G, Zhao Y. Human papillomavirus-negative cervical cancer: a comprehensive review. Front Oncol. 2021;10(3007):606335.
14. Stolnicu S, Barsan I, Hoang L, et al. International Endocervical Adenocarcinoma Criteria and Classification (IECC): a new pathogenetic classification for invasive adenocarcinomas of the endocervix. Am J Surg Pathol. 2018;42(2):214–26.
15. Roma AA, Fadare O. The pattern is the issue: recent advances in adenocarcinoma of the uterine cervix. Virchows Arch. 2018;472(6):897–905.
16. Bhatla N, Aoki D, Sharma DN, Sankaranarayanan R. Cancer of the cervix uteri. Int J Gynaecol Obstet. 2018;143(Suppl 2):22–36.
17. Salvo G, Odetto D, Pareja R, Frumovitz M, Ramirez PT. Revised 2018 International Federation of Gynecology and Obstetrics (FIGO) cervical cancer staging: a review of gaps and questions that remain. Int J Gynecol Cancer. 2020;30(6):873–8.
18. Ramirez PT, Frumovitz M, Pareja R, et al. Minimally invasive versus abdominal radical hysterectomy for cervical cancer. N Engl J Med. 2018;379(20):1895–904.
19. Melamed A, Margul DJ, Chen L, et al. Survival after minimally invasive radical hysterectomy for early-stage cervical cancer. N Engl J Med. 2018;379(20):1905–14.
20. NCCN Cervical cancer. 2021. https://www.nccn.org/professionals/physician_gls/pdf/cervical.pdf.
21. Cibula D, Pötter R, Planchamp F, et al. The European Society of Gynaecological Oncology/European Society for Radiotherapy and Oncology/European Society of Pathology guidelines for the management of patients with cervical cancer. Radiother Oncol. 2018;127(3):404–16.
22. Wright JD. Minimal risk for minimally invasive hysterectomy for stage IA cervical cancer? Int J Gynecol Cancer. 2021;31(8):1104–5.
23. Lécuru F, Mathevet P, Querleu D, et al. Bilateral negative sentinel nodes accurately predict absence of lymph node metastasis in early cervical cancer: results of the SENTICOL study. J Clin Oncol. 2011;29(13):1686–91.
24. Cibula D, Kocian R, Plaikner A, et al. Sentinel lymph node mapping and intraoperative assessment

in a prospective, international, multicentre, observational trial of patients with cervical cancer: the SENTIX trial. Eur J Cancer. 2020;137:69–80.
25. Favre G, Guani B, Balaya V, Magaud L, Lecuru F, Mathevet P. Sentinel lymph-node biopsy in early-stage cervical cancer: the 4-year follow-up results of the senticol 2 trial. Front Oncol. 2021;10(3423):621518.
26. Marnitz-Schulze S, Tsunoda A, Martus P, et al. 24 UTERUS-11 STUDY: a randomized clinical trial on surgical staging versus CT-staging prior to primary chemoradiation in patients with FIGO2009 stages IIB-IVA cervical cancer. Int J Gynecol Cancer. 2019;29(Suppl 3):A15.
27. Del Carmen MG, Pareja R, Melamed A, et al. Isolated para-aortic lymph node metastasis in FIGO stage IA2-IB2 carcinoma of the cervix: revisiting the role of surgical assessment. Gynecol Oncol. 2018;150(3):406–11.
28. Ramirez PT, Pareja R, Rendón GJ, Millan C, Frumovitz M, Schmeler KM. Management of low-risk early-stage cervical cancer: should conization, simple trachelectomy, or simple hysterectomy replace radical surgery as the new standard of care? Gynecol Oncol. 2014;132(1):254–9.
29. Schmeler KM, Pareja R, Lopez Blanco A, et al. ConCerv: a prospective trial of conservative surgery for low-risk early-stage cervical cancer. Int J Gynecol Cancer. 2021;31(10):1317–25.
30. Carneiro V, Batista T, Andrade M, et al. A proof-of-concept randomized phase 2 non-inferiority trial on simple versus modified radical hysterectomy in IA2-IB1 cervical cancer ≤2cm (LESSER). Gynecol Oncol. 2021;162:S36–S7.
31. Tseng JH, Aloisi A, Sonoda Y, et al. Less versus more radical surgery in stage IB1 cervical cancer: a population-based study of long-term survival. Gynecol Oncol. 2018;150(1):44–9.
32. Gupta S, Maheshwari A, Parab P, et al. Neoadjuvant chemotherapy followed by radical surgery versus concomitant chemotherapy and radiotherapy in patients with stage IB2, IIA, or IIB squamous cervical cancer: a randomized controlled trial. J Clin Oncol. 2018;36(16):1548–55.
33. Kenter G, Greggi S, Vergote I, et al. Results from neoadjuvant chemotherapy followed by surgery compared to chemoradiation for stage Ib2-IIb cervical cancer, EORTC 55994. J Clin Oncol. 2019;37(15_suppl):5503.
34. Costa SCS, Bonadio RC, Gabrielli FCG, et al. Neoadjuvant chemotherapy with cisplatin and gemcitabine followed by chemoradiation versus chemoradiation for locally advanced cervical cancer: a randomized phase II trial. J Clin Oncol. 2019;37(33):3124–31.
35. Mileshkin LR, Moore KN, Barnes E, et al. Adjuvant chemotherapy following chemoradiation as primary treatment for locally advanced cervical cancer compared to chemoradiation alone: the randomized phase III OUTBACK trial (ANZGOG 0902, RTOG 1174, NRG 0274). J Clin Oncol. 2021;39(18_suppl):LBA3.
36. Tewari KS, Sill MW, Penson RT, et al. Bevacizumab for advanced cervical cancer: final overall survival and adverse event analysis of a randomised, controlled, open-label, phase 3 trial (Gynecologic Oncology Group 240). Lancet. 2017;390(10103):1654–63.
37. Basu P, Mehta A, Jain M, et al. A randomized phase 2 study of ADXS11-001 Listeria monocytogenes-Listeriolysin O immunotherapy with or without cisplatin in treatment of advanced cervical cancer. Int J Gynecol Cancer. 2018;28(4):764–72.
38. Chung HC, Ros W, Delord JP, et al. Efficacy and safety of pembrolizumab in previously treated advanced cervical cancer: results from the phase II KEYNOTE-158 study. J Clin Oncol. 2019;37(17):1470–8.
39. Attademo L, Tuninetti V, Pisano C, et al. Immunotherapy in cervix cancer. Cancer Treat Rev. 2020;90:102088.
40. Tewari KS, Monk BJ, Vergote I, et al. VP4-2021: EMPOWER-cervical 1/GOG-3016/ENGOT-cx9: interim analysis of phase III trial of cemiplimab vs. investigator's choice (IC) chemotherapy (chemo) in recurrent/metastatic (R/M) cervical carcinoma. Ann Oncol. 2021;32(7):940–1.
41. Regalado Porras GO, Chávez Nogueda J, Poitevin Chacón A. Chemotherapy and molecular therapy in cervical cancer. Rep Pract Oncol Radiother. 2018;23(6):533–9.
42. Thaker PH, Salani R, Brady WE, et al. A phase I trial of paclitaxel, cisplatin, and veliparib in the treatment of persistent or recurrent carcinoma of the cervix: an NRG Oncology Study (NCT#01281852). Ann Oncol. 2017;28(3):505–11.
43. Klopp AH, Yeung AR, Deshmukh S, et al. Patient-reported toxicity during pelvic intensity-modulated radiation therapy: NRG oncology–RTOG 1203. J Clin Oncol. 2018;36(24):2538–44.
44. Chopra S, Gupta S, Kannan S, et al. Late Toxicity after adjuvant conventional radiation versus image-guided intensity-modulated radiotherapy for cervical cancer (PARCER): a randomized controlled trial. J Clin Oncol. 2021;39(33):3682–92.
45. Ajeet Kumar Gandhi DNS, Rath GK, Julka PK, Subramani V, Sharma S, et al. Long term clinical outcome and late toxicity of intensity modulated versus conventional pelvic radiation therapy for locally advanced cervix carcinoma. J Clin Diagn Res. 2019;13(3):XC09–13.
46. Huang J, Gu F, Ji T, Zhao J, Li G. Pelvic bone marrow sparing intensity modulated radiotherapy reduces the incidence of the hematologic toxicity of patients with cervical cancer receiving concurrent chemoradiotherapy: a single-center prospective randomized controlled trial. Radiat Oncol. 2020;15(1):180.
47. Chino J, Annunziata CM, Beriwal S, et al. The ASTRO clinical practice guidelines in cervical cancer: optimizing radiation therapy for improved outcomes. Gynecol Oncol. 2020;159(3):607–10.

48. Huang H, Feng Y-L, Wan T, et al. Effectiveness of sequential chemoradiation vs concurrent chemoradiation or radiation alone in adjuvant treatment after hysterectomy for cervical cancer: the STARS phase 3 randomized clinical trial. JAMA Oncol. 2021;7(3):361–9.
49. Serban M, Kirisits C, Pötter R, et al. Isodose surface volumes in cervix cancer brachytherapy: change of practice from standard (Point A) to individualized image guided adaptive (EMBRACE I) brachytherapy. Radiother Oncol. 2018;129(3):567–74.
50. Torre LA, Trabert B, DeSantis CE, et al. Ovarian cancer statistics, 2018. CA Cancer J Clin. 2018;68(4):284–96.
51. Kurnit KC, Fleming GF, Lengyel E. Updates and new options in advanced epithelial ovarian cancer treatment. Obstet Gynecol. 2021;137(1):108–21.
52. Siegel RL, Miller KD, Jemal A. Cancer statistics, 2019. CA Cancer J Clin. 2019;69(1):7–34.
53. Menon U, Gentry-Maharaj A, Burnell M, et al. Ovarian cancer population screening and mortality after long-term follow-up in the UK Collaborative Trial of Ovarian Cancer Screening (UKCTOCS): a randomised controlled trial. Lancet. 2021;397(10290):2182–93.
54. NCCN. Genetic/familial high-risk assessment: breast, ovarian, and pancreatic. Plymouth Meeting, PA: NCCN; 2021. https://www.nccn.org/guidelines/guidelines-detail?category=2&id=1503.
55. NCCN. Ovarian cancer including fallopian tube cancer and primary peritoneal cancer. Plymouth Meeting, PA: NCCN; 2021. https://www.nccn.org/guidelines/guidelines-detail?category=1&id=1453.
56. Fagotti A, Ferrandina MG, Vizzielli G, et al. Randomized trial of primary debulking surgery versus neoadjuvant chemotherapy for advanced epithelial ovarian cancer (SCORPION-NCT01461850). Int J Gynecol Cancer. 2020;30(11):1657–64.
57. Rauh-Hain JA, Melamed A, Wright A, et al. Overall survival following neoadjuvant chemotherapy vs primary cytoreductive surgery in women with epithelial ovarian cancer: analysis of the national cancer database. JAMA Oncol. 2017;3(1):76–82.
58. Fagotti A, Ferrandina G, Vizzielli G, et al. Phase III randomised clinical trial comparing primary surgery versus neoadjuvant chemotherapy in advanced epithelial ovarian cancer with high tumour load (SCORPION trial): final analysis of peri-operative outcome. Eur J Cancer. 2016;59:22–33.
59. Onda T, Satoh T, Ogawa G, et al. Comparison of survival between primary debulking surgery and neoadjuvant chemotherapy for stage III/IV ovarian, tubal and peritoneal cancers in phase III randomised trial. Eur J Cancer. 2020;130:114–25.
60. Harter P, Sehouli J, Lorusso D, et al. A randomized trial of lymphadenectomy in patients with advanced ovarian neoplasms. N Engl J Med. 2019;380(9):822–32.
61. Katsumata N, Yasuda M, Isonishi S, et al. Long-term results of dose-dense paclitaxel and carboplatin versus conventional paclitaxel and carboplatin for treatment of advanced epithelial ovarian, fallopian tube, or primary peritoneal cancer (JGOG 3016): a randomised, controlled, open-label trial. Lancet Oncol. 2013;14(10):1020–6.
62. Chan JK, Brady MF, Penson RT, et al. Weekly vs. every-3-week paclitaxel and carboplatin for ovarian cancer. N Engl J Med. 2016;374(8):738–48.
63. Clamp AR, James EC, McNeish IA, et al. Weekly dose-dense chemotherapy in first-line epithelial ovarian, fallopian tube, or primary peritoneal carcinoma treatment (ICON8): primary progression free survival analysis results from a GCIG phase 3 randomised controlled trial. Lancet. 2019;394(10214):2084–95.
64. Balieiro Anastacio da Costa AA, Baiocchi G, Guimarães APG. Progression-free survival in the ICON8 trial. Lancet. 2020;396(10253):756–7.
65. Falandry C, Rousseau F, Mouret-Reynier MA, et al. Efficacy and safety of first-line single-agent carboplatin vs carboplatin plus paclitaxel for vulnerable older adult women with ovarian cancer: a GINECO/GCIG randomized clinical trial. JAMA Oncol. 2021;7(6):853–61.
66. Gore M, Hackshaw A, Brady WE, et al. An international, phase III randomized trial in patients with mucinous epithelial ovarian cancer (mEOC/GOG 0241) with long-term follow-up: and experience of conducting a clinical trial in a rare gynecological tumor. Gynecol Oncol. 2019;153(3):541–8.
67. Armstrong DK, Bundy B, Wenzel L, et al. Intraperitoneal cisplatin and paclitaxel in ovarian cancer. N Engl J Med. 2006;354(1):34–43.
68. Walker JL, Brady MF, Wenzel L, et al. Randomized trial of intravenous versus intraperitoneal chemotherapy plus bevacizumab in advanced ovarian carcinoma: an NRG Oncology/Gynecologic Oncology Group Study. J Clin Oncol. 2019;37(16):1380–90.
69. van Driel WJ, Koole SN, Sikorska K, et al. Hyperthermic intraperitoneal chemotherapy in ovarian cancer. N Engl J Med. 2018;378(3):230–40.
70. Lim MC, Chang S-J, Yoo HJ, Nam B-H, Bristow R, Park S-Y. Randomized trial of hyperthermic intraperitoneal chemotherapy (HIPEC) in women with primary advanced peritoneal, ovarian, and tubal cancer. Proc Am Soc Clin Oncol. 2017;35:5520.
71. Spiliotis J, Halkia E, Lianos E, et al. Cytoreductive surgery and HIPEC in recurrent epithelial ovarian cancer: a prospective randomized phase III study. Ann Surg Oncol. 2015;22(5):1570–5.
72. Coleman RL, Spirtos NM, Enserro D, et al. Secondary surgical cytoreduction for recurrent ovarian cancer. N Engl J Med. 2019;381(20):1929–39.
73. Harter P, Sehouli J, Vergote I, et al. Randomized trial of cytoreductive surgery for relapsed ovarian cancer. N Engl J Med. 2021;385(23):2123–31.
74. Shi T, Zhu J, Feng Y, et al. Secondary cytoreduction followed by chemotherapy versus chemotherapy alone in platinum-sensitive relapsed ovarian cancer

(SOC-1): a multicentre, open-label, randomised, phase 3 trial. Lancet Oncol. 2021;22(4):439–49.
75. Tewari KS, Burger RA, Enserro D, et al. Final overall survival of a randomized trial of bevacizumab for primary treatment of ovarian cancer. J Clin Oncol. 2019;37(26):2317–28.
76. Pfisterer J, Joly F, Kristensen G, et al. Optimal treatment duration of bevacizumab (BEV) combined with carboplatin and paclitaxel in patients (pts) with primary epithelial ovarian (EOC), fallopian tube (FTC) or peritoneal cancer (PPC): a multicenter open-label randomized 2-arm phase 3 ENGOT/GCIG trial of the AGO Study Group, GINECO, and NSGO (AGO-OVAR 17/BOOST, GINECO OV118, ENGOT Ov-15, NCT01462890). J Clin Oncol. 2021;39(15_suppl):5501.
77. Tan DSP, Kaye SB. Chemotherapy for patients with BRCA1 and BRCA2–mutated ovarian cancer: same or different? Am Soc Clin Oncol Educ Book. 2015;35:114–21.
78. Chandrasekaran A, Elias KM. Synthetic lethality in ovarian cancer. Mol Cancer Ther. 2021;20(11):2117–28.
79. Penn CA, Wong MS, Walsh CS. Cost-effectiveness of maintenance therapy based on molecular classification following treatment of primary epithelial ovarian cancer in the United States. JAMA Netw Open. 2020;3(12):e2028620.
80. Banerjee S, Moore KN, Colombo N, et al. Maintenance olaparib for patients with newly diagnosed advanced ovarian cancer and a BRCA mutation (SOLO1/GOG 3004): 5-year follow-up of a randomised, double-blind, placebo-controlled, phase 3 trial. Lancet Oncol. 2021;22:1721.
81. Moore K, Colombo N, Scambia G, et al. Maintenance olaparib in patients with newly diagnosed advanced ovarian cancer. N Engl J Med. 2018;379(26):2495–505.
82. González-Martín A, Pothuri B, Vergote I, et al. Niraparib in patients with newly diagnosed advanced ovarian cancer. N Engl J Med. 2019;381(25):2391–402.
83. Akay M, Funingana I-G, Patel G, et al. An in-depth review of niraparib in ovarian cancer: mechanism of action, clinical efficacy and future directions. Oncol Ther. 2021;9(2):347–64.
84. Ray-Coquard I, Pautier P, Pignata S, et al. Olaparib plus bevacizumab as first-line maintenance in ovarian cancer. N Engl J Med. 2019;381(25):2416–28.
85. Coleman RL, Fleming GF, Brady MF, et al. Veliparib with first-line chemotherapy and as maintenance therapy in ovarian cancer. N Engl J Med. 2019;381(25):2403–15.
86. Pujade-Lauraine E, Ledermann JA, Selle F, et al. Olaparib tablets as maintenance therapy in patients with platinum-sensitive, relapsed ovarian cancer and a BRCA1/2 mutation (SOLO2/ENGOT-Ov21): a double-blind, randomised, placebo-controlled, phase 3 trial. Lancet Oncol. 2017;18(9):1274–84.
87. Poveda A, Floquet A, Ledermann JA, et al. Olaparib tablets as maintenance therapy in patients with platinum-sensitive relapsed ovarian cancer and a BRCA1/2 mutation (SOLO2/ENGOT-Ov21): a final analysis of a double-blind, randomised, placebo-controlled, phase 3 trial. Lancet Oncol. 2021;22(5):620–31.
88. Del Campo JM, Matulonis UA, Malander S, et al. Niraparib maintenance therapy in patients with recurrent ovarian cancer after a partial response to the last platinum-based chemotherapy in the ENGOT-OV16/NOVA trial. J Clin Oncol. 2019;37(32):2968–73.
89. NCI. Niraparib approved for women with recurrent ovarian cancer. Oncol Times. 2017;39(9):37.
90. Matulonis U, Herrstedt J, Oza A, et al. Long-term safety and secondary efficacy endpoints in the ENGOT-OV16/NOVA phase III trial of niraparib in recurrent ovarian cancer. Gynecol Oncol. 2021;162:S24–S5.
91. Wu XH, Zhu JQ, Yin RT, et al. Niraparib maintenance therapy in patients with platinum-sensitive recurrent ovarian cancer using an individualized starting dose (NORA): a randomized, double-blind, placebo-controlled phase III trial*. Ann Oncol. 2021;32(4):512–21.
92. Coleman RL, Oza AM, Lorusso D, et al. Rucaparib maintenance treatment for recurrent ovarian carcinoma after response to platinum therapy (ARIEL3): a randomised, double-blind, placebo-controlled, phase 3 trial. Lancet. 2017;390(10106):1949–61.
93. Penson RT, Valencia RV, Cibula D, et al. Olaparib versus nonplatinum chemotherapy in patients with platinum-sensitive relapsed ovarian cancer and a germline BRCA1/2 mutation (SOLO3): a randomized phase III trial. J Clin Oncol. 2020;38(11):1164–74.
94. Concin N, Matias-Guiu X, Vergote I, et al. ESGO/ESTRO/ESP guidelines for the management of patients with endometrial carcinoma. Int J Gynecol Cancer. 2021;31(1):12–39.
95. Pal N, Broaddus RR, Urbauer DL, et al. Treatment of low-risk endometrial cancer and complex atypical hyperplasia with the levonorgestrel-releasing intrauterine device. Obstet Gynecol. 2018;131(1):109–16.
96. Masciullo V, Trivellizzi N, Zannoni G, et al. Prognostic impact of hysteroscopic resection of endometrial atypical hyperplasia-endometrioid intraepithelial neoplasia and early-stage cancer in combination with megestrol acetate. Am J Obstet Gynecol. 2021;224(4):408–10.
97. Lee TY, Martinez-Outschoorn UE, Schilder RJ, et al. Metformin as a therapeutic target in endometrial cancers. Front Oncol. 2018;8:341.
98. Rossi EC, Kowalski LD, Scalici J, et al. A comparison of sentinel lymph node biopsy to lymphadenectomy for endometrial cancer staging (FIRES trial): a multicentre, prospective, cohort study. Lancet Oncol. 2017;18(3):384–92.
99. Cusimano MC, Vicus D, Pulman K, et al. Assessment of sentinel lymph node biopsy vs lymphadenectomy

for intermediate- and high-grade endometrial cancer staging. JAMA Surg. 2021;156(2):157–64.
100. Soliman PT, Westin SN, Dioun S, et al. A prospective validation study of sentinel lymph node mapping for high-risk endometrial cancer. Gynecol Oncol. 2017;146(2):234–9.
101. Persson J, Salehi S, Bollino M, Lönnerfors C, Falconer H, Geppert B. Pelvic sentinel lymph node detection in high-risk endometrial cancer (SHREC-trial)-the final step towards a paradigm shift in surgical staging. Eur J Cancer. 2019;116:77–85.
102. Hamilton CA, Pothuri B, Arend RC, et al. Endometrial cancer: a society of gynecologic oncology evidence-based review and recommendations. Gynecol Oncol. 2021;160(3):817–26.
103. Kandoth C, Schultz N, Cherniack AD, et al. Integrated genomic characterization of endometrial carcinoma. Nature. 2013;497(7447):67–73.
104. Talhouk A, McConechy MK, Leung S, et al. A clinically applicable molecular-based classification for endometrial cancers. Br J Cancer. 2015;113(2):299–310.
105. León-Castillo A, Boer SM, Powell ME, et al. Molecular classification of the PORTEC-3 trial for high-risk endometrial cancer: impact on prognosis and benefit from adjuvant therapy. J Clin Oncol. 2020;38(29):3388–97.
106. Vermij L, Horeweg N, Leon-Castillo A, et al. HER2 status in high-risk endometrial cancers (PORTEC-3): relationship with histotype, molecular classification, and clinical outcomes. Cancers (Basel). 2020;13(1):44.
107. Fader AN, Roque DM, Siegel E, et al. Randomized phase II trial of carboplatin-paclitaxel compared with carboplatin-paclitaxel-trastuzumab in advanced (Stage III-IV) or recurrent uterine serous carcinomas that overexpress Her2/Neu (NCT01367002): updated overall survival analysis. Clin Cancer Res. 2020;26(15):3928–35.
108. Slomovitz BM, Filiaci VL, Coleman RL, et al. GOG 3007, a randomized phase II (RP2) trial of everolimus and letrozole (EL) or hormonal therapy (medroxyprogesterone acetate/tamoxifen, PT) in women with advanced, persistent or recurrent endometrial carcinoma (EC): a GOG Foundation study. Gynecol Oncol. 2018;149:2.
109. Kooshkaki O, Derakhshani A, Safarpour H, et al. The latest findings of PD-1/PD-L1 inhibitor application in gynecologic cancers. Int J Mol Sci. 2020;21(14):5034.
110. Ott PA, Bang YJ, Berton-Rigaud D, et al. Safety and antitumor activity of pembrolizumab in advanced programmed death ligand 1-positive endometrial cancer: results from the KEYNOTE-028 Study. J Clin Oncol. 2017;35(22):2535–41.
111. Marabelle A, Le DT, Ascierto PA, et al. Efficacy of pembrolizumab in patients with noncolorectal high microsatellite instability/mismatch repair-deficient cancer: results from the phase II KEYNOTE-158 study. J Clin Oncol. 2020;38(1):1–10.
112. O'Malley D, Marabelle A, De Jesus-Acosta A, et al. 1044P - Pembrolizumab in patients with MSI-H advanced endometrial cancer from the KEYNOTE-158 study. Ann Oncol. 2019;30:v425–v6.
113. Makker V, Taylor MH, Aghajanian C, et al. Lenvatinib plus pembrolizumab in patients with advanced endometrial cancer. J Clin Oncol. 2020;38(26):2981–92.
114. Arora S, Balasubramaniam S, Zhang W, et al. FDA Approval Summary: Pembrolizumab plus Lenvatinib for Endometrial Carcinoma, a Collaborative International Review under Project OrbisFDA Approval: Pembrolizumab plus Lenvatinib; Project Orbis. Clin Cancer Res. 2020;26(19):5062–7.
115. van den Heerik ASVM, Horeweg N, de Boer SM, Bosse T, Creutzberg CL. Adjuvant therapy for endometrial cancer in the era of molecular classification: radiotherapy, chemoradiation and novel targets for therapy. Int J Gynecol Cancer. 2021;31(4):594–604.
116. de Boer SM, Powell ME, Mileshkin L, et al. Adjuvant chemoradiotherapy versus radiotherapy alone for women with high-risk endometrial cancer (PORTEC-3): final results of an international, open-label, multicentre, randomised, phase 3 trial. Lancet Oncol. 2018;19(3):295–309.
117. de Boer SM, Powell ME, Mileshkin L, et al. Adjuvant chemoradiotherapy versus radiotherapy alone in women with high-risk endometrial cancer (PORTEC-3): patterns of recurrence and post-hoc survival analysis of a randomised phase 3 trial. Lancet Oncol. 2019;20(9):1273–85.
118. Randall ME, Filiaci V, McMeekin DS, et al. Phase III trial: adjuvant pelvic radiation therapy versus vaginal brachytherapy plus paclitaxel/carboplatin in high-intermediate and high-risk early-stage endometrial cancer. J Clin Oncol. 2019;37(21):1810–8.
119. Matei D, Filiaci V, Randall ME, et al. Adjuvant chemotherapy plus radiation for locally advanced endometrial cancer. N Engl J Med. 2019;380(24):2317–26.
120. León-Castillo A, de Boer SM, Powell ME, et al. Molecular classification of the PORTEC-3 trial for high-risk endometrial cancer: impact on prognosis and benefit from adjuvant therapy. J Clin Oncol Off J Am Soc Clin Oncol. 2020;38(29):3388–97.
121. Eva LJ, Sadler L, Fong KL, Sahota S, Jones RW, Bigby SM. Trends in HPV-dependent and HPV-independent vulvar cancers: the changing face of vulvar squamous cell carcinoma. Gynecol Oncol. 2020;157(2):450–5.
122. Nooij LS, Ter Haar NT, Ruano D, et al. Genomic characterization of vulvar (pre)cancers identifies distinct molecular subtypes with prognostic significance. Clin Cancer Res. 2017;23(22):6781–9.
123. Olawaiye AB, Cotler J, Cuello MA, et al. FIGO staging for carcinoma of the vulva: 2021 revision. Int J Gynecol Obstet. 2021;155(1):43–7.
124. Te Grootenhuis NC, van der Zee AG, van Doorn HC, et al. Sentinel nodes in vulvar cancer: long-term follow-up of the GROningen INternational study

on sentinel nodes in vulvar cancer (GROINSS-V) I. Gynecol Oncol. 2016;140(1):8–14.
125. Oonk MHM, Planchamp F, Baldwin P, et al. European Society of Gynaecological Oncology guidelines for the management of patients with vulvar cancer. Int J Gynecol Cancer. 2017;27(4):832–7.
126. Olawaiye AB, Cuello MA, Rogers LJ. Cancer of the vulva: 2021 update. Int J Gynecol Obstet. 2021;155(S1):7–18.
127. Oonk MHM, Slomovitz B, Baldwin PJW, et al. Radiotherapy versus inguinofemoral lymphadenectomy as treatment for vulvar cancer patients with micrometastases in the sentinel node: results of GROINSS-V II. J Clin Oncol. 2021;39(32):3623–32.
128. NCCN. Vulvar cancer (squamous cell carcinoma). Plymouth Meeting, PA: NCCN; 2021. https://www.nccn.org/guidelines/guidelines-detail?category=1&id=1476.
129. Hemida R, Vos EL, El-Deek B, et al. Second uterine curettage and the number of chemotherapy courses in postmolar gestational trophoblastic neoplasia: a randomized controlled trial. Obstet Gynecol. 2019;133(5):1024–31.
130. You B, Bolze PA, Lotz JP, et al. Avelumab in patients with gestational trophoblastic tumors with resistance to single-agent chemotherapy: cohort a of the TROPHIMMUN Phase II Trial. J Clin Oncol. 2020;38(27):3129–37.
131. Cheng H, Zong L, Kong Y, et al. Camrelizumab plus apatinib in patients with high-risk chemorefractory or relapsed gestational trophoblastic neoplasia (CAP 01): a single-arm, open-label, phase 2 trial. Lancet Oncol. 2021;22(11):1609–17.
132. Gronchi A, Miah AB, Dei Tos AP, et al. Soft tissue and visceral sarcomas: ESMO-EURACAN-GENTURIS clinical practice guidelines for diagnosis, treatment and follow-up(☆). Ann Oncol. 2021;32(11):1348–65.
133. Comert GK, Turkmen O, Kar I, et al. Hormone therapy following surgery in low-grade endometrial stromal sarcoma: is it related to a decrease in recurrence rate? J Chin Med Assoc. 2019;82(5):385–9.
134. Hensley ML, Enserro D, Hatcher H, et al. Adjuvant gemcitabine plus docetaxel followed by doxorubicin versus observation for uterus-limited, high-grade leiomyosarcoma: a phase III GOG study. J Clin Oncol. 2018;36(15_suppl):5505.
135. Choi N, Jeong H-S. Precision surgery for cancer: a new surgical concept in individual tumor biology-based image-guided surgery. Precis Fut Med. 2019;3:116.

MIX
Papier aus verantwortungsvollen Quellen
Paper from responsible sources
FSC® C105338

If you have any concerns about our products,
you can contact us on
ProductSafety@springernature.com

In case Publisher is established outside the EU,
the EU authorized representative is:
Springer Nature Customer Service Center GmbH
Europaplatz 3, 69115 Heidelberg, Germany

Printed by Libri Plureos GmbH
in Hamburg, Germany